Crouch and Alers Occupational Therapy in Psychiatry and Mental Health

Crouch and Alers Occupational Therapy in Psychiatry and Mental Health

SIXTH EDITION

Edited by

Rosemary Crouch, Tania Buys, Enos Morankoana Ramano,
Matty van Niekerk and Lisa Wegner

WILEY Blackwell

Contents

8   Human Ecosystems and Other Disasters: The Impact on Health, Wellness and Human Occupation   123

Robin Joubert and Chantal Juanita Christopher

9   Occupational Therapy in Forensic Psychiatric Wards   135

Nicole Rautenbach and Matty van Niekerk

10   Occupational Therapy Assessments and Interventions: Priorities in Acute Mental Health   149

Annah Lesunyane, Lebogang Lefine, Rosemary Crouch and Catherine Shorten

13 Work and Mental Health – Facilitating and Sustaining Work Engagement   193

Lyndsey Swart, Tania Buys and Carol-lynn Andreitchenko

14 Psychiatric Occupational Therapy in the Corporate, Insurance and Medicolegal Sectors   211

Lee Randall

15 Spirituality and Mental Health: An Occupational Therapy Perspective   223

Thuli Godfrey Mthembu and Louise Fouché

25 The Assessment and Treatment of Eating Disorders in Occupational Therapy 384

Karlien Terblanche

26 Working with People with a Diagnosis of 'Personality Disorder' 400

Keir Harding and Hollie Berrigan

27 The Occupational Therapy Approach to the Management of Schizophrenia Spectrum and Other Psychotic Disorders 413

Kobela Veronica Ramodike, Iesrafeel Abbas and Rosemary Crouch[3]

**30 Care, Treatment and Rehabilitation
Programmes for Large Numbers
of Long-Term Mental Health Care
Users   460**

Daleen Casteleijn and Kobie Zietsman

Contributors

Iesrafeel Abbas – MSc Occ Ther (University of the Western Cape) and BSc Occ Ther (University of Cape Town) is a lecturer and clinical educator in the field of occupational therapy at the University of Cape Town (UCT). He has taught undergraduate and postgraduate courses at UCT since 2019. He heads the mental health cluster within the Occupational Therapy Division at UCT and is the Occupational Therapy Association of South Africa-student academic representative for UCT OT. Mr Abbas is an early career researcher, publishing in peer-reviewed journals and books and is a regular presenter at international and national conferences. His research interests focus on the impact of mental illness on occupational engagement and functioning (including student mental health and well-being).

Carol-Lynn Andreitchenko – Dip Voc Rehab (University of Pretoria), Dip Adv Occ Ther (University of the Witwatersrand) and BSc Occ Ther (University of the Witwatersrand) – is a clinician with extensive experience in the area of vocational rehabilitation spanning early intervention, case management and return to work. She has a special interest in chronic health conditions, persistent pain and mental health. She offers training in case management to colleagues and in a consultant capacity to the insurance sector. She has acted as an external examiner for postgraduate studies in vocational rehabilitation. She currently works as a rehabilitation consultant in Canberra Australia.

Hollie Berrigan – BSc (Counselling and Psychology) – is a Consultant Lived Experience Practitioner and Integrative Counsellor. She has experience in receiving a diagnosis of personality disorder, inpatient and community care, detention and a range of therapeutic interventions. She also has clinical experience in working with individuals who receive the 'personality disorder' label in hospital or live in the community. She has delivered a range of therapies. Hollie combines all of her experiences to provide a therapeutic environment where people can experience a level of understanding and validation that is often difficult to get in a typical clinician/patient relationship.

Susan Beukes – M Occ Ther (Stellenbosch University), BSc (Honours in Medical Science, Stellenbosch University), B Occ Ther (Stellenbosch University) and Head of the Division of Occupational Therapy (Stellenbosch University from 1988 to 2013) – is the former Chairperson of the Education Committee of the Professional Board for Occupational Therapy, Medical Orthotics and Prosthetics and Arts Therapy of the Health Professions Council of South Africa (2005–2008). She has extensive experience in psycho-social occupational therapy programmes and interventions in psychiatric hospitals, work rehabilitation programmes, workshops for the disabled and the establishment of service learning projects in communities.

Tania Buys – PhD (University of the Witwatersrand), M Occ Ther (University of Pretoria), B Occ Ther (Hons) (Revalidation/Vocational Rehabilitation) (University of Pretoria) and B Occ Ther (University of the Free State) – is a lecturer in the Department of Occupational Therapy at the University of Pretoria. Tania teaches in the area of vocational rehabilitation on an undergraduate and postgraduate level and was responsible for the implementation of the Postgraduate Diploma in Vocational Rehabilitation. Her other teaching areas include disability equity legislation, research methodology, ethics and interprofessional health management. She has published in the area of vocational rehabilitation and research methodology and is a regular presenter at workshops. Tania has extensive clinical experience in private practice focusing on clients with both physical and mental health limitations.

Daleen Casteleijn – PhD (OT), M Occ Ther, Dip Higher Education and Training, PG Dip Voc Rehab and B Occ Ther (Hons) – is an occupational therapy educator at the University of Pretoria in South Africa and a visiting professor at the University of Northampton. Her expertise lies in the field of outcome measurements and instrument development in healthcare. She developed the Activity Participation Outcome Measure (patented), which is based on the Vona du Toit Model of Creative Ability. This outcome measure is used nationally and internationally to track changes after occupational therapy intervention in several patient populations. She has a number of publications in national and international journals, is on the editorial committee of the *British Journal of Occupational Therapy*, acts as a reviewer of international journals in occupational therapy, is the chairperson of the Vona and Marie du Toit Foundation and is a regular presenter and trainer of the Vona du Toit Model of Creative Ability.

Chantal Juanita Christopher – MPhil Group Ther (University of KwaZulu-Natal), PG Dip (HIV Clinical Management, University of KwaZulu-Natal) and B Occ Ther (University of Durban-Westville) – is Lecturer within the discipline of occupational therapy at the University of KwaZulu-Natal. She is a critical reader of society, our world and the profession of occupational therapy. She believes that we, as a profession, need to ask the difficult question such as this: 'How do we work, think, engage, research and write to directly affect the pedestrian, inherited and oft oppressive conditions in society?' Chantal although based within academia, believes in taking the university into the streets and growing the streets within the university. She is a community practitioner.

Ray Anne Cook – M Occ Ther (University of Stellenbosch) and B Occ Ther (University of Stellenbosch) – has been an active occupational therapist in special schools and private practice for over 35 years. She is qualified in Ayres Sensory Integration® and was the director of Sensory Kidzone, specialising in children and adults with sensory integration difficulties, autism and ADHD. At present, she is focusing on mentoring and working with adults with ADHD and other challenges. Her passion is the misunderstood child, empowering parents in the upbringing of their child and developing the art of playfulness in all. She is involved in the South African Institute for Sensory Integration (SAISI) as a board member and lecturer, where she is the head for training Ayers Sensory Integration (ASI®) in South Africa. She also serves on the executive committee of the South African Association for Child and Adolescent Psychiatry.

Rosemary Crouch – PhD Occ Ther (Medical University of Southern Africa MEDUNSA), MSc Occ Ther with distinction (University of Witwatersrand), BSc Occ Ther (University of Witwatersrand) and Dip Occ Ther (University of Witwatersrand) – is Adjunct Professor of the School of Therapeutic Sciences, Faculty of Health Sciences, University of Witwatersrand, Johannesburg, South Africa. She was a senior lecturer in the Department of Occupational Therapy at the University of Witwatersrand from 1972 to 1989, a part-time senior lecturer at MEDUNSA and at the University of Pretoria and a practitioner in the private psychiatric field for 20 years. She was also Mellon Research Mentor at the University of Witwatersrand from 2007 to 2015. Rosemary is the Editor of the first two editions of *Occupational Therapy in Psychiatry and Mental Health* and co-editor with Vyvian Alers of the third, fourth and fifth editions. She has been granted the honour of being Honorary Editor of the sixth edition.

Shanay Davidson – MSc Occ Ther (University of Cape Town) and BSc Occ (University of Cape Town) – is an occupational therapist who specialises in mental health. Shanay has extensive experience in both public and private mental health sectors. With roles at Weskoppies and Valkenberg Psychiatric Hospitals, she has also contributed her expertise to student education through teaching, supervision and lectures. Currently, Shanay's research centres on supported education for health science students.

Marianne de Beer – PhD (University of Pretoria), PhD (MEDUNSA), M Occ Ther (University of Pretoria), Dip Ed Voc Ther (University of Pretoria) and Nat Dip Occ Ther (Pretoria College of Occupational therapy) – is Former Head of the Department of Occupational Therapy at the University of Pretoria, South Africa. She was a clinician and educator in the field of occupational therapy, mental health, psychiatry and group therapy. She has published her work in scientific journals and presented at international and national conferences.

Patricia de Witt – MSc Occ Ther and PhD (University of the Witwatersrand) – qualified as an occupational therapist in 1972 from the Vona du Toit College of Occupational Therapy. Pat is a retired Adjunct Professor with a post-retirement sessional appointment in the Department of Occupational Therapy at the University of Witwatersrand, where she was a member of the academic staff for 40 years including being Head of Department. While she has a wide occupational therapy interest, mental health and models of practice, especially the Vona du Toit Model of Creative Ability have been the focus of her interest, teaching and clinical work. Her personal research interests have been the education and training of occupational therapy students. She has published widely (40 publications in peer-reviewed journals and books) and has supervised the research of 30 students, both Masters and PhDs. She has done many oral and poster presentations both nationally and internationally. Pat has been a very active member of the professional Occupational Therapy Association of South Africa (OTASA) and has held many positions including President. She presented the Vona du Toit Memorial lecture in 2004.

Louise Fouché – B Occ Ther (University of Pretoria), M Occ Ther (University of Pretoria), PG Dip in Interpersonal relationships and groups (University of Pretoria), PG Cert in Higher Education (University of Pretoria), PG Cert in spiritual accompaniment (Jesuit Institute of South Africa) – has worked in numerous psychiatric settings, including Weskoppies Hospital, the acute psychiatric unit at Worcester Hospital, Louis Botha Children's homes, Huis Disa Old Age Home and the Baby Therapy Centre. She is also the owner of a private practice. Louise lectured at the University of Pretoria for eight years in group therapy and mental health. She presented the postgraduate diploma in group work at the University Pretoria and has been a guest lecturer at the University of Mauritius, the University of the Witwatersrand and the University of the Western Cape, for undergraduate and postgraduate students. She was instrumental in getting OTGrow launched in 2010 and has trained occupational therapists in group skills, both nationally and internationally. Her interests include groups, psychodrama, shadow work, spirituality and creative ability through which she helps others aspire to be their highest selves.

Pragashnie Govender – PhD (OT), University of KwaZulu-Natal, PGDip Health Professions Education and Leadership (FPD), MOT (University of KwaZulu-Natal), BOT (University of KwaZulu-Natal) is a Professor and practitioner with over

20 years of experience in occupational therapy, with a passion for early intervention and child health. She currently contributes to training of occupational therapy students up to post-doctoral level. She has published in peer-reviewed journals and presented at national and international conferences.

Zaakirah Haffejee – MSc Occ Ther (University of the Witwatersrand), PG Dip Voc Rehab (University of Pretoria), BSc Occ Ther (University of the Witwatersrand) and Highly Specialist Occupational Therapist-Acute Stroke Unit Team Lead (Kingston Hospital NHS Trust) – is a clinician in the field of occupational therapy, with a keen interest in neurological impairments, driving rehabilitation and vocational rehabilitation. She worked in the South African public health sector for six years in the field of mental health and neurology and was an active member of the Gauteng Vocational Rehabilitation Task Team. Zaakirah is currently a clinician and researcher in the United Kingdom, working in the field of stroke rehabilitation. Her research is due to be presented at stroke conferences.

Keir Harding – BSc Occ Ther and MSc (Working Effectively with 'Personality Disorder') – is an occupational therapist with 20 years of experience in mental health. He is a Dialectical Behaviour Therapist. He has worked in various mental health roles with the latter part of his career in specialist 'personality disorder' services. He has been fortunate enough to deliver the 50th Elizabeth Casson Memorial Lecture (Harding 2023) for the Royal College of Occupational Therapists where he shared his passions around the importance of therapeutic relationships, the impact of stigma and the social environment and the need for occupational therapists to explore the dark side of occupation.

Stephanie Homer – BSc Occ Ther (University of the Witwatersrand), Sessional Tutor (Department of Occupational Therapy, University of the Witwatersrand), Rural Rehab SA Executive Member and Office Co-ordinator Rural Doctor's Association of Southern Africa – is an educator for community-based rehabilitation in rural clinical fieldwork. Her interests are children and adults with chronic mental illness and advocating for better rural rehabilitation services through the NPO Rural Rehab SA (RuReSA), where she has served as an executive member for seven years. She is involved in ensuring rehabilitation policy is 'rural proof' and works with the committee for the annual Rural Health Conference to develop the conference programme, as well as being part of the RuReSA team promoting 'rural rehabilitation research' and analysing the results from the annual Community Service Exit Survey.

Elize Janse van Rensburg – M Occ Ther (University of the Free State) and B Occ Ther (University of the Free State) – is an occupational therapist in private practice and former Lecturer at the Department of Occupational Therapy at the University of the Free State. Elize is a private practitioner in the field of

paediatric occupational therapy, with a particular interest in autism and other neurodevelopmental conditions. She is trained in Ayres Sensory Integration® and is a lecturer and an executive committee member of the South African Institute for Sensory Integration (SAISI). She has published in peer-reviewed journals and books and presented at national and international conferences.

Robin Joubert – PhD (University of KwaZulu-Natal), M Occ Ther (University of Durban Westville), BA (University of South Africa) and Nat Dip Occ Ther (Pretoria College of Occupational Therapy) – is Honorary Associate Professor in the Department of Occupational Therapy at the University of KwaZulu-Natal (UKZN). Formerly, Robin was appointed as part of the team to start occupational therapy training at the University of the Free State and was later appointed to head the commencement of occupational therapy training at the University of Durban-Westville (UDW). She held the positions of academic leader in occupational therapy, University of KwaZulu-Natal; Vice Dean Faculty of Health Sciences (Education and Training portfolio) UDW; and Head of School of Audiology, Occupational Therapy and Speech and Hearing Therapy, University of KwaZulu-Natal. She is the past Vice-President and President of SAAOT (OTASA), an Honorary Fellow of OTASA, and Vona du Toit Memorial Lecturer (OTASA). She was awarded UKZN's Distinguished Teacher Award. She is the author/co-author of nine book chapters and 32 journal articles and presenter at 90 national and international conferences. Currently, she is semi-retired and is supervising postgraduate students at UKZN. She is also lay minister and lay preacher in the Anglican Diocese of KwaZulu-Natal.

Lebogang Lefine – M Occ Ther (Sefako Makgatho Health Sciences University) and B Occ Ther (University of Limpopo) – is Lecturer of the Department of Occupational Therapy at Sefako Makgatho Health Sciences University (South Africa). She is an educator in the field of occupational therapy, mental health and psychiatry. She is passionate about research with adolescents and substance abuse worldwide. As an educator in occupational therapy, she strives for excellence in her engagement with students. She has published her research and continues to challenge herself for greatness in her academic and professional path.

Annah Lesunyane – M Occ Ther (University of Limpopo-Medunsa Campus), B Occ Ther (Hons) (Medical University of Southern Africa) and B Occ Ther (Medical University of Southern Africa) – is Senior Lecturer at the Department of Occupational Therapy at Sefako Makgatho Health Sciences University, South Africa. Annah is an occupational therapist and has experience in acute psychiatry and community mental health. She currently teaches and supervises students in the field of psychiatry and mental health as well as supervises students conducting research in psychiatry and mental health. Annah is passionate about mental health challenges experienced by university students and is pursuing research in student wellness and support.

Thuli Godfrey Mthembu – BSc Occ Ther (University of the Western Cape), M Public Health (University of the Western Cape), PhD (University of the Western Cape) – is Associate Professor in the Department of Occupational Therapy, at the University of the Western Cape. His doctoral research explored how spirituality and spiritual care can be integrated into occupational therapy education. Professor Mthembu worked as a community service occupational therapist at Shongwe Hospital for a year and later became Chief Occupational Therapist. He also provided occupational therapy services as part of the community outreach programme and home visits to strengthen primary healthcare. Currently, he works with second-, third- and fourth-year occupational therapy and postgraduate students. Professor Mthembu's research focuses on spirituality, spiritual care, vulnerable youth, older adults with chronic diseases, occupational legacies in families, ageing and resilience and youth development. His recent research focuses on social transformation of youth not in education, employment or training.

Marie Clare (Mush) Perrins Gendron – BSc Occ Ther (University of Cape Town), M Occ Ther (Stellenbosch University) - worked for 18 years in government and more than 14 years at the Red Cross War Memorial Children's Hospital. Mush now runs her comprehensive paediatric private practice from home. She was a part-time lecturer/clinical supervisor for UCT's OT Department. She has presented papers on occupational therapy at international and national conferences. She has also presented many paediatric courses in South Africa as well as a few in neighbouring countries. Mush has attended many varied lectures and training courses over the past 41 years, from door gardening to music related to heart beats. Professionally, she has many tools in her toolbox, significantly neuro-developmental, sensory integration, sensory modulation and play therapy. Mush completed her MSc in occupational therapy in April 2021; her thesis title is *Exploring the Use of Play in Health Promotion: Perspectives Originating from the Continent of Africa.*

Enos Morankoana Ramano – PhD (University of Pretoria), M Occ Ther (University of Pretoria), PG Dip Voc Rehab (University of Pretoria) and B Occ Ther (Cum Laude) (Medical University of South Africa, MEDUNSA) – currently works as an occupational therapy clinician in private clinics in Soweto, Gauteng. The practice focuses on the treatment of individuals with mental health problems, group therapy and vocational rehabilitation.

Previously he worked as a senior lecturer in the Department of Occupational Therapy, University of Pretoria, in the field of occupational therapy, mental health, psychiatry and group therapy. His research interest is on individuals with major depressive disorders, bereavement, occupational therapy groups and vocational rehabilitation. He has published extensively in scientific journals. He regularly presents at international and national conferences.

Mpho Sylvia Ramano – M Occ Ther (University of Pretoria), PG Dip Voc Rehab with distinction (University of Pretoria) and B Occ Ther (Medical University of South Africa, MEDUNSA) – currently works as an occupational therapy clinician in private practice. The practice focuses on the treatment of individuals with mental health problems, group therapy and vocational rehabilitation. Her research interest is on major depressive disorders and vocational rehabilitation.

Kobela Veronica Ramodike – Master of Health Professions Education (Maastricht University, Netherlands), B Occ Ther (Hons) (Medical University of Southern Africa) and B Occ Ther (Medical University of Southern Africa) – is an educator at Sefako Makgatho Health Sciences University. Her area of teaching is mental health and psychiatry, with involvement in clinical education and supervision. She also teaches therapeutic media, with an interest in the use of problem-based learning as a teaching methodology in occupational therapy. Her research interest is in the education and development of assessment tools. She has published collaborative research and presented part of her study at one of the World Federation of Occupational Therapists conferences. She is currently in the process of completing her PhD.

Lee Randall – PhD (University of the Witwatersrand), MA (Boston School of Occupational Therapy, Tufts University, USA) and BSc Occ Ther (University of the Witwatersrand) – is a Private Practitioner and former Vice President of the Occupational Therapy Association of South Africa (OTASA). Her professional interests are medicolegal work, vocational rehabilitation, psychiatric disability, disability equity in the workplace and functional capacity evaluations (FCEs) for insurance purposes. She was awarded a Fulbright Fellowship to undertake her master's degree in Boston, Massachusetts, and spent a year working and studying in New Zealand in the 1990s. She has a keen interest in road safety, focusing on minibus taxi crashes for her PhD research through the Steve Biko Centre for Bioethics (Wits) and continuing with research into travel behaviour and road safety as a postdoctoral fellow at the SAMRC/Wits Centre for Health Economics & Decision Science-PRICELESS-SA. She co-founded the Road Ethics Project non-profit company, regularly presents at conferences and other events and has had many media engagements.

Tania Rauch van der Merwe – PhD (University of the Free State), M Occ Ther (University of the Free State) and B Occ Ther (University of the Free State) – is Senior Lecturer at the Department of Occupational Therapy, University of the Witwatersrand (South Africa) and former Chairperson of the Occupational Therapy Department at the University of the Free State (South Africa). Tania is an educator and supervisor in the fields of occupational therapy, research and mental health and psychiatry. Her research interests include critical discourse analysis and theory, and occupational therapy higher education. She was appointed as one of the members of the core organising committee for the 2024 World Conference on Qualitative Research, hosted in South Africa. She coordinated the Wits University 80th Celebration Symposium in 2023, publishes her work in international journals and books, and regularly presents her work at national and international conferences.

Nicole Rautenbach – BSc Occ Ther (UCT) – is a chief occupational therapist at Sterkfontein Psychiatric Hospital in Mogale City in the Gauteng Province of South Africa. She has experience working in the forensic psychiatric context as an occupational therapist and is involved in observations, assessment and treatment of forensic and long-term psychiatric inpatients. Nicole is currently completing an MSc in occupational therapy with her research focusing on occupational therapists' contribution to the assessment of children's criminal capacity.

Stephanie Redinger – PhD (Paediatrics and Child Health, University of the Witwatersrand), B Occ Ther (University of KwaZulu-Natal) is a Postdoctoral Research Fellow (Centre of Excellence in Human Development, University of the Witwatersrand) and has a research interest in mental health, parenting and child development. She is the co-author of UNICEF's mental health intervention, Caring for the Caregiver, and is currently conducting research to understand its effectiveness in a multi-country study.

Gina Rencken – M. Occ Ther (University of the Free State) and B Occ Ther (University of Pretoria) – is a lecturer and clinician in the field of paediatric occupational therapy at the University of KwaZulu-Natal, with a particular interest in neonatal care, early intervention, ADHD and neurodevelopmental conditions. She has a research and clinical interest in infant, child and maternal mental health. She is trained in Ayres Sensory Integration® and lectures in the South African Institute for Sensory Integration (SAISI)'s qualification course. She is an executive committee member of SAISI and serves on the International Council for Education in Ayres Sensory Integration (ICE-ASI). She has published in peer-reviewed journals and presented at national and international conferences.

Catherine Shorten – BA Socio-Cultural Anthropology (University of South Africa), Occupational Therapy Assistant (OTA) Diploma (Sandringham Gardens), Occupational Therapy Technician (OTT) (HPCSA), Fashion Design and Management Diploma with distinction (FDM College, Johannesburg) and Fashion Design and Pattern Cutting Diploma with distinction (City & Guilds Institute of London) – worked for many years in the garment industry as a designer, pattern cutter and grader before starting her OTA training. During her training, she worked in a number of old age homes and retirement facilities. Once qualified, she worked in an occupational therapy private practice for 16 years specialising in adult psychiatry, often including physical disability. She was awarded 'Top Academic Student' in her OTA training course (1994) and awarded 'OTA of the year' (2004). She has organised and presented training workshops for OTT's. Catherine has attended many national and international conferences and has presented papers at conferences in Madrid (Spain), Taipei (Taiwan), Mauritius, Bronkhorstspruit and Cape Town.

Olindah Silaule – PhD (University of the Witwatersrand), MSc Occ Ther (University of the Witwatersrand) and BSc Occ Ther (University of the Witwatersrand) – is a lecturer in the fields of occupational therapy, mental health and psychiatry at the Department of Occupational Therapy, University of the Witwatersrand. She coordinates a fourth-year student rural fieldwork placement, which is aimed at developing the students' knowledge and skills in rural health practice. Her expertise is in community-based mental health rehabilitation, with a focus on evidence-based practice for patients and families in rural communities. Her doctoral project focuses on developing strategies for alleviating caregiver burden among informal caregivers of persons with severe mental disorders in rural South Africa.

Mogammad Shaheed Soeker – BSc Occ Ther (University of the Western Cape), MSc Occ Ther (University of the Western Cape), Adv Dip Management (University of the Western Cape), PhD (University of the Western Cape) – is Professor and Chairperson of the Department of Occupational Therapy at the University of the Western Cape. He has extensive experience in the area of vocational rehabilitation and paediatric occupational therapy. He has published several articles and chapters in international peer-reviewed journals and books. Professor Soeker was awarded a National Research Foundation C3 researcher rating in January 2021 and has been called upon to be a keynote speaker at various international conferences.

Lyndsey Swart – M Occ Ther (University of the Free State), BSc Occ Ther (University of the Witwatersrand), PG Dip Voc Rehab (University of Pretoria), Certificate in Advanced Labour Law (University of South Africa) and Certificate in Occupational Health and Safety (University of Cape Town) – is a director at Ergonomics at Work, a consultancy offering ergonomics risk assessment and vocational rehabilitation services. She is also a session lecturer on the Postgraduate Diploma in Vocational Rehabilitation at the University of Pretoria. She has a keen interest in the legal aspects of medical incapacity and disability in the workplace and served on the drafting team of the Employment Equity Act's Code of Good Practice on the Employment of Persons with Disabilities (South Africa).

Zarina Syed – BSc Occ Ther (University of the Western Cape), M Occ Ther (Stellenbosch University) and PG Dip Addiction Care (Stellenbosch University) – has been involved in student education for the past 10 years. Her role includes clinical supervision of students, teaching undergraduate and postgraduate students as well as supervision of research. She began her career working as an occupational therapist at hospitals in Cape Town. Zarina is passionate about the field of mental health in occupational therapy, particularly the acute psychiatric setting and addiction care. She is currently exploring future studies around the role of the occupational therapist in addiction care.

Karlien Terblanche – M Occ Ther (Advanced Occupational Therapy) (University of Stellenbosch) and B Occ Ther (University of Pretoria) – is an occupational therapist in mental health, currently in private practice working with clients through individual and group therapy. She previously worked at Crescent Clinic, an acute mental health clinic, and at Lentegeur Hospital. She has 14 years of experience working within the field of mental health and seven years of experience working in private practice. She has offered clinical supervision to third-year students while working at Crescent Clinic and as a clinical supervisor for external placements. Her Master's thesis focused on the occupational life trajectories of young men in the Heideveld community. She has specific interest in the field of anxiety disorders and eating disorders.

Itumeleng Tsatsi-Mosala – M Occ Ther (Stellenbosch University) and BSc Occ Ther (University of Cape Town) – is an occupational therapist and researcher in psychiatry and mental health. She is a lecturer in the Department of Occupational Therapy at the University of the Witwatersrand. Her research niche includes promoting occupational justice with mental healthcare users. In 2018, Tumi was recognised as an influential young South African by the Mail and Guardian 200 Young South Africans for being a trailblazer in the occupational therapy field. In 2019, she received a 100 Young Mandela of the Future award by News24 for her contribution in occupational therapy mental health research. She is now serving in the Occupational Therapy Africa Regional Group (OTARG) executive committee as a social media coordinator and the Occupational Therapy Association of South Africa (OTASA) occupational science committee as secretary.

Marlene van den Berg – M Psych (University of North West) and B Occ Ther (University of Pretoria) – is Therapeutic Manager and Occupational Therapist at Akeso Montrose Manor in Cape Town and Founder and Group Therapist at Healing Spaces Wellness in Cape Town. She is an occupational therapist with more than 15 years of experience working in the field of mental health. She has worked with clients with acute and chronic mental health conditions, eating disorders, addiction concerns and personality disorders. She currently works in a specialist eating disorder unit and hosts an outpatient support community called Healing Spaces Wellness. She is a trained Gestalt and Play therapist, TRE and Enneagram practitioner and Yoga teacher. She has a specific interest in group intervention and holistic, healing processes.

Annamarie van Jaarsveld – PhD (University of the Free State), M Occ Ther (University of the Free State) and Dip Occ Ther (Vona du Toit College of Occupational Therapy) – is a semi-retired, former Senior Lecturer. She is currently Affiliated Lecturer at the Department of Occupational Therapy, University of the Free State. Her main fields of interest are paediatrics, sensory integration, and mental health. Her area of research is sensory integration. She has served on the board of the South African Institute for Sensory Integration (SAISI) for the past 35 years in various capacities, which includes chairperson and international liaison. In 2011, the Pediatric Therapy Network in Los Angeles awarded her the Sonia Martins Lopez International Award, recognising her as an outstanding individual from outside the United States for promoting sensory integration research and practice. In 2017, she received the Discovery Clinical Excellence Award 2017 at the IMFAR SAACAPAP, Congress with which SAISI recognised her contribution towards research within the field of sensory integration. In 2019, she received a rating as an established researcher from the National Research Foundation of South Africa. She has presented various papers nationally and internationally, which include keynote addresses. Her work has been published nationally and internationally.

Lana van Niekerk – PhD (University of Cape Town), M Occ Ther (University of the Free State) and B Occ Ther (University of the Free State) – teaches at bachelor's, masters' and doctoral levels; her fields of expertise include research methods, ethics and occupational science. Her research has focused on equitable participation of people facing disabling conditions in the world of work. She is a current member of the Expert Advisory Panel on Community Health and Transport (I-CHaT), which coordinates research on transport mobility; the Panel's current research is *linking people and activities through transport mobility* (LiPATTM). As an active researcher in the fields of work and disability equity, she is a C2-rated researcher with the National Research Foundation in South Africa.

Matty van Niekerk – MSc Med (Bioethics and Health Law, University of the Witwatersrand), PG Dip Health Professions Education and Leadership (Foundation for Professional Development), PG Dip Voc Rehab (University of Pretoria), B Occ Ther (University of Pretoria) and Baccalaureus Procurationis (University of the Free State) – is Head of the Department of Occupational Therapy, School of Therapeutic Sciences, Faculty of Health Sciences, University of the Witwatersrand, Johannesburg. She is a former Chairperson of the Professional Board for Occupational Therapy, Medical Orthotics and Prosthetics and Arts Therapy of the Health Professions Council of South Africa. Matty is an occupational therapy academic with a keen interest in the regulation of professions, the nexus between health/medical ethics and the law and health professions education. She publishes her work in accredited, peer-reviewed journals and is a regular presenter on professionalism, ethics and the law, and health professions education at national and international conferences.

Kerry Wallace – MSc Occ Ther (University of the Witwatersrand) and BSc Occ Ther (University of Cape Town) – Kerry is the Director of Therapy SPOT In Perth Australia, and a clinician in the field of occupational therapy, mental health and paediatrics. She has advanced training in Neurodevelopmental Therapy, Sensory Integration and DIR®:Floortime™ through Profectum Foundation, United States. She is also the Founder and Chairperson of SPOTlight Trust SA, which is a non-profit organisation that provides online and in-person training to health professionals, educators and parents.

Lisa Wegner – PhD (University of Cape Town), MSc Occ Ther (University of Cape Town) and BSc Occ Ther (University of the Witwatersrand) – is a Professor and the former Chairperson of the Department of Occupational Therapy at the University of the Western Cape (South Africa). She is an occupational therapist and educator in mental health and psychiatry. Her research interest is with vulnerable youth. She received the International Collaborative Prevention Science Award from the Society for Prevention Research (USA) in 2014. She is a C2-rated researcher with the National Research Foundation (South Africa), publishes her work in scientific journals and books and is a regular presenter at international and national conferences.

Minkateko Wicht – BSc Occ Ther (University of Cape Town) – is an occupational therapist based in Cape Town working in private and community practice. She has experience working in numerous settings in both urban and rural environments with individuals and groups across the lifespan. Currently, her practice is focused on trauma-informed approaches, enabling mental health and well-being and managing stress and burnout, at both an individual and a collective level. She works as an independent contractor facilitating transformation processes and trainings in various teams and organisations and sees individuals in her private practice. She is also completing a Master of Science in Occupational Therapy at the University of Cape Town and is exploring the role of context in emerging adults' experiences of occupational possibilities and occupational choices in a community in the Western Cape.

Elvin Williams – MPhil Infant Mental Health (Stellenbosch University) and BSc Occ Ther (Cum Laude) (University of the Western Cape) – is Lecturer in the Division of Occupational Therapy and Arts Therapies, School of Health Sciences, Queen Margaret University, Scotland. Elvin's professional interests include occupational therapy philosophy, mental health, identity and resilience, and leadership in the field of occupational therapy.

Kobie Zietsman – B Occ Ther (University of Stellenbosch) – is a retired occupational therapist who worked at the former Randfontein Care Centre from 1983 to 2013, being responsible for the development of rehabilitation programmes for 500 long-term mental healthcare users. She developed an outcome measure, the Functional Level Outcome Measure (FLOM) – to enable the multidisciplinary team to group each mental healthcare user according to a functional level. Under Kobie's supervision, appropriate rehabilitation programmes were developed according to the levels and presented by occupational therapy assistants and technicians. She also supervised numerous fourth-year occupational therapy students at Randfontein Care Centre.

Foreword

The sixth edition of *Occupational Therapy in Psychiatry and Mental Health* follows its fifth edition, published in 2014, by 8 years and the first edition by 34 years. I recall holding the first edition in my hands when it was published in 1989, thrilled by Rosemary Crouch's exceptional achievement in documenting the diverse practices of occupational therapists in mental health and psychiatry and in so doing, compiling the first textbook of its kind in South Africa for occupational therapy clinicians and students. Dr Crouch also edited the second edition published in 1992 and was joined by Vivyan Alers as co-editor of the third edition in 1997, the fourth edition in 2005 and the fifth edition in 2014. All the editions have significantly contributed to mental health occupational therapy practice, research and education in South Africa and internationally, each reflecting the contextual responsiveness of the profession to prevailing public mental health service challenges in low resource and culturally diverse settings.

Likewise, the sixth edition positions occupational therapy for relevance in a post-COVID, globalising and environmentally unstable world. It is a valuable addition to the current academic literature for occupational therapy practitioners, undergraduate and postgraduate students, and other members of the multi-professional team, most notably because of its overarching focus on human functioning, social inclusion and participation in real-world contexts. The high burden of mental, neurological and substance use disorders has major productivity and economic consequences, especially since their effect is felt more by disability than by mortality. Mental health disorders are projected to cost the global economy US$16.1 trillion by the year 2030, which is more than cancer, diabetes and respiratory diseases combined. This book foregrounds occupational therapy as a rehabilitation science concerned with preventing disability, building resilience and enabling adaptive participation in the activities of everyday life. It illustrates the interface between occupational science and occupational therapy and confirms the profession as an important human resource for mitigating the occupational causes and consequences of mental ill health.

Comprising 30 inter-related chapters written by expert practitioners and academics, the content of the book is aligned with contemporary international mental health nosology and sustainable development policy frameworks that advocate universal health access, human rights, deinstitutionalisation, community-based care and integration of mental health into general healthcare in accordance with the primary healthcare philosophy. The book considers how the social determinants of mental health and mental disorders affect human development and human occupation across the lifespan and provides occupation-focused practice guidelines for promoting mental health, identifying risk factors and preventative interventions for those at risk, and using recovery-orientated interventions for those with poor mental health. Each chapter draws on evidence-based research and practice-based evidence to describe the principles, processes and methods of psychosocial occupational therapy delivered across a range of intersectoral service platforms so that individuals, groups and populations benefit, not only in urban but also in rural areas. Readers will find the layout of the book accessible and the case examples and reflective questions at the end of each chapter useful for integrating theory with practice and for developing professional reasoning.

The editorial team, expertly mentored by Rosemary Crouch and guided by the academic and practice wisdom of lead editor Lisa Wegner, is congratulated for bringing the sixth edition to fruition in ways that reflect the diversity, innovation and client-centredness of occupational therapy in mental health and psychiatry.

MADELEINE DUNCAN
MSc OT (UCT), DPHIL (PSYCHOLOGY) (USTELL),
Emeritus Associate Professor,
Division of Occupational Therapy
Department of Health and
Rehabilitation Sciences
Faculty of Health Sciences,
University of Cape Town

Preface

We are delighted to present the sixth edition of Crouch and Alers Occupational Therapy in Psychiatry and Mental Health, named in recognition of the leadership of Rosemary Crouch and the late Vivyan Alers in previous editions of the book. The opportunity to update the fifth edition arose at a meeting of the Crouch Bursary Fund in October 2020 when Rosemary Crouch invited the board members to edit the book. The Crouch Bursary Fund is a registered non-profit organisation (2019/462842/08) and holds the accrued funds earned from the royalties from this book. The fund is used to support occupational therapy research in the psychiatric and mental health field.

The sixth edition of this book provides an up-to-date, informative, and practical guide for students and novice occupational therapists working in mental health and psychiatric settings and related contexts. Furthermore, we hope that the book stimulates critical, reflective practice by offering new, diverse insights and viewpoints. Although most authors are South Africans, we believe the book has relevance no matter the reader's context. Our intention was to build on the solid foundation and success of previous editions by incorporating contemporary research and recent developments in occupational therapy. Revision of the book took place in the context of unprecedented human ecosystem disruptions and unsettling world events that have exacerbated mental health distress, for example, the COVID-19 pandemic; global disasters caused by humans such as conflicts and wars; and natural disasters such as earthquakes, fires and flooding. We have taken cognisance of these global and regional events and the ways in which they have influenced psychiatry and mental health, and considered the role of occupational therapy in addressing them.

There are exciting new additions to the sixth edition. In Section 1 which considers theoretical concepts in occupational therapy, the first chapter focuses on theoretical perspectives for mental health care practice. Section 2 presents specific issues; here there are new chapters on occupational therapy groups in mental health, human ecosystems and other disasters, the model of occupational self-efficacy for returning individuals with brain injury to work, and spirituality and mental health. Section 3 deals with occupational therapy for children, adolescents and adults, and a new chapter focuses on maternal mental health concerns as a priority in occupational therapy.

The African concept of *ubuntu* means humanity for others or 'I am what I am because of who we all are'. This idea guided the editing process which was a collaborative team effort between the five editors and the authors. In the spirit of *ubuntu*, editors shared their reflections and insights, providing a glimpse into how the book was developed, and the choices we made along the way. Rosemary Crouch said, 'An exciting aspect is that so many young Whiz kid occupational therapists have come on board with their various postgraduate degrees, which means content is based on solid research – just what we need in our profession'. Tania Buys said, 'I stand in awe of occupational therapists who continue to develop and offer diverse services in the area of mental health and psychiatry. In doing so, they continue to strive for occupational justice for clients, many of whom have health related limitations invisible to many, but who face profound challenges in occupational performance as a result. I am privileged to have been part of this community who has produced a fabulous book to serve as an incredible reference for new and established practitioners'. Enos Morankoana Ramano mentioned that 'The growth and changes within occupational therapy are reflected in different chapters. I salute South African occupational therapists for their effort in shaping the profession and their commitment in research'. Matty van Niekerk said, 'I found it really interesting to see the diversity of opinions in our profession about fundamental aspects of occupational therapy and occupational science. This edition provides an excellent opportunity for established and novice practitioners to integrate occupational science knowledge and see the practical application thereof in the clinical/therapeutic space'. Lisa Wegner reflected, 'This sixth edition highlights the significant contribution of South African occupational therapists to occupational therapy practice, education and research globally'.

We thank all the contributing authors who worked so hard and dedicated their time to documenting their wealth of clinical and research expertise in the various chapters of this book. We are grateful to Madeleine Duncan for her valuable, expert assistance as guest editor. Finally, we acknowledge the nameless individuals, groups and organisations who contributed to the therapist–client engagements that have provided material for the book. Without all of you, this book would not have been possible.

Professor Lisa Wegner (PhD)
Professor Rosemary Crouch (PhD)
Dr Tania Buys (PhD)
Dr Enos Morankoana Ramano (PhD)
Mrs Matty van Niekerk (MSc Med Bioethics and Health Law)

Theoretical Concepts

Theoretical Perspectives for Mental Health Care Practice

CHAPTER 1

Tania Rauch van der Merwe and Itumeleng Tsatsi-Mosala

Department of Occupational Therapy, School of Therapeutic Sciences, University of the Witwatersrand, Johannesburg, South Africa

KEY LEARNING POINTS

- Occupational therapy theoretical constructs and concepts are powerful tools to explain what is observed and why occupational therapy interventions work.

- Occupational therapy philosophical underpinnings are foundational to the profession's identity of person-centred and occupation-centred care.

- Occupational therapy models (also referred to as occupation-based models) provide essential concepts in theoretical reasoning and inform the selection of appropriate theoretical frames of reference in order to realise theory into practice and achieve, explain and justify treatment.

- Theoretical frames of reference bring theory to practice.

- Techniques and activities/occupations in occupational therapy enable clients and families to see what occupational therapists do.

- Therapeutic principles are key elements needed to achieve a treatment aim/session goal and can be extracted from therapeutic approaches determined by a diagnosis, overarching theory and occupational therapy models, and theoretical frames of reference.

- Practical strategies/principles for a session in terms of handling, structuring of the environment and activity requirements can be extracted from practical occupational therapy models and theoretical frames of reference.

INTRODUCTION

Theoretical terms in occupational therapy and perhaps many disciplines are often seen as daunting and abstract constructs with little direct application in everyday practice. Yet, literature continues to point out the gap between occupation-based practice and available theory in the profession and occupational science (Gentry *et al.* 2018). The theory-practice gap in occupational therapy is not unique if this 'gap' at all can be argued as a real gap. Foucault (1998) highlights this in his historical analysis of how human thought gave shape to the formation of 'disciplines' such as psychology and psychiatry, and states that when there is a gap between theory and practice, this gap exists in practice (O'Farrell 2005). Perhaps then, an argument can be made for the value of conceptual clarity. If one knows the meaning of concepts in the theory (that undergirds our practice), we may know more about when and how we are 'doing' (Bullock & Trombly 1999) in occupational therapy. Moreover, the value/purpose of knowing theory is that it can explain what is observed and give form to why and how one's reasoning for treatment makes sense.

The aim of this chapter is to introduce and clarify the various concepts of theory related to occupational therapy practice in mental health, juxtapose their meanings and point out their relationships to one another as to serve as a guiding post in using them in 'thinking about occupational therapy-thinking'. The purpose of this content is therefore to ultimately assist readers to enhance conscious practice and enable practitioners

Crouch and Alers Occupational Therapy in Psychiatry and Mental Health, Sixth Edition.
Edited by Rosemary Crouch, Tania Buys, Enos Morankoana Ramano, Matty van Niekerk and Lisa Wegner.
© 2025 John Wiley & Sons Ltd. Published 2025 by John Wiley & Sons Ltd.

to articulate, explain and advocate conscious practice to patients and clients, their family members, as well as colleagues and other stakeholders. The main concepts that this chapter will be covering are philosophy/philosophical underpinnings, paradigms, theoretical frameworks and models; theoretical frames of reference; and techniques in occupational therapy, which include activities and occupations.

There are nuanced differences in literature on how certain theoretical concepts are defined. For example Kielhofner (2009) and Ikiugu *et al.* (2019) view theoretical frameworks and practice models as being less distinguishable from one another towards a 'theoretical reasoning' process to apply theory eclectically for best practice. On the other hand, authors such as Cole and Tufano (2020) and Duncan (2021a) and Ebrahim (2017) do differentiate between concepts such as theories, models and theoretical frames of reference. A similar phenomenon may exist in discerning conceptual models from practice models. From a critical theoretical point of view, it is important to note that theories are inevitably informed and supported by the ideologies and worldviews held by the theorists (Hammell & Beagan 2017; Murthi & Hammell 2021). However, in order to honour the purpose of this chapter for conceptual clarity, theoretical concepts are separated to illustrate their use in theoretical reasoning for clinical practice.

A TOOLBOX FOR CONSCIOUS OCCUPATIONAL THERAPY PRACTICE

The analogy proposed to consolidate the various terms in theory is a toolbox for reasoning and for practice. Imagine carrying this toolbox with you everywhere you go as an occupational therapist, including in a setting where you share the space with a colleague in a multi-disciplinary team. See Figure 1.1 below. (Note: Due to space constraints 'TFR' is the acronym for theoretical frames of reference, and 'Occ.' stands for occupation.) This toolbox consists of the basic concepts to assist in the articulation of theoretical thinking and reasoning.

PHILOSOPHICAL UNDERPINNINGS

The first, deepest and most weighted level of the box is the philosophy of the profession, which gave form (and function) to occupational therapy as a unique profession. These philosophical underpinnings and its initial paradigm of occupation filled a glaring gap in meaning-making of reality against the backdrop of the industrial revolution at the turn of the 19th century, and the subsequent two World Wars. It was during these times that occupational therapy's adopted philosophical underpinnings of humanism, pragmatism and holism were emphatically pushing back against the mechanisation associated with the industrial revolution; the confusion of immigrants not speaking the vernacular flocking to 'global north' cities in pursuit of wealth and work; and the devastation because of the World Wars. This is the level of the toolbox that constitutes the most weight of the container, forming an undetachable base and is the least visible. This level contains the profession's philosophical underpinnings: its philosophy, ontology, axiology (values and ethics), the historical markers of its previous paradigms, as well as its current contemporary paradigm, which will be explained under the relevant sections to follow.

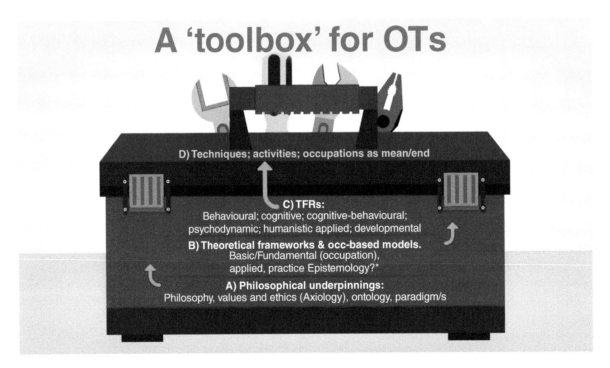

FIGURE 1.1   A 'toolbox' for occupational therapists.

OVERARCHING THEORETICAL FRAMEWORKS AND OCCUPATION-BASED MODELS

The second level is the overarching theoretical frameworks, occupation-based models and the second weighted level in the toolbox. This level (and the following ones) can be unpacked from the toolbox, allowing the practitioner to choose the best tool as the best goodness-of-fit for practice and reaching session goals and treatment outcomes. Overarching theoretical frameworks are the theories that are foundational to reasoning in occupational therapy and which may provide a language when engaging with members of the multi-disciplinary team on the occupation-centred foci of occupational therapy for health, healing, occupational participation and engagement. One such overarching theory is systems theory, which also underpins, for example the Model of Human Occupation (MOHO) (Kielhofner 2009). Systems theory explains why components of people's function and the context in which they live do not operate in isolation from one another but are rather irrevocably interdependent on one, or several other components, or even other systems. For example the contextual/environmental/occupational/functional components and their relationships to be considered in a treatment plan for a person with schizophrenia who happens to have a supporting family from a middle socio-economic status will differ from the considerations in reasoning for a person with the same diagnosis, even perhaps diagnosed at the same time, who does not have any familial, socio-economic or historical support. Embedded in systems theory is also complexity theory, which explains why seemingly small components, or actions, may have significant or major consequences, or the other way around. Closely linked with occupational therapy is occupational science, the allegorical 'mother borne from the daughter' as this foundational discipline historically originated from the applied science of occupational therapy in the 1980s (e.g. Duncan 2021b). Subsumed to the development of occupational science in the profession of occupational therapy is the critical decolonial theoretical framework. This framework may be an essential consideration in occupational therapy reasoning given the occupational therapy discipline's vital turn in reflection and awareness of the impact and relevance of the historical markers of the occupational therapy profession, and the occupational science discipline's Eurocentric origin (Hammell 2009a; Whiteford & Hocking 2012; Farias & Laliberte Rudman 2016; Galvaan et al. 2022). Another overarching theoretical framework worth mentioning is the International Classification of Function (ICF), which is a bio-psychosocial theoretical framework and a standardised tool that enables a common understanding and language across health professions about the impact of disease/disorder/injury/trauma on peoples' health, well-being and activity participation, given personal, societal and environmental factors. The socio-justice aim of this theoretical framework is to maximise humans' ability to fulfil their potential for participation in their environments to healthily thrive and actively participate in life rather than focusing on the health condition from the outset (World Health Organization 2002).

Models are a convergent depiction of theories describing, explaining and predicting the interactions between person/s, occupation and environment. However, when looking at a diagram of a model, one needs to familiarise oneself with the theory behind it to make full sense of the diagrammatic depiction. Theoretical models are typically unique to the discipline in which they are situated, and occupation-based models are no different. Models give the practitioner the terminology and concepts to understand observed/assessed behaviour and dynamics, as well as to posit a sound, justifiable clinical reasoning process towards the design of intervention and treatment plans. Occupation-based models can serve as a 'funnel' through which the selection of suitable theoretical frames of reference, as well as the extraction and generation of treatment principles, may be consolidated and contained. Models/frameworks that are put forward for the purpose of this chapter are Kielhofner's MOHO (Kielhofner 2008, 2009) which offers an encapsulated occupation-based view on dynamic systems theory, as well as its empirical development of assessment and treatment tools over time. A second model that will be presented for overview is the Vona du Toit Model of Creative Ability (VdTMoCA) (du Toit 1980; van der Reyden et al. 2019). This model was developed in South Africa in the 1970s by Vona du Toit, an iconic stalwart for the development of the profession in South Africa and its national representation in the newly found World Federation of Occupational Therapists in the second half of the 20th century. This model is particularly valuable as it serves fundamentally a practice model, giving detailed and systematic guidance for appropriate outcomes, aims, handling, presentation and activity requirements for each of the levels of creative ability. The levels of creative ability, based on the theory of human development, are in turn indicative of the level of volition, motivation and its associated level of action possible. The VdTMoCA is not only useful when working with individuals in mental health but also with large groups of people in psychiatric institutions. The applicability and utility of this model are increasingly gaining traction in community-based practice settings. A third model for overview is the Kawa model because of its collectivist, cultural view that is highly relevant for the majority/Global South population (Iwama 2006; Turpin & Iwama 2011; Iwama et al. 2009). Included for overview in this chapter is the theoretical organisation of concepts put forward by Galvaan and Peters' (2017): the Occupation-based Community Development (O-bCD) framework. This framework is included in the cluster of occupation-based models because of its highly relevant concepts in a majority world, such as belonging, the dialectic values of groups' rights and responsibilities as a drive towards self-determination as well as the value of drawing on existing social structures for the greater good of a community. The level of overarching theories and occupational-based models informs the way knowledge is regarded and generated in the profession, also referred to as epistemology.

THEORETICAL FRAMES OF REFERENCE (TFR)

The third level following theoretical frameworks and occupational therapy models is theoretical frames of reference. These theoretical tools are less weighted than the models but are key to connecting theory with practice. They are theoretical tools that originated typically outside the profession's theory-base in disciplines such as psychology or education. These frames of references have theoretical premises and principles from which occupational therapy practitioners can judiciously draw to design a treatment session with the scientific essences/ essential principles needed to reach treatment outcomes. Theoretical frames of reference relevant for occupational therapy practice in psychiatry include behavioural, cognitive behavioural, psychodynamic, existential and an adult learning theoretical frame of reference/principles. Spirituality as part of an existential theoretical frame of reference may be subsumed under the existential theoretical frame of reference, having its origin in the discipline of theology and philosophy. While spirituality has been employed as a concept in occupational therapy models or guidelines (e.g. Canadian Association of Occupational Therapy 1997; Mthembu 2017; Ramugondo 2017), it is still in the process of being developed as a theory standing on its own in occupational therapy. Theoretical frames of reference, together with principles associated with the specific diagnosis, practice guidelines from practice models and principles from occupational science, may be argued as tools that can be drawn on, and when crafted together through a theoretical reasoning process, make up the essential principles for successfully reaching treatment outcomes and session goals.

TECHNIQUES, ACTIVITIES AND OCCUPATION AS A MEANS AND/OR AN END

The fourth and final level of the theoretical toolbox is the top and most visible level. This level constitutes techniques, activities and the use of occupations as a means or an end. Occupation as means is, for example, when a therapist does a group cooking activity to improve socialisation and communication between the patients. Occupation as an end is when a cooking activity is done with a patient who has to return home and resume his/her role to cook for the family. If a colleague or client's family member observes an occupational therapist doing therapy, these actions are what is most visible, though the theory, models, theoretical frames of reference and theoretical reasoning behind what is viewed may not be visible for an observer from the outset.

The following sections contain more in-depth discussions about each of the levels of this toolbox.

THE RELATIONSHIP BETWEEN PHILOSOPHICAL UNDERPINNINGS, MODELS, THEORETICAL FRAMES OF REFERENCE AND PRACTICE

The analogy of the toolbox is extended (Figure 1.2) to show the relationship between philosophical underpinnings, models, theoretical frames of references (TFR) and practice.

Figure 1.2 shows how occupational therapy models/ frameworks represent the vehicle the practitioner chooses, based on the fieldwork setting, the patient/people's problems

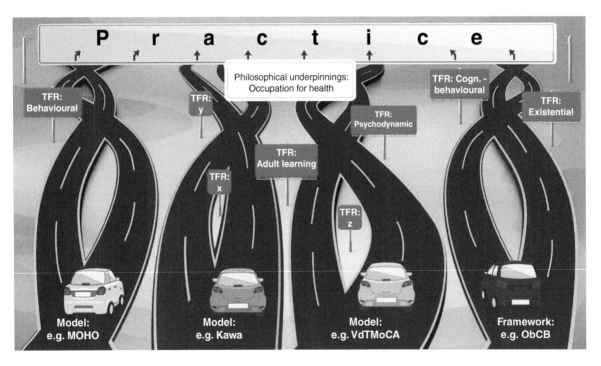

FIGURE 1.2 Depiction of relationship between philosophical underpinnings, occupation-based models/frameworks, theoretical frames of reference and practice.

and needs and their context. A theoretical model or framework serves as a figurative vehicle that provides the practitioner with the necessary tools (concepts) to start the clinical reasoning process in the artful crafting of necessary treatment principles for a treatment plan. This model/vehicle can access any of the roads, representing the various, appropriate theoretical frames of reference. In finding the best way towards successful practice, the vehicle/model can access more than one and the best roads/theoretical frames of reference, as well as moving between them. The roads/theoretical frames of reference, in this way, serve the purpose of bringing theory to practice.

PHILOSOPHY OF OCCUPATIONAL THERAPY

Seminal literature (e.g. Hagedorn 1995; Kielhofner 2009) suggests that there is fair consensus in occupational therapy about the meaning of an underpinning philosophy of the profession, its philosophy being the 'innermost core of knowledge in that it directly addresses the identity of occupational therapy' (Kielhofner 2009, p. 26). The occupational therapy profession's philosophical underpinnings are constituted by a view of human beings, the view of health, the view of the profession and a view of theory, the latter linking with the creation of knowledge (epistemology) and paradigms of the profession (Bryant *et al.* 2022). Both a personal (van der Merwe 2008) and therefore a professional philosophy may be argued as consisting of three kinds of views: how the world is viewed, how humankind is viewed and what is viewed as a good life. For example occupational therapists' professional philosophy about patients in this world who have a psychiatric condition still views people from this population as holistic, occupational beings (humankind) whose condition and environmental context (world) and therefore health and well-being are intrinsically linked with occupational opportunities, restrictions (Galvaan 2015) and participation. Occupational therapists' view of the world with humans (including people with mental health conditions) in it is anchored by the understanding that humans are biologically and neurologically wired with the need and desire to engage in a variety of occupations for various amounts of time, which provides the sense of gratification in mastery of occupational action; provides a sense of pleasure and a sense of restoration (Pierce 2003; Eklund *et al.* 2017; World Federation of Occupation Therapists 2012a). Occupational therapists' view of a good life is constituted by the premise of occupational balance and extends to occupational justice and occupational rights (Townsend & Wilcock 2004; Hammell 2008). These views are intertwined by the big 'ology'-words: ontology, epistemology and axiology. Though these concepts may appear abstract and difficult to articulate, they are useful, if not necessary, in consolidating consciously, a professional identity.

Ontology in the philosophy of a profession entails the view of reality and what it consists of. When working with persons who have a mental health/psychiatric condition, there are aspects that for example are universal because of a diagnosis of which the symptoms can be recognised in most contexts. Though there are also aspects of that person's function that are unique to a person or a population's historical, socio-economic, cultural and identity contexts. Both these universal and relativist views are part of the holistic ontology in occupational therapy.

Epistemology is about the scientific ways of generating knowledge about what the profession studies and views as true. The occupational therapy profession has a unique understanding of the array of complexities when working with individuals, groups and populations within various environments, and the associated occupations. For this reason, the profession epistemologically is quite proficient in generating qualitative research linked to a relativist ontological view and contexts (e.g. political, educational, socio-economic and ecological). However, for the occupational therapy profession to remain relevant, if not indispensable, in the biopsychosocial health realm, it must also epistemologically, generate scientific evidence of why and how what it does, works towards the improvement of people's mental health.

Axiology is basically the professional values and ethics inherent to occupational therapy, also when working with patients with mental health conditions. Examples of such values are altruism, equality, truth and justice. Examples of ethics inherent to occupational therapy, if not all health care professions, are ensuring non-maleficence, beneficence, dignity, confidentiality and respecting the autonomy of persons (e.g. World Federation of Occupation Therapists 2012b). An axiology, or core value of the occupational therapy profession, is its person-centred view of people as occupational beings. This means a person, group or population to whom occupational therapy service are rendered to always comes first. However, globally, there is an ever-growing neo-liberalist capitalist trend of converting/comparing all tangible and intangible qualities to a market value (e.g. Brown 2019). The equally increasing challenge for occupational therapy students and clinicians in this world is to maintain the core axiology of person- (in need of occupational-therapy) centredness. This means not to compare one's vulnerability, 'triggers', fragility and care needed with that of one's patients to the extent that a therapist can only provide a service to certain people barring certain conditions. Occupational therapists are humans and are not exempt from mental health challenges. However, these challenges must be addressed separately from one's service as a health care provider, and where possible, before engaging with persons needing therapy.

PARADIGM

Kielhofner (2009, p. 9) puts forward that a paradigm in occupational therapy is core to its knowledge and that a paradigm 'defines the nature, purpose, scope, and value of occupational therapy practice (meaning the) most basic nature of (occupational therapists') work'. A paradigm therefore gives form to culture of a profession and is the theoretical flow from the philosophical underpinnings of a profession.

A paradigm would typically change when its purpose crosses the threshold of inadequacy, and when it no longer has epistemic legitimacy. Hence, the occupational therapy profession has experienced several paradigm-shifts over its more than 100 years' existence (Kielhofner 2009; Duncan 2021a), an extraordinary though traumatic process for any profession as the core beliefs at that time are challenged and re-configured with consequences for its professional identity and culture. Such a shift can be analogically equated with a 'personality change', though it is also indicative of a dynamic nature and growth.

PARADIGMS AND PARADIGM SHIFTS IN OCCUPATIONAL THERAPY

The occupational therapy profession was established based on its original *paradigm of occupation* between the 1900s and the 1940s. The philosophy of humanism associated with Moral Treatment was also inclusive of the value of human dignity through meaningful occupations. Supporting philosophies were holism and pragmatism. Holism was the counter force to reductionism central to an industrial revolution which in contrast valued people to the extent they could contribute to production and the economy. Holism maintained the understanding that the whole is bigger than the sum of its parts.

Pragmatism, as an underpinning philosophy and paradigm was, and arguably remains, a strong theoretical influence in occupational therapy. Pragmatism was part of the social movement as a counter to industrialisation and was enacted by Jane Addams as a member of the Women Suffrage Movement and the first wave of feminism. She promoted social cohesion and human dignity of the working force, many of whom were immigrants and who were naturally exploited and marginalised in the throes of industrialisation and foreign social contexts. Pragmatism, theoretically, pursues practical and best ways of addressing problems. It was therefore central to the profession's strong base of know-how knowledge and a problem-solving focus (e.g. Morrison 2021).

The original paradigm of occupation was disrupted by the first crisis of epistemic legitimacy the profession was confronted with. While occupational therapy gained marked momentum as a needed profession that makes a difference, after the World Wars, it was also seriously questioned by the medical fraternity for not sufficiently substantiating its practice with theoretical evidence. This de-legitimisation led to the profession adopting a *mechanistic paradigm* (1960s–1970s) in its quest to provide positivistic evidence of its in-depth knowledge of systems, assessment and addressing human components situated in theoretical frames of reference (Rauch van der Merwe 2019; Cole & Tufano 2020; Duncan 2021a).

The second legitimacy crisis emerged when the occupational therapy profession, enabled by its innate reflexive posture and realised that in adopting the reductionistic mechanistic paradigm, it sacrificed its core philosophical construct of occupation, and therefore a core aspect of its identity.

Consequently, scholars at the University of Southern California in the 1980s called for doctoral proposals for the theorisation of the science of occupation, and the third and current *contemporary paradigm* (1980s henceforth) emerged (Duncan 2021a).

THEORY AND THEORETICAL FRAMEWORKS

Theoretical frameworks consist of a compilation of theories, which are an organised way of thinking about phenomena that draw together concepts, hypotheses and assumptions in order to describe, explain, and predict phenomena and behaviour. These latter characteristics are essential for a theory to qualify as a theory. Theory development does not occur overnight and is not only a re-iterative process but also a collaborative one. The development of theory can be reduced to six steps (Kielhofner 2009; Creswell & Creswell 2018; Gillen & Brown 2023):

1. Develop initial conceptual ideas.

2. Refine conceptual ideas.

3. Test theory in practice.

4. Develop tools for practice.

5. Increase evidence base for a conceptual model.

6. Externally verify conceptual model and tools for practice.

Theory development is not static but an ongoing and dynamic process. The following theories are overarching and foundational to occupational therapy and mental health care.

SYSTEMS THEORY

Systems theory is a central overarching theory of occupational therapy. Systems theory explains how various contextual factors interact with each other as well as their interdependence, while complexity theory explains how heterogeneity, or the variety between the various subsystems, determines a vast array of outcomes (Amagoh 2016). Systems theory was a significant point of departure and foundational framework for the development of Kielhofner's MOHO (Kielhofner 1978; Cole & Tufano 2020). Kielhofner adapted this model over the years to amongst other things, change the view of the person-occupation-environment system from a closed system where the components are hierarchical, to the view of an open system where the components operate and interact on a heterarchical level (Turpin & Iwama 2011). The Occupational Therapy Practice Framework (OTPF) IV (American Association of Occupational Therapy 2020) is also an example of a theoretical framework drawing on systems theory. Systems theory and complexity theory give occupational therapists a language to explain the many variables and their non-linear interdependent relationships when reasoning about the person-occupation-environment triad/system. However, complexity theory also explains why it is often difficult to equate maximum effort in clinical work with minimum outcomes or how a small action can have major effects. Hence, the importance of clinical reasoning (Chapter 6).

OCCUPATIONAL SCIENCE

The discipline of occupational science informs philosophy and theory in the profession of occupational therapy (Motimele 2022). Occupational therapy practice has its roots in the Global North. It is for this reason that many theoretical frameworks have been developed with a Global North perspective that may not suit a Global South practice. Scholars in the Global South have critically engaged the discourse and developed theories that do not only resonate with the Global South but are contextually relevant. Ramugondo (2015) explains occupational consciousness as an ongoing awareness of the dynamics of hegemony and recognition that dominant practices are sustained through what people do every day, with implications for personal and collective health. By subscribing to theories and practices of the west, the Global South unconsciously gives away power over everyday life, including practice. Therefore, the Global South needs to acknowledge its own theories and practices as valid and equally important.

Following Blau *et al.*'s (1956) conceptual framework on occupational choice, Galvaan (2015) acknowledged that occupational scientists in the Global North have not appreciated the complexities of its situated nature. In attempting to unpack such complexities, her work sought to critically investigate the factors shaping the occupational choices of marginalised young adolescents in a community in Cape Town, South Africa. Galvaan (2015) discusses the nature of occupational choice, emphasising how the social environment together with collective and contextual histories influence the manner and types of occupational choices made. This highlights how rich the Global South context is in culture and collective occupations. Individualism and independence in occupational therapy are often encouraged in the Global North. However, Tsatsi and Plastow (2021) found that in a group of male mental health care users residing in a hospital halfway house, the occupational need for interdependence was valued as it promoted collective occupational engagement while encouraging occupational independence. The occupational need for interdependence is the need to engage in occupations that keep individuals together and provide opportunities to rely on one another in working towards a common goal (Tsatsi & Plastow 2021).

This occupational need is present among various communities and is frequently encountered in practice. Similarly, Ramugondo and Kronenberg (2015) define collective occupations as occupations engaged in, by groups in ordinary environments with an intention towards social cohesion, or dysfunction, and may reflect an advancement of, or aversion to, a common good. It is such findings that encouraged

scholars in the Global South to name phenomena in their context and by doing so validate their everyday occupational therapy practices. This critical approach encourages a decolonial occupational therapy practice, making it more complex to apply Western theories without critical evaluation and relevance to the local context.

Occupational science constructs are widely used in the Global South with careful consideration of the contexts to which they are applied. Some are inspired by lived experiences in their given contexts. In occupational therapy education, some constructs are more understood than others, for example the experience of occupational injustice as a concept resonates with the history of apartheid South Africa. Occupational apartheid is when individuals, groups and communities are deprived of meaningful and purposeful activity through segregation due to social, political, economic factors and for social status reasons (Kronenberg et al. 2005). Exclusion and deprivation from participation in meaningful occupations due to race, socio-economic or political status are widely understood in the Global South. The majority of clients accessing public mental health care services experience some form of occupational apartheid.

CRITICAL THEORETICAL AND DECOLONIAL THEORETICAL FRAMEWORKS

Against the backdrop of the evolving development of knowledge of the occupational therapy profession (Hooper 2006) as well as its increasingly reflexive posture about its relevance and contextual responsiveness in and for a majority world/the Global South, the integration of a critical theoretical and decolonial epistemic framework may be argued as essential for the future development of the profession, in promoting epistemic justice (Fricker 2017) and collaboratively and collectively craft epistemic freedom (Ndlovu-Gatsheni 2018). It is therefore important to be constantly aware of how and where occupational therapy originated from, and which historical markers it may carry within. Historical markers may both enable or mitigate one's taken-for-granted assumptions about the ways of viewing, thinking and speaking about clients/patients from an array of diverse contexts. For example the subtle, albeit unintended ways one may 'other' a person who has different cultural views about illness and health, relationships and partners. Or one's assumptions about the occupational differentiations between activities for productivity, restoration and pleasure. Such awareness is anchored in both reflective (about one's own actions) and reflexive (about the effects of one's actions in a larger context) practice and should be the norm rather than the exception (e.g. Guajardo *et al.* 2015; Mignolo & Walsh 2018; Mthembu & Bell 2023). Much critical work has been done in occupational therapy and occupational science theory and students and practitioners should be strongly encouraged to acquaint themselves with these readings (which are too many to mention). In terms of overarching theoretical frameworks, examples of critical theoretical and decolonial theoretical frameworks include

Africana studies, critical race theory, post-colonial, and decolonial critical theory, queer theory and feminist theory (e.g. hooks 1988/2015; Butler 1990/2007; Said 1993; Rabaka 2009; Grosfoguel 2011).

CONCEPTUAL OCCUPATION-BASED MODELS

Occupational therapy occupation-based models form the theoretical foundation of occupational therapy assessment and intervention. They are useful for providing a comprehensive knowledge of clients, choosing appropriate outcomes for intervention and predominantly, ensuring that those outcomes are occupation based. The process of selecting an occupational therapy model should include knowledge of the client through in-depth assessment and occupational history taking.

Models ensure that occupational therapists stay within their scope of practice. Intervention planned outside of a conceptual occupation-based model runs the risk of not meeting the client's occupation-based needs. Conceptual occupation-based models can be likened to baking a cake; they constitute different ingredients and instructions that should strictly be amalgamated until they produce a masterpiece in the oven. The use of occupational therapy models in psychiatry and mental health should describe the interconnectedness of the person, the occupation, the environment within which the occupation takes place and how the three interact to facilitate occupational engagement or occupational performance.

In order to choose conceptual occupation-based models effectively, clinicians need to ask themselves the following questions:

- Who are the main theorists? This is important because the theorists hold a theoretical perspective that needs to be understood and appreciated within any given context.

- What are the primary assumptions and key concepts about the occupational human? Primary assumptions and key concepts are like the picture of the final cake product in the recipe book. It is what should entice a therapist to pick one model over the other.

- How are function and dysfunction understood? This should be a determining factor in picking a model. Some models define dysfunction as the inability to perform occupation, while others define it as a bodily impairment. The lens through which clients are viewed determines how function and dysfunction are understood.

- What are the postulates for change? What does the recipe promise as the final product? What are the measurements of the prescribed ingredients and how much of the ingredients are recommended to get a fluffy moist cake? Postulates for change are what each model promises to deliver when administered precisely well.

- Lastly, what are the principles for intervention that can be derived from each model? Principles are important to consider because they are building blocks for achieving any occupational therapy intervention. If a model is to be successfully implemented, it needs to prescribe principles that should guide intervention and practice. Principles of a model can provide guidelines on how to structure an environment, suggest activity requirements and how to handle the client to promote occupational engagement.

Having carefully considered the above guidelines, one can select a suitable model for intervention. There are various models that are suitable for guiding intervention in mental health practice. This could be attributed to their adaptability, applicability and relevance to the Global South context. This chapter follows the guidelines above in demonstrating how each model can be used in mental health practice.

MODEL OF HUMAN OCCUPATION (MOHO)

The MOHO is widely used for its belief that occupational performance must be understood within the context of emerging action and conditions (Kielhofner 2009). This model views humans as a system, using systems theory. It believes that the human system is constantly changing, unfolding and reorganising itself through engagement. The key concepts of this model acknowledge that human occupation is complex, that a person is made up of components and that the environment has an influence on these components. The fluidity of the MOHO to accommodate client-specific needs as well as permission to alter the environment makes it easier to understand and apply within any given context. The MOHO's intervention focus is on doing, rather than a person's impairment and encourages the acquisition of a new skill or role in therapy.

Occupational performance is said to result in health, well-being, development and change, therefore making it dynamic. This model understands occupational dysfunction to be the inability to perform occupations, any disturbance in role performance or the inability to meet both social and personal expectations. Intervention strategies of the MOHO should be client-specific and aim to change occupational performance. Intervention is not linear and may sometimes require environmental alterations to take place. MOHO is best suited for clients who lack enough motivation for occupational engagement.

Vona du Toit MODEL OF CREATIVE ABILITY (VdTMoCA)

The VdTMoCA was developed by Vona du Toit in the 1970s. The theory provides a framework to evaluate a client's occupational performance according to the skills attained in the personal, social, work and recreational occupational performance areas (de Witt 2014). Creative ability is one of the key concepts of the model. It is defined as the ability to present oneself without fear, anxiety, limitations and inhibitions (de Witt 2014). It is the client's preparedness to function at one's maximum level of competence. Creative ability develops through creative capacity. This is the maximum creative potential a client has with potential to develop under optimum circumstances. In order to grow one's creative capacity, one has to apply maximum creative effort, which is the exertion of creative effort at the boundary of creative ability to achieve growth. This maximum effort is dependent on creative response, creative participation and creative act. A further elaboration on how to use this model in practice is provided in the previous versions of this book.

Creative ability is valuable for its adaptability to mental health settings, particularly with practitioners who work with large groups and need to deliver evidence-based mental health services. The use of this model is evident in group settings regardless of the client's age, cultural group, language and diagnosis (de Witt 2014). It is an effective model to use with persons with intellectual disabilities, acutely and chronically ill mental health care users. It provides practice guidelines for each level of motivation and action and includes principles for structuring the environment, activity requirements and handing of the client. The Model of Creative Ability suggests that creative ability can be assessed. This includes assessment of a client's personal management, social ability, work ability and constructive use of time.

KAWA MODEL

The Kawa model was developed by Iwama (2006) as a response to the need for a contextually relevant occupational therapy model that considers diverse cultures and contexts of the Global South. This model embraces the issue of culture in occupational therapy (Iwama 2006). It focuses more on collective, shared interest and consensus between the client and the environment. For example the self is seen not as an individual, but a part of a larger whole, which could be a community, the environment or family (Iwama 2006; 2003). The metaphor of this model depicts life as a river, which represents life that flows through time and space. Water inside the river affects the life flow. The weakening of this water flow indicates a state of disharmony.

The applicability and relevance of this model in the Global South lies in its nonprescriptive nature. It encourages therapists to collaborate with clients in identifying challenges to be worked on within their context. It requires sensitivity to the client's circumstances in context. The river side walls represent the environment, which has enough power to affect the shape and boundaries through which the water can flow through.

This model is suitable for those clients who do not present with much symptomology but are hindered by their contexts to participate in meaningful occupations. It is for this reason that the depiction of the river constitutes rocks, which are problematic life circumstances that obstruct the life flow. Driftwoods are the assets that the client present with that may help us remove some of the rocks to encourage a smoother life

flow. Occupation is depicted as the spaces that have potential channels for life flow and they are opportunities for occupational therapists in collaboration with the client to consider outcomes for intervention.

OCCUPATION-BASED COMMUNITY DEVELOPMENT (O-bCD) FRAMEWORK

The O-bCD framework was developed to respond to the emerging need for occupational therapy in the Global South to articulate evolving community-based practice and to document principles that guide everyday practice (Galvaan & Peters 2017). This chapter will discuss the O-bCD framework concepts that are most applicable in mental health practice. Although the O-bCD framework is still in its development stage towards a model, we recognise its potential to be used as an advocacy tool for community mental health services. Community reintegration of mental health care users remains a challenge in the Global South regardless of contextual developments (WHO 2007). The health care system has battled with mental health care users who do not stay part of their community for long post discharge (Tsatsi & Plastow 2021). It is for this reason that we suggest a practical way of using this framework to promote successful community reintegration from psychiatric hospital settings into the community.

The O-bCD framework suggests four iterative processes: (i) initiating intervention, (ii) designing, (iii) implementation and (iv) monitoring reflection and evaluation (Galvaan & Peters 2017). Initiating interventions requires establishing and building relationships. According to Taylor et al. (2005), developing a deep understanding of social and occupational identities and occupational profiles within any given context establishes relationships with communities. Strong relationships provide opportunities to understand the context so much that goals of intervention and issues to be addressed are easily negotiated. To establish such relationships, occupational therapists in psychiatric hospitals should invest in taking time to understand the communities from which our clients come from and to bridge the gap between hospitals and the community. This may include conducting community appraisals, mental health awareness campaigns and assessments. Spending time in the community and neutralising power dynamics can also strengthen the relationships between the hospital and the community. In so doing, it becomes easier and more trustworthy for the community to be more accepting of mental health care users and to work in partnership with the hospital in identifying community members who need mental health care services and to support those who are already mental health service users.

According to the O-bCD framework, the design process is ongoing, dynamic and evolves through the initiation, implementation and monitoring and evaluation phases (Galvaan & Peters 2017; 2013). The use of occupational science theories that help us understand the occupational human as well as the needs they present informs the designing process.

Theories of occupational justice (Stadnyk *et al.* 2010; Whiteford & Townsend 2011), occupational choice (Galvaan 2015), occupational potential (Wicks 2005), occupational identity (Laliberte Rudman & Denhart 2008) and occupational consciousness (Ramugondo 2015), among others, together with the understanding of how occupations are performed and experienced in the relevant contexts, may be used to shape the design of the community reintegration intervention. Part of designing includes accessing resources necessary to realise the intervention. Participants together with the therapist should identify and then draw on a wide range of networks to ensure access to the necessary resources. This can be reinforced through community mapping and SWOT analysis. Resources may be human, financial, time or opportunities to access occupations and people skilled in specific occupations (Galvaan & Peters 2017; 2013). Resources may directly or indirectly support the performance of the occupation, for example job placements for vocational rehabilitation.

The implementation process is dependent on findings that emerged in the design process. This is where the applicable occupational science theories and resources identified are meant to work to achieve the identified goals of intervention. This is also a good place for the therapist to take stock of what is working and what needs improvement. This process precedes the monitoring, reflection and evaluation. It encourages the use of reflexive tools such as the Action reflection cycle by Taylor *et al.* (2005). This process should be monitored to inform how the intervention has evolved and to evaluate the outcome of the intervention.

The use of the O-bCD framework to advocate for mental health services in the community ensures continuity of occupational therapy mental health services from the hospital setting into the communities.

THEORETICAL FRAMES OF REFERENCE

Theoretical frames of reference (TFR) form an important part of the toolbox. Although it is borrowed knowledge, it provides a comprehensive view of the client that may otherwise not be provided by occupational therapy theory and practice. A theoretical frame of reference is a collection of ideas or theories that provide a foundation for practice (Mosey 1992; Duncan 2021b). Imagine you are wearing purple sunglasses while taking a stroll in the garden. It is not surprising that everything you see will be purple. This analogy can help us understand frames of reference better. They are the lens through which we view our clients. A frame of reference helps us link theory to practice (Mosey 1992; Duncan 2021b). There are different frames of reference that are applicable in mental health practice. This chapter discusses the following.

BEHAVIOURAL THEORETICAL FRAME OF REFERENCE

The behavioural frame of reference was developed by Stein (1983). This TFR emphasises the use of behavioural modification to shape behaviours. Maladaptive learned behaviours can be replaced by adaptive behaviours through reward of the desired behaviour (Stein 1983). The use of this TFR in mental health has become apparent as a lot of psychiatric clients present with maladaptive behaviours such as difficulty with following social norms, smoking, and aggressive behaviours, among others. The application of this TFR requires identification of the maladaptive behaviour, determining the baseline performance, selecting a reinforcer and working on using the reinforcer to encourage adaptive behaviour (Stein 1983). This should ultimately increase occupational performance in desired occupations. The use of this TFR is encouraged alongside numerous models like the MOHO and VdTMoCA. For example a client with an intellectual disability may be working on their social skills using the model of creative ability but may need a behavioural frame of reference to help address maladaptive behavioural patterns they present with.

A therapist using the behavioural TFR needs to provide objective feedback by mirroring and modelling desired behaviour. Dysfunctional behaviour needs to be disrupted in action through negative reinforcement, creating an immediate space where desired and adapted behaviour can be positively reinforced (Stein 1983). Attention should be given to observable actions. Activities selected to facilitate this TFR should give room for trying out desired behaviour and be broken down into manageable chunks that allow for the acquisition of the desired behaviour.

ADULT-LEARNING THEORETICAL FRAME OF REFERENCE

In the disposition of the acquisition of desired behaviour, and skills, the principles underlying adult learning are very useful when designing an intervention plan that requires a patient/client to (re)learn new skills. Adult learning is situated in the theoretical framework of learning theories. Vygotsky (1997), a constructivist, theorised that learning occurs often socially and that new knowledge is constructed not from a *tabla blanca* but also, and very significantly so, from existing knowledge. The following adult learning principles can be considered when crafting a goodness-of-fit for treatment outcomes that are skills related (e.g. Knowles 1984; Conner *et al.* 2018):

a. Promote autonomy

b. Promote goal-directedness

c. Facilitate motivation

d. Acknowledge prior learning/knowledge

e. Promote active involvement and co-decision making

f. Facilitate supporting structures

g. Facilitate evaluation and reflection

Using the principles of adult learning also requires seeing the person/patient/client as equally virtuous in his/her ability as a knowing person. The transactional posture of the therapist towards the client is from one adult to another, unconditional positive regard and egalitarianism, all of which are conducive to open and multi-lateral communication and constructive feedback. When adults are regarded as such, they are open to learning.

PSYCHODYNAMIC THEORETICAL FRAME OF REFERENCE

The psychodynamic TFR has its origins in the discipline of psychology. It focuses on the client's ability to view themselves realistically and to be aware of their strengths and weaknesses (Freud 1953). It considers the client's present behaviour and how their behaviour is influenced subconsciously by past events. Once a client masters past events and emotions associated with them, they can begin to direct their behaviour through recognition and coping (Freud 1953). It is used in mental health and psychiatric settings with mental health care users who are self-aware.

The use of the psychodynamic TFR in occupational therapy is beneficial. However, when using this TFR, therapists need to be able to support and contain the client while considering transference and counter transference. The therapist's actions may be misinterpreted or symbolised incorrectly. It is therefore important for the therapist to be cognizant of dysfunctional psychological behaviours such as defence mechanisms.

HUMANISTIC THEORETICAL FRAME OF REFERENCE

The humanistic TFR is centred on seeing the person as part of a whole (Maslow 1968; Rogers 1989). The person is seen within their context as being self-aware, reflective, able to exercise choice and be intentional. This TFR believes that when a client is shown unconditional positive regard and empathy, they are well able to resolve their own problems (Rogers 1989). The use of this TFR in practice includes the promotion of self-awareness and meaning for the client as the lack thereof results in illness. Therapists using this TFR need to handle clients with acceptance, unconditional positive regard, and empathy and not be judgmental. Furthermore, the client needs to be accepted as a human with creativity and difference, as able to make autonomous, self-aware decisions and able to direct their own treatment (Rogers 1989). Activities selected to apply this TFR should include activities that allow for self-reflection, prompt creative and active participation, allow for decision-making and honour the uniqueness of the individual. This TFR may be used with high-functioning clients as self-awareness requires insight and judgement.

COGNITIVE THEORETICAL FRAME OF REFERENCE

The cognitive behavioural therapeutic (CBT) TFR focuses on the relationship between thoughts, feelings, beliefs and behaviour (Beck 1963). This TFR challenges the client's negative thoughts and replaces them with positive ones. The core conception of this TFR is that unwanted thoughts are the most accessible and thus the client needs to manage negative thoughts by changing the way they think. Furthermore, thinking (i.e. automatic thoughts, beliefs, and core schemas) affects emotions, and emotions affect behaviour (Beck 1963). It is mostly used in mental health settings to treat clients presenting with anxiety, depression, substance abuse and panic attacks. It is an evidence-based practice TFR that leads to improvement in functioning. Techniques that are used alongside this TFR are the relaxation therapy techniques, activity diaries, and desensitisation, among others. The cognitive behavioural therapeutic TFR can be used alongside the MOHO in order to understand a client's occupational performance and identify occupational needs. Its core principles include learning better ways of coping with problems, recognising that psychological problems are a result of faulty and unhelpful ways of thinking, and learned unhelpful behaviour (Beck 1963).

A therapist using this TFR needs to focus on the client's presenting thought patterns and be able to model how to stop intrusive negative thoughts. The client needs coaching on how to disprove automatic negative thoughts (automatic, beliefs, or core schemas) and be able to replace them with positive ones, by for example questioning the rationality of these thoughts. Activities selected to facilitate this TFR need to be simple enough to allow the client to acquire alternative cognitive behaviours and facilitate experiential learning, and experimenting with desired cognitive behaviours.

EXISTENTIAL THEORETICAL FRAME OF REFERENCE

The existential TFR was founded by Kierkegaard (1980) and Frankl (2004). They believe that humans are spiritual beings who can transcend the self in search of meaning. Concepts that humans struggle to grasp with such as love, work, suffering and death are situated outside of the person and therefore, humans need to transcend the self to make sense of these concepts (Frankl 2004). The notion of doing deeds for others and self allows humans to find meaning. This maxim resonates strongly with Hammell's (2009b) and Motimele and Peters's (2017) critical argument for rethinking traditional occupational categories for the majority world where one of the occupational categories put forward is occupations cultivating a sense of belonging, interconnection and dependence, and contributing by doing with and for others. This TFR also postulates that humans become ill when they adopt self-centred values and thus lose perspective of their existence (Kierkegaard 1980) – a view that corroborates strongly with Mkhize's (2008) arguments of Ubuntu and Harmony as an African approach to morality and ethics. Self-awareness and acquiring meaning from life is seen as a cure for illness. Mthembu (2017) has theorised guidelines for the integration of spirituality and spiritual care in occupational therapy education, and from which many principles for designing a treatment plan in psychiatric occupational therapy practice can be extrapolated.

TECHNIQUES, ACTIVITIES/OCCUPATION AS A MEANS AND/OR AS AN END

Techniques, activities/occupation as a means and/or as an end are the treatment interventions that can be observed by the practitioner, the patient/client as well as family members of the clients, and MDT colleagues. Without the theoretical context, or clear communication from the practitioner about what the aim and purpose of the treatment modality is, these observations may often seem out of the ordinary or inexplicable in a medical setting, for example.

Techniques are chosen sensibly to meet the session goals and treatment outcomes and can be combined with an occupation-based activity. Examples of techniques are relaxation therapy; value clarification; the application of the group therapy process in occupational therapy; or trauma counselling in occupational therapy. Practitioners should ensure that they are proficient in the correct choice, as well as the application of techniques, and not chisel the session goal or treatment outcomes to fit available techniques in the occupational therapist's toolbox. The use of some techniques may implicate additional training such as using the group therapy process in occupational therapy effectively, and not merely treating patients together in a group.

Practitioners should also be well prepared to present activities or facilitate the experience of occupation as means or an end if they are not familiar with them. (See previous definition of occupation as a means or an end.) All planning and interventions should be able to be justified under an *occupation-centred* approach (Fisher 2013).

Activities, or an occupation as a means, such as playing cards, or doing gumboot dancing, or preparing a simple meal with patients in sub-acute or long-term settings are examples of *occupation-focused* activities (Fisher 2013) that improve a person's occupational performance. These activities may or may not form part of the person's everyday life when patients/clients return to their respective occupational environments/context.

Occupation-based interventions (Fisher 2013) are when an occupational therapist critically considers the conditions of function and form for an occupation presented as well as the subjective experience of the person about the meaning and purpose of this occupation. The meaning and contextual relevance of this occupation-based treatment session may be part of the person/s' need for the experience of satisfaction derived from a sense of productivity, sensory or complex pleasure experienced, or a sense of restoration and centredness (Pierce 2003; Fisher 2013).

USING THEORETICAL FRAMES OF REFERENCE AND CONCEPTUAL OCCUPATION-BASED MODELS TO EXTRACT PRINCIPLES

Core principles for the design of an intervention plan, as well as the practical strategies/ principles for a session, can be extracted from the best therapeutic approaches required by the diagnosis; theoretical frames of references judiciously considered, occupational therapy models and overarching theory, such as occupational science. The type of principle you are looking for will determine the theoretical tool you use. Core principles are the theoretical considerations, which through clinical reasoning are regarded as key to the achievement of a treatment aim. Core principles are often extracted from occupational therapy models. This is because they are the key to ensuring that the therapy one provides remains within occupational therapy parameters and that therapy remains occupation-centred. If we say that using occupational therapy models ensures that we provide occupation-centred/-based/-focused outcomes, then extracting principles from an occupational therapy model is the 'how' part of achieving those occupation-centred, -based or -focused outcomes. Not all occupational therapy models are overt in providing principles. Therefore, practitioners need to equip themselves with tools on how to extract principles from models but also from theoretical frames of reference, and for example from occupational science. An example of a core principle from the MOHO could be formulated as follows: 'By crafting an opportunity for the client to experience occupational competence so their occupational identity is affirmed, and internal motivation is enhanced'. An example of a core principle from occupational science could look like: 'By ensuring that occupational form and function is maintained despite of an activity simulated indoors as so allow for occupational engagement'.

Practical strategies are principles that ensure that while one is providing occupation-centred/-based/-focused therapy to a client, one remains therapeutic. Practical principles can be extracted from practice models such as the VdTMoCA, from which one can overtly infer handing, activity requirements and environmental structure principles. Practical strategies/ principles suggest how an aim or outcome is practically going to be achieved. Without these principles, it is hard to justify how you will structure the environment, select or design the activity and handle the client to ensure that the aim of your session is achieved.

Theoretical frames of reference may provide us with principles that realise theory into practice. Earlier in this chapter, it was explained that theoretical frames of references, when appropriately selected, can be adjacent to principles selected from an occupational therapy model towards achieving a treatment aim/session goal. Each TFR can provide practical ways in which to handle the client to ensure that the outcomes, goals and aims for the session are achieved. For example if one would extract a practical strategy from the behavioural TFR, it could be formulated as: 'by providing positive feedback when the client makes an effort or complete a step as to maintain external, and possibly enhance internal motivation'. Ideally, principles should start with 'by' because they answer the question 'how?'.

Let us look at Bontle's case study as an example of how to use core, practice, as well as TFR principles alongside each other to achieve a comprehensive treatment outcome.

CASE STUDY

Bontle is an 18-year-old admitted at Thabamoopo Psychiatric Hospital for attempted suicide. She was notorious for attempting suicide whenever she did not experience social support from her family. In all suicidal attempts, Bontle did not receive any therapy or treatment as she was never brought to the hospital. This is her first hospital admission and a Major Depressive Disorder diagnosis was made. When taking social history, you realise that her mother was absent from most of her teenage years and she felt neglected by her for this. She lives with her paternal grandmother in the nearby village together with her siblings. She feels partly responsible for depending on her grandmother's social grant for her survival. She often thinks about why her mother and father neglected her and her siblings and feels unloved. She's often consumed with feelings of guilt and resorts to overdosing on medication or cutting her wrists to kill herself. She admitted to attempting suicide for the third time, which led to her admission to the hospital. In her last suicide attempt, she messaged her teacher her last remarks and locked herself in her room to die. A multi-disciplinary team has come to the conclusion that Bontle is clinically depressed.

As part of your collateral information, you interviewed her teacher who mentioned that Bontle is a dedicated learner at school. The teacher hinted that Bontle needs love from her parents and that her suicide attempts are evident of that. She does not have friends at school to avoid peer pressures of having to buy things she cannot afford. She often sits in the teacher's class during break times and uses those times to speak about her social problems.

For the purpose of this case study, we will use the Kawa model as our occupation-based model, the VdTMoCA as our practice model and the cognitive behavioural TFR. We will extract one principle from each model and TFR to show an example of how principles can be extricated from each of these sources.

The Kawa Model is chosen for Bontle because the aim of occupational therapy will focus on removing problematic life circumstances that obstruct the flow of her life. We want to address the social circumstances that resulted in her suicide attempts and admission to the hospital. The Kawa model suggests many ways in which that can be done and those are the principles. Principles suggest the *how* part of achieving our aim.

Using the symbol of driftwood to remove the rocks, her teacher can be identified as an asset and therefore a driftwood. So, if we write this as a principle/strategy, we can say:

- By using her teacher as a driftwood post discharge, we can address the lack of family support by her mother.

This principle does not only provide a practical way in which to provide social support for Bontle in the hospital, but focus on how the intervention is cognizant of assets that exist in Bontle's environment that can be utilised as part of her intervention plan. The therapist can focus on how to empower the teacher to provide Palesa with social support so that she does not feel the gap between her parents and thus avoid suicidal attempts.

If we use one of her potential strengths, her dedication to school as a principle, we can say:

- By using her dedication to school as a distractor from her social environment, this can encourage her to do well in school and therefore get a bursary for her studies.

Just like the first principle, this principle provides core avenues in which Bontle's asset of performing well in school can be used to ensure that we reduce or eliminate her suicidal attempts. If Bontle performs well in school, she is likely to get her bursary and further her studies, which in turn may improve her social circumstances later in the years when she starts working.

The VdTMoCA is a good tool to use for how we can set up the environment, select or design our activities, and handle Bontle in a way that ensures that she is able to return to school. Let us assume that Bontle is on the imitative level of action. At this level, Bontle is able to do what is asked of her. (Please refer to the Model of Creative Ability chapter to find out how she is functioning in her personal management, social ability and her use of free time.) Her level of motivation is directed towards improving her need to attempt suicide and she is actively exploring alternative ways to deal with her depression. According to the VdTMoCA, these are the applicable principles.

Activity requirements and presentation of activity

- By presenting the activity logically to Bontle and emphasising the purpose of the activity in each session

- By ensuring that all the activities presented to Bontle encourage norm compliance and have imitative characteristics

Activity requirement and presentation of the activity, need to be more specific and further applied to the activity you are presenting. This ensures that the 'how' part of achieving your aim is clear in the activity you are presenting.

Handling

- By clearly stating the expectation of each session with Bontle, this will help her realise what is expected of her in the session.

- By providing Bontle with support when she fails to comply with imitative responses, this will allow her to explore different ways of ensuring success in a similar or different activity.

As you can see, principles derived from a practice model are more specific to a session than core principles/strategies are. While core principles may cut across the whole intervention plan, practical principles may be limited to one session and may need to be revisited in each session.

Environmental Structuring

The VdTMOCA does not provide environmental structuring principles for clients on the imitative level of action. However, it is beneficial to note that environment principles may be extracted from the client's diagnosis as well as TFRs. An example in Bontle's case, knowing her diagnosis of major depressive disorder can be:

• By structuring the session in a well-lit room, this will ensure that Bontle is able to engage with the activity at hand more clearly and improve her mood.

Cognitive Behavioural Therapy TFR

We chose the CBT TFR for Bontle for the main reason that she has recurring thoughts to commit suicide. It is for this reason that we want to challenge those thoughts in therapy. Let's assume that during an activity session with Bontle, you realise that she speaks negatively about herself. When using this TFR in practice, a principle of how you will practically use CBT may include:

• By challenging Bontle to say a positive thing about herself every time she speaks negatively about herself, this will encourage her to speak positively about herself in the session.

This provides a practical example of how a TFR can be used alongside occupation-based models in providing comprehensive treatment intervention.

CONCLUSION

This chapter provides an outline of the theoretical concepts, constructs and layers of theoretical perspectives. A toolbox was proposed in which the layers of these concepts are organised from the most weighted, and often less tangible to the more visible and practical layers. The philosophical underpinnings are the first layer which spoke to a professional worldview, its ontology, epistemologies and axiology. The concept of paradigm is also discussed in as much as it is a theoretical flow from the profession's underpinnings though it has changed several times over the existence of the profession to express best what the profession's focus and identity are. Overarching theoretical frameworks, such as systems theory, occupational science, as well as critical theoretical and decolonial theoretical frameworks, and occupational therapy models, are the next layer in this toolbox as they inform the profession's foundations for reasoning, as well as the development and application of theory and principles. Theoretical frames of reference are the following layer as these link theory with practice. The top and most visible layer are techniques, activities and occupations as a means and/or ends.

The chapter then proceeded by demonstrating how principles can be extracted and crafted from various sources. However, these were only demonstrative examples to serve as guidelines in thinking and should not be regarded as set in stone or to be followed without room to manoeuvre. Rather, the case study and suggestions can serve to ignite and guide systematic thinking and reasoning about the array of theoretical constructs and concepts in occupational therapy and ultimately affirm an articulated occupational therapy identity.

QUESTIONS

1. Define, in your own words, your understanding of occupational therapy's philosophical underpinnings and its overarching theoretical frameworks.

2. Discuss how the occupational therapy profession's worldview compares with your own.

3. Discuss with a partner, which occupational therapy models are more applicable in which settings, and why.

4. Argue why certain occupational therapy models need to be chosen in response to a client-centred approach and emerging clients' needs.

5. Differentiate between the terms 'occupation-centred', 'occupation-based' and 'occupation-focused'.

6. Explain the difference between occupation as a means and occupation as an end.

7. Choose a case study in your own practice and construct core principles for a treatment aim, as well as practical strategies/principles for handling, structuring of the environment and presentation of the activity for a session goal.

ACKNOWLEDGEMENT

Sincere thanks to Mr Spha Msimang, a Multi-Media Edu Content Designer from Wits School of Therapeutic Sciences for his assistance in the realisation of the design of Figures 1.1 and 1.2.

REFERENCES

Amagoh, F. (2016) Systems and complexity theories of organizations. In: A. Farazmand (ed), *Global Encyclopedia of Public Administration, Public Policy, and Governance*, pp. 1–7. Springer, Cham.

American Association of Occupational Therapy (AOTA) (2020) The occupational therapy practice framework, 4th edn. *The American Journal of Occupational Therapy*, **74** (**Suppl. 2**), 1–87.

Beck, A.T. (1963) Thinking and depression: I. Idiosyncratic content and cognitive distortions. *Archives of General Psychiatry*, **9**(**4**), 324–333. https://doi.org/10.1001/archpsyc.1963.01720160014002

Blau, P.M., Gustad, J.W., Jessor, R., Parnes, H.S. & Wilcock, R.C. (1956) Occupational choice: a conceptual framework. *ILR Review*, **9**(**4**), 531–543. https://doi.org/10.1177/001979395600900401

Brown, W. (2019) *The Rise of Antidemocratic Politics in the West*. Columbia University Press, New York.

Bryant, W., Fieldhouse, J. & Bannigan, K. (eds) (2022) *Creek's Occupational Therapy and Mental Health E-Book*. Elsevier Ltd, London.

Bullock, A. & Trombley, S. (1999) *The New Fontana Dictionary of Modern Thought*, 3rd edn, pp. 387–388. Harper Collins, London.

Butler, J. (1990/2007) *Gender Trouble: Feminism and the Subversion of Identity*. Routledge, New York.

Canadian Association of Occupational Therapists (1997) *Enabling Occupation: An Occupational Therapy Perspective*. CAOT Publications ACE, Ottawa, ON.

Cole, M.B. & Tufano, R. (2020) *Applied Theories in Occupational Therapy: A Practical Approach*. Slack Incorporated, Thorofare, New York.

Conner, L.R., Richardson, S. & Murphy, A.L. (2018) Teaching note: using adult learning principles for evidence-based learning in a BSW research course. *Journal of Baccalaureate Social Work*, **23**(**1**), 355–365.

Creswell, J.W. & Creswell, J.D. (2018) *Research Design: Qualitative, Quantitative, and Mixed Methods Approaches*. Sage Publications, London.

De Witt, P. (2014) Creative ability: a model for individual and group occupational therapy for clients with psychosocial dysfunction. In: R. Crouch & V. Alers (eds), *Occupational Therapy in Psychiatry and Mental Health*, 5th edn, pp. 3–32. Whurr Publishers, London and Philadelphia.

Duncan, E.A.S. (2021a) An introduction to conceptual models of practice and frames of reference. In: E.A.S. Duncan (ed), *Foundations for Practice in Occupational Therapy* 6th edn, pp. 38–44. Elsevier Limited, London.

Duncan, E.A.S. (2021b) Theoretical foundation of occupational therapy: internal influence. In: E.A.S. Duncan (ed), *Foundations for Practice in Occupational Therapy*, 6th edn, pp. 16–27. Elsevier Limited, London.

Du Toit, V. (1980) *Patient Volition and Action in Occupational Therapy*. Vona and Marie du Toit Foundation, Pretoria.

Ebrahim, A. (2017) Framing and understanding knowledge in occupational therapy. In: S.B. Dsouza, R. Galvaan & E.L. Ramugondo (eds), *Concepts in Occupational Therapy: Understanding Southern Perspectives*, pp. 122–138. Manipal University Press, Manipal.

Eklund, M., Orban, K., Argentzell, E. *et al* (2017) The linkage between patterns of daily occupations and occupational balance: applications within occupational science and occupational therapy practice. *Scandinavian Journal of Occupational Therapy*, **24**(**1**), 41–56.

Farias, L. & Laliberte Rudman, D. (2016) A critical interpretive synthesis of the uptake of critical perspectives in occupational science. *Journal of Occupational Science*, **23**(**1**), 33–50.

Fisher, A.G. (2013) Occupation-centred, occupation-based, occupation-focused: same, same or different? *Scandinavian Journal of Occupational Therapy*, **20**.

Foucault, M. (1998) So, is it important to think? In: J.D. Faubion (ed), *Aesthetics, Method and Epistemology. The Essential Works of Michel Foucault, 1954–1984, Volume 2*, pp. 454–458. Allen Lane, Penguin, Harmondsworth, Middlesex.

Frankl, V. (2004) *On the Theory and Therapy of Mental Disorders: An Introduction to Logotherapy and Existential Analysis*. Brunner-Routledge, NY and Hove.

Freud, S. (1953) The interpretation of dreams. In: J. Strachey (ed & Trans), *The Standard Edition of the Complete Psychological Works of Sigmund Freud*, Vols. **4–5**. Hogarth, London (Original work published 1900).

Fricker, M. (2017) Evolving concepts of epistemic injustice. In: I.J. Kidd, J. Medina & P. Gaile Jr (eds), *Routledge Handbook of Epistemic Injustice*, pp. 53–60. Routledge, New York.

Galvaan, R.2015) The contextually situated nature of occupational choice: marginalised young adolescents' experiences in South Africa. *Journal of Occupational Science*, **22**, 39–53. https://doi.org/10.1080/14427591.2014.912124

Galvaan, R. & Peters, L. (2013) '*Occupation-based community development framework*'. https://vula.uct.ac.za/access/content/group/9c29ba04-b1ee-49b9-8c85-9a468b556ce2/OBCDF/index.html (accessed 13 March 2024)

Galvaan, R. & Peters, L. (2017) Occupation-based community development: a critical approach to occupational therapy. In: S.B. Dsouza, R. Galvaan & E.L. Ramugondo (eds), *Concepts in Occupational Therapy: Understanding Southern Perspectives*, pp. 172–187. Manipal University Press, Manipal.

Galvaan, R., Peters, L., Richards, L.A., Francke, M. & Krenzer, M. (2022) Pedagogies within occupational therapy curriculum: centering a decolonial praxis in community development practice. *Cadernos Brasileiros de Terapia Ocupacional*, **30**, e3133.

Gentry, K., Snyder, K., Barstow, B. & Hamson-Utley, J. (2018) The biopsychosocial model: application to occupational therapy practice. *The Open Journal of Occupational Therapy*, **6**(**4**), 1–19. https://doi.org/10.15453/2168-6408.1412

Gillen, G. & Brown, C. (eds) (2023) *Willard and Spackman's Occupational Therapy*. Lippincott Williams & Wilkins, New York.

Grosfoguel, R. (2011) Decolonizing post-colonial studies and paradigms of political-economy: transmodernity. *Journal of Peripheral Cultural Production of the Luso-Hispanic World*, **1**(**1**), 1–38.

Guajardo, A., Kronenberg, F. & Ramugondo, E.L. (2015) Southern occupational therapies: emerging identities, epistemologies and practices. *South African Journal of Occupational Therapy*, **45**(**1**), 3–10.

Hagedorn, R. (1995) *Occupational Therapy: Perspectives and Processes*, 1st edn. Elsevier Limited, London.

Hammell, K.W. (2008) Reflections on . . . well-being and occupational rights. *Canadian Journal of Occupational Therapy*, **75**(**1**), 61–64.

Hammell, K.W. (2009a) Sacred texts: a sceptical exploration of the assumptions underpinning theories of occupation. *Canadian Journal of Occupational Therapy*, **76**(**1**), 6–13.

Hammell, K.W. (2009b) Self-care, productivity, and leisure, or dimensions of occupational experience? Rethinking occupational "categories". *Canadian Journal of Occupational Therapy*, **76**(**2**), 107–114.

Hammell, K.W. & Beagan, B. (2017) Occupational injustice: a critique. *Canadian Journal of Occupational Therapy,* **84**(**1**), 58–68.

Hooks, B. (1988/2015) *Feminism Is for Everybody*. Routledge, New York.

Hooper, B. (2006) Epistemological transformation in occupational therapy: educational implications and challenges. *Occupational Journal of Rehabilitation: Occupation, Participation and Health*, **26**(**1**): 15–24.

Ikiugu, M., Plastow, N.A & van Niekerk, L. (2019) Eclectic application of theoretical models in occupational therapy: impact on therapeutic reasoning. *Occupational Therapy in Health Care, 33*(**3**), 286–305. https://doi.org/10.1080/07380577.2019.1630884

Iwama, M. (2003) Toward culturally relevant epistemologies in occupational therapy. *American Journal of Occupational Therapy*, **57**(**5**), 582–528.

Iwama, M. (2006) *The Kawa Model: Culturally Relevant Occupational Therapy*. Churchill Livingstone, Edinburgh.

Iwama, M.K., Thomson, N.A. & Macdonald, R.M. (2009) The Kawa model: the power of culturally responsive occupational therapy. *Disability and Rehabilitation*, **31**, 1125–1135.

Kielhofner, G. (1978) General systems theory: implications for theory and action in occupational therapy. *The American Journal of Occupational Therapy: Official Publication of the American Occupational Therapy Association*, **32**(**10**), 637–645.

Kielhofner, G. (2008) *Model of Human Occupation: Theory and Application*, 4th edn. Lippincott Williams & Wilkins, Baltimore.

Kielhofner, G. (2009) *Conceptual Foundations of Occupational Therapy Practice*, 4th edn. F. A. Davis, Philadelphia.

Kierkegaard, S. (1980) *The Concept of Anxiety* (R. Thomte, Trans.). Princeton University Press, New Jersey.

Knowles, M.S. (1984) *Andragogy in Action. Applying Modern Principles of Adult Education*. Jossey Bass, San Francisco.

Kronenberg, F., Fransen, H., & Pollard, N. (2005). The WFOT position paper on community-based rehabilitation: a call upon the profession to engage with people affected by occupational apartheid. *World Federation of Occupational Therapists bulletin*, **51**(**1**), 5–13. https://doi.org/10.1179/otb.2005.51.1.002

Laliberte Rudman, D. & Denhart, S. (2008) Shaping knowledge regarding occupation: examining the cultural underpinnings of the evolving concept of occupational identity. *Australian Occupational Therapy Journal*, **55**, 153–162.

Maslow, A.H. (1968) Some educational implications of the humanistic psychologies. *Harvard Educational Review*, **38**(**4**), 685–696. https://doi.org/10.17763/haer.38.4.j07288786v86w660

Mignolo, W.D. & Walsh, C.E. (eds) (2018) *On Decoloniality: Concepts, Analytics, Praxis*. Duke University, Durham.

Mkhize, N. (2008) Ubuntu and harmony: an African approach to morality and ethics. In R. Nicolson (ed), *Persons in Community: African Ethics in a Global Culture*, pp. 35–44. University of KwaZulu Natal Press, Scottsville.

Morrison, R. (2021) Pragmatism in the initial history of occupational therapy. *Cadernos Brasileiros de Terapia Ocupacional*, **29**, e2147.

Mosey, A.C. (1992) *Applied Scientific Inquiry in Health Professions*. American Occupational Association, Rockville.

Motimele, M. (2022) Engaging with occupational reconstructions: a perspective from the Global South. *Journal of Occupational Science, 29*(**4**), 478–481. https://doi.org/10.1080/14427591.2022.2110659

Motimele, M. & Peters, L. (2017) Understanding human occupation. In: S.B. Dsouza, R. Galvaan & E.L. Ramugondo (eds), *Concepts in Occupational Therapy: Understanding Southern Perspectives*, pp. 1–15. Manipal University Press, Manipal.

Mthembu, T.G. (2017) *The sesign and development of guidelines to integrate spirituality and spiritual care into occupational therapy education using design-based research*. Doctoral thesis, University of the Western Cape, South Africa.

Mthembu, T.G. & Bell, T. (2023) Experiences and influences of COVID-19 confinement on the occupational engagement and mental wellbeing of adults in South Africa: a qualitative meta-analysis. *African Journal for Physical Activity and Health Sciences (AJPHES)*, **29**(**2**), 100–125. https://doi.org/10.37597/ajphes.2023.29.2.1

Murthi K. & Hammell, K.W. (2021) Choice' in occupational therapy theory: a critique from the situation of patriarchy in India. *Scandinavian Journal of Occupational Therapy*, **28**(**1**), 1–12. https://doi.org/10.1080/11038128.2020.1769182

Ndlovu-Gatsheni, S.J. (2018) *Epistemic Freedom in Africa - Deprovincialization and Decolonization: Rethinking Development*.

O'Farrell, C. (2005) *Michel Foucault*. SAGE Publications Ltd, London.

Pierce, D. (2003) *Occupation by Design: Building Therapeutic Power*. F.A. Davis Company, Philadelphia.

Rabaka, R. (2009) *Africana Critical Theory: Reconstructing the Black Radical Tradition, from WEB Du Bois and CLR James to Frantz Fanon and Amilcar Cabral*. Lexington Books, Lanham, Maryland.

Ramugondo, E.L. (2015) Occupational consciousness. *Journal of Occupational Science*, **22**(**4**), 488–501. https://doi.org/10.1080/14427591.2015.1042516

Ramugondo, E.L. (2017) Meaning and purpose in occupation. In: S.B. Dsouza, R. Galvaan & E.L. Ramugondo (eds), *Concepts in Occupational Therapy: Understanding Southern Perspectives*, pp. 16–31. Manipal University Press, Manipal.

Ramugondo, E.L. & Kronenberg, F. (2015) Explaining collective occupations from a human relations perspective: bridging the individual-collective dichotomy. *Journal of Occupational Science*, **22**(**1**): 3–16. https://doi.org/10.1080/14427591.2013.781920153-162

Rauch van der Merwe, T. (2019) *The political construction of occupational therapy in South Africa: a critical analysis of curriculum as discourse*. Doctoral thesis, University of the Free State, South Africa.

Rogers, C. (1989) *The Carl Rogers Reader*. Houghton Mifflin Harcourt, New York.

Said, E.W. (1993) *Culture and Imperialism*. Vintage Books, New York.

Stadnyk, R., Townsend, E. & Wilcock, A. (2010) Occupational justice. In: C. Christiansen & E. Townsend (eds), *Introduction to Occupation: The Art and Science of Living*, 2nd edn, pp. 329–358. Pearson Education, Upper Saddle River, New Jersey.

Stein, F. (1983) A current review of the behavioral frame of reference and its application to occupational therapy. *Occupational Therapy in Mental Health*, (**2**), 35–62.

Taylor, J., Marais, D. & Kaplan, A. (2005) *Action learning. A developmental approach to change CDRA nuggets*. http://www.cdra.org.za/ (accessed 12 March 2024)

Tsatsi, I.A. & Plastow, N.A. (2021) Optimizing a halfway house to meet mental health care users' occupational needs. *Canadian Journal of Occupational Therapy*, **88**(**4**), 352–364. https://doi.org/10.1177/00084174211044896

Townsend, E. & Wilcock, A.A. (2004) Occupational justice and client-centred practice: a dialogue in progress. *Canadian Journal of Occupational Therapy*, **71**(**2**), 75–87.

Turpin, M. & Iwama, M. (2011) *Using Occupational Therapy Models in Practice*. Churchill Livingstone Elsevier, Edinburgh.

van der Merwe, J.C. (2008) The relevance of worldview interpretation to health care in South Africa. In: T. Falola & M.M. Heaton (eds), *Health Knowledge and Belief Systems in Africa*, pp. 55–66. Carolina Academic Press, North Carolina.

van der Reyden, D., Casteleijn, D., Sherwood, W. & de Witt, P. (eds) (2019) *VdTMoCA, The Voca Du Toit Model of Creative Ability*. University of Pretoria, Pretoria.

Vygotsky, L. (1997) *Educational Psychology*. St. Lucie Press, Boca Raton, FL.

Whiteford, G.E. & Hocking, C. (eds) (2012) *Occupational Science: Society, Inclusion, Participation*. Blackwell Publishing Ltd, Oxford.

Whiteford, G.E. & Townsend, E. (2011) Participatory occupational justice framework: enabling occupational participation and inclusion. In: F. Kronenberg, N. Pollard & D. Sakellariou (eds), *Occupational Therapy Without Borders (Volume II): Towards an Ecology of Occupation-based Practices*, 2nd edn, pp. 65–84. Churchill Livingstone Elsevier, Philadelphia.

Wicks, A. (2005) Understanding occupational potential. *Journal of Occupational Science*, **12**(3), 130–139. https://doi.org/10.1080/14427591.2005.9686556

World Health Organization (2002) *Towards a common language for functioning, disability and health: ICF*. Geneva. http://www.who.int/classifications/icf/training/icfbeginnersguide.pdf (accessed 12 March 2024)

World Health Organization (2007) *Who-aims report on mental health system in South Africa ministry of health South Africa*. http://www.who.int/mental_health/evidence/south_africa_who_aims_report.pdf (accessed 10 March 2024)

World Federation of Occupation Therapists (WFOT) (2012a) *About occupational therapy*. https://wfot.org/about/about-occupational-therapy#:~:text=Occupational%20therapy%20is%20a%20client,the%20activities%20of%20everyday%20life (accessed 10 March 2024)

World Federation of Occupation Therapists (WFOT) (2012b) *Code of ethics for occupational therapists*. http://www.wfot.org/SearchResults.aspx?Search=code+of+ethics (accessed 11 March 2024)

Creative Ability

A Model for Individual and Group Occupational Therapy for Clients with Psychosocial Dysfunction

Patricia de Witt

Occupational Therapy Department, School of Therapeutic Sciences, Faculty of Health Sciences, University of the Witwatersrand, Johannesburg, South Africa

KEY LEARNING POINTS

- An introduction to the theory that supports the Vona du Toit Model of Creative Ability (VdTMoCA).

- Key concepts that underpin the VdTMoCA.

- The focus of volition and motivation at each level of action.

- Occupational behaviour and skills characteristic of each level of action.

- Assessment of creative ability.

- Treatment outcomes and intervention principles/guidelines to support and facilitate growth within the levels of action during occupational therapy for clients with mental health conditions.

This chapter aims to introduce the Vona du Toit Model of Creative Ability (VdTMoCA) and its application to adults with mental health conditions such as those listed in the ICD11 (WHO 2022) or the DSM V-TR (American Psychiatric Association 2022). This chapter is intended for students and novice occupational therapists working in a variety of mental health care settings.

Throughout this chapter, the term 'individual' or 'individuals' is used when referring to a person or people in general, and 'client' is used when referring to a mental health care user in a hospital or primary care setting during an occupational therapy process. Right through the chapter, the masculine pronoun is used, but the term also includes the feminine. All figures in this chapter and Table 2.2 have been included with the permission of the Vona and Marie du Toit Foundation.

INTRODUCTION

The VdTMoCA was initially described in South Africa in a series of academic texts between 1962 and 1974 (Watson & Coetzee 2019) but has received considerable international attention in the last decade (Sherwood & Wilson 2019). This model fits the practice model criteria initially described by Reed and Sanderson (Reed & Sanderson 1999) as the organising of profession's philosophy and scope into practice by describing the assessment tools, interventions and outcomes (Hussey *et al.* 2007, p. 288) and later by Turpin and Iwama (Turpin & Iwama 2011). The uniqueness of the VdTMoCA lies in the provision of a comprehensive framework to both assess and treat activity limitations and participation restrictions (WHO 2013), which result from or accompany a mental health condition using an occupational lens.

Crouch and Alers Occupational Therapy in Psychiatry and Mental Health, Sixth Edition.
Edited by Rosemary Crouch, Tania Buys, Enos Morankoana Ramano, Matty van Niekerk and Lisa Wegner.
© 2025 John Wiley & Sons Ltd. Published 2025 by John Wiley & Sons Ltd.

The VdTMoCA is particularly useful for occupational therapists working with individual clients but also with groups of clients as is common in acute and chronic mental health settings, where the client group is diverse in terms of age, gender, culture, language, educational background, life experiences, needs and health condition(s). The VdTMoCA is helpful in coping with such diversity as it enables the occupational therapist to group clients efficiently in terms of their occupational performance abilities, needs, phase of treatment and plan intervention to meet intervention outcomes that emerge from the occupational therapy process (American Occupational Therapy Association 2020) rather than just their mental health condition.

As an occupational therapist, Vona du Toit ascribed to the beliefs central to the profession's philosophy regarding the uniqueness and totality (bio-psycho-social-spiritual integration) of individuals and that occupational therapy actively engages a client in purposeful, meaningful and goal-directed therapeutic occupation in order to improve or maintain health and quality of life (du Toit 2009). Du Toit's professional interest was to understand the dynamic nature of interaction between an individual's volition, motivation and their unique and creative engagement in a variety of occupations within their specific context. These are the key components of the VdTMoCA (van der Reyden & Sherwood 2019). Du Toit described the domains of concern for an occupational therapist within the VdTMoCA as the motivation, action and quality of the product because of occupational engagement, as well as relational contact with materials and objects, people, situations, control of anxiety, ability to show initiative and exert effort (du Toit 2009).

The philosophical constructs that underpinned the development of the VdTMoCA are rooted in phenomenology and existential philosophy and theories of Husserl, van den Berg, Langeveldt Kluckholn, Piaget, Rogers and Frankl (Joubert 2019). Du Toit postulated that each individual, as a complex integration of mind, body and spirit, is motivated by their volition to determine their unique and creative interpretation of the meaning of their life through their interaction with and experience of the world through all that they do and engage with (du Toit 2009). This text does not allow for a comprehensive description of the philosophical and theoretic conceptualisation that underpinned the emergence of the model. This has been thoroughly described in other texts (Joubert 2019).

FUNDAMENTAL CONCEPTS IN THE THEORY OF CREATIVE ABILITY

The concepts of 'creativeness' and 'being creative' are not unique to occupational therapy. However, in the context of the VdTMoCA, they do not apply to a particular quality or quantity of creativity (du Toit 1991, p. 22) but are used to describe an individual's unique ability to alter or extend his occupational performance, thus being able to do some aspect of his daily occupations that he was not able to do before, to achieve

meaning and purpose and influence his occupational identity as a result of this engagement (Unruh 2004).

Creative ability was defined by du Toit as an individual's 'ability to form a relational contact with people, events and materials, and by his preparedness to function freely and with originality at his maximum level of competence' (du Toit 1991, p. 23).

According to du Toit, the development of creative ability occurs within the boundaries of an individual's 'creative capacity', which she defined as the creative potential each individual has and which could possibly develop under optimal circumstances (du Toit 1980). Creative capacity varies from one individual to another and is influenced by factors such as intelligence, personality structure and the human body's capacity to support participation in purposeful activities (du Toit 1980, p. 6). As with all other concepts that denote human potential, individuals seldom reach full potential and there is always some capacity in reserve for growth.

Creative ability is that part of an individual's creative capacity that has been realised and which the individual is able to use to engage in their daily life (du Toit 2009). An individual's ability to translate creative capacity into participation in purposeful activity is consistent with his level of creative participation and is facilitated or limited by contextual factors such as opportunities or challenges and contextual support for purposeful engagement (du Toit 2009, p. 7).

Du Toit used a slightly different taxonomy from the Occupational Performance Areas to that used in the Occupational Therapy Practice Framework: Domains and Process IV (OTPF IV) (American Occupational Therapy Association 2020). The terms used include:

- personal management to include 'activities of daily living (ADLs)' as well as 'instrumental activities of daily living (IADLs)' and health management.

- social ability to include 'social participation.'

- work ability to include education and work.

- 'constructive use of free time' was used instead of 'leisure' (du Toit 1980).

Rest and sleep as occupations were not included (du Toit 1980; American Occupational Therapy Association 2020).

To grow or develop in a creative ability sense, the individual must exert considerable effort to overcome the challenges presented by the demands of occupational engagement or the context where achievement requires extension of existing capacities (physical, mental, social, or spiritual). Sherwood described four zones of effort: no effort, minimal effort, effortful participation and maximum effort (Sherwood 2016). However, maximum effort, which is very energy intensive and thus of short duration, refers to the motivated exertion of 'creative effort' in the harnessing of all capacities at the boundary of an individual's current creative ability to achieve growth (see Figure 2.1) (du Toit 1991, p. 28).

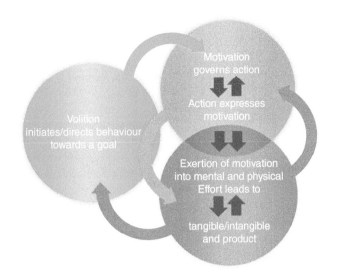

FIGURE 2.1   Relationship between volition, motivation, and action.
Source: With permission from the Vona and Marie du Toit Foundation.

However, to exert maximal effort, three other aspects need to be present for this to occur:

1. Creative response which reflects the positive attitude or response an individual displays towards any opportunity offered to him associated with occupational engagement. It reflects the individual's preparedness to use all his capacities to participate for anticipated pleasure, gain or acknowledgement, despite some anxiety about his capabilities and the success of the outcome. It precedes creative participation (du Toit 1980, p. 6; de Witt 2014).

2. Creative participation is the process of being actively involved in activities and occupations concerned with 'the doing' of the components of everyday living appropriate to the individual's level of development and context. This concept refers to taking an active, rather than a passive role and engaging in such a way that it challenges his abilities and internal resources (du Toit 1980, p. 7).

3. Creative act is the result of an individual's creative response and creative participation, in terms of producing a change in activity participation, which may be tangible or intangible but demonstrates growth in creative ability (du Toit 1980). See Figure 2.2.

Therefore, in summary to behave creatively and extend the level of creative ability, a client has to have a positive attitude towards an occupational opportunity offered to him by a therapeutic activity despite some anxiety (creative response) and be actively engaged in 'doing' the activity which offers an appropriate 'just right' challenge. The 'just right challenge' is a key concept in occupational therapy (Christie 1999), in the intersection of person-activity-environment (creative participation) and the creation of a 'product 'as a result of active engagement or outcome that denotes some activity participation change, be it tangible or intangible (creative act). These have also been termed the growth factors (van der Reyden & Sherwood 2019) (see Figure 2.3).

Furthermore, du Toit defined 'volition', central concept within creative ability theory, as the will to be and direct one's own life. Van der Reyden and Sherwood explain that volition governs the preparedness to act and assigns meaning and purpose to that action (van der Reyden & Sherwood 2019). Du Toit described volition as giving rise to two intrinsically linked components: motivation and action. The motivational component represents the energy source for motives (needs, wants and desires) for occupational behaviour and the action component translates the motivational energy into occupational behaviour; thus, motivation governs action since it is only possible to express the motivation that exists within the individual into action (du Toit 1980).

Inspired by the work of Coleman, du Toit defined motivation as the inner condition of an organism that initiates or directs behaviour towards a goal (Coleman 1960), which remains consistent with current literature. Du Toit described this as meaning 'being in becoming' (du Toit 2009, p. 53). Motivation is both intrinsic and extrinsic (Ryan & Deci 2020). Intrinsic motivation denotes an internal locus of control and relates to motivation to engage in activities and occupations for personal interest, enjoyment from the participation and

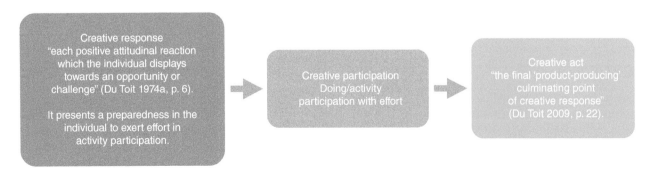

FIGURE 2.2   Creative ability growth factors.
Source: With permission from the Vona and Marie du Toit Foundation.

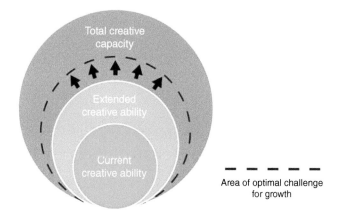

FIGURE 2.3 Growth of creative ability.
Source: With permission from the Vona and Marie du Toit Foundation.

Area of optimal challenge
for growth

personal capacity building (Ryan & Deci 2020). Literature described four levels of extrinsic motivation with a locus of control varying from external to more internal. The levels are external regulation to achieve external rewards and compliance, introjection with ego involvement for approval by others, identification linked to endorsement of goals and achievements by others, and integration that is congruency and constancy of identification with others (Ryan & Deci 2020). It has been suggested that intrinsic motivation is the most relevant to the occupational therapy process (Wu 2001; Taylor 2017).

Du Toit believed that the volition and motivation that directed creative ability had a different focus at each stage in the development of creative ability. Du Toit described nine sequential levels of motivation, each with its own qualities that directed activity participation, thus creating specific creative ability developmental milestones. These levels indicate what 'motivates' an individual to engage or participate in everyday activities. They also indicate changes in the nature and strength of motivation and the factors that facilitate motivation as it develops through the levels of creative ability.

Action is defined as 'the exertion of drive, or mental and physical effort which results in the creation of a tangible or intangible product' (du Toit 2009). Like motivation, action can also be ordered into ten levels. These levels of action describe the sequential differences in the nature and quality of the individual's engagement in occupations and activities and competencies required to support these that are described in terms of the ability to form relational contact with others, events, materials and objects in the environment, as well as the characteristics of engagement.

The levels of creative ability, both motivation and action, emerge as an interlinking spiral created from the dynamic relationship between the person, the occupation and environment (see Figure 2.4). An individual develops his creative ability within the confines of his creative capacity by demonstrating a creative response, creative participation, the exertion of maximal effort so as to produce a creative act, which is the demonstration of growth (van der Reyden & Sherwood 2019).

DEVELOPMENT OF CREATIVE ABILITY THROUGH EMERGING LEVELS OF MOTIVATION AND ACTION

The development of creative ability describes how activity participation develops along a continuum from mere existence and egocentrism to contribution to the community and society at the highest level, which only a few extraordinary individuals achieve. Development starts at birth and continues throughout life. Although development is usually sequentially progressive following the expansion of the levels of creative ability, regression in creative ability can also occur following a sequential restriction in creative ability. Development is not always consistent from day to day, with growth often taking place in spurts followed by periods of consolidation, while the individual remains in a relative 'comfort zone' for varying periods of time.

As indicated in Figure 2.4 a dynamic relationship exists between the external environment and the development of creative ability in any individual. While the external environment provides challenges and opportunities for growth, new opportunities and both positive and adverse circumstances may create stress that may lead to regression. Development of creative ability is therefore dependent on 'the fit' between the readiness of the individual to grow creatively (i.e. creative response, creative participation and creative act) and the appropriate 'just right' challenge that occupations and their environmental context provide (Christie 1999; de Witt 2002).

Like all other human developmental models, the emergence of creative ability is subject to the following theoretical assumptions (du Toit 2009): development occurs in an orderly fashion throughout life and the steps within the developmental process are sequential and none can be omitted. Individuals have an innate drive to encounter their world and master its challenges to grow and change in a creative ability sense, but confronting change creates tension, disequilibrium and stress, which represent a developmental opportunity that needs to be overcome. Change can result in adaptation, mastery and growth, while an inability to adapt results in maintaining the current developmental level or regression and dysfunction. The ability to master developmental tasks is influenced by the individual's internal human capacities, physical, mental, social and spiritual; life experiences; activity/occupational demands; resources availability and opportunity within the occupational context. Mastering a developmental opportunity successfully leads to adaptation. This can be the achievement of a developmental step, self-satisfaction and societal approval and promotes confidence in meeting future challenges in creating the belief that 'I can' (Krupa et al. 2016).

Creative ability has two main characteristics:

- *Sequential development*: the growth, regression and recovery of creative ability follow a constant and sequential pattern (see Figure 2.3). This means that growth and recovery of both the motivation and action components follow a stable, predictable and sequential pattern in which no level or phase may be omitted (de Witt 2014, p. 7).

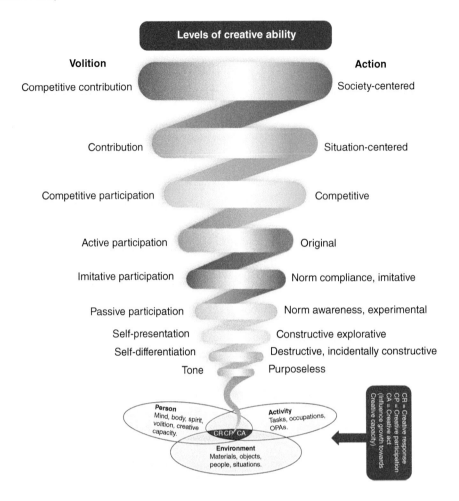

FIGURE 2.4 Levels of creative ability.

Source: With permission from the Vona and Marie du Toit Foundation.

• Action is a direct manifestation of the motivational component of an individual's creative ability and this is evident in the nature and quality of an individual's activity participation and occupational behaviour (de Witt 2014, p. 7).

As creative ability is dynamic and varies with the individual's circumstances, inner resources, confidence, anxiety level and the demands that occupations, activities and their context place on a person's human system, there is often a gentle forward and backward flow within, and sometimes between, the levels of creative ability, which is related to feelings of security and of being in control in the former and stress in the latter. However, if the individual is devastated by trauma, illness, disability or adverse environmental circumstances (natural disasters, socio-political unrest and poverty), the movement across the continuum of the creative ability levels is more marked.

Creative ability is applicable to the activity participation of all individuals. However, in occupational therapy, it is mostly used with clients with activity limitations and participation restrictions due to or associated with one or more health conditions. A mental health condition, experienced at any time across the life span, may limit or disrupt, either temporarily or

permanently, the client's creative ability, which may lead to a delay in development, regression or disability (Global Burden of Disease 2019; Mental Health Collaborators 2022).

It is well described that mental health conditions affect functioning (American Psychiatric Association 2022) and the International Classification of Function Disability and Health (ICF) defines functioning in terms of activity restrictions and participation (WHO 2013), which are similar domains as those used by du Toit (du Toit 2009) and are listed above. Mental health disorders disrupt the domains of creative ability due to difficulties within the human system and an unconducive environment that fails to support previous levels of occupational behaviour.

In each level of motivation and action, a wide range of competencies and occupational behaviours are accomplished directed by changes in volition and motivation. In an occupational therapy process, it is important to distinguish if the client's activity participation is consistent with the beginning, the middle of a level or moving towards the next level. Du Toit described the following phases that can be applied at each level of both motivation and action to describe the position of client within a particular level (du Toit 1980). The therapist-directed phase describes the first phase of the level. The client is demonstrating skills and occupational behaviour characteristics of both the previous and current levels. However, he is not able to maintain the activity participation characteristic of this current level and activity participation will easily regress to that of an earlier level. Thus, the client needs continuous therapeutic facilitation to practice the competencies and occupational behaviours consistent with the beginning of the current level. Client-directed is the second phase of a level and indicates that the client's occupational behaviour is generally characteristic of the requirements of that level. He can maintain this occupational behaviour relatively independently provided the context is supportive and the activity demands are within his available competencies. Transitional is the final phase of each level and the client's occupational behaviour is consistent with the characteristics of the current level but can demonstrate some occupational behaviour and characteristics of the next level under optimal conditions.

The application of VdTMoCA and its associated theory within mental health occupational therapy practice is based on the principle of the client's active engagement through the process of doing, not talking about doing. The VdTMoCA does not dictate specific activities or occupations for clients during assessment and intervention, but only describes the characteristics that therapeutic activities and occupations should meet to be appropriate to the client's creative ability level. This model presupposes that occupational therapists use their professional competencies, clinical reasoning, knowledge of activities and occupations and skill in activity analysis to select activities to be used as a therapeutic means or ends (American Occupational Therapy Association 2020). Therapeutic activities must be appropriate to the client's individual profile and be considered meaningful, purposeful and goal-directed in the context of the client's life, needs, values, interests and environment and be executed in a manner which is culturally appropriate.

Coping with, and recovering from, both mild and severe mental health conditions is complex, multi-layered, difficult, takes time and effort and is sometimes uncertain. It requires a team of skilled health practitioners who collectively contribute to the process. However, the VdTMoCA provides occupational therapists with a comprehensive process with clear and practical guidelines to assess and provide effective care for clients with mental health conditions. The desired outcome is to facilitate activity and participation to gain the highest level of independence in personal, social and work ability and constructive use of free time domains so as to enable mental health and well-being.

ASSESSING AND RECORDING THE LEVELS OF CREATIVE ABILITY

The client's level of creative ability can be determined from any comprehensive occupational therapy assessment but requires three sequential steps related to the clinical reasoning or interpretation of the assessment information in relation to VdTMoCA theory.

Step 1: *Evaluation of occupational skills and behaviour.* This should be part of the client's initial assessment and the ongoing monitoring of his condition as well as changes in his creative ability in all facets of intervention. The assessment of a client's current level of creative ability should be based on observation and clinical evaluation of occupational skills and behaviour in a variety of situations considering all domains of VdTMoCA. While the client's occupational history is pertinent in trying to establish treatment outcomes and goals, the assessment must confirm what the client is currently able to do. This can only be achieved by involving the client in an activity or variety of activities and critically observing the nature of his engagement and the quality of performance to determine his level of action. The occupational therapist in consultation with the client, considering his interests and aptitudes, should select an activity(ies) which have purpose, relevance and meaning to the client but also can elicit satisfactory assessment information. The activity should be within his frame of reference but not a habituated skill or routine unless it is in the domain of basic personal care like washing and dressing. The activity should require that the client must think and process the activity which should be completed within approximately 45 minutes. It should have a defined end product and encourage active participation. The assessment activity may be done alone or alongside other clients.

Understanding a client's level of creative ability is facilitated by taking careful note of his attitude and ability to make relational contact with the materials, objects, people and events in the environment; ability to plan, initiate and sustain effort until the activity is complete or to continue at the same level of performance over time if the activity or task is repetitive; observe the quality of performance and ability to evaluate what has been done and the standard set for himself; the supervision and assistance required, the environmental structure required for adequate participation, his ability to read environmental cues and meet norms that are both overt and covert; ability to control anxiety when faced with obstacles or challenges; ability to act with originality, to solve problems and to make and act on decisions made; the emotional response to engagement, performance and the end product. Most of these factors illicit the nature of the client's action rather than his motivation, the quality of which is more difficult to directly observe and is commonly deduced from the nature of his action.

Step 2: *Establishing the level of action.* Each level of action defines the occupational skills and behaviour characteristics of that level; thus, by analysing the information gathered about the client's occupational skills and behaviour, the occupational therapist can determine his level of action in each domain of occupation that du Toit described (du Toit 1991). The level of action can be recorded through one of two recording methods: the grid system (Table 2.1) described by de Witt or the Creative Participation Assessment (CPA) described by van der Reyden (see Table 2.2) (de Witt & Sherwood 2019). Using the grid system as an example, make a cross in the grid in the appropriate column, positioning it to

Table 2.1 Creative ability assessment grid.

Level of motivation	Levels of action	Phases of action	Personal management	Social ability	Work ability	Constructive use of free time
Tone	Purposeless and unplanned action	Therapist directed				Group1 Development for constructive action
		Client directed				
		Transitional				
Self-differentiation	Destructive	Therapist directed				
		Client directed				
		Transitional				
	Incidentally constructive	Therapist directed				
		Client directed				
		Transitional				
Self-presentation	Constructive explorative	Therapist directed				
		Client directed				
		Transitional				
Passive participation	Norm awareness experimental	Therapist directed				Group 2 Development for Norm compliance
		Client directed				
		Transitional				
Imitative participation	Norm-compliant imitative	Therapist directed				
		Client directed				
		Transitional				
Active participation	Original	Therapist directed				Group 3 Development for Self-actualisation
		Client directed				
		Transitional				
Competitive participation	Situation centred	Therapist directed				
		Client directed				
		Transitional				
Contribution	Competitive centred	Therapist directed				
		Client directed				
		Transitional				
Competitive contribution	Society centred	Therapist directed				
		Client directed				
		Transitional				

Source: de Witt. PA and Sherwood (2019) / Vona and Marie du Toit Foundation.

indicate the phase of the action. If there are marked variations across a number of levels, review the assessment data to ensure that it represents the client's overall pattern of activity participation rather than his past or habituated skills.

Where there is clustering in all occupational domains, determining the overall level of action is straightforward, as shown in the example in Table 2.3. Table 2.3 shows that the client's occupational skills and behaviours are consistent with a level of constructive exploration but in the client-directed phase in three domains (social, work and free time). In one domain (personal management), the phase has been rated as being transitional. This indicates that although occupational behaviour and skills are all characteristics of the constructive explorative level, there are some skills and behaviours that are associated with the norm awareness experimental level of action under optimal circumstances. Thus, using the principle of majority rules, the client's overall level of action is constructive explorative client-directed phase.

Table 2.4 indicates that although all the client's skills are within the norm awareness experimental level, personal management and social ability fall within the patient-directed phase, while work and leisure fall within the therapist-directed phase. When there are two domains in one phase and two in another, the following principles can be applied: social ability has the most impact on occupational performance, followed by work ability. Since the social domain has a

Table 2.2 Creative participation assessment (CPA).

Patient name:		Date:		Therapist:		
LEVELS OF CREATIVE ABILITY						
	Tone	**Self-differentiation**	**Self-presentation**	**Passive participation**	**Imitative participation**	**Active participation**
Action	Undirected and unplanned. Purposeless.	Incidentally constructive or destructive. (1–2 step task)	Constructive explorative. (3–4 step task)	Fairly product-centred. Norm awareness experimental. (5–7 step task)	Product centred. Follows the norm. (7–10 step task)	With originality – transcends norm/expectations.
Volition	Egocentric. To maintain existence.	Egocentric. To differentiate self from others.	Seems willing to try to present self; unsure.	Robust. Directed to attainment of skill.	Directed to produce a good product. Acceptable behaviour.	Directed to improvement of product, procedures or systems.
Handle tools and materials	Not evident; unaware.	Only simple everyday tools (e.g. spoon). Poor handling	Basic tools for activity participation – poor handling.	Appropriate; limited skill.	Appropriate, good use and care.	With initiative, skill evident.
Relate to people	No awareness.	Fleeting awareness.	Selective identification. Responds and tries to communicate, superficial interpersonal relations.	Communicates, initiates contact, conversation. Spectator role.	Communicates / Interacts; open to others' views; may be assertive.	Close interpersonal relations. Intimacy evident. Can assist others.
Handle situations	No awareness of different situations.	No or fleeting awareness, no ability shown to cope, inappropriate.	Partial awareness, stereotypical handling. Makes effort, but unsure or timid.	Follower/spectator. Manages fairly in a variety of situations. Participates in passive way.	Comprehends and manages variety of situations. Appropriate behaviour.	Can interpret, evaluate, adapt and adjust, according to need or plan.
Task concept	No task concept. Basic concepts	No Task concept. Basic and elementary concepts	Partial Task Concept (developing). Compound concepts.	Full Task Concept. Extended compound concepts (abstract element).	Consolidated Task concept. Integrated abstract concepts.	Abstract reasoning. Organisation, planning, individualisation.
Product	None.	No product.	Simple – familiar activities or part thereof. Process orientated. Poor quality product.	Product fair quality. Aware of expectations / norms; needs direction.	Product good quality. Norms internalised; with norm compliance; meets expectations.	Open labour market quality. Can adapt, modify, evaluate.
Assistance/supervision needed	Total assistance including physical assistance. Supervision, assistance, needs (24 h) nursing care constant supervision.	Physical assistance and constant supervision. Requires full-time care.	Constant supervision needed for task completion.	Regular supervision.	Guidance needed. Regular supervision for new activities and tasks; occasional supervision for known activities.	Occasional guidance needed in training for new skills. Takes full responsibility and helps to supervise others.

(continued)

Table 2.2 (*Continued*)

Patient name:		Date:		Therapist:		
			LEVELS OF CREATIVE ABILITY			
	Tone	Self-differentiation	Self-presentation	Passive participation	Imitative participation	Active participation
Behaviour	Haphazard, disorientation and bizarre behaviour.	Little or inappropriate reaction, disorientation and bizarre behaviour.	At times inappropriate or strange behaviour. Hesitant, unsure but willing to try out.	Follower, participates passively, occasionally inappropriate or hesitant behaviour.	Socially acceptable behaviour. Symptoms generally controlled.	Socially acceptable behaviour. Shows originality. May decide to act contrary to norm with appropriate and original behaviour.
Norm awareness	None noted.	None noted.	Starts to be aware of norms for appearance and behaviour, but not for task or product norms.	Norm awareness for appearance, behaviour, task and product.	Norm compliance. Does as expected, meets required standard for product, procedure and social behaviour.	Norm Transcendence (does better or more, adapts). Transcend norms in activities as well as situations.
Emotional responses and anxiety	Limited responses: positive/negative.	Limited, uncontrolled basic emotions displayed (positive or negative). Shows fleeting comfort and discomfort, satisfaction, or dissatisfaction.	Broader range of emotions, intensity, frequency and duration not always appropriate. Low self-esteem and anxiety present.	Refined nuances of emotions evident. Prone to immobilising effects of anxiety. Low self-esteem. Intensity, frequency and duration better controlled in known situations.	Full range of emotions mostly controlled and makes effort to control emotions. Maybe immobilised by anxiety.	Shows compassion, picks up subtle differences in emotions. ↑ Self-awareness. Anxiety used positively.
Initiative and effort	None noted.	No initiative. Fleeting, minimal. Effort not sustained.	Initiative usually inappropriate. Effort inconsistent, not sustained. Low frustration tolerance.	Hesitant to use initiative and put own ideas forward. Courage to exert effort but needs guidance or assistance when problems are encountered.	Initiative seldom used, prefer to follow the norm. Sustained effort in known task, able to handle occasional failures.	Initiative is original and frequently used. Exert maximum effort over extended period of time.
Total per level						

Level of creative ability:

Phase within level:	Therapist directed
	Client directed
	Transitional

Source: de Witt. PA and Sherwood (2019) / Vona and Marie du Toit Foundation.

governing influence, the overall level of action would in this case be constructive explorative patient-directed phase.

Where there is variation in the client's level of action in the four domains of creative ability, determining the level of action is more complicated. Table 2.5 indicates a variation in the level of occupational skills and behaviours in four domains: the social ability is constructive exploration on the patient-directed phase; in both the work and constructive use of free time areas, skills are characteristic of the norm awareness experimental action level, but in the work domain, there are a few indications of skill and behaviours of the imitative norm-compliant level (transitional phase); in the personal management, although skill and behaviours are predominantly imitative norm-compliant in nature, some norm awareness experimental behaviour are still evident (therapist directed).

Table 2.3   An example of a clustered level of action.

Level of action	Phasee	Personal management	Social ability	Work ability	Use of free time	Level of motivation	Phase
Constructive explorative	Therapist directed					Self presentation	Therapist directed
	Client directed		X	X	X	X	Patient directed X
	Transitional	X					Transitional

Table 2.4   An example of a split action grid.

Levels of action	Phases	Personal management	Social ability	Work ability	Use of free time	Levels of motivation	Phase
Constructive explorative	Therapist directed					Self-presentation	Therapist directed
	Client directed						Client directed
	Transitional			X	X		Transitional
Norm awareness experimental	Therapist directed	X	X			Passive participation X	Therapist directed X
	Cient directed						Client directed
	Transitional						Transitional

Table 2.5   An example showing a variable level of action.

Levels of action	Phases	Personal management	Social ability	Work ability	Use of free time	Levels of motivation	Phases
Constructive explorative	Therapist directed					Self-presentation	Therapist directed
	Client directed		X				Client directed
	Transitional						Transitional
Norm awareness experimental	Therapist directed				X	Passive participation	Therapist directed
	Client directed						Client directed
	Transitional			X			Transitional
Norm-compliant imitative	Therapist directed	X				Imitative participation	Therapist directed
	Client directed						Client directed
	Transitional						Transitional

Thus, the client's overall level of action is norm aware-ness experimental – fluctuating between therapist-directed and transitional phases. Clustering usually occurs within the level or across two levels, so the example in Table 2.5 would be unusual. As stated earlier, when marked variations occur, the occupational therapist should review the assessment data to ensure that the current activity participation has been assessed correctly at the same time taking note of habituated skills.

Variations in the different activity participation domains within one or across two levels of action must be accounted for in planning intervention. The occupational therapist there-fore uses the assessment grid as a guide to mix and match the principles and guidelines of treatment so that they fit the client's needs and reflect the assessed variation.

Step 3: *Establishing the level of motivation*. As motiva-tion is difficult to observe and measure directly, the occupational therapist must assume the client's level of motivation from the quality and nature of his observable occupational skills and behaviour. It has already been discussed that there is a stable relationship between the levels of motivation and the levels of action (see Table 2.1). Using the data recorded on the level of action grid completed in Step 2, a presumption can be made about the client's level of motivation.

The completion of the CPA Table 2.2 follows the same assessment steps as the Activity Participation Outcome Mea-sure (APOM) developed by Casteleijn (Casteleijn 2010). The APOM is an occupation-based outcome measure that has been based on the VdTMoCA. The APOM can be used to track changes in a client's creative ability (Casteleijn 2013). The construct validity of the APOM as well as the reliability and responsiveness has been established with mental health disor-ders. The APOM is licenced, and additional training is required to ensure the standardised use of the tool (de Witt & Sherwood 2019).

APPLICATION OF CREATIVE ABILITY IN OCCUPATIONAL THERAPY FOR CLIENTS WITH PSYCHOSOCIAL DYSFUNCTION

Mental health conditions have a negative influence on the client's well-being and occupational component of health resulting in disturbances in occupational performance in the domains of caring for self, relationships and socialising, education and work and constructive use of leisure time. Some mental health conditions have a more disorganising effect on occupational performance than others. Occupational therapy aims to improve or maintain the client's skills and abilities in occupations through engagement in purposeful and meaningful therapeutically selected activities. The purpose is to facilitate independent living as far as this is possible, improve health and well-being, facilitate quality of life (health promotion) and reduce the chances of regression and disability (secondary and tertiary prevention).

Creative ability theory can be applied to any of the mental health conditions listed in the ICD11 (WHO 2022) or in the DSM V-TR (American Psychiatric Association 2022) and can be aligned to the ICF. It can be applied to both acute and chronic conditions and can also be used equally effectively in hospital- and community-based treatment settings. The VdTMoCA is applied using five sets of principles, which differ at each level: those relating to the therapeutic relationship and how to interact with the client; how the environment should be structured, the most therapeutic way to present the activity; the activity requirement for the level and the grading that should be considered. Addressing the client's level of creative ability is only an aspect of occupational therapy but forms the platform from which the occupational therapist can focus on specific occupational performance deficits as well as the client factor and performance skill problems.

THE LEVELS OF CREATIVE ABILITY

As described previously, creative ability represents a continuum of occupational behaviour, which is divided into levels of motivation, each with its corresponding levels of action. Due to similarities in the overall volitional purpose of levels, they can be divided into three quite distinct groups (see Table 2.1):

Group 1: *Preparation for constructive action*. This is where the overall purpose of these levels is for the development of functional body use as a prerequisite for engagement in activities and occupations.

Group 2: *Behaviour and skill development of norm compliance*. Both concentrate on developing the occupational behaviours necessary to live and be productive in the community and comply with the prescribed norms of the context, society and group within which one lives.

Group 3: *Behaviour and skill development for self-actualisation*. Concentration is on developing leadership skills and occupational behaviours that are novel in any aspect of life. It may involve developing new products, methods of doing things, use of advanced technology, problem-solving processes or solutions to complex problems, challenges and situations.

Motivation and action are directed towards the benefit of self in groups 1 and 2, and in group 3 – towards others in a specified group of people initially and then towards society at large. These levels demand personal dedication, self-motivation, continuous critical reflection and self-evaluation. People functioning in the last group do not need to see the results of their efforts immediately and they may wait many months, years and even a lifetime to see the results of their work.

DESCRIPTION OF THE LEVELS OF MOTIVATION AND ACTION

GROUP 1

Tone

Volition on this level is directed at establishing and maintaining the will to live, which du Toit called 'positive tone' (du Toit 1980). This refers to self-directedness to survive (van der Reyden & Sherwood 2019, p. 72), which is the starting point for the development of all human systems that are required to enable occupational performance. The motivation is directed towards developing the human system sufficiently to survive/exist.

Purposeless and Unplanned Action

Action on this level is purposeless and unplanned and clients have no occupational skills other than developing the performance skills related to survival and early development (American Occupational Therapy Association 2020). Individuals on this level are defenceless, dependent and incapable of caring for themselves. They need protection, care and nurturing. They lack awareness of themselves and their bodies as being separate from the world around them. Their 'actions' are mainly automatic, appear purposeless and not goal-directed, but these 'actions' contribute to the development of the internal human systems to achieve 'biological tone'. Individuals have very little or no control over their bodies and bodily functions. They have little awareness of others. They communicate basic needs of discomfort, hunger or thirst, but this is non-specific, for example they may cry, grunt or shout, but this seldom identifies the problem or the extent of their distress. Language is frequently absent or, if present, is often only monosyllabic and is mostly incoherent. They usually respond positively to nurturing and may recognise daily caregivers as familiar. They appear to be unable to identify different situations other than a momentary awareness of strangeness or familiarity, have some awareness of routine and daily patterns, and are distressed by changes in these.

These clients are totally non-productive in an occupational sense and have no concept of 'doing'. There is little evidence of intention or effort. They can focus their attention momentarily on stimuli. Their physical movements are uncoordinated, often reflexive and haphazard. They need to be washed, dressed, toileted, fed, cared for and protected. They have no concept of free time. Clients with mental health conditions, such as the late stages of dementia, catatonic schizophrenia and patients who are unconscious can regress to this level. They are usually severely disordered and impaired in all the client factors and performance skills, which incapacitates them. They are usually found in frail care centres and institutions that care for the chronically ill.

The treatment outcomes on the purposeless and unplanned level of action are:

- To encourage positive tone and biological tone.

- To stimulate the client maximally via all his sensory modalities.

To achieve these outcomes, all members of the multidisciplinary team must adopt a uniform approach. Clients on this level are so occupationally incapacitated that a specific programme of activities is not practical; however, all interactions with the client should focus on stimulating awareness of his own body, making him aware of things and others in the environment, and stimulating the sensory and motor systems to promote biological tone.

The occupational therapist or occupational therapy assistant (OTA) or occupational therapy technician (OTT) is responsible for the initiation and maintenance of the therapeutic contact as a relationship is not yet possible. The occupational therapist must give everything in the relationship and talk to the client, expect nothing in return, not even recognition of himself as an individual. The client and his behaviour must be accepted unconditionally and should not be reprimanded for accidents. Interaction with the client should be warm and caring, and the client should be treated with dignity and respect. Caregivers should also be patient and persistent, making regular contact with the client to try to bring him into contact with the here and now, even if only momentarily. This is done by continuously talking to him, in a slightly raised voice (not shouting) to attract his attention, making use of physical contact (but with discretion), calling him by his given name and by describing the environment, objects and events to the client without expecting a verbal response. All staff should be encouraged to verbalise the processes involved in caring for the client and should never talk about him in his presence.

These clients are usually treated in their room or a familiar room in the ward if they can be moved. The treatment area should be stimulating but not be distracting or overwhelming. The external stimuli should be changed from time to time to prevent habituation, and his attention should be drawn to the changes. If practical, clients should not sit in the same place all day even if immobile; they should be seated in places with different environmental stimuli. If possible, clients should be actively encouraged to move around and be taken out of doors regularly, although this should be supervised. If the client is very mobile, he should be contained within the ward area as he may get lost. Draw the client's attention to the objects and people in the environment. Therapy should be divided into a few short sessions (five minutes), spread throughout the day, but also included in caregiving interventions.

The client although unable to engage in any constructive activity must be encouraged to engage and make contact with safe objects and materials from the environment. These should be presented singly in a consistent manner, with much repetition. Objects or materials should be placed in his hands and their basic concepts (shape, form, size and texture) and these properties should be verbalised to him, encouraging him to focus attention whilst in contact with the object/material. The objects and materials should stimulate all the senses, allow for physical handling, interaction within his capabilities and should be non-toxic in case he puts them into his mouth. They should be non-breakable should the client handle them in an uncoordinated manner. Do not expect him to be able to use the object or materials during this stage unless it is habituated. The only purpose is for him to focus his attention on it momentarily, and once his concentration is exceeded, the object or material will probably be discarded.

If the client shows signs of becoming more receptive to stimulation, it should be gradually upgraded by the following: increasing the frequency of the stimulatory sessions, the duration, the number of objects and materials to which he is exposed, both in a session and over a period and encouraging him to focus his attention on the object or material more frequently and for longer. If the client shows signs of becoming less receptive to stimulation, the programme can be downgraded by reversing the principles listed earlier.

There are three criteria that should be used to evaluate whether a client is ready to move to the unconstructive level, which is the next level of action: increasing receptiveness to environmental stimuli, ability to focus and maintain attention more than fleetingly (one to two minutes) and indications that the nature of his interaction with materials and objects is becoming unconstructive.

The second level of motivation in Group 1 is self-differentiation. There are two levels of action associated with this level of motivation, namely destructive and incidentally constructive action.

Self-differentiation

Clients who deteriorate to the self-differentiation level show evidence of severe, incapacitating client factors and performance skills. Frequently, the disturbances in client factors and performance skills are more evident because the client is more active and more verbal than on the level of tone.

Disorganisation of thinking, language impairments, aggressive and bizarre uncontrolled behaviour are common. Clients on this level are usually found in chronic institutions, which provide habilitation and rehabilitation programmes. The patients have serious debilitating mental health conditions such as schizophrenia, dementia, severe intellectual disabilities and autism.

Volition is directed at the development and delineation of the sense of self in the world. The motivation is directed at three areas: (i) establishing and maintaining awareness of self as a separate entity from the environment, the objects and people in it; (ii) achieving primary control over the body including bladder and bowel, self-soothing and feeding and (iii) learning the basic skills involved in using the body to interact with the world and integrating these into coordinated behaviours and learning basic social behaviours such as person recognition, basic culturally appropriate greetings, making requests and complying with commands.

Destructive Action

This is the first level of action to appear in the self-differentiation level. It represents the most primitive interaction that the client has with the world. Destructive action aims to assist the client to define his body boundaries and to practise the basic skills necessary for material and object handling. He is not destructive in an aggressive sense but handles materials and objects non-constructively in order to examine the basic properties of materials and to help develop the basic client factors and performance skills needed to enable occupational performance on later levels. These skills include focusing of attention; basic concept formation (such as form, shape and texture); basic elements of thinking, deciding and planning; body concept; sensory perception; coordination; balance; movement; hand function and communication. These in turn stimulate primary intention and construction that occurs coincidentally on the next level of action.

Destructive action has the following characteristics: clients are receptive to external stimulation and are prepared to make contact with the environment using their bodies; action is of short duration (2–5 minutes), and the client shows an inability to sustain effort; action is nonconstructive in that no end product is produced, other than fragments or a change in the form, volume or position of the material or objects owing to his non-productive interaction with it. This interaction is generally unplanned, non-specific and does not take the properties of the materials or objects into account during the interaction. It is, however, the first step in the exploration of materials and objects and his ability to interact with them.

In all domains of occupation, the client remains incapable, dependent and defenceless. He is still not able to do any personal care tasks independently or even assist with them. However, because the client is more receptive to environmental stimuli, the interaction between the environment and the body in activities related to bathing, dressing and feeding makes him aware of his body and its functions. Verbal reinforcement facilitates this. For example when the client is bathed, the contact with the water, the facecloth, soap and the towel makes him aware of his body and its boundaries. He can use his hands to splash the water and hold the soap.

In the social environment, clients are more open to social contact. They can recognise the caregivers as familiar or unfamiliar and develop a preference for some caregivers over others. They respond positively to nurturing. Communication remains difficult with only familiar caregivers able to understand. They have difficulty communicating their needs effectively, even though language may be present. They sometimes use simple words and gestures to communicate and may resort to slapping and physical withdrawal if distressed. Clients have no concept of social norms. They are still unable to recognise situations as being different, and consequently, behaviour is not differentiated from one situation to another. There may be evidence of bizarre behaviour resulting from psychotic phenomena, disturbed concepts and the need for self-stimulation such as rocking, head banging and genitalia stimulation. They start to respond to simple commands such as 'sit here', 'lift your arms' and 'take that out of your mouth'. There is a differentiation between the expression of positive and negative emotions, negative emotions are often more obvious than positive ones, and anger and unhappiness are often expressed through shouting and sometimes hitting out. Anxiety is apparent if the client is distressed or frightened, but if distracted, like all other emotions, it dissipates quickly.

Clients tend to be more active and mobile than on the previous level, but they seldom venture out of their immediate environment. Their action remains destructive in a non-constructive sense, but there is evidence of conscious direct physical interaction with materials and objects in the environment. This results in a change of volume, shape or fragmentation of materials and change of position of objects with interaction sustained for short periods. Material and object handling do not appear to reflect any active thinking, although clients tend to be attracted by colour and shape, indicating a developing awareness of basic concepts. The destructive interaction with materials and objects like banging, tearing, throwing and pulling is the first step in the development of the part–whole concept. As the client's basic concepts are developed, he can recognise shapes, colours, size and textures of objects and materials, but he usually cannot name them until the next level. Clients still have no concept of the use of free time.

Clients with serious debilitating mental health conditions such as schizophrenia, dementia, severe intellectual disabilities and autism can revert to this level.

Treatment outcomes for clients on the destructive level are to:

- Consolidate body awareness, especially body boundaries.

- Stimulate the physical awareness of people and objects in the environment and the sense of familiarity/non-familiarity.

- Stimulate focusing of attention for at least five minutes.

- Facilitate the primary client factors and performance skills needed for basic interaction with the environment.

As with clients on the previous level, for treatment to be successful, all multidisciplinary team members should be involved in the treatment programme regardless of their discipline. All should be actively involved in the planning of the treatment so that principles are consistently applied in all caregiving activities, even though they might take more time. Stimulation does need to be applied according to a specific plan so that stimulation is changed regularly to avoid habituation and both under- and over-stimulation are prevented.

Incidentally Constructive Action

This is the second level of action to develop the self-differentiation motivation level. This level is characterised by unplanned, unintentional, constructive action that results, by chance, in an immediate, recognisable end product. This one-task activity stimulates the consolidation of the part–whole concept and of 'making something' that is different from the parts used. There is a tendency for incidentally constructive action to be repeated in both the same and other situations, which stimulates generalisation. Du Toit (1980) saw this as the essential precursor to constructive activity participation.

Although clients on this level remain dependent on others for care, nurturing, safety and security, they establish the basic skills necessary to care for themselves, although they are not yet able to do this without supervision. As the client's body concept becomes consolidated, he is able to learn the basic skills and behaviours involved in care and control of his body, hygiene, dressing, feeding and toileting. During this level, the client achieves basic competence in the practical skills involved in these activities but continues to have difficulty with the following: timing and control of toileting, putting shoes on the correct feet and coping with fastening, selecting appropriate clothes and carrying out all of the aforementioned tasks independently and at an acceptable level of performance. Clients learn to do these basic personal activities within a specific routine set by caregivers. This stimulates the start of the concept of temporal organisation of activities and routines and performance patterns (American Occupational Therapy Association 2020). Clients often get distressed when the routine is disturbed as it provides a sense of security and predictability to their lives.

In the social situation, the awareness of familiar people is extended to those other than caregivers, which helps to extend their orientation to the person although the naming of people remains inconsistent. They can be very demanding, wanting immediate gratification of needs.

Communication becomes more coherent, and they can communicate their needs more efficiently, although this is egocentric and simple. Clients continue to have little awareness of social norms, although they do start to differentiate between right and wrong from the response of the caregiver.

For example they may be praised for eating their food but reprimanded for spitting on the floor. Behaviour continues to be undifferentiated from one situation to another and bizarre behaviour again may be evident in response to psychotic phenomena. Tantrums may occur if the client's needs are not met as soon as he would like or if he is restricted or refused something he desires.

The client can focus his attention more easily and concentrate on his activity for longer, initially five minutes and extending to ten minutes of active concentration towards the end of the level. He can interact with materials and objects, usually more than one or two at a time, unintentionally producing an immediate, clearly recognisable end product, which is a direct result of his interaction with the world. Although he demonstrates no desire to do anything with what he has produced, he might practise this incidentally constructive response several times, not always immediately, but within a few hours or days. Basic concepts are usually consolidated in the therapist-directed phase with clients able to name objects and verbalise the basic properties (naming objects by their properties, e.g. woof for a dog (van der Reyden & Sherwood 2019) that need consideration when interacting with the objects or materials. Elementary concepts (properties and purpose of things) (van der Reyden & Sherwood 2019) also develop and by the transitional phase, clients can use most of the common objects within their environment, although they may still have difficulty in describing these verbally and may have personal names for them.

These clients are often mobile and may be reluctant to sit for long periods of time. They appear to want to be of help and can-do simple tasks or chores directed by the caregiver, for example fetch your shoes, take this. They are more aware of the environment. They can recognise the different people and can identify the different rooms where activities take place. They can identify their own bed area and become very possessive about their possessions. Their orientation to person and place is improved, but they are quite sensitive to changes in the environment, although they often cannot identify the nature of the change. Clients on this level continue to have no concept of free time, but often enjoying leisure activities like singing, clapping to music as well as basic ball games and activities with balloons.

The **treatment outcomes** for clients on the level of incidentally constructive action are:

- Consolidation of body concept by making clients aware of their body parts, shape, size and functions by using sensory stimulation during hygiene and other tasks involving movement and interaction with materials and objects. Improvement of their awareness of the physical presence of others in the environment by exposing them to people other than caregivers, for example other clients and staff, and focusing their attention on others during the treatment process in small groups.

- Development or improvement of the occupational patterns, client factors, performance skills necessary for constructive action by encouraging incidentally constructive interaction, with possibilities for practice and repetition.

- Basic orientation to person, place and time, as well as basic skills of personal care.

Occupational therapy programmes for these clients must be planned, designed and monitored by an occupational therapist in consultation with a trained OTA/OTT. The caregivers should also be actively encouraged to use the critical principles of treatment effectively, even if this is more time-consuming. A specific programme of therapeutic activities prescribed by the occupational therapist should be introduced into a ward programme, and specific therapy sessions can be introduced as well so that treatment is now extended beyond caregiving activities. This treatment can be implemented by an OTA or OTT.

These clients should also be handled in a caring and dignified way. Positive and appropriate behaviour should be rewarded and unacceptable behaviour, such as defecating on the floor, screaming, or biting or hitting others, should be reprimanded in a kind and non-punitive manner. It is important to talk to the client clearly, in a slightly raised voice to attract his attention, but not to shout. Continuously orientate the client in terms of person, place and time making him aware of others and the occupational patterns and routines in the day. He should be called by name and actions verbalised, made aware of the environment and the different activities that occur there. Stimulate orientation to time by orientating him to the day, date, year, time of day and seasons and the events that take place regularly, and as well as those that are more irregular like a birthday. The occupational therapist should verbalise the client's activity and movement to encourage the development of basic and elementary concepts and body concept and keep his attention when stimulating him. He should be encouraged to look at the occupational therapist, if it is culturally appropriate, which assists with contact with reality and the 'here and now'.

The treatment situation should be stimulating, but there should be no external stimuli that unduly overwhelm or distract the client. External stimuli can be increased as his active concentration improves. Clients should be contained within the ward area as they are often disorientated, especially on the level of destructive action, but should be moved to different areas within the ward for different activities: bathroom for personal hygiene activities, dining room to eat and the lounge for stimulation activities. The various wards and rooms should be stimulating but not overwhelming or distracting. Colour and labels should be used to facilitate orientation, and clients should be made aware of changes in the environment, for example a new flower arrangement. Encourage them to extend their world by looking out of windows, creating an awareness of the objects and people outside. If the weather is good, clients should be taken out of doors for short walks or just to sit in the garden for a short period.

Treatment time should be broken up into several short sessions of between 10 and 20 minutes. There should be at least two to four sessions during the day. Treatment programmes can start to incorporate activities from different areas of occupations and may also be part of some of the caregiving processes, such as bathing, washing, dressing and eating. Some clients on this level may require habit training associated with personal care skills and routines. This should be negotiated with the nursing staff until the skill has been achieved. The daily execution should be managed by the nursing staff with the occupational therapist responsible for checking that the skill is maintained. Treatment will only be effective if it occurs daily.

Intervention and treatment principles for both levels of action, that is the destructive level and the incidentally constructive level, at the self-differentiation (level of motivation).

Although there may be slight differences in approach, most principles are similar on this level. Those that are different will be indicated.

These clients should be interacted with in a caring, nurturing and dignified way. Caregivers should not talk to them as though they are children or use a patronising approach. On this level, the client should be accepted unconditionally including his behaviour, which may not always be socially acceptable. Greet clients regularly and talk to them about what is happening in the environment to raise their level of awareness about what is happening around them. Verbalise all activities, in order to stimulate basic orientation to person and place, all basic concepts and to start the stimulation of elementary concepts (exploring the properties of objects, e.g. it is texture, size, shape colour) (van der Reyden & Sherwood 2019). Call all objects and people by their correct names. Ensure that you have the clients' attention and encourage them to look at you if that is appropriate. This will help to bring them into contact with reality. Physical contact to gain their attention should be used with discretion. Encourage cooperation in all caregiving activities and facilitate body action to assist them to participate in these activities, for example lift arms when dressing or open mouth when feeding, and positively reinforce this.

Clients should be treated in small groups with clients on the same level of action for short stimulation groups – usually only a single session a day and no more than about 15 minutes. The group should consist of no more than six group members, and the group leader needs to be consistent in approach. Group treatment assists in developing awareness of others and the environment but expects little interaction. The occupational therapist should encourage introductions and an awareness of the characteristics and activities of each member of the group.

The treatment situation must be well organised before the clients arrive so that the session can start immediately. Materials and equipment must be at hand, and the workplace should be carefully structured, taking safety and ergonomic factors into account. Where possible, no tools should be used and clients must be encouraged to make direct contact with the materials and objects with their hands. Remember to include time for basic hygiene such as hand washing and regular toileting. The ward areas should be planned or structured to promote orientation. This is particularly important during the later phases of the incidentally constructive level. Calendars and clocks should be correct and clearly displayed. All doors should be clearly marked, especially the toilet.

Clients must be given clear, simple, direct, verbal step-by-step instructions. Instructions should be repeated frequently in the same way every time, so that they do not have to deal with new elements that were not present earlier. Treatment materials should be presented one at a time and the client should be made familiar with the basic (destructive action) and elementary concepts (incidentally constructive action) of the material and objects. They should stimulate the part–whole concept wherever possible. Objects and materials should not require fine coordination, skilled action or require physical resistance. Verbalise the texture, form, shape and size of the material or object while encouraging clients to make relational contact with it via their senses. The clients should look at, hold, feel, taste, listen to and smell the item in question, verbalising the movement of involved body parts and the physical action involved, for example rolling, patting, squeezing and so on. Encourage destructive action actively at this early stage as clients interact with the materials. Praise and positively reinforce them for any effort. Do not expect constructive action. Objects and materials used should, where possible, come from the natural material group. They should demand no prior knowledge for clients to interact with them and should be edible, nontoxic and safe if mishandled. They should fall within their frame of reference and be part of their environment.

Grade physical demands of activities by increasing the range of movement required from small to larger as well a more coordination being expected during interaction with objects and materials. Although coordination will still be poor, grade the movement from very slow to a little faster and increase the control of their actions. Grade psychological demands of activities in the following way: extending the period for which clients can keep their attention focused; stimulating memory by encouraging them to name objects, materials and people by increasing the need for awareness of objects and people in the environment, and upgrading the amount and quality of cooperation required from the client in caregiving activities.

In the unconstructive action level, the following criteria need to be met before a client is ready to move onto the next level if the client: shows interest in interacting unconstructively with all materials and objects; shows some indication for intention, basic concepts are evident and he is showing some interest in elementary concepts; and he is more aware of immediate environment and is orientated to familiar persons who interact with him.

If the above criteria are met, then he is ready to move to the next level.

When facilitating incidentally constructive action, demonstrate by physically moving his body through the desired movements, until he has the idea. Repeat the action until he can do it alone. Remember that the quality of what he does will be poor and he will still need help, support and structure.

Incidentally, constructive activities representative of all occupational domains should be planned, prepared and structured for the client. All that should be required of him is to interact with the materials and objects in the activity to produce an end product/outcome that he did not expect. Activities must give immediate gratification. An edible end product often has more impact. Activities should clearly show the impact of his effort and the difference between the parts and the whole. All that can be expected is that he should interact with materials and objects. The activities should be concrete, simple and should facilitate the client's knowledge and control of his body as well as pre-functional physical and psychological factors and performance skills. The activities also need to help to develop basic self-care skills and encourage verbal communication.

The following aspects need to be graded: therapy centred on all caregiving activities to the introduction of specific therapy sessions; treatment only within the ward setting to therapy in occupational therapy department and outside; client cooperation in basic self-care activities to more independence in these skills but still requiring supervision; increasing the physical demands of activities; increasing rate, control and range of movement, coordination, duration and physical effort; increasing the psychological demands of activities on body concept by grading from body awareness to identification of body parts and their function to more functional use of the body and control of body processes within the activity; extending the client's active and passive concentration span by extending the concentration demands of the activity, and as his level of distractibility improves, so more external stimuli can be introduced; grading from minimal awareness of self and familiar others to more consistent awareness of both self and others; grading the temporal and spatial relationship to the client by discussing 'before and after tea' and spatial concepts, such as 'sitting next to', 'in front of' or 'on the left or right' of a person sitting next to him. Increasing the orientation expected from orientation to person, place and then a basic sense of the flow of time and patterns of occupations.

Should the client show indications of deterioration, the above principles can be reversed to accommodate this.

The client is ready to move onto the next level when body concept is consolidated and when toileting is independent with only rare accidents. He must have the skill to carry out hygiene tasks with some supervision of safety, although the quality of performance may be poor. The client should be aware of self and others and the temporal and spatial relationship between them. The client should be able to interact with materials and objects in an incidentally constructive manner and should show interest in more constructive exploration. He should also be orientated to person and place and have some orientation to time.

GROUP 2

Self-presentation

On this level, Volition is focused on the presentation of the self to and within the world, motivation is directed towards the development of the sense of 'individualness', but at the same time, a sense of belonging to a group. The development of the basic components of self-concept are evident as well as the presentation of self to others. The most fundamental skills involved in social interaction and interpersonal relationships (social awareness, social judgement, basic social skills, relating to others and socially acceptable behaviour) are also developing. The client's motivation is directed to the exploration of his ability to influence the environment, to be constructive and to begin to discriminate interests, likes and dislikes. Basic elements of constructive activity participation in all domains of occupations are emerging (achieving task concept, an awareness of pre-vocational skills and a concept of leisure). Throughout this stage, clients demonstrate a readiness to present the newly differentiated self to others and to explore the world and define its reality and their place within it. Exploration of the world is a co-requisite for constructiveness and productivity, which develop in this and subsequent levels.

Constructive Explorative Action

Constructive explorative action can be defined as the intentional investigation of materials, objects and others in the environment in search of understanding a person's occupational identity (Kielhofner 2002; Hansson *et al.* 2022), basic occupational competencies and occupational efficacy through 'doing'. This exploration is directed towards establishing the properties of materials and objects and the way in which they can be influenced through purposeful engagement and interaction. It is also their reaction to the materials, objects and others in the environment to the client that adds to this first step towards constructiveness and productivity. The more he interacts with others and objects in the environment, the more he learns and affirms about his basic effectiveness as an occupational being, similar to what Kielhofner referred to as personal causation During this level, the client also learns many of the fundamental occupational skills, but the need for structure, encouragement and support as well as external organisation precludes him from using these skills independently.

Clients with mental health conditions such as schizophrenia, mood disorder, moderate intellectual disability, chronic anxiety disorders, autism spectrum disorders (ASDs) to name a few often regress to this level of action during periods of acute illness and may plateau on this level in the chronic phase. During this level, limitations are placed on activity participation by symptoms in all of the psychosocial client factors and performance skills that impact on a client's ability and limit occupational performance throughout the constructive explorative level. Although the mental health conditions symptoms are less severe than on the earlier levels, psychopathology remains of moderate intensity. Clients on

this level can be found in acute units, mental hospitals and Non-Governmental Organisation (NGO) care centres. When the mental health condition is controlled, they can also live in supportive living environments, within a protective family unit, provided the context has the resources to cope with the burden of care. They can seldom work in the open labour market unless the job is simple, undemanding and highly supervised.

In the therapist-directed phase, clients consolidate their basic hygiene, which had to be supervised on the previous level. The quality and efficacy of occupational performance in this domain become more socially acceptable. However, they cannot organise these skills into a routine and need reminders to carry them out, but can execute them independently. Clients can dress themselves efficiently and can select clothes, but they may not consider the appropriateness for the situation or the weather. The fewer choices there are available, the more appropriate their clothes tend to be. In the client-directed phase, the clients learn basic care for their clothes, personal belongings and their immediate surroundings. They develop some awareness of the need to be presentable and so, for example, learn to wash, iron, sew on a button if this is a cultural expectation, and keep personal belongings safe and orderly. Despite this, they still may wear clothes for several days, but recognise that they should change. They often like to have their own belongings and develop preferences for clothes, which reflect their developing individuality. Choice may still not be socially appropriate. All these tasks need supervision and assistance should be given where needed. In the transitional phase, clients develop an interest in and start to explore refined forms of self-care and grooming. They also develop some basic skills for independent living, for example making their bed, making tea and sandwiches, sweeping, structured yard work and washing dishes. Clients usually change their clothes more regularly. If facilities are available, clients can do their own washing, although relatives frequently do this if he is hospitalised or if this is not part of their prescribed social role. Care of clothing and belongings is more regular, but socially appropriateness varies. However, they often manage themselves poorly when not supervised and need external structure as they have difficulty organising their activities into a routine, using their time effectively and organising their resources, and therefore, living independently is often not successful. They find it difficult to be persistent, organised and disciplined.

Clients come into the constructive explorative level with an awareness of the physical presence of others. This is further refined in the therapist-directed phase as they recognise other clients from their ward and can sometimes name them. They can differentiate between staff and other clients. In the client-directed phase, they become aware that others in the environment have needs and feelings. During the transitional phase, their recognition of the needs and feelings of others becomes more accurate as their social judgement improves, but they have difficulty in responding to these cues appropriately.

Throughout this level, the client develops basic social skills. The quality and appropriateness of verbal and non-verbal skills improve towards the transitional phase. Conversation remains superficial and egocentric throughout the level. Conversation also tends to reflect the client's psychopathology, and they have difficult in dealing with interpersonal anxiety. In the patient-directed and transitional phases, clients tend to form egocentric, superficial, childlike and transient relationships with people within their immediate environment and they develop dependency relationships with caregivers. These 'buddy' relationships with others tend to be short-lived, tend not to tolerate absences and differences of opinion. Social behaviour in the relationship is often inconsistent and they often disregard the feelings of others. Relationships with family members may be strained especially if there is a history of aggression, conflict about delusions and other behaviours associated with their illness. The insight of the family into the client's condition often influences their support and tolerance of him and his illness. Clients often have a disturbed sense of belonging to groups. Either they feel quite detached from family and secondary groups or overdependent on one or another group.

The most important development at this level is the emergence of the task concept and the nature of engagement, which is essential for doing activities independently and for being productive (de Witt 2003).

The task concept has two interacting concepts, firstly:

- Understanding the process of the activity, which is similar to understanding the activity as a whole described by du Toit (2009). This is initially a conscious process in developing competency in activity participation which becomes more automatic but can revert to being more conscious when the activity is very unfamiliar or very complex.

- Task identification, which is the understanding the influence of his effort, having a sense of engagement in the activity and that the activity is the product of his effort. Du Toit (2009) described this as identifying with the task – see Figure 2.5.

These two concepts are influenced by a client's interest in, recognition and ownership of the task at hand. This implies that the development of an understanding of the process of the task is more likely to be facilitated when the activity is both within his range of interests and frame of reference. Thus, a therapeutic activity should also meet his personal needs and environmental demands, be sanctioned by the sociocultural group, be goal directed in the sense that the activity should have a purpose and goal, which is both valued and meaningful, and the activity should provide the just right challenge to stimulate interest and fully engage energy levels and resources (Christie 1999; Reed & Sanderson 1999).

The third concept is the nature of a client's engagement in the activity. The following five aspects describe the process of a client's engagement essential for productive action:

1. Task selection relates to the client's decision 'to engage'. Task selection appears to imply that the decision 'to do or engage' needs to be made first and this is followed by deciding between the options that the environment

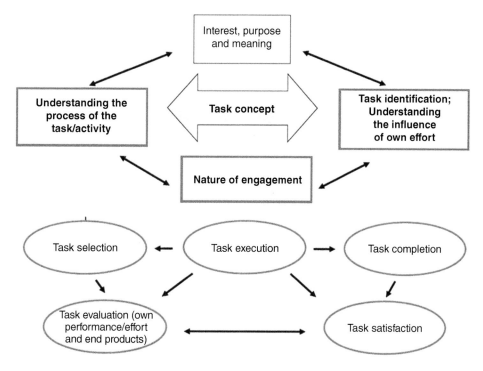

FIGURE 2.5 Task concept and its components.
Source: With the permission of the Vona and Marie Foundation.

offers. Task selection is the most difficult aspect of the therapist-directed phase. However, throughout the constructive explorative level, the occupational therapist should offer clients the opportunities and resources to engage in therapeutic activities that are potentially meaningful, purposeful and goal directed and within their abilities. However, a client must make the decision to engage even though he may need structure, support and some gentle persuasion to do this.

2. Task execution relates to how a client goes about the process of the task. This includes how he interacts with the activity resources and uses his internal capacities (client factors, performance skills) to work through the steps of the activity, as well as the level of motivation required to keep to the task at hand and sustain effort until the task is complete. This is poor at the beginning of the constructive explorative level and improves considerably towards the end.

3. Task completion indicates that a client is aware that the end of the activity has been reached and no more work is needed or desired. In the therapist-directed phase, clients want an end product, but cannot conceptualise the end. They often believe that the activity is complete after only one step. In the patient-directed phase, they seem more concerned with the process than the end product, while in the transitional phase, the client knows what is needed for completion, although he does not necessarily act on this, but acknowledges that more could be done.

4. Task evaluation indicates a client's capacity to evaluate the quality of what has been done, as well as the effort that is needed. This evaluation is not robust or accurate; rather, it is the capacity to look at what has been done in a reflective manner. Thus, a client exercises his interpretative and evaluative skills in relation to his performance in order to develop his sense of personal causation and occupational identity. This is often influenced by psychopathology such as depression, manic or a low self-esteem, which may colour the evaluation.

5. Task satisfaction usually implies a client gains a positive emotional response from engagement that should reinforce his engagement. However, emotions in relation to engagement are quite conflicting, for example frustration if the client found engagement challenging and disappointment when the end product is not exactly what was expected, but pleasure at the fact that something was achieved even though the quality is poor. Clients on this level seldom achieve realistic task satisfaction due to their inadequate self-concept, resultant low self-esteem and unrealistic judgement and poor occupational identity (de Witt 2003).

Throughout this level, the client's participation is goal-directed and the components of the task concept should be developing and evident by the transitional phase although efficient use of these continues to develop in the subsequent levels. Although an end product is usually produced, the emphasis during this level is on the process of exploring how the client can interact with and influence the materials, objects and people encountered during the process, rather than on end product itself. However, the production of a reasonable end product is important to support personal causation, the fragile self-esteem and the developing occupational identity. This constructive exploration is also directed to the way in which the client can influence or affect other situations and things in the world to find out about himself and his abilities and use this knowledge to enhance his occupational engagement and occupational competency development or re-emergence.

Throughout this level, occupational performance is influenced by a poorly developed self-concept and difficulty (hesitant or without consideration) in making a concrete decision where there are more than two or three options or where the options are very similar (positive to positive) or equally poor (negative to negative). Clients also have difficulty with all abstract decisions and working at an acceptable rate. They either work too fast and impulsively or too slowly. Due to inadequacy in some or many of pre-vocational skills (personal and social presentation and work competency skills) the quality of their work is usually poor. In addition, they have difficulty in delaying gratification for long periods of time and their ability to confront and cope with obstacles/challenges in the activity process is poor.

On this level, clients start to develop leisure interests. This is facilitated by their discrimination of activities into those they are attracted to and those they are not, based on their experience and interests. At the same time, they develop the understanding that some activities are for the purpose of work or survival, while others are only for pleasure and recreation or leisure. In the client-directed phase, the concept of leisure is firmly established and in the transitional phase they develop or regain a few isolated interests, but are not able to pursue them or leisure activities independently. They often intend to participate, but they need structure and support to do so.

Throughout the constructive explorative level, unique characteristics of the client's personality and his background are more evident and need to be considered more specifically in the activities selected in the treatment programme. Clients may have some awareness of their occupational incapacity but seldom realise the reason for it or what needs to be done to improve it. This limited insight into their occupational performance problems often limits clients' understanding of the value of occupational therapy in their overall treatment. This influences their ability to cooperate fully and they need continual encouragement to do so.

Intervention and Treatment Principles for the Level

There are three main outcomes for treatment for clients on this constructive explorative level:

- Presentation of self to others in different situations to facilitate awareness of others, to practise both verbal and non-verbal social skills, to gain an impression of ability to interact with and react to others and to form fundamental relationships.

- Exploration of ability to influence the materials and objects in the environment to gain an impression of his abilities, and this will help develop the concept of self and feelings of competence as an occupational being (personal causation).

- Explorative engagement in all activities and occupations and consolidation of the task concept components. In the context of this chapter consolidation of the task concept means that all aspects of the task concept are present in the client's activity participation. It does not assume that the client is able to use all components effectively and efficiently, which are capacities that develop further in the higher levels of creative ability, which is the criteria used by some other authors (Casteleijn & Holsten 2019, p. 94).

The occupational therapist needs to be encouraging and supportive of the client because of his poor self-concept, as he frequently feels insecure about his ability. As a result, engagement and effort in activity are often inconsistent, resulting in too much or too little activity. Patience is needed as this insecurity is usually reflected in all behaviours. The client's individuality should be facilitated and emphasised in all interactions. This can be done by asking the client for his opinions and ideas and acting on these if practical; sharing the client's contribution and pointing out his achievements to others as this helps to develop the external feedback system needed in the development of self-esteem and effective occupational performance; executing the client's wishes if they are realistic and fall within therapeutic goals and discussing those that do not; and giving the client the opportunity to make decisions concerning his activities and actions and encouraging him to take responsibility for them if this is realistic. Expectations for behaviour and occupational performance should be made clear to the client. Covert norms need to be made overt, but the expectation for compliance remains low. These overt norms should be used to help his judgement of performance and of situations. Clients should be made aware of inappropriate and unacceptable behaviour in a non-punitive and accepting manner with the suggestion of more appropriate actions. However, actions that may be harmful to others must be firmly handled. Clients who are reticent to be involved in occupational therapy should be gently encouraged but not forced. Involvement can be facilitated by using a roundabout method of inclusion and by sharing the responsibility for the activity with the client initially. A clear simple explanation about the role of occupational therapy within his total treatment and the setting of session outcomes that measure improvement may also help.

The occupational therapist should actively encourage the client to present himself to others in an appropriate way. He should be given many opportunities to do this and the occupational therapist should facilitate communication between him and others, and group activities may facilitate this. The occupational therapist should also enable constructive exploration of his ability by giving him the opportunity to make relational contact with materials, objects and others and should focus his attention on the effect of and result of his actions. The occupational therapist should help the client to direct his energy towards active engagement in a wide variety of activities and interactions to facilitate the development of the task concept and the nature of his engagement so as to explore his ability to be constructive. Throughout this level, pre-vocational skills should be stimulated to develop awareness rather than to actively improve these skills.

In a hospital setting clients require a half-day treatment programme where sessions are spread throughout the day with adequate rest periods in between. The client should be given a copy of his treatment programme. Initially, he will need reminders to attend, but towards the transitional phase, he should be encouraged to be more independent and be expected to report if he is unable to attend. In community settings, this may not be feasible, but regular sessions and a structured, practical and negotiated home programme should be planned with the client and his caregivers.

The programme should include both individual sessions and activity groups, both structured and spontaneous. Sessions should be approximately 45 minutes. The occupational therapist should always be at hand to give assistance, encouragement and support and to dissipate anxiety that the situation or activity may provoke. Treatment situations should be varied, sufficiently structured so that the client feels safe and secure and should be appropriate to an activity. The treatment situation should be stimulating, but external stimuli should be adjusted to the client's level of distractibility. Special care must be taken to orientate the client to a new treatment environment and the expectations for behaviour should be made clear to him. The treatment situation should be well organised with set locations for tools and materials. It is important as this gives the client security and helps organise his actions in relation to the environment. Other clients should be included in the treatment environment, but they should be involved in their own activities. This is important to promote interaction, to give feedback and to help the client to learn to share the time and attention of the occupational therapist. The occupational therapist should prepare the selected therapeutic activity appropriate to the client's phase and should structure the workplace to promote pre-vocational skills, safety and ergonomics. In the transitional phase, the client should be encouraged to assist with this. The occupational therapist should initially clear up and pack away after the treatment session but can direct the client to do some aspects of the clearing up to promote awareness of a tidy area and care of resources. Clients should be encouraged to label and store their own activities in a safe place.

On this level, all activities should be presented in a way that evokes a feeling of anticipation and competence. Clients tend to use verbal instructions more effectively than other types, and these should be given in a stepwise manner. Presentation and teaching should facilitate the development of the task concept and nature of engagement, facilitating what the client thinks should happen during each step. Written and verbal instructions should be introduced only after facilitating the client's thinking about the activity process so as to guide the processes or steps to be followed to complete the task. Demonstration should be used with discretion so as not to form a model for interaction with materials, others and objects and thus reduce constructive exploration. Evaluation of performance should be facilitated on a concrete level. The client should be encouraged to recognise the point at which the activity or his participation is complete and that the purpose of the activity is reached. Throughout treatment, emphasis should be placed on the client's effort and involvement with the materials and processes and not on the end product. In spite of this, it is important that the results of the client's interaction be positive; therefore, the occupational therapist should direct the client's participation to important aspects of the activity (key points of control) in order to ensure success. In the therapist-directed phase, no norms should be set for quality or rate of performance. In the patient-directed and transitional phases, clients should be made aware of the norms relating to quality of performance, but compliance to these should be facilitated but not be expected.

All activities should enable the client to constructively explore objects, materials, tools and equipment and the way he can influence them to enhance his occupational engagement. As the client's task concept is not consolidated, it is acceptable for him to do only some aspects of an activity, with the occupational therapist doing most of the planning and preparatory steps. The client should do the execution and completion steps. Each task can consist of between four and seven steps. Activities should assist in the development of components task concept and facilitate engagement, and he should be encouraged to make concrete decisions about the end product in terms of such aspects such as colour or what will be done with it; be within the interests and frame of reference of the client, be purposeful and meaningful to him and also be sustainable in the context of his life and not be childish or demean the client in any way; encourage tool and material handling and should be infallible or easily controlled with a good end product; be unfamiliar so that client cannot compare current ability with any previous skill (especially important if the client has insight into his loss of competency); be unique so performance cannot be compared to that of others and that copying does not reduce exploration; not include elements of competition or actively compare the client's skills or

performance with that of others; always be concrete and straightforward so as not to unduly raise the client's anxiety.

Grading should take place in the following areas: interpersonal contact: Social situations should be concrete and structured, but the people to whom he is exposed and with whom interaction is facilitated should vary from known selected people to known unselected people to unknown and unselected people, attendance: In the therapist-directed phase, the client needs to be fetched for treatment, in the patient-directed phase the client should be encouraged to attend treatment with other client's, even if he needs reminding. In the transitional phase, the client can usually attend treatment independently but needs to have the time and venue clearly stated, and frequent reminders are needed. Inconsistencies in punctuality must be tolerated; engagement needs to be actively facilitated throughout the level. In the therapist-directed phase, exploration should be actively facilitated, whilst in the patient-directed phase, the client should be given the opportunity to direct his own exploration and in the transitional phase. Some opportunities for experimental action should be introduced into activities that are predominantly consistent with the constructive explorative level; initially in the therapist-directed phase all behavioural disturbances should be tolerated, but the client should be tactfully and supportively made aware that his behaviour is not socially appropriate or acceptable and should be given some alternative suggestions for more acceptable behaviour while in the two later phases, the client should be given the opportunity to try out and explore the alternative behaviours suggested. Should the client show signs of deterioration, the grading principles mentioned earlier can be reversed.

The criteria which mark the movement to the passive participation level are as follows: all aspects of the task concept are evident and clients demonstrate an interest in being involved in all aspects of the activity, particularly showing concern around the end product; an interest in the rules or norms which govern behaviour and activity participation, an ability to work through an activity without constant supervision and individual attention and consolidation of basic social skills and an increase in awareness of people and social situations and an interest in the norms governing social behaviour.

Passive Participation

This is the first of the four levels of participation. Volition is directed at participation with norm compliance, while motivation on this level focusses on establishing the rules and norms accepted by the social setting in which the client finds himself and according to which occupational behaviour is judged and developing the occupational behaviours to achieve compliance. Motivation is more extensive and goal-directed as the client shows interest in the totality and purpose of activities. He has some difficulty initiating activities that are not habitual and independently organising them into a routine but does demonstrate the ability to sustain interest and effort in activities. Effort, ability and behaviour are characteristically erratic over time. The client is easily influenced by others whom he perceives as 'accepted' demonstrating behaviour that makes them acceptable to a desired group. During this level, ideals and morals are more evident. Clients on this level become aware of the interpersonal, social, political and economic factors influencing their immediate environment. This awareness leads to the identification of potentially threatening environmental stressors. Their poor anxiety control and limited behavioural resources negatively influence spontaneous participation, particularly in unfamiliar situations. Throughout this level, the client's emotional repertoire is extended. More refined emotions such as regret, pride, sympathy and loyalty become evident, and he has more control of his emotional response. If provoked, threatened or stimulated strongly, emotional control is tenuous. The client still has unconsolidated self-esteem demonstrated as either hesitance to engage in unfamiliar occupations and contexts that are viewed as challenging or impulsively engaging without due consideration.

Norm Awareness Experimental Level of Action

Occupational skills and behaviour tend to be both passive and erratic. Clients on this level tend to be the followers, doing what others do and say, and they want to blend into and be accepted by the crowd. However, on a psychological level, despite their engagement seeming passive, they watch and listen to everything going on around them to establish those occupational behaviours and skills that are both acceptable and unacceptable and the effects of compliance and non-compliance. They actively experiment with their own behaviour by following what others do. This is to establish how society will react and how acceptable their behaviour will be within specific contexts.

In this level of action, the client is developing and achieving a number of skills essential for independent living. He has a well-ordered, independent and efficient hygiene routine. The skills acquired on the previous level such as the care of clothing and belongings are further developed. However, the quality of performance is negatively influenced by undeveloped pre-vocational performance skills, erratic effort and the lack of ability to organise these skills into a practical routine. Clients need structure to be organised, or they often leave the chores until they are pressurised into doing them. An example is only doing washing and ironing when they have no more clothes to wear or shopping when there is no more food. They show an interest in socially acceptable refined forms of self-care, grooming and fashion. In the therapist-directed phase, their interest needs to be focused on these issues, while in the patient-directed phase, they actively experiment with them when encouraged. In the transitional phase, clients tend to experiment more independently. Throughout the level, clients show a hesitancy to initiate tasks. The ability to budget time and funds are limited, and there is a tendency not to be able to organise time effectively, to be 'crisis-driven' and to be impulsive or reticent. There is some disorganisation of personal business such as budgeting, paying accounts and

income tax. Throughout the level, clients express the desire for independence, but they need outside supervision and structure to achieve this successfully.

Interpersonal activity is directed towards being accepted and belonging to a group. Communication is usually rational and logical, and they can discuss a wide range of subjects, although clients demonstrate a reluctance to give their opinion if they are unsure of the opinion of the group. Conversation can be maintained effectively if other parties take most of the responsibility. They are able to form interpersonal relationships, but relationships tend to be egocentric. They have a tendency to form intense, sometimes inappropriate, relationships, which often are short-lived. Clients on this level find groups anxiety provoking. They like to be involved with the group but not to be singled out to give an individual opinion or make a suggestion. They tend to take on a spectator role but are actively involved in the group process, although they offer little, unless specifically invited to do so. Due to their desire to be 'one of the crowd', they have difficulty in being assertive, in dealing with a difference of opinion and resolving conflicts. Assertive skills tend to start developing during this level.

Occupational behaviour becomes progressively more product-centred. The consolidated task concept facilitates his desire to work through an activity from beginning to end. Although clients are eager to participate, they have difficulty initiating activities. Once started however they work reasonably effectively but are reluctant to participate in any activity where success is not ensured. They need less supervision, but they still need to have the steps and sequence confirmed. Throughout this level, they are concerned with the pre-vocational competency skills required to make their activity acceptable. Judgement of performance remains inconsistent, although it improves towards the transitional phase. They tend to judge their performance in terms of good or bad and tend to blame the materials, tools or environmental factors rather than how they contributed to the problem or have an unrealistic desire for perfection and excellence which they are not able to meet. Clients are able to sustain effort and quality of performance over time, although this tends to be inconsistent. They are able to deal with some obstacles during the course of the activity but are unable to demonstrate initiative. Quality of performance tends to improve towards the transitional phase.

Domestic or survival (IADL) skills are encouraged on this level. In the therapist-directed phase, the client can be responsible for caring for his bed area and personal possessions. He is able to take care of his room, clean up and pack things away, but the quality varies and the organisation of these activities is often poor or inconsistent. He can make nutritious meals with encouragement and structure. However, motivation to do this on a regular basis is inconsistent.

Clients who have achieved this level can work in the open labour market, but the work environment must be very structured, routine and organised and supervision is required. The job should be such that variations in quality and rate of performance should not be too important to job security.

A greater range of interests in recreational/leisure develops throughout this level, although discrimination of interests is largely dependent on others. Clients will actively participate if organised and encouraged. If others are not available to encourage them, they tend to use their time unproductively or passively.

High-functioning individuals can regress to norm awareness experimental action because of an acute relapsed or chronic mental health condition. The health condition is usually of mild to moderate in severity, and the psychopathology has an individualised presentation. These clients may be hospitalised in acute- or medium-term units and are often in a pre-discharge phase. Several clients on this level with well-controlled mental health conditions such as mood disorders, personality disorder, substance use disorders and anxiety disorders to name a few, may also be found in the community, participating in day-care or other rehabilitation facilities.

The Intervention and Treatment Principles for the Level

The main outcomes of treatment at this level are as follows.

Awareness of norms and experimentation with those occupational behaviours and skills will make them acceptable to the society in which they live and carry out their daily occupations and with socially accepted norms for healthy occupational engagement.

Clients should be handled with patience and the occupational therapist should be tolerant of their inconsistent effort and inability to produce behaviour and work of a consistent standard. Clients should continuously be made aware of the norms, both overt and covert, and they should be encouraged to evaluate the acceptability of their own and the group's occupational behaviour and performance. They should be encouraged to participate in their treatment, remembering that their participation will be passive and will need extra support to initiate activities. Encouragement will be needed from time to time until the activity is complete, especially if it takes time and they need to overcome challenges to complete it. They will need to read cues for socially appropriate behaviour and understand why behaviour is both appropriate and inappropriate. Assist clients with assertiveness, conflict resolution, problem-solving, value clarification as well as the understanding of the consequences of inappropriate or socially unacceptable behaviour, especially if the group is involved in activities that do not support health and well-being and engage in 'dark activities' (Twinley 2013; Kramer 2022). They need to be given opportunities and facilitated in developing healthy acquaintance relationships into a more meaningful relationship.

During this level, pre-vocational performance skills should be actively trained or retrained, although compliance is likely to be erratic.

Clients should be included in a full-day programme, especially if vocational rehabilitation is required, which should be negotiated if not hospitalised. The programme should be extended beyond the time for occupational therapy and should help them structure their free time in the late afternoon, evening and weekend. The programme should include both individual and group activities (both task centred and discussion).

Any occupation-appropriate treatment area can be used. However, for group work, the atmosphere needs to be accepting and permissive, while for individual activities, a work-related atmosphere should be created, allowing for norm awareness experimentation. Others should be included and involved with work-orientated or work-related activities. The treatment area should be structured in keeping with the client's concentration. Preparation of the activity and workplace should be done together with the client. He should be given the responsibility for cleaning up, packing away and storage of the tools, materials and activities. The occupational therapist should, however, direct and check this in order to comply with safety and risk concerns.

The client should be given comprehensive instructions that clearly define the sequence and the contents of the steps of an activity. He should be given practice at following all types of instruction (verbal, written, diagrammatic). The occupational therapist should ensure that he grasps what needs to be done and how it should be done before starting. He should be given some guidelines on how to check his progress. A client should be allowed to decide when the activity or step is complete and should be encouraged to work without continuous supervision and to ask for assistance only after trying to solve the problem first. The occupational therapist must help them to evaluate their effort, quality and progress in work as well as the reasons for success or failure. In the therapist-directed phase, clients find this difficult and it is necessary to focus the evaluation on the properties of the activity such as the neatness, size, colour or texture. They may be given an example against which to evaluate their work. In the client-directed phase, the evaluation should be done at the end of the activity because of the client's inability to tolerate negative feedback and their fear of failure. In the transitional phase, evaluation of quality can be introduced during the steps of the activity.

The activities used in treatment should make clients aware of the norms and be mainly concrete, but introducing some abstract elements. The clients should be involved in all the steps. The activities must be successful and give clients the opportunity to improve their pre-vocational performance skills initially and later their vocational skills, but initiative should not be expected. Activities should enable a client to learn and practise higher-order social skills such as assertiveness and conflict resolution and be given the opportunity to form relationships with people who were previously acquaintances.

On this level, the treatment is graded as follows: increase the expectation for more consistent pre-vocational performance skills and effort; initiation of familiar activities independently as the client moves towards the transitional level; increase the complexity of the activities; abstract elements and can also be introduced into activities on the client-directed phase; some specific vocational skills can be introduced on the transitional phase.

The client should meet the following criteria before moving to the next level:

- Start to initiate familiar activities consistently.

- Demonstrate the desire to comply with the norms of all situations or activities.

- Should become less dependent on environmental structure to direct actions and activities.

- Pre-vocational performance skills should be consolidated.

Imitative Participation Level of Motivation

During this level, volition is directed towards productive participation with norm compliance, while motivation is predominantly directed at complying with the norms set by society in an imitative manner. The client actively develops the competencies and behaviours that enable him to belong to selected groups and contexts and does not wish to be identified as being different from others, although individuality is evident within the client. Motivation is product-centred and directed towards productiveness, but there is little evidence of initiative and there is a reluctance to actively compete and compare skills with those of others. Clients on this level are stressed by the unknown and unfamiliar as well as any situation where the norms are unclear. The major developmental task that takes place during this particular level is the establishment of an independent, self-supporting and self-sustaining lifestyle, and activity participation, which is defined by the group(s) and context in which he functions.

Imitative Norm-compliant Level of Action

At this level, individuals may have been successfully treated and are now integrating back into society. They probably will no longer be in a hospital setting but may be attending clinics as out-patients and private appointments on a regular or infrequent basis. These clients may be seen in some specialised units for substance abuse or eating disorders. They may also be seen in the community when transitioning from a hospital to community and returning to work after a period of illness.

This level of action indicates that clients do what is asked of them, no more and no less. Although there are individual and socio-cultural variations in what is considered to be norm-compliant, there are some general trends.

In personal management, behaviour concerning hygiene and care of clothes and belongings is usually consistent and efficient. Refined forms of self-care and grooming are usually appropriate with the client developing awareness of fashion and suitability of dress for a wide variety of situations and occasions. There may, however, be a tendency to follow fashion, which may not be totally appropriate, that creates a sense of belonging or being part of the group. Clients on this level are mature enough to look after others: pets, children

and parents. While they can deal with their practical needs, they may still have difficulty in dealing effectively with their emotional needs. Management of personal business usually improves, but there may be impulsive spending on things that will improve their social acceptability, for example clothing, a car and the latest craze object.

All social behaviour is directed towards belonging. More mature, intimate relationships tend to develop during this level, but egocentric needs are still evident. Communication is usually efficient and basic social skills are good. However, assertiveness skills are not yet consolidated. Clients tend to function well socially in familiar situations but poorly in unfamiliar situations and in situations where the norms are not very clear. They tend to be followers rather than leaders and acceptance by others is important. They are very susceptible to group pressures and sensitive to acceptance or rejection by group members.

Independent living and productivity are the focus of attention on this level. This includes setting up and maintaining a home within financial and other resource restraints. In the therapist-directed phase, the client experiences difficulty in coping with the stresses of being responsible for himself and in managing the chores in an orderly and effective manner, but this tends to improve towards the transitional phase.

In the domain of work, the client's participation is goal-directed and norm-compliant. He is able to do what is asked of him efficiently, provided that the activities are straightforward, do not have any unexpected hitches and do not demand any initiative and complex problem-solving on his part. Pre-vocational performance skills are good and vocational skills develop either due to formal or informal vocational training. While work tolerance and endurance are more robust, clients often feel overwhelmed by their workload, even if it is not extensive and find it difficult to manage their time appropriately.

In the recreational/leisure sphere, they tend to be involved in activities which are in vogue with other members of the group.

As with the previous level, psychopathology, characteristic of the condition, usually has an individualised presentation. Psychopathology may be of mild to moderate intensity, influencing social, occupational and recreational/leisure performance, but the client is not usually occupationally incapacitated.

Intervention and Therapeutic Principles for the Level

The outcomes of treatment expected are as follows:

Compliance with norms within all domains of occupation that are healthy and support well-being and are appropriate to the group and society in which they function.

The ability to look after themselves independently complying with community norms and pressures.

To be productive and be able to work effectively and efficiently and to use leisure time in a health-promoting constructive manner.

The therapeutic relationship should have more qualities of maturity than previously, being based on mutual trust and respect, with elements of both give and take. The client should be considered a partner in the treatment. The occupational therapist should handle the client firmly in terms of norm compliance while being sensitive to the anxiety this may cause. Expectations should be negotiated, be clearly stated and generalised to as many situations as possible. The client should be given recognition for imitative norm-compliant responses. If he is unable to comply, be supportive, help him to explore the reasons for failure and explore alternative behaviours that may increase the possibility of success.

Plan the programme with the client and establish the goals and norms towards which he should be working. Where practical, the client should have a full-day programme of activities within his usual context and should be given the responsibility for compliance or lack thereof. The treatment programmes should be balanced and include the following: IADL-related activities and work-related or work-simulated activities for approximately half the time; sport and recreational/leisure activities for approximately one-sixth of the time.

Group activities for the rest of the time

All treatment should emphasise the following: personal independence and effective living; mature relationships where loyalty, cohesion and conformity to group norms are reinforced but at the same time supporting individuality and assertiveness and the development of a sound support system; consolidation of pre-vocational performance skills and development of vocational skills; and stress management, problem-solving, conflict resolution, value clarification and other coping skills.

The therapeutic value of all activities to health and well-being should be carefully explained.

The client should use all types of instructions from resource material, although technical skills may need to be demonstrated. Instructions should emphasise the purpose for undertaking the activity and the sustainability of the activity/occupation in the context of the client's life. Instructions should outline the technique and method to be used and give tips for success and clearly indicate the norms against which performance will be judged. A completed, high-quality end product can be used to rate or compare performance. All activities must facilitate norm compliance.

As the client moves from the therapist-directed phase, the demands of the activities should be graded: increasing the number of steps, the elements of fallibility, the complexity of the method and decreasing the completion time; elements of abstract thinking, decision-making and problem-solving can also be introduced when the client-directed phase has been achieved; upgrade the demands for norm compliance in all required occupational domains; decrease the structure and support and increase demands for independent personal management and lifestyle within the contextual opportunities and constraints;

increase the demands for productive and vocational ability; increase demands for constructive and healthy use of leisure time; increase demands for effective use of coping skills in the face of environmental demands.

The following are the indications that the client is ready to move to the next level: should be able to structure and execute familiar activities consistently meeting the norms set efficiently; should be prepared to meet the challenge of unfamiliar situations despite some anxiety; should become aware of shortcomings within the current method of an activity or behaviour and have an interest in exploring possibilities for improvement or change.

GROUP 3

The levels in this group are least well described in the VdTMo-CA (see Table 2.6). This does not mean that individuals on the levels within the group are immune to mental health conditions, but they require occupational therapy assistance less frequently and only in targeted areas of activity participation. There may be some regression in their occupational performance from their premorbid state; these individuals are seldom occupationally dysfunctional. For this reason, the levels falling in the group will not be described in this chapter. Information on these levels is to be found in du Toit (2009).

CONCLUSION

The purpose of this chapter is to provide introductory information about the VdTMoCA and its application to clients with mental health conditions. It is intended for students and novice occupational therapists working in a variety of mental health care settings. Research and development into VdTMo-CA and its application to various health conditions is ongoing in a number of countries but predominantly in South Africa. There has been some refinement and further deliberations about core concepts in VdTMoCA, so there is greater clarity

Table 2.6   Group 3 Levels of action and motivation.

Volition	Levels of motivation	Levels of action	Group
Transcending the self within the personal and productivity context	Active participation	Original	Group 3
Self-actualisation transcending the self	Competitive participation	Situation centred	
Commitment to developing and managing systems or organisations for the benefit of others	Contribution	Competitive centred	
Realisation of altruistic convictions to the benefit of society	Competitive contribution	Society centred	

and understanding. A strong team of experienced and dedicated occupational therapists in South Africa and the United Kingdom have joined forces to develop this exciting theory further. The material in this chapter offers a useful set of guidelines for occupational therapists working in various areas of occupational therapy. It is of particular value in the mental health field of occupational therapy, where the VdT-MoCA is widely used and many occupational therapists in this field have contributed to its development over the years.

QUESTIONS

1. Define the following in your own words and the relationship between these concepts: creative capacity, creative response, creative participation and creative act.

2. Define in your own words the concept of 'creative ability'.

3. Define in your own words the term 'maximal creative effort' and state its relationship to creative ability.

4. Define the terms therapist-directed phase, client-directed phase and transitional phase. Discuss the value of these terms for the levels of motivation and action.

5. Make a table indicating the relationship between the levels of motivation and action.

6. Describe the steps in the assessment of creative ability.

7. Make a table indicating the similarities and differences in occupational performance between each of the levels of action.

8. Make a table indicating the similarities and differences in the principles required for handling, structuring the treatment situation, presentation and teaching of the activity, activity requirements and grading of treatment that would be used in the first four levels of action.

REFERENCES

American Occupational Therapy Association (2020) Occupational therapy practice framework: domain and process (4th ed.). *The American Journal of Occupational Therapy*, **74**(2), 1–87. https://doi.org/10.5014/ajot.2020.74S2001

American Psychiatric Association (2022) *Diagnostic and Statistical Manual of Mental Disorders VTR*, 5th edn. American Psychiatric Publishers Inc. https://doi.org/10.4135/9781412964500.n104

Casteleijn, D. (2010) *Development of an outcome measure for occupational therapists in mental health care practice.* Master thesis, University of Pretoria.http://upetd.up.ac.za/thesis/available/etd-02102011-1433032/ (23 August 2023)

Casteleijn, D. (2013) Stepping stones from input to outcome: an occupational perspective 22nd Vona du Toit lecture. *South African Journal of Occupational Therapy*, **43**(1), 1–9.

van der Reyden Casteleijn, D., Sherwood, W., *et al* (2019) The Vona du Toit Model of Creative Ability: origins, constructs and applications in occupational therapy. Vona du toit foundation, Pretoria, 1–325 (chapter 4106-147).

Christie, A. (1999) A meaningful occupation: the just right challenge. *Australian Journal of Occupational Therapy*, **46**(2), 52–68.

Coleman, J. (1960) *Psychology and Effective Behaviour.* D B Taraporevata Sons and Co.

du Toit, V. (1980) *Volition and Action in Occupational Therapy.* Vona and Marie du Toit Foundation, Pretoria.

du Toit, V. (1991) Creative ability, *Patient Volition and Action in Occupational Therapy*, 2nd edn. Vona and Marie du Toit Foundation, Hilbrow.

du Toit, V. (2009) *Patient Volition and Action in Occupational Therapy*, 4th edn. Vona and Marie du Toit Foundation, Pretoria.

de Witt, P.A. (2002) The occupation in occupational therapy: 19th Vona du Toit Memeorial Lecture. *South African Journal of Occupational Therapy*, **32**(3), 2–7.

de Witt, P.A. (2003) Investigation into the criteria and behaviour used to assess task concept. *South African Journal of Occupational Therapy*, **33**(1), 4–7.

de Witt, P.A. (2014) Creative ability: a model for individual and group occupational therapy for client with psychosocial dusfunction. In: R. Crouch & V. Alers (eds), *Occupational Therapy in Psychiatry and Mental Health*, 5th edn, pp. 3–32. 495. Wiley, Chichester.

Global Burden of Disease 2019 Mental Health Collaborators (2022) Global, regional, and national burden of 12 mental disorders in 204 countries and territories, 1990–2019: a systematic analysis for the Global Burden of Disease Study 2019. *The Lancet Psychiatry*, **9**(2), 137–150. https://doi.org/10.1016/S2215-0366(21)00395-3

Hansson, S.O., Björklund Carlstedt, A. & Morville, A.-L. (2022) Occupational identity in occupational therapy: a concept analysis. *Scandinavian Journal of Occupational Therapy*, **29**(3), 198–209. https://doi.org/10.1080/11038128.2021.1948608

Hussey, S.M., Sabonis-Chafee, B. & O'Brien, J.C. (2007), *Introduction to Occupational Therapy*. Elsevier Health Sciences TW, 301 pages.

Joubert, R.W.E. (2019) Theoretical paradigms and influences underpinning the development of the Vona du Toit model of creative ability. In: D. van der Reyden *et al* (eds), *The Vona du Toit Model of Creative Ability: Origins, Principles and Application in Occupational Therapy*, 1st edn, pp. 46–56. Vona and Marie du Toit Foundation, Pretoria.

Kielhofner, G. (2002) Motives, patterns and performance in occupations: basic concepts. In: G. Kielhofner (ed), *Model of Human Occupation: Theory and Application*, 3rd edn, pp. 11–27. Lippincott Williams & Wilkins, Philadelphia.

Kramer, P. (2022) Illuminating the dark side of occupation: International perspectives from occupational therapy and occupational science. *Occupational Therapy in Mental Health*, **38**(2), 211–213. https://doi.org/10.1080/0164212x.2022.2061671

Krupa, T., Kirsh, B., & Pitts, D. *et al* (2016) *Bruce and Borg's Psychosocial Frames of Reference: Theories, Models and Approaches for Occupation Based Practice*, 4th edn. Slack, Thorofare.

Reed, K. & Sanderson, S. (1999) *Concepts of Occupational Therapy*, 4th edn. Lippincott Williams & Wilkins, Philadelphia.

Ryan, R.M. & Deci, E.L. (2020) Intrinsic and extrinsic motivation from a self-determination theory perspective: definitions, theory, practices, and future directions. *Contemporary Educational Psychology*, **61**, 101086. https://doi.org/10.1016/j.cedpsych.2020.101860

Sherwood, W. (2016) *An investigation into the theoretical construction of effort and maximal effort as a contribution to the theory of creative ability*. Doctoral thesis. University of the Witwatersrand.

Sherwood, W. & Wilson, S. (2019) International perspectives: an illustration of the VdTMoCA beyond South Africa. In: D. van der Reyden *et al.* (eds), *The Vona du Toit Model of Creative Ability: Origins, Principles and Application in Occupational Therapy*, 1st edn, pp. 248–264. Vona and Marie du Toit Foundation, Pretoria.

Taylor, R. (2017) *Kielhofner's Model of Human Occupation: Theory and Application*, 5th edn. Wolters Kluwer, Philadelphia.

Turpin, M. & Iwama, M. (2011) Introduction. In: *Using Occupational Therapy Models in Practice: A Field Guide*, pp. 1–12. Churchill Livingston Elsevier, Edinburgh.

Twinley, R. (2013) The dark side of occupation: a concept for consideration. *Australian Occupational Therapy Journal*, **60**(4), 301–303. https://doi.org/10.1111/1440-1630.12026

Unruh, A. (2004) Reflections on: so . . . What do you do? Occupation and the constructing of identity. *Canadian Journal of Occupational therapy*, **71**(5), 290–295. https://doi.org/10.1177/000841740407100500

van der Reyden, D. & Sherwood, W. (2019) The Vona du Toit model of creative ability core constructs and concepts. In: D. van der Reyden *et al.* (eds), *Vona du Toit Model of Creative Ability: Origins, Constructs, Principles and Application in Occupational Therapy*, 1st edn, pp. 59–105. 325. Vona and Marie du Toit Foundation, Pretoria.

Watson, L. & Coetzee, Z. (2019) Back ground and origins of Vona du Toit model of creative ability 1962–1974. In: D. van der Reyden *et al.* (eds), *The Vona du Toit Model of Creative Ability: Origins, Principles and Application in Occupational Therapy*, 1st edn, pp. 26–43. Marie and Vona du Toit Foundation, Pretoria.

WHO (2013) *How to Use the ICF: A Practical Manual for the International Classification of Function, Disability and Health ICF*. WHO Press, Geneva.

WHO (2022) *International Statistical Classification of Diseases and Related Health Problems 11*. WHO Press, Geneva.

Wu, C. (2001) Facilitating intrinsic motivation in individuals with psychiatric illnesses: a study on the effectiveness of occupational therapy. *Occupational Therapy Journal of Research*, **21**(3), 142–167.

The Relevance of Occupational Science to Occupational Therapy in the Field of Mental Health

CHAPTER 3

Lana van Niekerk

Division Occupational Therapy, Stellenbosch University, Tygerberg, South Africa

KEY LEARNING POINTS

- Developments in occupational science and benefits for occupational therapy mental health practice.

- Broadening of occupational therapy practice to address occupational needs of mental health service users.

- Occupational science perspectives in addressing social determinants of mental health.

- Potential of occupational science to facilitate inter-professional research and practice development.

- Exploration of occupation as a unifying lens for inter-professional and cross-disciplinary approaches to address the occupational needs of individuals, groups and populations.

INTRODUCTION

The relationship between occupational science and occupational therapy, once much debated, has revealed itself as mutually beneficial and enriching. Benefits of occupational science include an impetus for occupation-based practice, provision of an inter-professional interface platform and press for practice development across service sectors and system levels. Arguably, the most important outcome has been an increased focus on the development of occupation-based practice, an approach that resonates strongly with a focus on social determinants of health. For mental health practice, the relevance of occupational science in recovery and community integration also requires consideration. This chapter will discuss how occupational science provides the language required to foreground occupation *as an end* in real-world contexts and thus stimulate the broadening of occupational therapy practice beyond traditional institution-based programmes. As such, occupational science provides the conceptual underpinning for prevention and promotion programmes that address social determinants of mental health.

Sharon[1] was a research participant in an interpretive biography study undertaken to explore the influences impacting the work-lives of persons with psychiatric disability (Van Niekerk 2009). The biography included below was developed as part of the narrative analysis that was conducted; it captures Sharon's remarkable awareness of the impact that participation in work had on her recovery and reintegration into society.

Excerpt from Sharon's biography:

> When I first met her, Sharon struck me as a little socially awkward; she started to speak rapidly - covering the twelve years from her first experience of schizophrenia (as a first-year student at university studying English literature); she focussed on key events - getting

[1]Sharon is not her real name. A pseudonym is being used for confidentiality.

Crouch and Alers Occupational Therapy in Psychiatry and Mental Health, Sixth Edition.
Edited by Rosemary Crouch, Tania Buys, Enos Morankoana Ramano, Matty van Niekerk and Lisa Wegner.
© 2025 John Wiley & Sons Ltd. Published 2025 by John Wiley & Sons Ltd.

married, becoming a mother, having her daughter placed in foster care and many failed attempts to obtain work. She painted a picture of personal disorganisation, reduced ability and lost dreams. This picture changed after she accessed a community-based mental health programme and was referred for occupational therapy. Sharon commenced supported employment and was placed as an administrative assistant in a public library.

Sharon highlighted the need to earn money as a strong driver in her seeking work: '. . . *we really desperately needed the money, so I was forced to stand up as I say, from the dead, and go back to work, you know?'*

She had good insight into the work requirements with which she would be able to cope: '*I said I would like to sit down, I would like to be out of the mainstream and please, I don't want to speak on the telephone, or handle money, because I still have a problem counting, I can't count very well. And I don't mind talking to people but I don't want a desk job'.*

As time progressed, Sharon consciously improved her competencies at work by setting clear goals that were aligned with the development of new skills. She engaged in constant appraisal of her own performance and knew when to ask for help. She reflected on her work tasks, weighing the demands against her own performance enablers and deficits in order to optimise her performance:

. . . I do funnily enough have problems reading, which it is how wonderful it is that I can do this job. I can read essays, magazines, letters, computer briefs, but in the last eight years, I've only read about two books. I find also I can't watch television very easily. So, it's like minutia . . . focussing in on something small. . . . I can work with excerpts or cuttings . . . small subject matter, and this I can manage easily, but I cannot read whole books anymore.

Sharon also started to draw explicitly on skills, competencies and experience obtained at work to improve the way she managed challenges at home:

So, I'm trying actually to re-structure my life. As my mind is becoming restructured through routine and discipline at work, everything has to be filed consecutively and numerically, so it's a very good exercise for the mind.

I have to work twice as hard at it. . . . establishing relationships or preparing a meal, you know, I work at it.

I read recipe books for five years when I wasn't working, to teach myself how to cook. It's actually a lot more complex. . . . what appears to come . . . naturally, I have to reasonably work out, which I do with a recipe. If I make chicken Kiev, which is a very complicated thing, I've got to simplify it to a few steps. So that it won't be as exotic as it was, but . . . the only way I can explain it is, cut down the recipe to three or four ingredients and . . . make it into a practical experience, instead of an art experience. In fact, that is how I learn to cope in most situations. . . . You know, you've got to think before you act.

Sharon equated the transformation she underwent because of the opportunity to work as '*returning from the dead . . . step by step'.* Her story will be used throughout the chapter to elucidate the potential contribution of occupational science in shaping services for mental health users.

THE CHARACTER OF OCCUPATIONAL SCIENCE AND IMPLICATIONS FOR OCCUPATIONAL THERAPY PRACTICE

> Occupational science is a basic science devoted to the study of the human as an occupational being. As a basic science, it is free to pursue the widest and deepest questions concerning human beings as actors who adapt to the challenges of their environments via the use of skill and capacities organised or categorised as occupation. (Yerxa, 1993, p. 5)

By putting forward the working definition above, Yerxa (1993) emphasised the character of occupational science as a basic science that cannot be 'constrained in its development by preconceptions of how its knowledge will be applied in occupational therapy clinical practice' (p. 5). Yerxa (1993) identified the following assumptions:

- Skill is an essential capacity of human beings and is a vital component of occupation.

- People's experience of engagement in occupations influences both their satisfaction with performance and intrinsic motivation.

- Occupation is engaged in by whole human beings that may not be reduced to cells or organ systems (holism).

- The occupational human is a complex living system that interacts with multiple environments.

- Occupational science represents an important focus of study and, as such, a legitimate scholarly resource.

Each of the occupational science assumptions highlighted above has the potential to shape occupational therapy practice in meaningful ways. The first two are firmly embedded in occupational therapy mental health practice, evidenced by the centrality of these assumptions as a focus for occupational therapy interventions and in the conceptual frameworks that inform occupation therapy reasoning. Increased recognition of the health-enhancing characteristics of occupation confirms a continued focus on mastery of essential skills through participation in a range of occupations in mental health practice (Silaule & Casteleijn 2021; Sammells *et al.* 2023). The third assumption holds an imperative for holistic occupational engagement in real-world contexts, thus avoiding potential tendencies to underestimate the capacity of persons with mental illness to participate meaningfully. The fourth assumption legitimises occupational therapy practice outside traditional health sectors and calls for interventions that support occupational engagement in real-world contexts. The last assumption reinforces evidence-based practice and practice-based evidence. This chapter will focus on the role of occupational science in shaping occupational therapy practice in line with assumptions three to five.

FOREGROUNDING ENVIRONMENT

Because occupations are more than an abstraction of the mind, occupations occur in real-life contexts grounded in real time and real places, using real equipment, materials, and supplies with real people. Furthermore, occupations occur in a context of invisible occupational determinants and forms that determine possibilities and limits for occupational participation. (Townsend & Wilcock 2004, p. 256)

Occupational scientists concern themselves with studying the impact of the environment, within which occupation occurs, on the occupational behaviour of people and populations. Thus, insight is gained into the impact of macro influences, for example the effect of poverty, on the occupational behaviour of people. Occupational risk factors, such as occupational alienation, deprivation, marginalisation and imbalance, are a result of negative environmental impacts on occupational opportunities (Townsend & Wilcock 2004). Social and economic factors, such as poverty, human rights, high unemployment, food insecurity and access to quality education at societal and community levels have a fundamental effect on participation in occupations. Importantly, stigma and discrimination associated with mental health conditions amplify the risk of marginalisation or exclusion because these often involve questioning the abilities or competence of persons with mental illness (Van Niekerk 2010). Persons with mental illness continue to more readily face exclusion from work, school and social activities (Henderson & Gronholm 2018; Patel *et al.* 2018).

The occupational therapy profession has done well to develop techniques with which to address performance deficits associated with mental illness in rehabilitation, for example life skills training, development of coping strategies and supported employment. In their review of the complexity of science in occupational therapy and occupational science, Fogelberg and Frauwirth (2010) placed the bulk of published research at the individual level. The need to shift focus towards higher levels foregrounded the argument that 'like individuals, collective entities such as groups, communities and populations also engage in occupational behaviours, and that occupation produced at each of these levels represents a legitimate unit of analysis for occupational science' (Fogelberg & Frauwirth 2010, p. 136). Since the review, valuable contributions have paved the way for decolonial perspectives (Hammell 2011) conceptualisation of collectivist occupation (Ramugondo & Kronenberg 2015; Lee 2019; Adams & Casteleijn 2023), examples showing macro-analyses of occupational patterns at a societal level (O'Halloran *et al.* 2018) and guidance on how to apply occupation in public health environments (Duncan *et al.* 2021). The priority in terms of further development for mental health is to explore and address social determinants of mental health in keeping with the direction provided by Duncan *et al.* (2021).

AN OCCUPATIONAL JUSTICE PERSPECTIVE

We need to establish ourselves as advisers at all levels of society to increase awareness and understanding. (Wilcock 2001, p. 416)

With the introduction of occupational science, occupational therapists' concern is broadened to include analysis of the impact of positive and negative environmental influences on the occupational opportunities and behaviour of so-called healthy persons and groups, but who are exposed to factors that predispose them to ill-health; referred to as upstream social determinant factors in public health (Naik *et al.* 2019). Promotive and preventive programmes, based on occupational science foundations, inform advocacy for occupational engagement in the form of advocacy work. Scrutiny of policies that affect occupational engagement of persons throughout the life span is required to identify potential pitfalls for occupational risk and opportunities for occupational enrichment. Inclusion of persons with mental illness has been a policy directive for social justice; however, occupational science also makes it an occupational justice imperative.

Occupational science is not limited by a focus on illness and health; instead, it encompasses a study of occupation in its broadest sense. Occupational justice provides a lens with which to recognise and address occupational risk factors that usually prevail when prejudice and/or stigma is experienced, something persons with mental illness have been shown to confront in contexts of community living as well as residential facilities (Kearns Murphy & Shiel 2019).

Occupational science theory has shown rapid development – with more recent thinking emphasising the centrality of environment, social and moral factors on the occupations of individuals, groups and communities (Venkatapuram 2023). Occupational justice gives prominence to economic, political and social forces in that these create, or restrict, opportunity and the means to choose, organise and perform occupations that people find useful or meaningful. Townsend (1999, p. 154) situated occupational justice as 'economic, political and social forces which create equitable opportunity and means to choose, organise and perform occupations that people find useful or meaningful in their environment'.

Occupational justice, as a domain of concern for occupational therapists, is of particular relevance in lower- and middle-income countries. This is because macro-environmental influences such as poverty, high unemployment, educational inadequacies and food insecurity add to the vulnerability of persons with mental illness. In addition, stigma and discrimination experienced by persons with mental illness are major contributors to occupational injustice and have been described a 'wicked problem' (Henderson & Gronholm 2018, p. 1) with multi-layered effects on community living and key occupational domains, including employment and education. The tendency to internalise stigma further exacerbates the problem (Alemu *et al.* 2023). The realisation of human rights for persons with mental illness continues to be a problem in all countries, particularly in low-income and middle-income countries (Patel *et al.* 2018).

A focus on occupational justice will guide the profession in its positioning to better address current and anticipated occupation-related macro influences that impact occupational opportunities, thus providing direction on how to address the negative impact of restrictive environments, which deny opportunities for equal participation in work, leisure, learning social interaction and play. Interventions that are suitable for addressing occupational risk factors usually occur in real-world contexts, outside the traditional health domain and should continue to benefit from developments in occupational science.

Sharon's biography illustrates many positive spin-offs that came from being able to work in a real-world setting. She captured the transformative experience of participation in work in her own words:

> 'You know, even my physical appearance has changed. I now have money to buy suitable clothing, and for my husband and my daughter. So . . . this has helped so much in my life, being a useful, productive member of society. But now, like I'm getting into routine, because I can see . . . I don't . . . when I was ill, I'd lie in bed all day, [small pause] and just cry and scream, and drink 16 cups of tea, and you know, I was a basket case'.

Sharon extrapolated lessons from her experiences at work to apply at home. A natural shift from participation in work to integration in other aspects of society is evident in Sharon's narrative. She seamlessly drew lessons from work to apply to other contexts. A similar tendency to draw explicit links between participation in occupation and ability was evident in the narratives of other participants in the same research (Van Niekerk 2009) and service users shown to recognise the wellness-enhancing impacts of work in their lives (Black *et al.* 2019). It should however be noted that Sharon's attempts to work were unsuccessful until she joined a supported employment programme. Persons with disability often require support in finding and maintaining work because of the marginalisation experienced.

INTEGRATION AND PARTICIPATION OF PEOPLE WITH DISABILITIES IN SOCIETY

Persons who experience disability as a result of psychiatric or intellectual impairments confront many barriers when they attempt to participate in a world that is constructed by, and for, people without disabilities. In such a world, those with disabilities are often assumed to be 'second-class' citizens, that is less worthy and/or less competent, without seeking evidence for such assumptions. This is particularly true for persons with psychiatric disability because of the fear and stigma that are often associated with psychiatric impairments. Barriers confronted by persons with psychiatric impairment are therefore not limited to the restrictions imposed by a particular impairment but are multiplied as a result of society's inability to ensure integration and accommodation of those with special needs. While some attention is being given to the removal of obvious environmental barriers, usually those that limit the participation of people with physical disabilities, not enough is done to confront attitudinal barriers that prevent the participation of people with psychiatric disability. To assist people with psychiatric disability in achieving integration and participation, occupational therapy practice will have to be better situated to address occupational needs across those public service sectors that influence these. Occupational therapy practice continues to flourish in the traditional health sector, where service delivery is focused on alleviation of symptoms. Considering the centrality of a systems approach in occupational science, research and service could be guided to better understand and remove the barriers that hinder occupational behaviour at all system levels within society. Society, with the systems that operate within it, should be scrutinised to ensure the removal of barriers and to find strategies that will foster the participation of persons with disability within real-world occupational contexts, in accordance with their own needs.

Strategic drivers for occupational therapy practice with mental health service users in real-world settings build on human rights, equity and justice imperatives that call for meaningful and equitable participation of persons with disability. Such drivers take shape in policies that can be used by occupational therapists to optimise their services. Working alongside mental health service users in a quest to achieve optimum participation in real-world contexts necessitates good knowledge of policy and legislative environments (Van Niekerk *et al.* 2020).

Both the necessity for and the complexity of achieving participation of persons with mental illness in real-world occupations are heightened by the level of disorganisation in occupational environments. Such disorganisation can be the result of systemic poverty, short- or long-term human rights violations, civil unrest, climate crises, pandemics or the consequences of war. However, even in environments with progressive policies (with good implementation) and relative stability, occupational therapists require good knowledge of relevant policies and legislation that serve as drivers that can promote or hinder the participation of persons with mental illness in real-world contexts. Occupational science provides the conceptual foundation to guide occupational therapy practice in real-world settings.

SERVICES IN REAL-WORLD ENVIRONMENTS

> As occupational science expands, new insights concerning the nature of occupation and the manner in which it enriches people's lives are expected to emerge; such insights will spur the development of improved therapeutic techniques and thereby generate important yields both to the profession and to the clients whom it serves. (Clark *et al.* 1993, p. 184)

Yerxa (1993, p. 4) observed that 'the profession may not be fully achieving its rich potential in making a difference in people's lives', stating the reason for this dilemma being that many occupational therapists still 'practice in hospitals and clinics in which the traditional medical view of illness and disability predominates' (Yerxa 1993, p. 4). With the medical model's priority concern being the alleviation of symptoms, it fosters a singular focus that does not include the occupational engagement of people within their real-world contexts.

The most exciting and important application of occupational science in mental health practice is the conceptualisation of real-world occupations. For the purpose of this argument, the term 'real-world occupations' are those that are performed in naturalistic contexts and that currently form part of the occupational repertoire of service users or are envisaged to become a part of their occupational repertoire. Occupational repertoire is used here to refer to occupations a person would generally perform when not undergoing treatment or rehabilitation. Conversely, constructed occupations, often occupation as a means, are more readily used to meet particular therapeutic outcomes within occupational therapy practice settings, including hospitals, residential facilities and rehabilitation centres. As such, real-world occupations are differentiated from constructed occupations that are generally used within health or rehabilitation contexts as part of an intervention. Examples include participation in competitive work, socialising with friends, participating in sport and shopping. When occupations used as part of an intervention end up in the occupational repertoire of a service user, the obvious advantage will be that of achieving a continued effect. When real-world occupations are introduced, or re-introduced, by occupational therapists during intervention, support might be required during the occupational transitions expected to ensue during the incorporation of such occupations into the occupational repertoires of service users.

Real-world occupations should increasingly be the focus of occupational therapists because such developments will inform and guide occupation-based practice that has direct follow-through for users of occupational therapy services. Interventions designed to enhance the goodness of fit between occupational environments, opportunities for participation and the abilities of people with mental illness hold obvious advantages. One example is the placement of persons with psychiatric disability in work, usually through supported employment, which constitutes a 'place and train' approach. As such, the potential pitfall of 'train and place' approaches, which tend to remain focused on identified performance deficits without follow-through into real-world occupations, is avoided. Importantly, a focus on real-world occupation, as opposed to simulated occupation in therapeutic contexts, will also lead the development of occupational therapy and occupational science in ways that will meet policy imperatives. Such a focus will direct occupational therapy to meet the real needs of the people they work with and harness benefits from the interrelatedness of participation in occupation and the achievement of health and wellness.

INTERFACING RELEVANT THEORIES TO INFORM INTERPROFESSIONAL PRACTICE

The way I see it, occupational scientists study people's occupational natures across a broad spectrum of concern, that is, they explore any other perspective, philosophy or idea from the point of view of the human need for occupation. So, for example, they reconsider, research and advise on politics, spirituality, education, social structures, science and technology, the media, work, growth, development and creativity, and health from an occupational perspective. If they are thorough, that will encompass reductionist as well as holistic perspectives and exploratory methods. (Wilcock 2001, p. 416)

Occupational science provides a lens through which scientists from varied backgrounds can look at occupation. Occupational science can thus serve as an interface theory for practitioners from varied professional and disciplinary backgrounds. As such, it offers a unifying occupational lens, one that will focus attention and efforts on achieving occupational outcomes for occupational therapy service users.

Fogelberg and Frauwirth (2010) confirm occupational science as interface theory by stating, 'just as occupation-based frames of reference provide a shared world-view for occupational therapists across multiple practice arenas, so can the framework provide a shared world-view for researchers, both within the discipline and across disciplines' (Fogelberg & Frauwirth 2010, p. 137). Zemke (1996) defended concerns that occupational science overlaps with other sciences by sharing a view that it is the unique subject matter with an emphasis on the occupation that sets it apart. Wilcock (2001, p. 416) agreed, suggesting that 'we need to establish ourselves as advisors at all levels of society to increase awareness and understanding'. She adds, 'for the discipline to grow and develop most effectively and quickly, it would be best for it to be studied internationally across many disciplines' (Wilcock 2001, p. 416). It is the focus on occupation that makes occupational science distinct, rather than the use of particular research methodologies or the delineation of particular domains of concern. The flexibility of approaches used to generate knowledge situates it to allow an easy interface between different theories and disciplines. This is different from other social sciences that historically 'establish their distinctiveness not by their formal description but by their emphases and traditions' (Zemke 1996, p. ix). What this means is that occupational scientists could draw on a range of theories and disciplines to inform their study that focuses on better understanding the occupational behaviour of people within the mental health field. Furthermore, research and practice dilemmas in mental health tend to be complex, as such a combination of quantitative and qualitative research paradigms and the cooperation of varied diverse disciplines would provide the best answers.

SOCIAL DETERMINANTS OF MENTAL HEALTH

Yerxa (1993, p. 3) was discussing the dilemmas of occupational therapy practice when she identified 'a major question confronting societies', namely 'what is the relationship between human engagement in a daily round of activity (such as work, play, rest and sleep) and the quality-of-life people experience including their healthfulness?' This question would suggest occupational therapists' concern with the goal of restoring the occupational engagement of people who lost their ability to do, due to the experience of impairment or disability. It also implies a concern for people who have reduced opportunity to participate in occupation due to macro contextual influences such as high unemployment, limited access to education, discrimination (including gender restrictions), inequality and deprivation (including issues associated with living in poverty).

The World Health Organisation conceptualised social determinants of health as the conditions in which people are born, grow, live, work and age (Commission on Social Determinants of Health 2008). The identification of these determinants brought recognition of the bidirectional influence between social factors and health and led to a broadening of focus for health professionals. Mounting research evidence confirms the impact of 'upstream factors' on poor mental health outcomes for certain segments of populations exposed to factors such as, for example income inequality, adverse early life experiences, food insecurity and experiences of racism (Shim & Compton 2018). The Lancet Commission on global mental health and sustainable development call for 'broader conceptualisation of mental health and disorder and to position this agenda as an integral element of the SDGs' (Patel et al. 2018, p. 1561). Lovell and Bibby (2018) provided a quick reference summarising social determinants of health in eight domains, namely family as well as friends and community, good work, money and resources, education and skills, housing, transport, our surroundings and food we eat. Their quick guide was further developed by Giljam-Enright et al. (2020) into a checklist included below.

The dimensions included in Table 3.1 demonstrate the potential for a focus on occupation within public health in real-world contexts. By positioning occupations as determinants of health, their health-enhancing qualities are recognised, for example *work with good wages*. The spin-off effects between various occupations are recognised, for *example education and skill development to find good work*. Contexts within which occupations are performed are highlighted throughout, for example *vibrant spaces which are accessible*, thus recognising occupational environments as much more than placeholders for occupation; in fact, the environments within which occupations are performed contribute directly and significantly to the health and wellness related consequences of such participation. Occupations that foster social interaction and involve caring for self and the environment feature strongly with direct connections to wellness. Duncan *et al.*

Table 3.1 Social determinants of health framework (Giljam-Enright *et al.* 2020), derived from the health foundation's quick guide on what makes us healthy: an introduction to social determinants of health (Lovell & Bibby 2018).

Family, friends and community	Positive family life	0/1
	Supportive relationships	0/1
	Feeling part of a community	0/1
	Taking part in community life	0/1
Money and resources	Enough money to access support and services needed for participation in society	0/1
	Enough money to access support and services needed for participation in health	0/1
	A monetary safety net is available to reduce stress	0/1
	Investment for the future	0/1
Housing	Homes that are affordable	0/1
	Homes that are warm and stable	0/1
	Homes offering safety and space within which to develop	0/1
	Homes with running water, electricity and sanitation	0/1
Education and skills	Education and skill development to access opportunities for the maintenance of healthy habits	0/1
	Education and skill development to find good work	0/1
	Education and skill development to afford to live and work in a safe environment	0/1
	Education and skill development to feel empowered and valued	0/1
Good work	Work comprises regular work	0/1
	Work with good wages	0/1
	Work in a safe environment with good working conditions	0/1
	Work which matches competence and interest	0/1
Transport	Safe and well-designed transport system available	0/1
	Transport system that is accessible	0/1
	Transport system that is affordable	0/1
	Transport system that is efficient	0/1
Our surroundings	Vibrant spaces which are accessible	0/1
	Good places which allow people to feel safe and be active	0/1
	Easy access to important facilities	0/1
	Sustainability of these spaces	0/1
The food we eat:	Enough food	0/1
	Healthy food	0/1
	Food for healthy living that is easily accessible	0/1
	Food for healthy living that is affordable	0/1

Table 3.1 (*Continued*)

Productivity:	Self-care	0/1
	Domestic tasks (cleaning, cooking, laundry etc)	0/1
	Home maintenance (gardening etc)	0/1
	Caring for family	0/1

Binary categories: No = 0; Yes = 1.

(2021) provide further guidance for occupational therapy on how to upstream occupation.

The connection between creating opportunities in real-world occupations for persons with disability, as a strategy to alleviate occupational injustice, is an easily recognised across professions, especially in the field of rehabilitation. Service users themselves tend to recognise the spin-offs of participation and inclusion.

Sharon was transferring new skills and routines obtained at work to enhance her performance as homemaker and mother and used the income she earned to improve her fit into her religious community and broader society. Her story demonstrates the relative sophistication with which she reflected on the 'goodness of fit' between her competencies and the activities she was required to perform at work. She continued to appraise her performance and set goals for herself:

> But like, I still make mistakes, not at work but just generally, but maybe I don't dress properly, or my hairstyle is inappropriate, you know, I would like somehow rehabilitating myself to dress properly for work and you know, so that I don't sit there and look like, you know [small pause]. . . the village idiot in an environment that is quite up-market, because it's a very nice library, you know, it's very smart.

The inter-relatedness of identity and participation in occupation is clearly evident in Sharon's narrative that shows identity construction as a central process in managing demands and transitions brought by participation in occupation.

THE ROLE OF OCCUPATION IN IDENTITY CONSTRUCTION

Much has been written on the interrelatedness of occupation and identity. From the earliest occupational therapy models, exploration and mastery in activity have been tied to positive gains in self-esteem or improved confidence (Fidler & Fidler 1978). Maersk (2021) drew on 'an assemblage of theories positioned in psychodynamic theory, personality psychology, and narrative theory' (p. 469) in his postulation of occupation as a source of self-continuity (Maersk 2021). He provides an overview of occupational therapists' work in conceptualising identity and occupation. He emphasises the power of occupation in 'personal transformation and becoming a self' (Maersk 2021, p. 469) and concludes that 'occupation is a source of self-continuity underpinning the occupation-identity' (Maersk 2021, p. 476).

The Occupational Spin-Off Model was developed from research undertaken to provide empirical evidence to close the gap between 'the use of occupation as means and a research/knowledge base to support its continued use in mental health practice' (Rebeiro & Cook 1999, p. 177). This model illustrates the central position of accomplishments in occupational engagement in appraisal of own worth, a central component of identity construction and mental health.

Munro's conceptualisation of 'punctualized identity' (Munro 2004) provided an explanation for results of an interpretive biography ($n = 17$), which suggested that participants who were more flexible in their accommodation of the impact of impairment on self-identity seemed better able to continue participation in occupation (Van Niekerk 2016). It provides a theoretical underpinning to explain how both context and occupation can lead to revealing of identity and illustrates inter-directionality of identity, performance, occupation and context (Van Niekerk 2016). As such, the value of providing support and opportunities for participation in real world occupations is demonstrated.

CONCLUSION

The boundaries between occupational therapy and occupational science should be drawn thoughtfully and remain flexible so as to steer and support research and development. Occupational science offers freedom to occupational therapists and occupational scientists alike to study occupation; the findings obtained in such studies are available to inform the practice of occupational therapists. The generation of knowledge that explores and explains 'what people do', 'how they do it' and the 'impact of such doing on the human system and the environment' is fostered within the discipline of occupational science. Knowledge obtained should be drawn on to strengthen occupational therapy programmes that support and facilitate participation in real-world occupations.

Whilst evidence for occupation-based practice is growing, more research is required to explore the potential for, and effect of, occupation-based interventions in real-world contexts. The voices and involvement of mental health service users in research through the use of participatory methodologies are proposed. When the users of occupational therapy services recognise the link between participation in chosen occupations and the impact on health and wellness, they are better able to appraise the value of intervention for themselves. Wider dissemination of research evidence on occupation-based interventions to service users is thus proposed in order to foster partnerships with persons facing mental health issues.

Social determinants of health brought acknowledgement of the bi-directional influence of environments within which people live and their health. As such, health professions and other stakeholders who have the power to influence social determinants of health can work together in a more focussed manner. Because occupational science provides language with which to convey the prominence of occupation in meeting people's needs, it provides a unifying lens for multi-professional intervention and building of therapeutic partnerships with service users.

QUESTIONS

1. Provide reasons why occupation-based programmes in real-world contexts should be available for mental health service users.

2. Explain why occupational science can assist in addressing the social determinants of mental health.

3. Explain how occupational science could promote inter-professional collaboration in addressing the social determinants of mental health.

4. Provide a rationale for using occupational science in the development of mental health promotion programmes.

REFERENCES

Adams, F. & Casteleijn, D. (2023) Assessment of participation in collective occupations: domains and items. *South African Journal of Occupational Therapy, 53*, 86–94.

Alemu, W.G., Due, C., Muir-Cochrane, E., Mwanri, L. & Ziersch, A. (2023) Internalised stigma among people with mental illness in Africa, pooled effect estimates and subgroup analysis on each domain: systematic review and meta-analysis. *BMC Psychiatry, 23*, 480.

Black, M.H., Milbourn, B., Desjardins, K., Sylvester, V., Parrant, K. & Buchanan, A. (2019). Understanding the meaning and use of occupational engagement: findings from a scoping review. *British Journal of Occupational Therapy, 82*(5), 272–287.

Clark, F., Zemke, R., Frank, G. *et al* (1993) Dangers inherent in the partition of occupational therapy and occupational science. *The American Occupational Therapy, 47* (2), 184–186.

Commission on Social Determinants of Health (2008) *Closing the Gap in a Generation: Health Equity through Action on the Social Determinants of Health. Final Report of the Commission on Social Determinants of Health*. World Health Organization, Geneva.

Duncan, M., Sinclair, K. & Creek, J. (2021) Upstreaming occupational therapy: reflections on sustaining contextual relevance in a globalising world. *WFOT Bulletin, 77*, 85–92.

Fidler, G.S. & Fidler, J.W. (1978) Doing and becoming: purposeful action and self-actualization. *American Journal of Occupational Therapy, 32*, 305–310.

Fogelberg, D. & Frauwirth, S. (2010) A complexity science approach to occupation: moving beyond the individual. *Journal of Occupational Science, 17*, 131–139.

Giljam-Enright, M., Statham, S., Inglis-Jassiem, G. & Van Niekerk, L. (2020) The social determinants of health in rural and urban South Africa: a collective case study of Xhosa women with stroke. In: Q. Louw (ed), *Collaborative Capacity Development to Complement Stroke Rehabilitation in Africa*, pp. 307–349 [Internet]. AOSIS, Cape Town.

Hammell, K.W. (2011) Resisting theoretical imperialism in the disciplines of occupational science and occupational therapy. *British Journal of Occupational Therapy, 74*, 27–33.

Henderson, C. & Gronholm, P.C. (2018) Mental health related stigma as a 'wicked problem': the need to address stigma and consider the

consequences. *International Journal of Environmental Research and Public Health, 15*, 1158.

Kearns Murphy, C. & Shiel, A. (2019) Institutional injustices? Exploring engagement in occupations in a residential mental health facility. *Journal of Occupational Science, 26*, 115–127.

Lee, B.D. (2019) Scoping review of Asian viewpoints on everyday doing: a critical turn for critical perspectives. *Journal of Occupational Science, 26*, 484–495.

Lovell, N. & Bibby, J. (2018) *What Makes Us Healthy? An Introduction to the Social Determinants of Health*. Health Foundation, London.

Maersk, J.L. (2021) Becoming a self through occupation: occupation as a source of self-continuity in identity formation. *Journal of Occupational Science, 28*, 469–478.

Munro, R. (2004) Punctualizing identity: time and the demanding relation. *Sociology, 38*, 293–311.

Naik, Y., Baker, P., Ismail, S.A., *et al* (2019) Going upstream – an umbrella review of the macroeconomic determinants of health and health inequalities. *BMC Public Health, 19*, 1678.

O'Halloran, D., Farnworth, L., Innes, E. & Thomacos, N. (2018) An occupational perspective on three solutions to unemployment. *Journal of Occupational Science, 25*, 297–308.

Patel, V., Saxena, S., Lund, C., *et al* (2018) The Lancet Commission on global mental health and sustainable development. *The Lancet, 392*, 1553–1598.

Ramugondo, E.L. & Kronenberg, F. (2015) Explaining collective occupations from a human relations perspective: bridging the individual-collective dichotomy. *Journal of Occupational Science, 22*, 3–16.

Rebeiro, K.L. & Cook, J.V. (1999) Opportunity, not prescription: an exploratory study of the experience of occupational engagement. *Canadian Journal of Occupational Therapy, 66*, 176–187.

Sammells, E., Logan, A. & Sheppard, L. (2023) Participant outcomes and facilitator experiences following a community living skills program for adult mental health consumers. *Community Mental Health Journal, 59*, 428–438.

Shim, R.S. & Compton, M.T. (2018) Addressing the social determinants of mental health: if not now, when? If not us, who? *Psychiatric Services, 69*, 844–846.

Silaule, O. & Casteleijn, D. (2021) Measuring change in activity participation of mental health care users attending an occupational therapy programme in rural South Africa. *South African Journal of Occupational Therapy*, **51**, 63–73.

Townsend, E. (1999) Enabling occupation in the 21st century: making good intentions a reality. *Australian Occupational Therapy Journal*, **46**, 147–159.

Townsend, E. & Wilcock, A.A. (2004) Occupational justice and client-centred practice: a dialogue in progress. *Canadian Journal of Occupational Therapy*, **71**, 75–87.

Van Niekerk, L. (2009) Participation in work: a source of wellness for people with psychiatric disability. *Work: A Journal of Prevention, Assessment & Rehabilitation.*, **32**, 455–465.

Van Niekerk, L. (2010) Disability stereotypes defied by life stories. *South African Journal of Occupational Therapy*, **40**, 15–22.

Van Niekerk, L. (2016) Identity construction and participation in work: learning from the experiences of persons with psychiatric disability. *Scandinavian Journal of Occupational Therapy*, **23**, 107–114.

Van Niekerk, L., Casteleijn, D., Govindjee, A., Holness, W., Oberholster, J. & Grobler, C. (2020) Conceptualising disability: health and legal perspectives related to psychosocial disability and work. *South African Journal of Bioethics and Law*, **13**, 43–51.

Venkatapuram, S. (2023) Occupational science, values and justice. *Journal of Occupational Science*, 1–10.

Wilcock, A.A. (2001) Occupational science: the key to broadening horizons. *British Journal of Occupational Therapy*, **64**, 412–417.

Yerxa, E.J. (1993) Occupational science: a new source of power for participants in occupational therapy. *Journal of Occupational Science*, **1**, 3–9.

Zemke, R. (1996) Preface. In: R. Zemke & F. Clark (eds), *Occupational Science: The Evolving Discipline*, pp. vii–xviii. FA Davis, Philadelphia.

CHAPTER 4

Law, Human Rights and Ethics in Mental Health Care Practice

Matty van Niekerk

Department of Occupational Therapy, School of Therapeutic Sciences, Faculty of Health Sciences, University of the Witwatersrand, Johannesburg, South Africa

KEY LEARNING POINTS

- Awareness of the substance and significance of human and patient rights as fundamental to all aspects of care.

- A basic understanding of legislation and policy as relevant for this area of practice with awareness of implications for practice and conduct.

- Basic understanding of ethics and professionalism in relation to the field of mental health.

- Conceptualisation of a framework in which to situate ethics, law, mental health and mental health service provision.

- Be able to demonstrate greater awareness of selected everyday practice issues and how to deal with these in a professional, ethical and legally appropriate manner.

- Apply a step-wise approach to solving legal and ethical dilemmas.

INTRODUCTION

One of the purposes of legislative frameworks, human rights and ethics is to protect the vulnerable. The 2016 South African Life Esidimeni tragedy (see Chapter 3), resulting in the deaths of 144 chronically ill and vulnerable mental health care users (MH-CUs), is a stark reminder of the consequences of failures of legislative frameworks, human rights and ethics (Ferlito & Dhai 2017, 2018; South African Depression and Anxiety Group [SADAG] 2023). Despite a greater awareness of mental health globally, COVID-19 has underscored the multiplicity of vulnerabilities of persons with psychiatric diagnoses and mental ill-health (Hossain *et al.* 2020). Thus, occupational therapists practicing in mental healthcare and psychiatry must have sound knowledge and understanding of legislative frameworks, human rights, ethics and the interrelationships between these concepts.

In order to better equip (student) occupational therapists to navigate ethical and legal dilemmas surrounding mental health care practice, this chapter presents a conceptual framework situated in human rights, (health) legislation, morality and ethics. This framework will assist practitioners' understanding of the complex interrelationship between ethics, morality, human rights and health law, which in turn will better equip them to identify whether a dilemma is of a moral, ethical or legal nature and thus will facilitate sound decision-making.

The World Federation of Occupational Therapy (WFOT) included human rights in its Minimum Standards for the Training of Occupational Therapists (World Federation of Occupational Therapists [WFOT] 2016); however, little has been written about human rights in occupational therapy generally, and mostly in its application to occupational science concepts. For this reason, the chapter will at times take on a more generalist approach but will use examples from mental health and psychiatry.

The chapter starts by briefly discussing sources of law, laws and legislative frameworks, followed by a discussion of medical and health law, as well as professionalism (which this chapter argues is more a question of law than ethics). The chapter then turns to discussing all four generations of human rights, which is also a departure from most texts in health sciences, followed by a brief explanation of ethics and morality in the mental healthcare context. The chapter ends with an application of all of the above-mentioned concepts to a case. Because it is impossible to describe all possible pieces of legislation for all countries in a short text such as this, most of the reference sources are United Nations (UN) documents. Although not uniformly ratified, signed or assented to, UN documents provide a foundation from which to discuss what most of the world agrees to be worthy values of human rights for all, and specifically for MHCUs.

LAW

There is an ever-increasing number of laws outside of medical/ health-related law of which healthcare practitioners, and occupational therapists in particular, must be cognisant (Van Niekerk 2019). This ever-expanding pool of laws gradually codifies ethical values/principles such as confidentiality and increasingly clarifies human rights. Simultaneously, these laws make the legislative and policy context within which occupational therapists practice progressively complex. Consequently, this chapter's discussion about law, occupational therapy, and psychiatry and mental health starts with a broad general introduction to law and its sources, followed by a discussion of the legalities around the care, treatment and rehabilitation of MHCUs, human rights and professionalism.

GENERAL BACKGROUND

Sources of law

Before delving into some of the legalities specific to mental health care, a succinct overview of the sources of law is necessary, as it will further assist non-law practitioners to understand the chapter. Generally, there are five sources of law (du Plessis 1999):

Common Law Common law has been defined as the law that is communal within a specific geographical area and/or a group of people. Most Western countries have Roman law as part of their historical roots; thus to some extent, Roman law forms part of the common law of many countries. Colonised countries, such as South Africa, will have historical legal underpinnings from the colonising countries, for example, the Netherlands and England. South African common law includes principles of both Roman-Dutch law and English law, which influenced different parts of its legal system.

Statutory Law Statutory law refers to written laws that codify principles from the common law. English law is mostly uncodified common law, but as the world modernises, it becomes increasingly difficult to apply historical common law principles

without any form of modernisation or modification – one example is matrimonial (property) law. In ancient times, women could not own property, and everything belonged to the husband. This is no longer the case. Additionally, some modern societies recognise marriages or civil unions between same-sex partners, which was not the case in the 16th and 17th centuries when some of the common law principles/rules originated.

Statutory law is hierarchical in nature (Figure 4.1, which uses South African legislation as an example). In constitutional democracies where the country's constitution is the highest law, such as in South Africa, statutes, or parts thereof, can be struck down if it does not comply with the Constitution. In South Africa, with human rights incorporated into its Constitution, there is also a large body of Constitution-specific case law that has developed. Although many legal scholars consider Constitutional law a separate source of law, such a level of technicality is not necessary for a text such as this; thus, it is included in statutory law in general for our purposes.

Next in the hierarchy would be statutes, but often statutes need additional documentation to clarify how they must be enforced. This usually is in the form of promulgated Regulations, or Codes of Good Practice. Codes of Good Practice do not have the same legal standing as Regulations and Statutes, but in South African law, they must be consulted in decision-making about interpreting and applying a relevant Statute. Another explanatory document is Technical Assistance Guidelines, which has a similar standing as Codes of Good Practice.

Case Law Case law is also known as law of precedent, which means that one court is absolutely bound by the reasoning and ruling of a higher court, or of a larger court on its own level in the hierarchy, in that order, unless the decision was rendered without due consideration of a statute or a previous relevant, binding decision of another court. Case law provides important (and often interesting) interpretation and application of statutory, common and customary law, as can be seen below, for example in the discussion about the standard regarding informed consent.

Customary Law In countries with diverse cultural and religious groups, customary law often includes indigenous law. It does not have general application because it is the unwritten laws from specific cultural or religious groups. These laws are known to all members of that particular cultural or religious community, who all act in accordance with these rules.

Legal Writings In some jurisdictions, such as South Africa, the writings of historical Roman-Dutch legal scholars, such as Hugo de Groot (Grotius) (1583–1645) and Johannes Voet (1647–1713), are considered part of the sources of law, and thus worthy of citation in judgements and heads of argument. Modern legal texts, however, do not have the same *gravitas* as these Roman-Dutch scholars, although the courts may from time to time consult such modern texts.

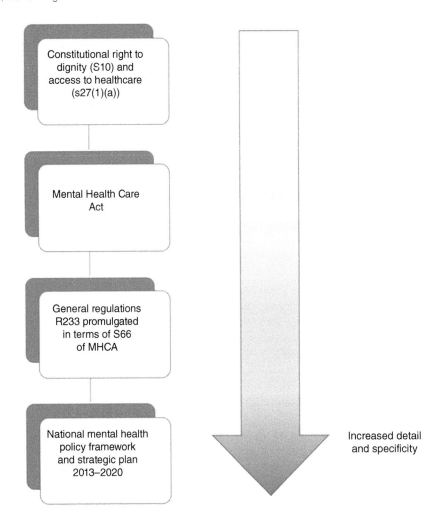

FIGURE 4.1   Hierarchical nature of statutory law.

WHAT IS RELEVANT TO OCCUPATIONAL THERAPY?

Because of the centrality of the Person-Environment-Occupation relationship to occupational therapy practice (World Federation of Occupational Therapists [WFOT] 2016), occupational therapists should at least be aware of a number of non-medical laws, such as labour laws, which affect both occupational participation and the environment(s) in which occupations occur. Expanding on Van Niekerk's (2019) argument, Table 4.1 depicts the range of legislation that potentially affects occupational therapy practice in general and in mental health specifically and its interrelationship with human rights. It is impossible to present an exhaustive list of laws in every context or country of which occupational therapists should be aware. Thus, Table 4.1 provides examples with some application to the South African context.

Knowledge of legislation in these three categories: (i) enables practitioners to comply with statutory and regulatory requirements, for example, lawful processing of personal information, (ii) enables occupational therapists to render intervention such as vocational rehabilitation that is contextually appropriate and (iii) better prepares occupational therapists to advocate for patients/clients and the profession.

For the purposes of this chapter, the focus will only be on the first column of laws, that is medical and health-related laws and policies codifying patients' (healthcare users') rights and practitioners' duties. As was the case in previous editions of this textbook, the emphasis will be on specific principles derived from the legislation, rather than on specific Acts. These principles are applicable to a greater or lesser extent in most jurisdictions, irrespective of how, or the extent to which, these are incorporated into law in various countries. This section will emphasise legalities about the care treatment and rehabilitation and legal status of MHCUs, and the regulation of healthcare practitioners.

Singh (2017) distinguishes medical law as the law that relates to doctors and their interaction with patients, as well as their interaction with other health professionals. This view differs from the more inclusive stance that the Health Professions Act and the Health Professions Council of South Africa (HPCSA) have taken post-1994; thus, the focus in this chapter

Table 4.1 Categories of legislation relevant to occupational therapy.

	Traditional/typical health professions (medical) and health-related legislation codifying, *inter alia* patients' rights and practitioners' professional duties	(General) legislation, often based on human/consumers' rights, that affects HOW we practice	(General) legislation affecting occupations and/or the environment in which occupations occur
Examples	• Laws and policies which affect the registration of healthcare practitioners • Laws and pertaining to mental healthcare users • Laws and policies pertaining to adults' and children's rights to access healthcare services including reproductive services, provide informed consent, etc.	• Where applicable, a country's constitution • Laws and policies protecting consumers • Laws and policies protecting privacy and data security • Competition laws and policies.	• Labour laws and policies • Laws and policies pertaining to accessibility of public buildings/ facilities • Laws and policies pertaining to accessible education • Disability equity
South African application*	• Constitution of South Africa (Bill of Rights in chapter 2) • Health Professions Act 56 of 1974 (as amended) • Mental Healthcare Act 17 of 2002 • National Health Act 61 of 2003 • Termination of Pregnancy Act • Aspects of the Children's Act 38 of 2005	• Consumer Protection Act • Promotion of Access to Information Act 2 of 2000 (PAIA) • Protection of Personal Information Act 4 of 2013 (POPIA) • Competition Act	Work • Employment Equity Act, • Labour Relations Act, Environment/ civic participation • Promotion of Equality and Prevention of Unfair Discrimination Act

Source: Van Niekerk M. 2024. Unpublished PhD research proposal. Used with permission.
*Only legislation referred to in the remainder of the chapter is cited in full and included in the table of legislation.

is on health professions law incorporating what Singh (2017) considers medical law, and not the narrower view juxtaposing doctors against the rest of the health professions fraternity.

Legalities About the Care Treatment and Rehabilitation of Mental Health Care Users

In 2020, the World Health Organisation (WHO) reported that 57% of their 194 member states had a standalone mental health law, and 75% of their member states had a standalone mental health policy or plan for mental health (World Health Organisation 2020). This means that it is virtually impossible to describe every potential version of mental health care legislation. Nonetheless, most of these standalone laws or policies are founded on the United Nations (UN) Principles for the Protection of Persons with Mental Illness and the Improvement of Mental Health Care (General Assembly Resolution 46/119) (United Nations 1991), which provides some common ground for a discussion about mental health law. For the purposes of this chapter, therefore, the UN Principles will be discussed in conjunction with the South African Mental Health Care Act to illustrate its potential application to law, but also how it affects healthcare provision and occupational therapy services. To facilitate consistency in terminology, the term MHCUs from the South African Mental Health Care Act will be used, rather than the word 'patient' which is used in the UN Principles.

Legal Status of Mental Health Care Users The UN Principles differentiate between voluntary and involuntary MHCUs, and it also speaks of persons who are unable to attend to their own affairs needing representation. Many mental health–related statutes also include a category of assisted MHCUs. While the UN Principles neither define involuntary MHCUs (it only defines the word patient) nor refer to assisted MHCUs, the South African Mental Health Care Act defines both. An assisted MHCU is defined as a person who is not capable of making an informed decision due to their mental health status **and** is not refusing health interventions. An involuntary MHCU is also incapable of making an informed decision due to their mental health status, is refusing health interventions, but requires such interventions/services for their own safety or the safety of others, according to the Act. Voluntary MHCUs are those who have consented to care, treatment and rehabilitation.

It is important to differentiate accurately between voluntary, assisted and involuntary MHCUs because MHCUs have the right to informed consent and informed refusal of treatment (United Nations 1991; Grobler & Van Staden 2022), and their status determines the way in which their consent or refusal is sought and regarded.

Rights of MHCUs MHCUs have the right to the best mental health care, as part of the health and social care system(s).

They have the right to be treated in the least restrictive way as far as possible, which means that the presumption should be against institutionalised care (United Nations, 1991). They also have the right to be treated within, or as close as possible to, their own communities. This last right was one of the justifications for the deinstitutionalisation and move of almost 2000 low-functioning chronic MCHUs to community-based residential facilities in the Life Esidimeni tragedy, although the community-based residential facilities did not meet the standards required by governmental Regulations mentioned in Figure 4.1, nor were they appropriately registered with either of the authorities (National Department of Health and Department of Social Development) required by South African law (Dhai 2017; Ferlito & Dhai 2017, 2018; South African Depression and Anxiety Group [SADAG] 2023).

All MHCUs, including those who lack the capacity to make decisions independently or to govern their own affairs, must be treated with dignity and respect as human beings. Lack of capacity does not mean that MHCUs should not be allowed to somehow participate in decisions about themselves or to exercise other rights due to human beings. Persons who lack capacity have the right to be represented by legal counsel in the decision about their capacity, and should a representative be appointed to manage the MHCU's personal affairs (*curator bonis*), such a representative also has the right to be consulted in decisions about the MHCU (United Nations 1991).

In terms of the UN Principles, MHCUs have the right to exercise civil, political, social, cultural and economic rights, as per UN instruments discussed below. Two important principles that speak to these rights are highlighted here, namely Principle 9, referring to MHCUs' right to freedom of movement, and Principle 11: Informed consent.

Because they have the right to freedom of movement, *where* MHCUs are treated must be carefully considered, having regard for their own health needs, as well as the need to protect their own and others' physical safety (United Nations 1991, para. 9(1)). Thus, MCHUs should preferably be treated in the least restrictive environment and with the least restrictive or intrusive treatment approaches, unless institutionalised care is necessary. All MHCUs have the right to informed consent or informed refusal, except if they do not have the capacity to make informed decisions. Read together, these two principles mean that only when an MHCU is unreasonably withholding consent that jeopardises their own or others' safety may they be held as an involuntary patient. Treatment must always be in their best interests (United Nations 1991, para. 11(6)(b)).

Table 4.2 explains the important principles and rights related to care, treatment and rehabilitation (hereafter intervention) in relation to MHCUs' legal status. For comprehensiveness' sake, children are included, but only insofar as their consent pertains to treatment, care and rehabilitation. Legislation such as the South African Children's Act has specific

Table 4.2 MHCUs' status and rights.

Rights and principles	Voluntary	Assisted	Involuntary	Children
Right for the decision regarding capacity to be reviewed	n/a	Decisions regarding capacity and the need for a personal representative shall be reviewed at reasonable intervals prescribed by domestic law. The person whose capacity is at issue, his or her personal representative, if any, and any other interested person shall have the right to appeal to a higher court against any such decision.		n/a
Informed consent (which inherently entails a right to refuse intervention)	• MHCU themselves give consent. • Information must be provided in an understandable way, preferably, but not necessarily, their home language. • MHCUs' *refusal* of intervention must be respected, even if it differs from the opinion of the healthcare practitioner.	• The MHCU has not refused intervention. Their consent must be respected because they lack capacity but still need intervention for their own or others' protection. • If they have a representative (e.g. *curator bonis*), the representative must be consulted in decisions about the MHCU.	• Disregard a refusal if any delay in intervention will result in irreversible harm or death of the MHCU, or the MHCU is likely to inflict serious harm on themselves or others, or the MHCU will cause serious damage or loss of property belonging to them or others, *because of a mental illness.* • If an independent institution-based review board or a court of law determines that the MHCU poses a risk to themselves and others, their refusal cannot be respected. • If a representative has been appointed, the representative must be informed and where possible consulted. • All decisions must be in the best interests of the MHCU.	• Children over 12 years and who have sufficient maturity and have the mental capacity to understand the benefits, risks, social and other implications of the treatment, may consent to (and refuse) treatment on their own behalf. • Children under 12 years, or over 12 years who do not meet the above-mentioned criteria must be assisted by a parent or guardian, or in emergencies by a caregiver. • Information must be provided to children in an understandable way, and due consideration must be given to the needs of disabled children.

Table 4.2 (*Continued*)

Rights and principles	Voluntary	Assisted	Involuntary	Children
Confidentiality	Information may not be disclosed to a third party without the consent of the MHCU, unless such a disclosure is obligatory because of a court order, an Act of Parliament, or disclosure is necessary for the defence of a healthcare practitioner in a criminal, civil or disciplinary matter, or the disclosure is necessary for the medical management of the MHCU.	Information may only be disclosed to a third party if the disclosure is: • With the consent of the MHCU's representative, or an institutional review board, or • In the MHCU's best interests, or if a court orders such disclosure, e.g. because it is necessary for their medical management, or • Obligatory because of a court order, or an Act of Parliament, or • Necessary for the defence of a healthcare practitioner in a criminal, civil or disciplinary matter Where there is knowledge of a sexual crime against a person with intellectual development disorder, there is a statutory duty to report the information to the relevant authority.		In addition to the aforementioned conditions, children also have the right to confidentiality of their parents', caregiver's or family member's health status (Slabbert 2004). Furthermore, there is a statutory obligation to disclose information about the ill-treatment of children, or of the sexual abuse of children to a social worker, or a police official or the commissioner of child welfare. In the UK and Australia, in terms of the Gillick-competency test (from the case of *Gillick vs West Norfolk and Wisbech Area Health Authority*), a competent child under 16 years 'may consent to medical treatment when he or she has "sufficient understanding and intelligence to understand fully what is proposed". It follows that if a child may legally consent to medical treatment, he or she should also be able to consent to disclosures about his or her medical treatment to third parties' (Slabbert 2004, p. 5/21), and thus also refuse their parents access to their records. The situation regarding children refusing their parents' access to their information is not so clear-cut in South Africa (Slabbert 2004).
Privacy	All persons have freedom from intrusion into their personal matters, their personal information and have the right to control the extent of information they share, as well as the timing and circumstances of sharing such information about themselves. This includes written information, or verbal, behavioural information or information pertaining to their opinion or intellectual information. For the various legal statuses, it means that:				
	The MHCU can decide how much information they share, as well as the nature of the information they share. Healthcare practitioners should gather only so much information as is necessary for intervention.	Because the MHCU lacks the capacity to decide, healthcare practitioners should gather information only to the extent that it is necessary for the diagnosis and intervention of the MHCU. Where there is a representative, the representative should only disclose information that is necessary for the diagnosis, care, treatment and rehabilitation of the MHCU.	Where a MHCU is admitted for observation of their behaviour to determine their status, 'involuntary admission or retention shall initially be for a short period as specified by domestic law for observation and preliminary treatment pending review of the admission or retention by the review body' (United Nations 1991, sec. 16(2)), thus observation should be for the purpose of gathering necessary information to assist in determining the best course of action regarding the MHCU's legal status and required intervention.	Healthcare practitioners should gather only so much information as is necessary for intervention, from either the child themselves, or in the case of children under 12, or 12 and older but unable to understand the consequences of disclosure, from a parent, guardian or caregiver.

(*continued*)

Table 4.2 (*Continued*)

Rights and principles	Voluntary	Assisted	Involuntary	Children
Access to health records	In terms of freedom of information legislation, such as the South African PAIA, all persons have the right to access their own information that is held by a private or public body. Where the private or public body believes that the information will cause harm to the person's physical or mental health or well-being, a person over the age of 16 may then nominate a healthcare practitioner of their choice to determine whether this is indeed the case (Van Niekerk 2021).	In addition to the aforementioned right, the MHCU's representative, where applicable, may also access the information in terms of PAIA, because they are trying to exercise or protect a right on behalf of the MHCU.		The situation is not clear-cut in South Africa (see above regarding confidentiality and Slabbert [2004]), but presumably, where there is no perceived harm to the child based on the disclosure, children over the age of 12 years, with the necessary maturity and understanding of the consequences of their decision, may access their medical records. Where there is perceived harm, all children under the age of 12, and children over the age of 12 without the necessary capacity to understand the consequences of their decision, must be assisted by a parent, guardian or caregiver.

provisions pertaining to interventions such as surgery, which are not covered here.

Informed consent is an important concept to understand, specifically related to how much information is enough to enable a person to make an informed decision about whether to accept medical intervention or choose between interventions. Two standards have developed in the case law over the years: the prudent practitioner (doctor) standard and the prudent patient standard, as explained in Box 4.1.

Human Rights

The WFOT in its 2016 revision of the Minimum Standards for the Training of Occupational Therapists (World Federation of Occupational Therapists [WFOT] 2016) included knowledge of human rights in its essential areas of knowledge, skills and attitudes for competent occupational therapy practice. Importantly, occupational therapists and other rehabilitation practitioners may be involved in realising human rights for MHCUs, such as the right to work; thus, it is imperative that occupational therapists receive training in human rights.

The interaction between ethics and human rights provides an important backdrop for the compassionate provision of (mental) healthcare services and advocacy (Dhai & McQuoid-Mason 2020). This section does not aim to create the impression that achieving a human right is a 'static endpoint' (Yamin 2020, p. 164), but all rights, including civil and political rights, are progressively realised and aligned to a country's available resources (Yamin 2020).

Numerous human rights conventions, covenants and declarations exist. The most important of these documents were adopted by the United Nations (UN), such as the Universal Declaration of Human Rights (UDHR, which is not a treaty that binds any state) (United Nations General Assembly 1948), the International Covenant on Civil and Political Rights (1966) (ICCPR) (United Nations General Assembly, 1966), the International Covenant on Economic, Social and Cultural Rights (1966) (ICESCR) (United Nations, 1966), and the Convention on the Rights of Persons with Disabilities (2006) (CRPD) (United Nations, 2006). Although not all countries have ratified these documents, countries such as South Africa, Canada and Hungary have written some of these rights into legislation such as the Constitution of South Africa Act 106 of 1996 and the Canadian Charter of Rights and Freedoms 1982 (Robertson 2004), which means that in those contexts, there will be a country-specific interpretation of the rights in accordance with its specific legal system. The UN documents provide a common basis from which to start a discussion about human rights in the context of mental health, and psychiatry and occupational therapy.

Human rights development has historically been closely linked to health, amongst others because of the interlinked nature of human rights. In fact, the UDHR describes the right to health in Article 25 as a right for everyone to:

'a standard of living adequate for the health and well-being of [themselves], and of [their] family, including food, clothing, housing and medical care and necessary social services, and the right to security in the event of unemployment, sickness, disability, widowhood, old age or other lack of livelihood in circumstances beyond [their] control'. (United Nations General Assembly 1948, para. 25)

BOX 4.1

How does a practitioner know how much information is enough to enable a person to make an informed decision about whether to accept medical intervention, or to choose between interventions?

Two standards have developed in the case law over the years: the prudent practitioner (doctor) standard, and the prudent patient standard.

Prudent doctor/practitioner (reasonable doctor) standard

- Doctor decides what information to disclose or withhold

- Decision is based on what a **reasonable doctor**, having regard to all the circumstances of the particular case, should or should not do

- Formulated in the case of *Richter & another v Estate Hammann*

Prudent patient standard

- Patient must fully comprehend the extent of risks involved in an assessment or procedure
- Doctor must disclose information pertaining to **material risk**
- Knowing what/how much information the patient would have wanted to know
- Formulated in the case of *Castell v De Greef*

What is material risk?

The Castell case at 426 has defined a risk to be material if:

a. A reasonable person, ***in the patient's position***, if warned of the risk, would attach significance to it; and
b. The healthcare practitioner should reasonably be aware that the patient, if warned of the risk, would attach significance to it.

This does not mean that a practitioner must point out every possible complication that could occur, but where a patient may consider a risk material, the practitioner must explain it to the patient, even if the practitioner considers the likelihood of the risk occurring to be remote (Dhai & McQuoid-Mason (2020)/Medical Association of South Africa).

Thus, human rights violations may have a significant impact on the health and well-being of individuals, groups and communities. Additionally, when health policies/legislation, practices and research violate human rights, it affects not only the well-being of people, but also the integrity of a health system and its practitioners (Dhai & McQuoid-Mason 2020). One example is from South Africa during Apartheid, when the South African occupational therapy fraternity came under intense scrutiny by the WFOT due to human rights abuses and discriminatory systems in South Africa at the time. This culminated in a delegation from WFOT visiting South Africa in 1986 to investigate whether the South African Association of Occupational Therapy must be evicted from WFOT, despite South Africa being a founding member of WFOT. Although South Africa remained a member of the WFOT, South African occupational therapists and academics were isolated, not being able to publish in international journals nor attend international occupational therapy congresses, including the WFOT congresses (Crouch, 2016).

Human rights seemed to have developed in phases, as societies object to historical atrocities (Lauren 2011). This has given rise to a notion of 'generations' of human rights. The first Secretary-General of the International Institute of Human Rights in Strasbourg, Karl Vasak, initially introduced a theory of generations of human rights in 1979. He aligned the three generations to the ideals of the French Revolution, namely liberty, equality and fraternity. Thus, three broad categories or generations of human rights, i.e. civil and political rights (e.g.

the right to vote), economic and social rights (e.g. the right to have a job and be economically active), and environmental and cultural rights (referred to by Vasak as solidarity rights, e.g. the right to a healthy environment) were described. There is some controversy about the use of the word 'generations' when referring to groups of human rights because the first generation of human rights is not necessarily the 'parent' of the second generation of human rights, etc. (Wellman 2000). While this chapter continues to use the word generation, it is not intended to create the impression that one generation 'births' another, but to classify them as discrete sets of rights that develop from individual to collective rights. These rights also develop from relatively inexpensive rights to rights that increasingly require economic investment from governments (e.g. by making health care services available), or economic sacrifices (through a commitment to a clean environment, which necessarily may curtail the use of 'dirty' energy that pollutes).

Recently, an argument has been put forth that a fourth category of human rights is emerging, that is epistemic rights in digital lifeworlds (Risse 2021; White House Office of Science and Technology Policy 2022).

Health law textbooks usually only discuss the first two of these categories, likely because their main focus is on doctors. However, because of occupational therapy's concern with the person-environment-occupation interaction, we need to be cognisant of more than just the first two categories; thus, all four categories will be discussed along with foundational principles and truths about human rights.

Human rights are considered universal – that is they apply to all human beings, irrespective of where they live, or their medical and socio-economic status. Human rights are inalienable, that is one cannot give up one's human rights and are indivisible and interdependent. Importantly, though, not all human rights are absolute, which means that sometimes rights can be limited or might need balancing when two (or more) parties' rights are in conflict (Currie & De Waal 2013; Dhai and McQuoid-Mason 2020). The Siracusa Principles (United Nations Economic and Social Council 1985) describe basic considerations for when it will be justifiable for governments or courts to limit or balance human rights. These principles for limitation have been adopted by most governments and have influenced, for example, section 36 of the South African Constitution (commonly known as the limitations clause):

- A limitation must be prescribed by 'a national law of general application which is consistent with the' ICCRP.

- Limitations may not be arbitrary or unreasonable, or discriminatory.

- Limitations may not impair the democratic functioning of a society, or a society which recognises and respects the human rights contained in the United Nations Charter and the UDHR.

- Limitations must be necessary for the democratic functioning of a society. 'Whenever a limitation is required in the terms of the Covenant to be "necessary", this term implies that the limitation:

  a. Is based on one of the grounds justifying limitations recognised by the relevant article of the Covenant,

  b. responds to a pressing public or social need,

  c. pursues a legitimate aim, and

  d. Is proportionate to that aim'. (United Nations Economic and Social Council 1985, p. 6)

- Limitations must be applied according to their intended purpose.

Most human rights rest on the principle of the inherent dignity of the person. Although dignity is not described as a separate right in the ICCPR (United Nations General Assembly 1966), Article 1 of the UDHR (United Nations General Assembly 1948) states that all persons are born free and equal in dignity and rights. In the preamble of the CRPD (United Nations 2006), signatories recognise 'that discrimination against any person on the basis of disability is a violation of the inherent dignity and worth of the human person' (United Nations 2006, p. 1). Some countries, for example South Africa's Constitution, expressly include the right to dignity. Thus, dignity underpins all of these rights and freedoms, including second-, third- (Currie & De Waal 2013) and likely also fourth-generation rights. In the South African case of *Greunen and Another v. McGovern* Judge Daffue defined dignity as follows:

> 'Dignity is defined as a "valued and serene condition" in a person's social or individual life which may be violated, either publicly or privately, by another through "offensive and degrading treatment", or when the person "is exposed to ill-will, ridicule, disesteem or contempt"'. (*Greunen* at paragraph 18)

A distinction must be made at this point between a Human Rights–based Approach to rights such as the right to life and right to health, and a legally enforceable right. A Human Rights–based Approach to rights recognises the need for intersectoral and often international cooperation to create an environment of accountability, transparency, non- or anti-discrimination, participation and an acknowledgement that nobody (person or government) is above the law (i.e. the rule of law). A justiciable, or legally enforceable, right is that right, which is distilled to its essence without subsuming other rights (and then becoming unenforceable) (Yamin 2020). In this section, the intention is to describe succinctly the essence of the justiciable rights rather than a Human Rights–based Approach, which is an application and thus better suited to the discussion of justice in the ethics section of this chapter.

First-Generation Human Rights (Also Known as Civil and Political Rights) First-generation human rights have arisen from a variety of revolutions and wars in the 17th and 18th centuries. Although homo sapiens have existed for centuries, all members of the species were not necessarily regarded as 'fully human' (Lauren 2011, p. 37) for a very long time. Some of the people who were not regarded as 'fully human' included first peoples, slaves, the bourgeoisie and women. These humans were denied some of the basic human rights included under civil and political rights to various extents, e.g. dignity, freedom and suffrage.

One should not be lured into the misconception that breaches of these rights stopped after the revolutions and wars of the 17th and 18th centuries. At the heart of the transgression of these basic rights is othering. Unfortunately, othering (alterity/discrimination) on the grounds of religion, nationality, race, ethnicity etc. still abounds, as evidenced by the practices of the Nazis in the Second World War, the genocide in Rwanda in 1994 and more recently, reports of rape and torture during the Russian invasion of Ukraine in 2022 and 2023. As long as humans, governments and societies do not respect all humans as equal, othering or alterity, and thus denial of basic human rights will continue, which is all the more reason why occupational therapists and other healthcare practitioners must be knowledgeable about basic human rights.

The United Nations has two primary instruments that pertain to first-generation human rights and human rights in general, namely the UDHR, adopted in 1948, and the ICCPR adopted by the General Assembly in 1966. Article 2 of the ICCPR requires signatories to respect the rights of all individuals in its territory, not to discriminate on any grounds, and to make legislation and adopt measures that will give effect to political and civil rights. Some of the rights provided for in the Covenant include:

- The right to vote and participate in civic activities.

- The right to (human) dignity.

- The right not to be subjected to medical or scientific experimentation without (informed) consent.

- The right to freedom from torture.

- The right to freedom from slavery.

- The right to security and liberty of the person, and thus not to be arbitrarily arrested or detained.

- The right to life, which in all UN instruments is qualified to mean that governments may not arbitrarily allow or perpetrate the death of its citizens or residents. This is not meant to automatically abolish the death penalty, but the ICCPR places certain restrictions on the death penalty. In the context of the ICCPR, the UDHR and the ICESCR, this right has not been written to cover the topic of termination of pregnancy, beyond prohibiting carrying out the death penalty on a pregnant woman.

- The right of citizens to access public services (United Nations General Assembly 1966).

Some first-generation rights that are of importance to healthcare practitioners and occupational therapists specifically are described in Table 4.3.

When considering limitations of first-generation rights, one can then see that in the case of (temporarily) depriving an acute mental healthcare user of their right to freedom of movement, it may be a fair limitation of their right because of a 'pressing public or social need', in pursuit of a legitimate aim, that is the safety, treatment, care and rehabilitation of such a person.

Second-Generation Rights (Also Known as Economic and Social Rights) The recognition of the need for another set of human rights, now known as second-generation human rights' developed from events such as the socialist and Marxist revolutions in the 19th and early 20th centuries (Lauren 2011). These events highlighted that one's ability to live a decent life is dependent on the protection of basic rights such as the right to health, food and water. Flowing from these events, is the realisation that these rights must be protected for everyone, including marginalised people.

The United Nations' Committee on Economic, Social and Cultural Rights has described and commented on a number of economic and social rights. The Committee, in explaining the rights from the ICESCR, often implements a framework to interpret the right and to assess the extent to which the right has been implemented (Dugard *et al.* 2020), which is described below. For the purposes of this chapter, the focus is on the right to work, right to social security, right to health, right to education, the right to food, the right to adequate housing and the right to water and sanitation. These have

Table 4.3 Implications of first-generation human rights to occupational therapy in psychiatry and mental health.

Basic right described in the ICCPR	Implication for occupational therapists in the field of mental health and psychiatry
No one shall be subjected without his free consent to medical or scientific experimentation (Article 7)	Occupational therapists, when conducting research among mental health care users, must ensure that participants have enough information to make an informed decision about their participation. Where mental health care users do not have the capacity to consent: a. The research must be necessary to meet the needs of these mental healthcare users (or people in similar circumstances), and b. That a lawfully appointed proxy has provided informed consent to participate.
Everyone has the right to liberty and security of the person and not to be arrested or detained without knowing why and without just cause (Article 9), and persons deprived of their liberty shall be treated with humanity and with respect for the inherent dignity of the human person (Article 10)	Prisoners and forensic patients have the right to healthcare services without discrimination. Prisoners and forensic patients must be treated with dignity and respect.
Everyone in a country has the right to freedom of movement, provided that they are legally in the country/territory (Article 11)	This right is not absolute and may be limited as per the Syracuse Principles described below. That means that it may be lawful to restrict the right to freedom of movement of a person who is a danger to themselves or others, such as an acutely psychotic mental health care user, by means of involuntary admission to a mental health care facility. However, every case must be determined on its own merits.
No one shall be subjected to arbitrary or unlawful interference with his privacy, family, home or correspondence, nor to unlawful attacks on his honour and reputation (Article 17)	MHCUs have the right to privacy and confidentiality. Nobody may demand information from or about a person unless it is necessary for the care treatment and rehabilitation of MHCUs. Occupational therapists and other healthcare practitioners may not share information about a person without the person's or their lawful proxy's (where the person themselves cannot consent) consent.

been referred to as social determinants of health; thus, it is important for occupational therapists to have a basic understanding not only of the rights, but also of their potential to help MHCUs (and other clients/patients) to realise these rights that are so closely linked to the ability to be healthy.

Framework to Interpret Second-Generation Human Rights

The Committee adopted the 4-A scheme, originally described by Tomaševski in 2004 in relation to education (Veriava & Paterson 2020), namely availability, accessibility, acceptability and adaptability. Over time, these have evolved into five criteria to describe whether a right has been met, namely availability, accessibility, quality, affordability and acceptability (Dugard *et al.* 2020). Notably, not all four of the original criteria are included in the later five; thus, for comprehensiveness' sake, all six criteria will be described.

Availability: For a right to be *available*, it must meet people's needs now and in the future, and it must be enough (De Albuquerque & Roaf 2020).

Accessibility: For a right to be accessible, there must be sufficient infrastructure to facilitate engagement in the right, which could include roads, a public transport system (e.g. to allow children from low socioeconomic environments to get to school), or pipes to deliver potable water (Dugard *et al.* 2020). Accessibility also relates to non-discrimination in one's ability to access the right, and non-discrimination, for example in the treatment of people with disabilities, refugees, women and in the context of this textbook, MHCUs, when they want to exercise social and economic rights (Veriava & Paterson 2020).

Quality: Usually refers to safety, for example in relation to food and water, which both should be free from harmful microorganisms (De Albuquerque & Roaf 2020).

Affordability: Is closely related to accessibility, in that expensive goods such as food and education are inaccessible to those who cannot afford to pay for it. Additionally, the cost of meeting some of one's basic needs, for example food and water, must not limit one's ability to meet other basic needs such as housing (De Albuquerque & Roaf 2020, Committee on Economic Social and Cultural Rights 1991).

Acceptability: People will not use basic goods and services, including food, water, sanitation and education, that do not meet their social and cultural standards (Dugard *et al.* 2020; see also Chapter 5 of this textbook).

Adaptability: In the context of education, this means that children have different needs and an education system must be sufficiently inclusive and flexible to cater to individual scholar's needs. This is based on the principle of always acting in a child's best interests (Veriava & Paterson 2020). The 'best interests principle' has been expanded to also apply in healthcare situations to all patients (Dhai & McQuoid-Mason 2020). In relation to MCHUs, it means that work systems, social security systems etc. must be sufficiently flexible to meet the needs of MHCUs, who also have the right to work (United Nations 2006).

What Is Relevant to Occupational Therapy? Occupational therapists obviously have a role in advocating for MHCUs' social and economic rights (see, for example how final-year occupational therapy students attempted to advocate for the safe housing and treatment, care and rehabilitation of profoundly disabled MHCUs at the time of the closing of the Life Esidimeni facilities [Politics Web 2017]). However, occupational therapists also have a clinical role to enable MHCUs to access basic goods such as water and food and education, for example by improving community mobility or making reasonable accommodations in the school and workplace to ensure participation in education and work. Table 4.4 describes the implications of second-generation human rights for occupational therapy, beyond advocacy, using the six criteria described above.

In conclusion, occupational therapists have a role clinically to ensure that persons with disabilities and other vulnerable persons are able to access and realise their social, economic and cultural rights in a variety of ways that are not restricted to advocacy only.

Third-Generation Rights Third-generation rights are also referred to as solidarity rights (Wellman 2000), and are 'group' or 'collective' rights. The recognition of these rights stem among others from World War II and subsequent anti-colonialist revolutions (Lauren 2011). When Vasak first introduced solidarity rights specifically, it was in response to highlighting the fact that first- and second-generation rights were mostly pertaining to the individual, i.e. freedom from mistreatment (tyranny) by the State, and a demand that the State creates programmes that will benefit the individual, e.g. education, housing etc. However, Vasak recognised that humans cannot thrive if they do not participate in communal activities – lives 'worthy of human beings requires fraternity as well as liberty and equality' (Wellman 2000, p. 642). Nonetheless, there is some contention in legal circles about the existence of a third generation and the possibility of its enforcement in international law (Wellman 2000). The legal debate as enunciated by Wellman is not within the ambit of occupational therapy; however, in the context of decoloniality, occupational justice and other occupational science concepts, it would be remis not to include the possibility of collective or solidarity rights in this broader discussion.

Some of the rights included under solidarity rights include the right to self-determination, a healthy environment, subsistence and development, peace and freedom from violence and war, and the right of peoples to control their natural resources. Realising these rights requires a concerted effort not only from the individual, but also a variety of actors such as the government, public and private groups, and even the entire international community. Solidarity applies because these rights must be group rights, not reducible to the individual rights of the members of these groups (Wellman 2000). Again, the occupational therapist's role extends beyond advocacy, to ensuring that rehabilitation services facilitate or enable individuals

Table 4.4 Second-generation human rights and occupational therapy.

Human right	Application for occupational therapy

Right to work and rights at work.
 	
People with disabilities have the right to work, irrespective of the extent of their disability (United Nations 2006). Everyone has the right to the opportunity to gain their living by work that they freely choose or accept, which means that governments must also make technical and vocational guidance and training programmes increasingly available and accessible to all people (United Nations 1966). The right also includes fair remuneration without discrimination, as well as safe working conditions and fair conditions of employment (e.g. working hours, leave provisions, etc.), and the right to form and/or join trade unions and protection from unemployment (Bras Gomes 2020).
	• Occupational therapists must ensure that mental healthcare users are able to engage in productive activities of their choosing, aligned with their abilities.
	
	• Work practice and vocational rehabilitation services should be designed to ensure that MHCUs are able to work in integrated, stigma-free environments, receive due benefits from their labours, and where possible are able to engage and advance in employment.
	
	• Providing vocational rehabilitation/work practice services, e.g. supported employment, that will enable MHCUs to live productive lives
	
	• This presupposes that occupational therapists must be *au fait* with:
	
	  • Enabling labour legislation, to ensure appropriate recommendations and return-to-work processes.
	  • Job analysis techniques, including understanding the physiological and psychosocial demands of work and thus to make *reasonable* accommodations for MHCUs to access acceptable work.
	  • Contextually appropriate adaptive and reasonable accommodations to ensure that MHCUs can participate and advance in employment.

Right to social security Social security flows from human dignity, and has been seen as a critical tool to reduce poverty and ensure that people/communities are developed. Thus, social security has a strong link to the Sustainable Development Goals. Social security includes (but is not limited to) benefits for children and families, benefits related to maternity, unemployment, injury resulting in unemployment, sickness, old age, disability and health protection. Social security is achieved in two ways, namely by means of contributory and non-contributory schemes. Contributory schemes, also referred to as social insurance, means that beneficiaries themselves contribute to their own insurance, whereas non-contributory schemes are tax-funded and are also referred to as social assistance (Sepulveda, 2020). This is a progressive right – i.e. states must make it progressively attainable; it has been found that states cannot discriminate on the basis of nationality when giving access to social assistance; see, e.g. the cases of *Ahmad Shah Ayubi v Bezirkshauptmannschaft Linz-Land* (2018; Court of Justice of the European Union) which facilitated refugees' access to social assistance, irrespective of their status as temporary or permanent residents. *Khosa and another v Minister of Social Development and others* (2004; South African Constitutional Court) held that excluding permanent residents on the basis of nationality from receiving social grants was an unreasonable restriction on the right to social security, AND denying children who are South African citizens on the basis of their parents' nationality (non-South African citizens), is also discriminatory and unfair. This has resulted in a change in South African regulations, which means that citizens, permanent residents and refugees are entitled to receive non-contributory social protection benefits, e.g. children's grants, disability grants and old-age pensions (Sepulveda, 2020).	• In many countries occupational therapy to refugees and other displaced persons is an emergent field of practice. Many of these people may experience pre-existing mental illness but might also have trauma and other mental health sequelae arising from their displacement (see also Chapter 8). Occupational therapy services therefore must be culturally sensitive (see also Chapter 5) • Occupational therapists need to leverage appropriate social security mechanisms to ensure people's access to services that will support their health and well-being, as well as their human dignity. • Occupational therapists may render services to MHCUs in facilities that are linked to the social security system, e.g. orphanages, old-age homes and residential facilities for MHCUs with severe or profound (psychiatric) disabilities. Occupational therapists must then ensure age-appropriate, productive and restorative/pleasurable activities for the residents that ensure their dignity and prevent boredom and facilitate their development and optimal engagement in society. • Occupational therapists must collaborate with key role players, e.g. social workers, to ensure access to social security, which may be an important determinant for other basic needs such as food, water and health.

(continued)

Table 4.4   (*Continued*)

Human right	Application for occupational therapy

Right to health
 	
Article 12 of the ICESCR (United Nations 1966) describes the right to health as follows:
 	
1. The States Parties to the present Covenant recognise the right of everyone to the enjoyment of the highest attainable standard of physical and mental health.
 	
2. The steps to be taken by the States Parties to the present Covenant to achieve the full realization of this right shall include those necessary for:
 	
   a. The provision for the reduction of the stillbirth-rate and of infant mortality and for the healthy development of the child;
   b. The improvement of all aspects of environmental and industrial hygiene;
   c. The prevention, treatment and control of epidemic, endemic, occupational and other diseases;
   d. The creation of conditions which would assure to all medical service and medical attention in the event of sickness. (United Nations, 1966, para. 12)
 	
Importantly, it does not define health, but includes public health preconditions, such as environmental and occupational health and sanitation.
 	
General Comment 14 of the UN's CESCR acknowledges that health is dependent on a number of other social and economic rights and factors (or social determinants of health), such as food and nutrition, housing, access to safe and potable water and adequate sanitation, safe and healthy working conditions, and a healthy environment (Committee on Economic Social and Cultural Rights 2000, para. 14; Yamin, 2020).
	• Although it is silent about rehabilitation, rehabilitation (occupational therapy in particular) is crucial for the 'highest attainable standard of physical and mental health'
	
	• Occupational therapists must know the communities from which MHCUs come, and also the extended health system (including traditional health practitioners) in those communities.
	
	• Applying community-based rehabilitation principles is key to stop the revolving door in mental health and psychiatry.
	
	• Occupational therapists must have preventative and promotive programmes in these communities, not only rehabilitative programmes.
	
	• Discharge-planning is an important part of occupational therapy services, which was not done adequately in the case of Life Esidimeni.
	
	• Accurate and adequate record-keeping is important to ensure continuity of care. Furthermore, where services are delivered at multiple levels (e.g. primary, secondary and tertiary facilities), integration of rehabilitation services is important (see Maseko, Adams & Myezwa in print).

Right to education At its most basic, the right to education means that basic, primary school education should be free. There remain barriers to education for marginalised groups, such as children with disabilities, undocumented children and children from minority groups such as the Roma (Veriava & Paterson 2020). The best interests of the learner are always paramount, and this includes the best interests and rights of marginalised and vulnerable learners (Veriava & Paterson 2020).	• Occupational therapists should assist with ensuring functional and safe ablution facilities for disabled children, including girls during menstruation. • The right of children with disabilities to enjoy equal access to education, means that occupational therapists must be involved in designing and developing reasonable accommodations and individualised support strategies should be implemented to support children in accessing not only basic, but also secondary, tertiary and vocational education and training. • Provide clinical interventions that ensure that children, adolescents and adults with mental health conditions are able to participate effectively in educational pursuits at all levels of education
Right to Food The Committee on Economic, Social and Cultural Rights in its General Comment 12, explained that the right to food entails: 'The availability of food in a quantity and quality sufficient to satisfy the dietary needs of individuals, free from adverse substances, and acceptable within a given culture; and the accessibility of such food in ways that are sustainable and that do not interfere with the enjoyment of other human rights'. (Committee on Economic Social and Cultural Rights 1999, para. 8).	• Accessibility is an important consideration for occupational therapists. Some of the Life Esidimeni MHCUs passed away, not because they did not have food, but because they were unable to feed themselves. Thus, food was available, but inaccessible (South African Depression and Anxiety Group [SADAG] 2023). • In the Global South, food gardening is an important activity used in occupational therapy community-based practice (and even in institutions), as it uses the occupation as a means and an end. Food gardening often helps to make food available to vulnerable MHCUs in communities where stigma may make it harder for them to get food.
Right to Adequate Housing The right to housing is more than just a structure, or the proverbial roof over one's head; it also should provide the necessary privacy, enough space, adequate security, sufficient ventilation and light, adequate basic infrastructure, an appropriate (adequate) location in relation to one's work at basic amenities, and should come at a reasonable cost. General Comment 4 (Committee on Economic Social and Cultural Rights 1991) provides seven conditions that must be considered when determining whether housing meets the right	• Housing that allows all MHCUs to live in safe, stigma-free environments, where they are able to attain the highest level of independent participation in all of the occupations that are meaningful to them. This could include occupational therapists training caregivers in communal housing facilities to prevent learnt helplessness and to facilitate participation.

Table 4.4 *(Continued)*

Human right	Application for occupational therapy
Rights to water and sanitation Although not originally included in the UDHR or the ICESCR, these two rights were recognised as separate rights by the UN's General Assembly in 2015. As has already been seen, other rights, such as the right to education and the right to adequate housing are dependent upon access to potable drinking water and safe sanitation. Everyone should have access to sufficient, safe, acceptable, physically accessible and affordable water for personal and household use (De Albuquerque and Roaf 2020). There must be enough sanitation facilities to make sure that everyone's needs are met. Shared facilities must not result in long lines. Governments must ensure that human waste is collected, transported, treated, disposed and/or reused with due regard for the associated hygiene.	• In the Global South, access to water is often more difficult than in the Global North. Decolonised occupational therapy descriptions of occupations must therefore take cognisance of the fact that (often women's) occupations such as instrumental activities of daily living would include the task of fetching water (and fuel such as firewood). • Occupational therapists must understand what this productive occupation entails, including what it takes to render water collected from sources such as streams and rivers, potable. • In societies where MHCUs are marginalised, what does it take for them to collect (potable) water? • Educating persons with disabilities and/or their caregivers on disposing of menstrual care products and infants' waste products (e.g. soiled disposable nappies, infants' faeces) in a safe and hygienic way.

and groups to participate in the concerted efforts to secure and realise their collective rights. Care should be taken not to create isolated 'communities' of MHCUs who are separated from their cultural and family communities. The idea is to facilitate solidarity, not new separated 'communities'.

Fourth-Generation Rights Arising from technological advances resulting in increased data gathering, data surveillance and 'surveillance capitalism', Risse (2021) has argued for a fourth generation of human rights, namely epistemic rights in digital lifeworlds. Humans increasingly inhabit a digital lifeworld, where much of our human occupation leaves digital marks, or digital footprints, both in the form of overt/visible data and in the form of metadata of which most people are largely unaware. These human occupations are not necessarily restricted to our interaction with digital devices and applications, but also include digital records of our physical movement, such as surveillance camera footage in shopping malls. Much of our digital data provide information 'about what humans do, think or feel', thus

> 'digital lifeworlds engage humans much more as *epistemic actors* – as *knowers* and *knowns* – than ever was possible in the analog (sic) world, with its limited capacities for storing, sorting, or processing information. Accordingly, it is regarding their epistemic rights, rights as knowers and knowns, that humans need especially high levels of protection in the late stage of Life 2.0, with its colossal possibilities of epistemic intrusiveness'. (Risse 2021, p. 3) (original emphasis)

In these digital lifeworlds, Risse (2021) argues that humans have four roles:

• Individual epistemic subjects: we gather information (to learn and to know) and are expected to respect standards of inquiry (e.g. what is the best way of gathering information) – there are norms within the episteme to which we must adhere (e.g. not to plagiarise)

• Collective epistemic subjects, in which we help establish and maintain standards of inquiry, or the various norms and rules of the current episteme – people contribute to, or sustain, the information environment.

• Individual epistemic objects – getting to be known by others, according to the rules about what information you may or may not share with others – to be known, but simultaneously to manage privacy, which is increasingly complicated. This role is determined largely by those with whom we interact: there are limits to the information we are allowed to share with others in various contexts: a healthcare practitioner will share less information about themselves to their patients than what they expect the patients to share with them. Importantly, though, what we believe or feel 'increasingly is data that can be gathered or inferred from other things we do, such as clicks' (Risse 2021, p. 6), which have important implications for privacy. By merely clicking, we are already giving information away that might affect our privacy in the longer term.

• Collective epistemic objects, as a contributor to data patterns, giving 'rise to known patterns of human behaviour, (sic) thought, and feeling' (including metadata), which would not have been possible to the same extent in an analogue world. (Risse 2021, p. 6)

What ought MHCUs' rights be in respect of digital lifeworlds? Because human rights in respect of digital lifeworlds is an emerging field, there is little clarity and certainty about human rights beyond exiting first-generation human rights (e.g. right to privacy in a digital lifeworld and the right to equality or non-discrimination between users of platforms and owners of platforms), second-generation human rights (e.g. the right to have quality information in digital classrooms) and third-generation rights (e.g. the right to engage freely with [real] people of one's choosing in online communities). The White House Office of Science and Technology

Policy in 2022 published a set of rights of Americans in relation to automated systems (thus speaking to our rights as collective and individual epistemic subjects and objects) based on five principles, namely

1. Safe and effective systems

2. Algorithmic discrimination protections

3. Data privacy

4. Notice that an automated system is being used, and explanation of the reasons for its use and how the outcomes thereof might impact people.

5. Human alternatives, consideration and feedback (i.e. the ability to opt out of automated systems and access to a human person who can resolve one's issues)

Digital lifeworlds have some emergent implications for occupational therapy, which include:

- How using social media and other digital lifeworlds affect occupational performance. At what point is it considered a sub-set of, for example, communication and social participation?

- Occupational therapists and MHCUs must also know that their privacy is affected not only by the content they share, but also by the platforms they use, the people with whom they interact, as well as the sites they access. It is harder to manage responsible citizenship in a digital lifeworld than in an analogue lifeworld.

- Where laws and regulations exist about data privacy, occupational therapists must be careful about the platforms they use to communicate with clients, or with fellow healthcare practitioners about clients. The onus is on the practitioner to make sure that data are secure.

Closing Remarks About Human Rights

In conclusion, all four generations of human rights have important implications for MHCUs and occupational therapists. Second-generation rights are closely linked to the social determinants of health and occupational therapists, because of their knowledge of and skills to affect the human–environment–occupation interaction of MHCUs, are uniquely positioned to help MHCUs realise and exercise their human rights.

PROFESSIONALISM

In many countries, professions, and thus professionalism, are governed by statutory regulators, such as the Health and Care Professions Council of the UK (HCPC), the HPCSA and the Occupational Therapy Board of New Zealand (OTBNZ). Statutory regulators derive all their power from the empowering legislation – in the case of the HPCSA, it is the Health Professions Act of 1974 (as amended) (Burns 2013).

The requirements statutory regulators place on healthcare practitioners regarding professional behaviour thus fall within the bounds of medical and health law, as they usually follow regulations and guidelines that are promulgated and published in terms of the empowering legislation. This has necessarily resulted in some confusion about professionalism and its relationship to ethics and law – it is no longer purely one or the other, and the rule-boundedness of research and medical/health professions ethics means that there are now defined answers to questions unlike previously when answers used to be philosophical and purely ethical.

A variety of definitions of professionalism exist, the most succinct of which is that from Williams (2009), who importantly, linked professionalism to professions, that is arising from an occupation being considered a profession and thus having to adhere to (uniform) professional standards. He defined a healthcare profession as 'an occupation that is characterised by high moral standards, including a strong commitment to the well-being of others, mastery of a body of knowledge and skills, and a high level of autonomy' (Williams 2009, p. 48). Correspondingly, professionalism is defined as referring 'to the characteristics of a profession' (Williams 2009, p. 48). Most of the professional moral standards highlighted in the literature include 'integrity, respect, competence, honesty, trustworthiness and accountability' (Nortjé & De Jongh 2017, p. 41).

For the purposes of this chapter, two components from Williams' definition are important, namely 'moral standards' and 'mastery of a body of knowledge and skills'.

Moral Standards

Morality and moral values are not universal because these are influenced by culture, religion and other societal values as is evidenced by the growing body of literature about topics such as African moral values and ethics (see Figure 4.1). Importantly, in occupational therapy there is a recognition that much of the professionalism literature is written from a Western perspective (Hordichuk *et al.* 2015). Some international occupational therapy regulators, such as the OTBNZ overtly include indigenous cultural values in their professional standards (Occupational Therapy Board of New Zealand 2022). Apart from having to comply with regulatory requirements, understanding clients' culture is important, particularly in mental health and psychiatry because MHCUs have the right to be treated in a way that respects and supports their culture (United Nations 1991; Chapter 5 of this textbook). Two examples thereof can be found in African philosophy and Māori episteme, beliefs and values.

In African philosophy, communal interdependence plays an important role. According to Ubuntu, for example, an individual is characterised by their relationships with others. In Africa, this often finds expression in the extended family (Letseka & Ganya 2017). It is therefore important for practitioners practicing in these contexts to understand the importance of the extended family to a person, as this has implications for institutional care of MHCUs – both for the client and their family and only adhering to Western professional/moral standards will not be sufficient. Additionally, in some cultures such as the isiZulu and isiXhosa cultures in South Africa, psychosis and mental health disturbances may likely have a different cultural meaning (Van Niekerk *et al.* 2014), and could *inter alia* relate to a calling from the ancestors to become a traditional health practitioner (van der Zeijst *et al.* 2021). Merely applying Western professional values in these contexts will unlikely result in an MHCU being treated in a way that respects and supports their culture.

The OTBNZ requires occupational therapists to apply their knowledge and skills to work for equitable outcomes of Māori health and well-being, and to respect and support the episteme, values and beliefs related to the Māori world, culture, spirit, healthy family and wealth (Occupational Therapy Board of New Zealand 2022). This necessarily impacts institutional care, treatment and rehabilitation, as well as the outcomes and nature of interventions occupational therapists choose when treating Māori MHCUs. Only adhering to Western professional values will not serve the interests of Māori MHCUs optimally.

Mastering a Body of Knowledge

Mastering a body of knowledge means that a practitioner must practice skilfully and competently. Many occupational therapy regulatory bodies' practice and ethical standards regulations/guidelines prescribe what it means to practice competently. Among others, competence relates to the mastery and application of the occupational therapy process and its component parts (e.g. assessment, intervention and evaluation), evidence-based practice (Occupational Therapy Board of Australia 2018; Alberta College of Occupational Therapists 2019; Royal College of Occupational Therapists 2021; Occupational Therapy Board of New Zealand 2022) and keeping appropriate records, including communicating one's findings competently to fellow healthcare practitioners, as well as the MHCUs and their caregivers and/or family members (Occupational Therapy Board of Australia 2018; Alberta College of Occupational Therapists 2019; Royal College of Occupational Therapists 2021; Health Professions Council of South Africa 2022). This requirement necessitates profession-specific professional guidelines (Hordichuk *et al.* 2015).

No profession is static in its knowledgebase. Evidence-based practice requires practitioners to produce contextually relevant evidence for practice, and to keep up with new developments in the profession and field. Practicing competently also means that practitioners need to be aware of situations and conditions that might affect a practitioner's (or student-practitioner's) 'competence, attitude, judgement or performance' (Health Professions Act no 56 of 1974, sec. 1), such as a mental or physical medical condition or abuse/dependence on substances. Countries such as South Africa require practitioners to report themselves or fellow practitioners and student-practitioners if their practice is compromised by such an impairment (Health Professions Council of South Africa 2023).

Professionalism, then, rather than being purely based on ethical philosophy, is rule-bound and practitioners must familiarise themselves with the rules and norms in their contexts. In occupational therapy specifically, professionalism also includes cultural awareness and sensitivity (see Chapter 5). In the mental health care context, this includes incorporating culturally and contextually appropriate occupations and activities in intervention, and rendering services in contextually appropriate environments and including culturally appropriate members of the community in intervention.

MORALITY AND ETHICS

Morality and ethics are discrete and separate fields, but over time, they do influence each other. Morality is situated in how a society behaves and what it values. Morality uses some philosophical thought to answer moral questions, which can be influenced by cultural, religious and sometimes even political values. One only has to look as far as the United States of America to see how culture, religion and politics influence how moral questions about issues such as abortion and gun control are answered. Ethics, on the other hand, is a branch of philosophy that uses clear, reflective and systematic philosophical reasoning to answer similar questions (Van Niekerk 2017). Ethical reasoning must be coherent and congruent with the ontology, epistemology and axiology underpinning the ethical theory being applied to answering the question. Importantly, the distinction between morality and ethics lies in the answer to the questions 'what do people actually do (morality) and what do they think they ought to do (ethics)?' (Van Niekerk 2017).

MORALITY, WORLDVIEW AND THE 'GOOD MORAL STANDARDS' OF SOCIETY

Over time, a society's common worldview, its common values, and how it understands or creates knowledge (among others), also influence societal values and thus, eventually, also long-standing customs and traditions that develop into a set of unwritten do's and don'ts that contribute to a society's sense of right and wrong. The Romans referred to this as the society's *boni mores*, which at its core refers to the 'good morals' or 'good moral standards' of society (Sharp 2014). In essence, the *boni mores* of a society captures a society's sense of lawfulness – what is lawfully right or wrong, but not necessarily codified. Although the concept of *boni mores* emanates from Roman society and Roman law, all societies have a notion of what is good and right to do – a sense of morality – which is demonstrated in how the society is organised and how it behaves. Over time, the *boni mores* of a society become captured in (long-standing) traditions and customs and become the society's rules. Societal morals are influenced by a variety of factors, including culture, worldview, values, religious or spiritual beliefs, to name but a few. These influences help to explain why different societies have differing *boni mores* and why *boni mores* of a society influences its common law.

There exists a cyclical process between morality/*boni mores* and a society's ontology (worldview, or *weltanschauung*) axiology (values) and epistemology (the limits and validity of knowledge), as is demonstrated in Figure 4.2. These long-standing customs and traditions, over time, could result in people expecting to be treated in a specific way, which, if codified, could result in rights. *Boni mores* and human rights can be codified into international instruments, for example the United Nations' UDHR, or captured in local policies and legislation, as discussed above.

Society has undergone many changes over the past 200 years or so, with women being 'emancipated' and overt slavery being abolished, which is also evident in society's changing attitude towards mental (ill) health. Contemporary literature and popular culture provide evidence of some of the changes in attitude towards mental (ill) health in keeping with the *zeitgeist* – after all, contemporary literature and popular culture have the 'power to drive a narrative' (Shemilt 2022). Nonetheless, pervasive stigma and prejudice still surround persons with psychiatric diagnoses and/or mental ill-health.

When communities have deep-rooted prejudices, for example related to worldview (holding a Western worldview, with a bias or prejudice against Eastern or African worldviews, that results in a specific way in which a society is organised and how it operates), this could give rise to systemic discrimination, because these instinctual ways of handling life, make access to systems hard for people who do not hold the same view or understand that way of thinking/operating (Bras Gomes 2020). It is usually hard for people within to recognise or understand how this gives rise to systemic discrimination and injustice, because these 'ways' or rules coincide with their own worldview and they often are unaware of other worldviews.

MHCUs often face systemic injustice because pervasive stigma about mental ill health and mental disability makes it harder for MHCUs, especially those with chronic debilitating conditions, to access systems and services. Occupational therapists have a role to not only educate and empower MHCUs, but also members and structures of society, such as employers, governmental officials, etc.

ETHICAL PERSPECTIVE

Ethicists have long held that ethics and the law are distinct and should be treated as discrete but separate fields (Van Niekerk 2017). Nonetheless, many (bio)ethical principles have been recorded into legislation and policies, which complicates an attempt at a hard distinction. This section of the chapter tries to highlight only the ethical applications of these principles, although they are quite rule-based rather than purely philosophical.

A variety of ethical theories exist, including Kant's Deontology, virtue ethics, and utilitarianism. Each of these has a unique approach to ethical dilemmas, which is situated in their ontology and epistemology. More recently, bioethics has developed as a discrete, inter-disciplinary (academic) field,

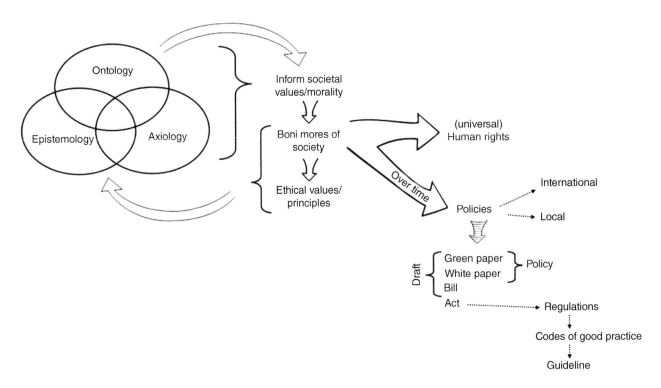

FIGURE 4.2　Interrelationship between world view, *boni mores*, human rights and the law.

incorporating medical ethics, animal ethics and environmental ethics. Bioethics is concerned with ethical, social and legal issues in biomedicine and biomedical research, and there is some overlap between the principles it applies to research and clinical practice, as well as between the three fields of medicine, animals and the environment (Gordon n.d.).

Four of the most important bioethical principles that apply to psychiatry and mental health are respect for persons, beneficence, non-maleficence and justice. What follows is a brief explanation of these principles and their application to occupational therapy in the field of mental health and psychiatry.

RESPECT FOR PERSONS

In the 2002 edition of its ethical guidelines for biomedical research, the Council for the International Organisations of Medical Sciences (CIOMS) explained respect for persons as follows:

> 'Respect for persons incorporates at least two fundamental ethical considerations, namely:
>
> a) respect for autonomy, which requires that those who are capable of deliberation about their personal choices should be treated with respect for their capacity for self-determination; and
>
> b) protection of persons with impaired or diminished autonomy, which requires that those who are dependent or vulnerable be afforded security against harm or abuse'. (Council for the International Organizations of Medical Sciences 2002, p. 17)

In the context of MHCUs, this means that persons capable of making informed choices should be allowed to do so and that in the case of persons who are not able to make informed choices for themselves, they are treated in a way that respects and upholds their best interests.

Worldview plays an important part in practitioners' and ethicists' understanding and application of autonomy. In Western worldviews, individuality takes precedence over collective decision-making in most instances. In occupational therapy, however, respect for persons means that the practitioner must respect cultural and religious worldviews where individuality is not pre-eminent and treat all (M)HCUs in such a way as to give effect to their choices, and cultural values and expression in a dignified manner.

Vulnerability is an important concept in mental healthcare because a variety of factors render (some) MHCUs vulnerable. Some persons, for example those with Intellectual Developmental Disorder, or those who have treatment-resistant forms of psychotic conditions that constantly impair their reality orientation, are vulnerable due to the condition itself, which makes independent living difficult and results in an inability to make sound, judicious decisions about finances, healthcare, etc. In some instances, vulnerability arises from stigma and lack of access to mental healthcare services. Despite increased awareness about mental health during and post-COVID-19, researchers have found that persons with mental ill-health pre-pandemic did not benefit from this increased awareness in the same way as those who developed mental ill-health during the pandemic. In fact, persons with pre-existing mental ill-health were more likely to be worse off due to the inability to access treatment, the prolonged adverse effects of lockdowns etc. (Snider & Flaherty 2020). Respect for persons then means that occupational therapists need to ensure that vulnerable people are protected from exploitation and harm.

Beneficence

The notion of beneficence is not new and refers to the ethical obligation to seek or maximise the benefit to healthcare users and society (Council for the International Organizations of Medical Sciences 2002; Beauchamp & Childress 2019; Dhai & McQuoid-Mason 2020). An important aspect of beneficence is acting in the patient's/client's best interests. Much of the literature on the topic of patients' best interests situates the discussion in the context of end-of-life decisions, particularly for those persons in a persistent vegetative state (PVS). Best interests have been described as relating to experiencing pain and pleasure on one hand, and issues concerning judgement and dignity on the other (Ellis 1996; Beauchamp & Childress 2019). These remain abstract concepts that are difficult to define. On a more practical level, with reference to MHCUs who lack capacity, some considerations that have been mentioned include considering the person's own 'past and present wishes, feelings, values and belief' (Saunders 2020, p. 680), whether expressed by themselves, for example, in the form of an advance directive, or knowledge of other people about their wishes, such as family members or significant others (Health Professions Council of South Africa 2021b). Other factors to consider include their cultural, religious and employment background, as well as intervention options that 'least restricts the patient's future choices' (Health Professions Council of South Africa 2021b, p. 10).

While occupational therapists will not regularly be called upon to provide input regarding end-of-life decisions, they have an important role to play in promoting and working towards enhancing the quality of life of all their clients, which is a key tenet when determining best interests.

Dual loyalties and paternalism raise the question as to whose interests are being served (Ellis 1996; Beauchamp & Childress 2019; Dhai & McQuoid-Mason 2020). The Life Esidimeni tragedy provides some examples of dual loyalties and paternalism. Family members' concerns about moving the MHCUs into community-based facilities were discounted by paternalistic officials who because of their supposedly superior training and knowledge and their governmental authoritative positions, were in an authoritative position to decide what was in the best interests of these chronically ill and incapacitated patients (Beauchamp & Childress 2019; Dhai & McQuoid-Mason 2020). Healthcare practitioners, such as psychiatrists, who were employed by the Provincial health department were placed in a position of dual loyalties – needing to advocate for patients' rights and best interests but needing to toe the company line or lose their jobs (Dhai & McQuoid-Mason 2020). Occupational therapy students who questioned the move and tried to advocate for the patients (Politics Web 2017) were accused by officials at facility-based meetings that they were only interested in losing a clinical practice learning placement and thus were advocating for their own interests rather than patients'. It is therefore important when determining patients' best interests, that occupational therapists and other decision-makers are clear and document the various role-players who were consulted about a person's best interests, especially when that person has diminished capacity and cannot advocate for themselves.

Non-Maleficence

To some beneficence incorporates non-maleficence (Council for the International Organizations of Medical Sciences 2002), but others such as Beauchamp and Childress describe non-maleficence as a separate ethical principle because they view the obligation not to harm someone (non-maleficence) as different from the obligation to help others (beneficence) (Beauchamp and Childress 2019). Importantly, according to Beauchamp and Childress, the duty to avoid harm includes the duty to avoid the risk of causing harm. This is notable because placing someone at risk of harm often is unintentional, but usually can (and should) be avoided. An important standard that is related to non-maleficence, is that of duty of care. This standard holds that there is a duty to take the necessary due care to avoid causing harm and risk of harm. Negligence is a consequence of failing to meet the standard of duty of care. In bioethics, negligence can arise from intentionally taking an unnecessary risk (i.e. being reckless) or from unintentionally placing a patient at risk of harm (Beauchamp & Childress 2019), but caselaw presents other measures for negligence, for example failing to meet the due care that a reasonable person in the same position as the practitioner (or student-practitioner) would have taken (reasonable man test).

Another important consideration regarding non-maleficence is that of nontreatment decisions. This is usually presented in the light of withholding or withdrawing life-sustaining treatment for persons in a PVS. This rarely applies to occupational therapy, but there are examples of practitioners who choose not to treat some psychiatric clients because they are too psychotic or low functioning, or practitioners are afraid of MHCUs or feel ill-equipped. When making a decision to withhold treatment, occupational therapists should consider that depriving another person of the 'goods of life' (Beauchamp & Childress 2019, p. 159) also breaches the duty not to harm someone.

Justice

The principle of justice takes on a broader lens than merely looking at how an individual should be treated. Instead, it considers whether people as members of a society, or particular group (e.g. pregnant women accessing public healthcare) are treated fairly (Beauchamp & Childress 2019; Dhai & McQuoid-Mason 2020).

Typically in medical ethics, justice is primarily described in terms of distributive justice. However, it has been argued that justice has three obligations: legal justice, rights-based justice and distributive justice (Moodley *et al.* 2017), but a fourth approach is described, that is justice as a capabilities approach.

Legal Justice Legal justice requires practitioners to respect morally acceptable laws. In this sense, practitioners need to have a fair understanding of laws that affect healthcare service-delivery (Moodley *et al.* 2017). In this text, it is not possible to describe these in detail, but the framework is described in Table 4.1. Helps practitioners to understand and apply legal justice to their own countries/contexts.

Rights-based Justice Rights-based justice is concerned with entitlements, and importantly also the nexus between rights and obligations/duties. Rights are valuable and create duties. The right to healthcare, for example, creates a number of duties. Healthcare practitioners have a duty to provide competent healthcare services to patients to allow them to exercise their right to healthcare. Patients have a duty to follow the instructions of healthcare providers (i.e. comply with prescribed treatment), and to maintain whatever health records they have in their possession. Governments must provide a health system that (progressively) allows access to healthcare services to the whole population (Moodley *et al.* 2017).

Distributive Justice Distributive justice is concerned with ensuring that the benefits and risks/burdens in research and/or healthcare are equally distributed (Council for the International Organizations of Medical Sciences 2002; Beauchamp & Childress 2019; Dhai & McQuoid-Mason 2020).

In this sense, then, it is concerned with ensuring that scarce healthcare resources are fairly allocated. From an occupational therapy perspective, this means that practitioners in the public sector particularly, must be mindful, and careful, of how they spend their resources and budgets. Occupational therapists need to ensure that the largest number of (mental) healthcare users will benefit from occupational therapy services and activities, and thus avoid acquiring expensive activities/resources that will only benefit a small proportion of healthcare users served in a particular facility.

Capability Theory of Justice The difficulty with the bioethics perspective and the four principles is that it poorly accounts for pluralism. Autonomy, non-maleficence and beneficence are essentially individual rights, and the principle of justice does not adequately account for fairness across groups – while it is good for people within a group to be treated fairly, how does justice ensure that various groups are treated fairly and equally/equitably? Take a two-tiered health system, such as that of South Africa, for example. Roughly 80% of the South

African population is served by the public health system, which only receives about 20% of the funding in the country that is spent on healthcare. The remainder of the 20% of the population access the private healthcare sector, which receives the other 80% of healthcare expenditure. While rights-based justice and even distributive justice will ensure that people accessing the public health system have equitable access to services in the public sector, it does not account for ensuring distributive justice for all people accessing all healthcare in South Africa. This is not unique to South Africa but illustrates the limitations of bioethics in pluralistic societies and in the global context.

Another ethics theory that arose from the recognition that there is a need to practice global ethics, which transcends cultural, religious, ethnic, gender, race, class, sexuality, global location, historical experience, environmental and even nationalist borders, is the capabilities approach. Two main theorists, Amartya Sen and Martha Nussbaum, are the proponents of this approach.

Essentially, the capabilities approach differs from other ethical approaches, such as utilitarianism which focuses on subjective well-being, by focusing on 'the moral significance of individuals' capability of achieving the kind of lives they have reason to value' (Kleist n.d.).

While an understanding of the four principles of bioethics is important to assist occupational therapists in communicating with other healthcare practitioners, Nussbaum's list of central capabilities enhances our vocabulary because it is a much better natural fit to the ethos and episteme of occupational therapy (see Box 4.2).

SOLVING ETHICO-LEGAL DILEMMAS

It is inevitable that ethical dilemmas will occur. The preceding sections of this chapter presented a broad overview of relevant legal, human rights, professional and ethical theoretical knowledge, which will be used in a step-wise, procedural framework, adapted from the HPCSA (2021) and Moodley (2017) (Table 4.5) to solve the ethico-legal questions arising from the case of Mr Bhengu. It is important to reiterate that the preceding information is not context-specific; thus, it is imperative that students and practitioners consult local, contextual sources for specific legislative and regulatory prescriptions.

BOX 4.2   NUSSBAUM'S JUSTICE AS CAPABILITIES

Among philosophers who influenced Nussbaum, she recognises Karl Marx, whose ideas about human occupation have influenced occupational therapy also (see, e.g. Drolet [2014]). Nussbaum describes 10 human capabilities, which are essential for human functioning and justice serves to realise the potential of these capabilities into actual functioning.

1. *Life:* Capability to live to the end of a normal length human life, living a life that is worth living, that is with quality of life.
2. *Bodily health:* Capability of good health, through accessing adequate housing, participating in employment, accessing good quality nourishing food.
3. *Bodily integrity:* Being able to move freely and safely from place to place (which means being free from violence/assault, and also having opportunities for sexual satisfaction, having occupational justice).
4. *Senses, imagination and thought:* Able to use one's senses to imagine, think and reason in a 'truly human way'– informed by an adequate education. Furthermore, the ability to produce self-expressive works and engage in religious rituals without fear of political ramifications. The ability to have pleasurable experiences and avoid unnecessary pain. Finally, the ability to seek the meaning of life.
5. *Emotions:* Able to have attachments to things outside of ourselves; this includes being able to love others, grieve at the loss of loved ones and be angry when it is justified.
6. *Practical reason:* Able to form a conception of the good and critically reflect on it.

7. *Affiliation:*
   A. Able to live with and show concern for others, empathise with (and show compassion for) others and the capability of justice and friendship. Institutions help develop and protect forms of affiliation.
   B. Able to have self-respect and not be humiliated by others, that is, being treated with dignity and equal worth. This entails (at the very least) protections against being discriminated on the basis of race, sex, sexuality, religion, caste, ethnicity and nationality. In work, this means entering relationships of mutual recognition.
8. *Other species:* Able to have empathy for and live with other animals, plants and the environment at large; to improve one's spirituality.
9. *Play:* Able to laugh, play and enjoy recreational activities.
10. *Control over one's environment:*
    A. *Political:* Able to effectively participate in the political life, which includes having the right to free speech and association. To speak up for yourself.
    B. *Material:* Able to own property, not just on paper, but materially (that is, as a real opportunity, thus being able to live as independently as possible in your own environment). Furthermore, having the ability to seek employment on an equal basis as others, to participate in employment as independently as possible with or without reasonable accommodations.

Source: Adapted from Mousavi *et al.* (2015).

Table 4.5   Step-wise framework to solve ethical dilemmas.

Step-wise framework	Application to the case
1. The problem • Identify and formulate the problem. Consider whether there is a better/different way of understanding it.	• Mrs Bhengu wants the occupational therapist to breach Mr Bhengu's privacy and confidentiality by sharing information about his care, treatment and rehabilitation.
2. Information • Gather all the relevant information (clinical, personal, social etc.) data.	Scientific and medical information Mr Bhengu suffers from PTSD. The most recent incident triggered flashbacks and nightmares. Legal information Mr Bhengu is an adult. Mr Bhengu has not been found to lack the capacity to make decisions. The psychiatric hospital must adhere to the POPI Act, thus needing his consent to *inter alia* share information with other parties, e.g. his mother. Mr Bhengu is a voluntary MHCU. Ethical information Healthcare practitioners must act in their best interests. Mr Bhengu has the right to being respected as a person, including his choices about practitioners.
3. Analyse the information Weigh the ethical content of each option by asking questions such as: • Which of the rights, legal duties and principles best give effect to the MHCU's best interests? • Which of the rights, legal duties and principles allow the MHCU to express their cultural and socioeconomic rights and needs?	• Mr Bhengu has the right to privacy. • Mr Bhengu has the right to care treatment and rehabilitation. • Mr Bhengu has the right to care that considers his culture and his ability to engage with values, including traditional healing, that give expression to his identity as a Zulu male. • Although Mrs Bhengu is paying for her son's care, that does not entitle her to directing the care and she must respect her son's rational, informed decisions even though she disagrees with him.
4. Options • Consider all reasonable options, choices or actions in the circumstances	• Consider having Mr Bhengu transferred to the public psychiatric hospital where the occupational therapists collaborate with a THP. • Ask Mr Bhengu to consider allowing you to share some information about his care, treatment and rehabilitation with his mother. He must be explicit about what you may and may not share. • Continue treating Mr Bhengu with Western methods only, thus refusing his request to involve a THP in his care. • Collaborate with the occupational therapists at the public hospital and start incorporating some of the intervention approaches they have learnt from the THP. • Recommend a support group for Mrs Bhengu for families affected by suicide.
5. Moral assessment Weigh the ethical/legal content of each option by asking: • What are the likely consequences of each option? • What are the most important values, duties, and rights? Which weighs the heaviest? • What are the weaknesses of your view? • How would you want to be treated in the circumstances of the case? That is, apply the *Golden Rule* (always do good and avoid harm)	• Sharing Mr Bhengu's information not only is a breach of POPIA in the South African context, but will also damage your therapeutic rapport and therapeutic alliance with him. • Not considering the possibility of collaborating with a THP denies Mr Bhengu the right to have culturally sensitive care, treatment and rehabilitation. • Transfer to the public hospital means that he is able to access more affordable care that is likely also more culturally sensitive to Mr Bhengu's needs. However, there are currently no available beds. • One weakness of the view to allow the THP to engage is that Mr Bhengu's and his mother's values are clashing; thus, it might result in friction in their relationship. THPs can be expensive, but he is on paid sick leave and could be able to afford at least a couple of sessions to ease his mind.

Table 4.5 *(Continued)*

Step-wise framework	Application to the case
6. Discuss • Discuss your proposed solution with those whom it will affect (e.g. the MHCU)	• Invite Mrs Bhengu to a family meeting with MR Bhengu and the MDT in which boundaries regarding care, treatment and rehabilitation are reaffirmed. • Since there is no space at the public hospital, collaborate with Mr Bhengu and the occupational therapists from the public hospital regarding more culturally sensitive interventions. Facilitate telephonic consultations with the THP in the interim.
7. Act • Act on your decision with sensitivity to others affected	• Remain sensitive to Mrs Bhengu's role in her son's life, but be firm about legal and professional boundaries.

8. Evaluate
 	
  • Did the solution result in upholding the MHCU's best interests?
 	
  • Did the case result in the need for a policy change at the facility? Whose responsibility is it to formulate or amend policies at the institution?
 	
  • Are there standardised information/documents that could flow from this solution, e.g. educational videos, new/amended information sheets and informed consent forms?
	• What must the occupational therapy department at your hospital do in future regarding THP involvement in care?
	
	• Are the hospital's policy documents regarding privacy clear enough?

CASE STUDY   MR BHENGU

Mr Bhengu is a 38-year-old former policeman. He resigned from the South African Police Services after he found that his diagnosis of Post-Traumatic Stress Disorder (PTSD) affected his ability to be promoted. He started working at a private security company, Cobra Security Services (Cobra) as a reaction officer. Cobra renders services such as neighbourhood patrols and armed response services to an affluent neighbourhood in the north of Johannesburg, a big city in South Africa. A reaction officer is an armed security officer who accompanies a patrol vehicle and enters residential or commercial premises to whom Cobra is contracted to render security services when an alarm on the premises is triggered.

Approximately six months ago, Mr Bhengu sustained compound fractures of his right femur when his patrol vehicle collided with the 'get-away car' used by suspected robbers following an armed robbery at a local shopping centre to which Cobra renders services. Although his femur healed well and he is able to walk as before, he is plagued by nightmares and flashbacks, not only of this incident, but others from his days in the police services as well. He returned to work three months ago and is still on desk-duty.

After he was discharged from the orthopaedic hospital, he went to stay with his mother, a 65-year-old retired theatre nurse, who was to help him with his wound care post-discharge. Four weeks ago, Mr Bhengu attempted suicide by overdosing on prescription painkillers because the nightmares were causing him considerable distress. This was his second attempt since the accident. After being medically stabilised, he agreed to be admitted to a private psychiatric hospital. You are his treating occupational therapist.

Understandably, Mrs Bhengu is very worried about her son and calls you, the occupational therapist, demanding that you share all the details of her son's current admission, treatment and prognosis with her. She is responsible for most of the costs of this admission because his medical aid (insurance) benefits have been depleted. Mr Bhengu refuses to provide consent, but Mrs Bhengu is worried that he will attempt suicide again after discharge and feels she is entitled to information because she is helping to pay for his treatment.

Mr Bhengu, who has been investigating traditional health practitioners (THP) as an option to help him deal with the nightmares, wants to know if you are willing to work with a THP to help with his sleep. You know that the occupational therapist at a Johannesburg-based public psychiatric facility does work with a THP. When Mrs Bhengu, who is a devout Christian, gets wind of her son's enquiries about traditional healing, she phones you again, adamant that he must not get involved in what she feels is un-Christian care and demands that her pastor be allowed to attend to him for healing prayers and religious counselling.

How do you handle Mrs Bhengu's demands and requests? What choices do you make regarding Mr Bhengu's enquiries about traditional healing?

CONCLUSION

Healthcare practice is becoming increasingly regulated. Through a framework (Figure 4.2) based on the interrelationship between morality, (societal) values, worldview, human rights and law, this chapter has provided an overview of the concepts related to a legislative framework, human rights, professionalism, ethics and morality to help occupational therapy practitioners identify the nature of the dilemma they face and how to go about solving them.

REFERENCES

CASE LAW

Ahmad Shah Ayubi v Bezirkshauptmannschaft Linz-Land Case C-713/7 (Court of Justice of the European Union, 21 November 2018)

Castell v De Greef 1994 (4) SA 408(C)

Equal Education v Minister of Basic Education [2018] ZAECBHC 6; 2019 (1) SA 421 (ECB)

Gillick vs West Norfolk and Wisbech Area Health Authority [1984] QB 581, [1984] 1 All ER 365; on appeal [198] AC 112, [1985] 1 All ER 533; review [1986] AC 112, [1985] 3 All ER 402 (HL)

Greunen and Another v McGovern (5395/2022)[2023] ZAFSHC 104

Khosa and Others v Minister of Social Development and Others, Mahlaule and Another v Minister of Social Development and Others (CCT 13/03, CCT 12/03) [2004] ZACC 11; 2004 (6) SA 505 (CC); 2004 (6) BCLR 569 (CC) (4 March 2004)

Richter and another v Estate Hamman 1976 (3) SA 226 (C)

Tripartite Steering Committee v Minister of Basic Education [2015] ZAEC-GHC 67; 2015 (5) SA 107 (ECG)

TABLE OF LEGISLATION

South Africa. Children's Act no 38 of 2005

South Africa. Choice on Termination of Pregnancy Act no 92 of 1996

South Africa. Competition Act no 89 of 1998

South Africa. Constitution of South Africa. Act no 108 of 1996

South Africa. Consumer Protection Act no 68 of 2008

South Africa. Employment Equity Act 55 of 1998

South Africa. Health Professions Act no 56 of 1974

South Africa. Labour Relations Act no 66 of 1995

South Africa. Mental Healthcare Act no 17 of 2002

South Africa. National Health Act no 61 of 2003

South Africa. Promotion of Access to Information Act no 2 of 2000

South Africa. Promotion of Equality and Prevention of Unfair Discrimination Act no 4 of 2000

South Africa. Protection of Personal Information Act no 4 of 2013

REFERENCES

Alberta College of Occupational Therapists (2019) *Standards of practice.* https://doi.org/10.2307/30146882

Beauchamp, T.L. & Childress, J.F. (2019) *Principles of Biomedical Ethics,* 8th, edn. Oxford University Press, Oxford.

Bras Gomes, V. (2020) The right to work and rights at work. In: J. Dugard, B. Porter, D. Ikawa & L. Chenwi (eds), *Research Handbook on Economic, Social and Cultural Rights as Human Rights,* pp. 227–249. Edward Elgar Publishing, Cheltenham.

Burns, Y. (2013) *Administrative Law,* 4th edn. LexisNexis, Durban.

Committee on Economic Social and Cultural Rights (1991) *General comment no. 4.* Geneva. https://tbinternet.ohchr.org/_layouts/15/treatybodyexternal/Download.aspx?symbolno=INT%2FCESCR%2FGEC%2F4759&Lang=en (accessed 22 April 2023)

Committee on Economic Social and Cultural Rights (1999) *General comment no. 12.* Geneva. https://tbinternet.ohchr.org/_layouts/15/treatybodyexternal/Download.aspx?symbolno=E%2FC.12%2F1999%2F5&Lang=en (accessed 22 April 2023)

Committee on Economic Social and Cultural Rights (2000) *General comment no. 14.* Geneva. https://doi.org/10.2307/2752479

Council for the International Organizations of Medical Sciences (2002) *International Ethical Guidelines for Biomedical Research Involving Human Subjects.* Council for the International Organizations of Medical Sciences, Geneva.

Crouch, R. (ed) (2016) *OTASA - A Remarkable Story.* Shorten Publishers, Cape Town.

Currie, I. & De Waal, J. (2013) *The Bill of Rights Handbook.* 6th edn. Juta & Company Ltd, Cape Town.

De Albuquerque, C. & Roaf, V. (2020) The human rights to water and sanitation. In: J. Dugard, B. Porter, D. Ikawa & L. Chenwi (eds), *Research Handbook on Economic, Social and Cultural Rights as Human Rights,* pp. 202–226. Edward Elgar Publishing, Cheltenham.

Dhai, A. (2017) After Life Esidimeni: true human rights protections or lip service to the constitution? *South African Journal of Bioethics and Law,* **10**(1), 2–3. https://doi.org/10.7196/sajbl.542

Dhai, A. & McQuoid-Mason, D.J. (2020) *Bioethics, Human Rights and Health Law: Principles and Practice,* 2nd edn. Juta & Company Ltd., Cape Town.

Drolet, M.J. (2014) The axiological ontology of occupational therapy: a philosophical analysis. *Scandinavian Journal of Occupational Therapy,* **21**(1), pp. 2–10. https://doi.org/10.3109/11038128.2013.831118

Dugard, J., Porter, B., Ikawa, D. & Chenwi, L. (eds) (2020) *Research Handbook on Economic, Social and Cultural Rights as Human Rights.* Edward Elgar Publishing, Cheltenham.

Du Plessis, L.M. (1999) *An Introduction to Law.* 3rd edn. Juta & Company Ltd., Cape Town.

Ellis, P. (1996) Exploring the concept of acting "in the patient's best interests". *British Journal of Nursing*, **5**(17), 1072–1074. https://doi.org/10.12968/bjon.1996.5.17.1072

Ferlito, B.A. & Dhai, A. (2017) The Life Esidimeni tragedy: a human-rights perspective. *South African Journal of Bioethics and Law*, **10**(2), 52–54. https://doi.org/10.7196/sajbl.2017.v10i2.00627

Ferlito, B.A. & Dhai, A. (2018) The Life Esidimeni tragedy: some ethical transgressions. *South African Medical Journal*, **108**(3), 157. https://doi.org/10.7196/SAMJ.2018.v108i3.13012

Gordon, J.-S. (n.d.) *Bioethics*. Internet Encyclopedia of Philosophy. https://iep.utm.edu/bioethics/ (accessed on 11 April 2023)

Grobler, G. & Van Staden, W. (2022) Algorithmic assessments in deciding on voluntary, assisted or involuntary psychiatric treatment. *Diagnostics*, **12**(8), 1–12. https://doi.org/10.3390/diagnostics12081806

Health Professions Council of South Africa (2021a) *General Ethical Guidelines for the Healthcare Professions. Booklet 1.* HPCSA, Pretoria. https://www.hpcsa.co.za/Uploads/professional_practice/ethics/Booklet_1_Guidelines_for_Good_Practice_vDec_2021.pdf (accessed 10 March 2024)

Health Professions Council of South Africa (2021b) *Seeking patients' informed consent, the ethical considerations booklet 4.* https://www.hpcsa.co.za/Uploads/professional_practice/ethics/Booklet_4_Informed_Consent_vDec_2021.pdf (accessed 10 March 2024)

Health Professions Council of South Africa (2022) *Guidelines on the Keeping of Patient Records, Booklet 9.* HPCSA, Pretoria. http://www.hpcsa.co.za (accessed 10 March 2024)

Health Professions Council of South Africa (2023) *Ethical Rules of Conduct for Practitioners Registered under the Health Professions Act 1974.* Health Professions Council of South Africa, Pretoria. https://www.hpcsa.co.za/Content/upload/professional_practice/ethics/ETHICAL_RULES_OF_CONDUCT_FOR_REGISTERED_HEALTH_PRACTITIONERS.pdf (accessed 10 March 2024)

Hordichuk, C.J., Robinson, A.J. & Sullivan, T.M. (2015) Conceptualising professionalism in occupational therapy through a Western lens. *Australian Occupational Therapy Journal*, **62**(3), 150–159. https://doi.org/10.1111/1440-1630.12204

Hossain, M., Tasnim, S., Sultana, A. *et al* (2020) Epidemiology of mental health problems in COVID-19: a review. *F1000Research*, **9**, 636. https://doi.org/10.12688/f1000research.24457.1

Kleist, C. (n.d.) *Global ethics: capabilities approach.* https://iep.utm.edu/ge-capab/#H2 (accessed 6 May 2023)

Lauren, P.G. (2011) *The Evolution of International Human Rights Visions Seen*, 3rd edn. University of Pennsylvania Press, Philadelphia.

Letseka, M.M. & Ganya, W. (2017) African philosophy and medical ethics. In: *Medical Ethics, Law and Human Rights: A South African Perspective*, 2nd edn, pp. 41–51. Van Schaik Publishers, Pretoria.

Moodley, K. (2017) Resolving ethical dilemmas: an approach to decision making. In: K. Moodley (ed), *Medical Ethics, Law and Human Rights: A South African Perspective*, 2nd edn, pp. 183–197. Van Schaik Publishers, Pretoria.

Moodley, K., Moosa, R. & Kling, S. (2017) Justice. In: K. Moodley (ed), *Medical Ethics, Law and Human Rights: A South African Perspective*, 2nd edn, pp. 91–104. Van Schaik Publishers, Pretoria.

Mousavi, T., Forwell, S., Dharamsi, S. & Dean, E. (2015) Do Nussbaum's ten central human functional capabilities extend occupational thera-py's construct of occupation? A narrative review. *New Zealand Journal of Occupational Therapy*, **62**(1), 21–27.

Nortjé, N. & De Jongh, J. (2017) Professionalism - a case for medical education to honour the societal contract. *South African Journal of Occupational Therapy*, **47**(2), 41–44. https://doi.org/10.17159/231-3833/1017/v47n2a7

Occupational Therapy Board of Australia (2018) *Occupational therapy competency standards.* https://www.occupationaltherapyboard.gov.au/documents/default.aspx?record=WD18%2F24856&dbid=AP&chksum=R3g7rsrtvyNroIMQcl%2BESQ%3D%3D (accessed 20 May 2023)

Occupational Therapy Board of New Zealand (2022) *Competencies for registration and continuing practice for occupational therapists.* https://www.otboard.org.nz/wp-content/uploads/2018/01/Competencies-Handbook.pdf (accessed 20 May 2023)

Politics Web (2017) *Life Esidimeni: the wits students' warning to Makhura & Co.* Politics Web Newsletter, 12 February. https://www.politicsweb.co.za/documents/life-esidimeni-the-wits-students-warning-to-makhur (accessed 10 March 2024)

Risse, M. (2021) The fourth generation of human rights: epistemic rights in digital lifeworlds. *Moral Philosophy and Politics*, **8**(2), 351–378. https://doi.org/10.1515/mopp-2020-0039

Robertson, D. (2004) *A Dictionary of Human Rights.* Europa Publications, London and New York. https://doi.org/10.4324/9780203486887

Royal College of Occupational Therapists (2021) *Professional standards for occupational therapy practice, conduct and ethics.* Royal College of Occupational Therapists UK. https://www.rcot.co.uk/publications/professional-standards-occupational-therapy-practice-conduct-and-ethics (accessed 10 March 2024)

Saunders, K.E. (2020) Considerations in the assessment of capacity. *Medicine*, **48**(10), 680–682. https://doi.org/10.1016/J.MPMED.2020.07.003

Sepulveda, M. (2020) The rights to social security. In: J. Dugard, B. Porter, D. Ikawa & L. Chenwi (eds), *Research Handbook on Economic, Social and Cultural Rights as Human Rights*, pp. 89–112. Edward Elgar Publishing, Cheltenham.

Sharp, M. (2014) *A critical analysis of the role of the boni mores in the South African law of contract and its implications in the constitutional dispensation.* University of KwaZulu-Natal. https://ukzn-dspace.ukzn.ac.za/bitstream/handle/10413/13591/Sharp_Marie_2014.pdf?sequence=1&isAllowed=y#:~:text=boni%20mores%20was%20said%20to,the%20morals%20of%20the%20community.&text=Aquilius%20stated%20that%20morals%20have,became%20crystallised%20into%20legal%20principles (accessed on 7 April 2023)

Shemilt, J. 2022 *Tracing the portrayal of mental disorders in literature over time, through five books.* CrimeReads. https://crimereads.com/mental-disorders-in-literature/ (accessed on 10 April 2023)

Singh, J.A. (2017) Law and the health professional in South Africa. In: K. Moodley (ed), *Medical Ethics, Law and Human Rights: A South African Perspective.* 2nd edn, pp. 129–165. Van Schaik Publishers, Pretoria.

Slabbert, M.N. (2004) Parental access to minors' health records in the South African health care context: concerns and recommendations. *Potchefstroom Electronic Law Journal*, **7**(2), 21. https://doi.org/10.17159/1727-3781/2004/v7i2a2854

Snider, C.J. & Flaherty, M.P. (2020) Stigma and mental health: the curious case of COVID-19. *Mental Health: Global Challenges Journal* **3**(1), 27–32. https://doi.org/10.32437/mhgcj.v3i1.89

South African Depression and Anxiety Group (SADAG) (2023) *Life Esidimeni*. Never Again. https://www.lifeesidimeni.org.za/ (accessed 10 March 2024)

United Nations (1966) *International covenant on economic, social and cultural rights.* https://doi.org/10.4324/9781315236674-25

United Nations (1991) *Principles for the protection of persons with mental illness and the improvement of mental health care.* General Assembly Resolution 49/119. New York. https://doi.org/10.1163/9789004479890_025

United Nations (2006) *Convention on the rights of persons with disabilities.* https://treaties.un.org/doc/Publication/CTC/Ch_IV_15.pdf (accessed 22 April 2023)

United Nations Economic and Social Council (1985) *Siracusa principles on the limitation and derogation provisions in the international covenant on civil and political rights.* U.N. Doc. E/CN.4/1985/4, Annex.

United Nations General Assembly (1948) *The Universal Declaration of Human Rights.* United Nations General Assembly, New York.

United Nations General Assembly (1966) *International covenant on civil and political rights.* Geneva. https://www.ohchr.org/sites/default/files/ccpr.pdf (accessed on 22 April 2023)

Van der Zeijst, M., Veiling, W., Makhathini, E. M. *et al* (2021) Ancestral calling, traditional health practitioner training and mental illness: an ethnographic study from rural KwaZulu-Natal, South Africa. *Transcultural Psychiatry*, **58**(4), 471–485. https://doi.org/10.1177/1363461520909615

Van Niekerk, A. (2017) Ethics and philosophy. In: K. Moodley (ed), *Medical Ethics, Law and Human Rights: A South African Perspective*, 2nd edn, pp. 7–17. Van Schaik Publishers, Hatfield.

Van Niekerk, M. (2019) Providing claimants with access to information: a comparative analysis of the POPIA, PAIA and HPCSA guidelines. *South African Journal of Bioethics and Law*, **12**(1), 32–37. https://doi.org/10.7196/sajbl.2019.v12i1.00656

Van Niekerk, M. (2021) Promotion of access to information act: key issues for occupational therapists. *South African Journal of Occupational Therapy*, **51**(2), 4–10. https://doi.org/10.17159/2310-3833/2021/vol51n2a2

Van Niekerk, M., Dladla, A. & Gumbi, N. (2014) Perceptions of the traditional health practitioner's role in the management of mental health care users and occupation: a pilot study. *South African Journal of Occupational Therapy* http://www.scielo.org.za/scielo.php?script=sci_arttext&pid=S2310-38332014000100005 (accessed on 10 March 2024)

Van Niekerk M. 2024. *Unpublished PhD research proposal.* University of the Witwatersrand. Johannesburg. Used with permission.

Veriava, F. & Paterson, K. (2020) The right to education. In: J. Dugard, B. Porter, D. Ikawa & L. Chenwi (eds), *Research Handbook on Economic, Social and Cultural Rights as Human Rights*, pp. 113–136. Edward Elgar Publishing, Cheltenham.

Wellman, C. (2000) Solidarity, the individual and human rights. *Human Rights Quarterly*, **22**(3), 639–657. https://doi.org/10.1353/hrq.2000.0040

White House Office of Science and Technology Policy (2022) *Blueprint for an AI bill of rights: making automated systems work for the American people.* Washington DC. https://www.whitehouse.gov/wp-content/uploads/2022/10/Blueprint-for-an-AI-Bill-of-Rights.pdf (accessed 12 August 2023)

Williams, J.R. (2009) The future of medical professionalism. *South African Journal of Bioethics and Law*, **2**(2), 48–50. https://www.ajol.info/index.php/sajbl/article/view/50243 (accessed 10 March 2024)

World Federation of Occupational Therapists [WFOT] (2016) *Minimum standards for the education of occupational therapists revised 2016.* https://wfot.org/resources/new-minimum-standards-for-the-education-of-occupational-therapists-2016-e-copy (accessed 10 March 2024)

World Health Organisation (2020) *Mental health atlas 2020.* Geneva. https://www.who.int/publications/i/item/9789240036703 (accessed 12 August 2023)

Yamin, A.E. (2020) The right to health. In: J. Dugard, B. Porter, D. Ikawa & L. Chenwi (eds), *Research Handbook on Economic, Social and Cultural Rights as Human Rights*, pp. 159–179. Edward Elgar Publishing, Cheltenham.

Enhancing Mental Health and Wellness

A Cultural Approach in the Provision of Occupational Therapy Services in Psychiatry and Mental Health

CHAPTER 5

Rosemary Crouch[1] and Annah Lesunyane[2]

[1]School of Therapeutic Sciences, Faculty of Health Sciences, University of the Witwatersrand, Johannesburg, South Africa

[2]Department of Occupational Therapy, School of Health Care Sciences, Sefako Makgatho Health Sciences University, Pretoria, South Africa

KEY LEARNING POINTS

- Understand culture and how cultural humility can be addressed in occupational therapy.

- Understand considerations of culture and understand the relevance in occupational therapy practice.

- Understand help-seeking behaviour and attitude to mental illness that can occur in different cultures.

- Describe the cultural factors associated with the concept of occupation and performance in the occupational intervention process.

- Describe the cultural factors associated with the use and experience of activities in occupational therapy intervention.

INTRODUCTION

This chapter begins with a description of culture and related concepts. This aims to provide insights into the relevance of understanding these concepts and their implications for occupational therapy practice. The attitudes of different cultures about mental illness and cultural factors associated with occupational therapy intervention are discussed. The chapter concludes by describing how occupational therapists working with people with mental illness can be culturally responsive.

Culture is a core concept in understanding determinants of health, illness experience, and provision of healthcare (Monteiro 2015). Knowledge of health matters, meanings attached to illness, and help-seeking behaviours are learned through cultural backgrounds and teachings. Available literature emphasises how health and illness are perceived in different ways in many cultures (Iwama 2007; Gopalkrishnan 2018).

The field of mental health is a complicated socially constructed area of health concern, which is partly dictated by cultural and religious norms. In mental health, practitioners inevitably encounter clients from cultures other than their own. Mental health issues commonly have a strong cultural connotation that may have adverse effects on the health and well-being of those affected. Although mental illness is universal across cultures, this universality may be hidden by how mental health conditions are understood and interpreted in different cultures. Mental illness carries with it a host of different theories and beliefs, which differ in their conceptualisation of the illness according to societies, groups, cultures, institutions, and professions (Crouch 2014). Cultural diversity as indicated by Gopalkrishnan (2018, p. 2) '. . . has significant impacts on the many aspects of mental health, ranging from how health and illness are perceived, help-seeking behavior, attitudes of clients and practitioners' and mental health systems'.

Crouch and Alers Occupational Therapy in Psychiatry and Mental Health, Sixth Edition.
Edited by Rosemary Crouch, Tania Buys, Enos Morankoana Ramano, Matty van Niekerk and Lisa Wegner.
© 2025 John Wiley & Sons Ltd. Published 2025 by John Wiley & Sons Ltd.

Occupational therapists render services to diverse populations in different multicultural practice settings, including mental health care settings. The need to demonstrate cultural responsiveness when working in cross-cultural settings is a global obligation for healthcare professions including the occupational therapy profession (Sonn & Vermeulen, 2018). The World Federation of Occupational Therapy's (WFOT) Diversity and Culture Position Statement endorses the need for occupational therapists to focus on the cultural diversity, lifestyle, and perspectives of clients receiving occupational therapy services (WFOT 2010). The ethnicity, training, culture, class, political and religious backgrounds of professionals will dictate what intervention, if any, is appropriate and which methods will be applied during treatment. The profession of occupational therapy considers cultural factors in the provision of care, including selection and interpretation of assessment instruments, interpersonal communication, intervention, and outcome expectations (McGruder 2009; Padilla 2015).

UNDERSTANDING CULTURE AND RELATED CONCEPTS

Understanding culture, including how cultural factors can be addressed in occupational therapy practice, is necessary for culturally responsive caring in occupational therapy (Muñoz 2007). Iwama (2007) asserts that culture is a fundamental concept in the occupational therapy profession because occupational therapy services are rendered in diverse contexts. The understanding of culture varies and consensus on a definition is not yet established. The complexity and broadness of the concept pose difficulty in definition; thus, 'culture' cannot be easily defined and may be dependent on the personal perspectives and experiences of an individual (Sonn & Vermeulen, 2018). Iwama (2007, p. 184) states that: 'Culture cannot be universally defined and there are no static, definitive explanations of culture in occupational therapy'. He cautions that understanding culture should be viewed beyond the issues of diversity and inclusion and should include the creation of knowledge, theories and the structures and contents of occupational therapy practices to align with diverse cultural perspectives. Although opinions regarding the importance of various definitions of culture vary, the common understanding is that culture is a learned, intergenerational, patterned, shared experience among a particular group that is localised geographically (Scaffa *et al.* 2010).

Culture is relevant to occupational therapy practice because perceptions of health and illness are determined by it (Whiteford & Wilcock 2000). People attach importance to tasks and norms that are associated with the use of occupations brought on by cultural practices, standards, morals, and ways of life that are different from their own cultural beliefs, for example the value that is attached to occupations such as work and play (Padilla 2015). Culture is viewed as a concept that is made up of an ever-changing awareness of how we view and interpret the world, enabling people to relate to others within their environments (Gopalkrishnan 2018).

Padilla (2015:346) stated that '. . . culture affects performance of occupations in many ways and . . . prescribes norms for the use of time and space, influences beliefs regarding the importance of various tasks, and transmits attitudes and values regarding work and play as well as what people are expected to do at different phases of their lives'.

Occupational therapists need to develop cultural awareness to be sensitive in their practice. Hopton and Stoneley (2006) suggest that cultural awareness involves a three-part process that includes awareness by the occupational therapist of the culture of the client, their own culture, and the particular culture of the occupational therapy profession in the country or area where the practice is situated.

CULTURE IN MENTAL HEALTH AND MENTAL ILLNESS

'Cultures may influence and contribute to the causation of mental illnesses, mould symptoms, render certain sub-groups more vulnerable as well as modify beliefs and explanations of illnesses. This demonstrates that cultural beliefs and values represent a crucial factor in mental illness'. (Bhugra *et al.* 2021, p. 2)

Consideration of culture is important when providing mental health services. The provision of mental health services may be challenged by the relationship between cultural factors and knowledge about mental health issues, especially in developing countries. Cultural awareness and sensitivity are necessary for the provision of all quality health care, but it has particular importance for the mental health field because of the nature of the practice (Grandpierre *et al.* 2018). Perceptions of aetiology and treatment of mental illness can be different across cultures. In Africa and other countries such as India and China, mental health problems are usually understood and perceived within traditional health systems and religious contexts (Crouch 2014; Gopalkrishnan 2018). The mentally ill client may express himself/herself within the cultural norms, for example a paranoid patient from a Western culture may explain that someone is trying to harm him through radar waves or traditional African beliefs may influence a patient who subscribes to the beliefs to presume that he has been bewitched or cursed (Shange & Ross 2022). The onset of mental illness in some cultures may be ascribed to the possession of ancestral spirits, magical powers, and bewitchment or breaking of taboos, thus placing interventions within the responsibility of traditional healers, faith healers, and significant elders within the family or community (Lesunyane 2010; Gopalkrishnan 2018).

Religion and spirituality are central to the interpretation of mental illness experiences within traditional health systems. Gopalkrishnan (2018) states that people experiencing mental health issues often associate the experience of hardships with punishment from a higher order and visit healing temples and religious pilgrimages as a way of finding solutions.

Mental health literacy and interpretation of symptoms complicate the differentiation of the illness experience between physical and mental health. Cultural meanings of mental illness have implications for coping with the illness, patterns of family, and social support networks. These will influence the choice of seeking treatment either from psychiatrists, clinics, religious leaders, or traditional healers. Gopalkrishnan (2018) explains that people from diverse cultures may not make a clear distinction between body and mind health as in Western therapeutic systems, which may influence help-seeking and diagnosis. Biswas *et al.* (2016) observed that in India, those seeking help from mainstream health systems tended to present with somatic symptoms, whereas those in the United States of America (US) tended to present with cognitive symptoms. Research conducted by Nguyen and Bornheimer (2014) in high-income countries including the United States, Australia and Canada reported that these cultures tend to seek treatment much later and present with acute stages of mental distress. This may be attributed to the stigma associated with mental illness as compared to African cultures, which may be influenced by traditional beliefs and perhaps low mental health literacy. Beliefs amongst people may also be influenced by factors such as the socio-economic status, the environment, and the educational standard of a person. Even within the most educated societies, strong traditional beliefs and healing systems can influence a person's perception of mental illness (Padilla 2015). Lesunyane (2010:290) describes clients being 'diagnosed differently by different diagnostic systems', giving the example of a client 'being diagnosed as schizophrenic by the local hospital and the biomedical system, described as bewitched by the traditional healer and possessed by the devil by the Pentecostal church'. This is indeed confusing for all concerned! Lesunyane (2010) also discusses the fact that treatment in Africa is often sought in the following order: the traditional healer, then a church, and lastly, the hospital when the condition is out of control. Language barriers contribute to the difficulties of interpreting what the patient's symptoms and problems are, frequently making a diagnosis difficult.

In countries such as South Africa, psychiatric patients access both indigenous healers and services rendered by psychiatric facilities (Zabow 2007; Musyimi *et al.* 2016). Although the belief that traditional practices may affect the treatment outcomes, it should be noted that traditional practices often serve cultural and therapeutic purposes (Lesunyane 2010). The services practiced by traditional healers include the provision of informal counselling and support in improving family, community or work relationships. These services can help to relieve distress associated with mild symptoms of common mental disorders like depression and anxiety (van Niekerk *et al.* 2014; Musyimi *et al.* 2016).

They therefore should not be disregarded, especially since professional mental health care services are scarce, particularly in a rural community. Indigenous healers are still widely consulted, especially for mental illnesses and some clients still opt for traditional healing even if modernised health care resources are available to them (Zabow 2007; van Niekerk *et al.* 2014). It is therefore important for health care providers to have an understanding of the systems of indigenous healing

(Musyimi *et al.* 2016). Lesunyane (2010) also stresses that Western-trained professionals should recognise good traditional healers and their contribution to dealing with mental health problems within the broader context of the sociocultural context of their clients.

Culture has long been defined with respect to its underlying influence on individual views, or in terms of its artistic or scientific expression. It is, however, unfortunate that culture in today's society is often immediately replaced with the idea of race or ethnicity, as well as the pre-judgments that may accompany those ideas. It is important to note that neither race nor ethnicity is synonymous with culture (Townsend & Polatajko 2007:52). Culture also plays a very important role in the interpretation of the cause of a mental illness. A modern-day approach attributes a mental illness to stress, viruses and chemical causes such as drugs and alcohol, family background, living conditions and genetic disposition (Monteiro 2015). The client and family may attribute mental illness to ancestors' dissatisfaction, witchcraft and magic spells in which hate, envy or jealousy may exist (Mkize 2003). These beliefs often lend comfort to them. People who still believe and practice traditional health beliefs experience these contributing factors as real as modern epidemiology is to health care providers (Musyimi *et al.* 2016). Mkize (2003) affirms that the African view of mental ill health encompasses a wide spectrum of factors including, ancestral influences, folk belief in witchcraft, to modern medical science.

In some cultures, options are not communicated directly, and feelings are not expressed verbally. People are conservative in acting out or talking about their problems, and as a result, body reactions and somatic symptoms are common. Cross-cultural work must be approached with open-mindedness, acceptance, and positive attitude towards different cultures (McGruder 2009). The stigma of mental illness continues to exist in most cultures but is greatly influenced by education and familiarity with the reality and the nature of the illnesses. In some ways, the media has helped in this regard in educational films and programmes. However, in other cases, the media promotes a negative stereotyping of mental illness and reports on crimes as being related to conditions such as personality disorders, conduct disorders in young people, schizophrenia, hypomania and drugs, thereby worsening negative stigmatizing attitudes toward mental illnesses (Crouch 2014). A lack of mental health policy, as well as social stigma, has meant that in much of Africa, mental illness is a hidden issue (Ehiemua 2014; van Niekerk *et al.* 2014). Ignorance and inadequate knowledge about mental illness contribute to abuse, discrimination, and human rights violations both from those in the field of health care and the community. The Mental Health Gap Action Programme (mhGAP) Intervention Guide can act as a guide to the projects that are in place to try to combat this problem (WHO 2019). The intervention guides approaches are directed towards interventions for the prevention and management of priority services for people affected by mental, neurological and substance use (MNS) disorders in low- and middle-income countries (WHO 2019). Ehiemua (2014) points out that stigma and discrimination can exacerbate the suffering and disability associated with mental disorders. Social movements attempting to increase understanding of mental health problems and challenge social exclusion are important advocates for minimizing stigma and creating a more positive focus on mental illnesses.

Hechanova and Waelde (2017) identify five cultural components that have implications for the provision of mental health services, namely:

- Emotional expression and mental distress.

- Shame and stigma affect help-seeking and access to professional help.

- Power relations regarding differences in power that may exist between the clients and practitioners influence clients' autonomy in the therapeutic relationship.

- *Ubuntu* or collectivism as a supportive factor to resilience and coping. '*Ubuntu*' is a concept that emanates from humanist African philosophy and is focused on principles of community survival, a spirit of solidarity, compassion, respect and dignity (Ngubane & Makua 2021).

- Spirituality and religion regarding coping with the illness.

OCCUPATIONAL THERAPY AS RELATED TO CULTURE AND MENTAL ILLNESS

The cornerstone of occupational therapy is 'occupation', and within any occupation, there is a multitude of activities. It is one of the reasons why the profession is intimately involved with the culture with which the client is most familiar. Whether at work, in the home, socialising with others, or at the birth or death of someone in the community, activities are in line with cultural norms, and occupational therapists must recognise the ethnic culture of the person with whom they are working. The use of activity as therapy is very powerful and relates directly to that which is identified to be within that social and cultural context (Lesunyane 2010; AOTA 2020).

In urban areas, occupational therapists in the mental health field may be treating clients from many different cultures; however, when working in a rural community, it is far less complicated because the local people are usually from one culture, and cultural norms are firmly set. One of the earliest proponents of cultural influences in occupational therapy is Hocking (1994). She has researched the subject of the historical impact of objects and occupation on culture and emphasises the meaning of objects rather than the physical manipulation of them. Of great importance is the fact that sharing an activity with a patient is often a basic manner of communication and developing an interpersonal relationship through which treatment is facilitated. Punching a ball of clay with a child with anxiety who does not speak the same language, kneading dough with a disturbed woman from a rural community, and sharing computer knowledge with a depressed businessman are activities that could be culturally appropriate and that facilitate the start of the intervention and also provide information on the functional aspect of the person. Another proponent of cultural influences on occupational therapy intervention is Iwama (2007), who focuses on the subtle and complex cultural beliefs of clients that influence their lives – in other words, the meanings, ideals, and values that they have. His culturally sensitive assessment called the 'Kawa Model' is widely used and accepted in countries across the world.

Another important aspect of cultural awareness is the fact that occupational therapists are trained and socialised into the culture of the society in which they live. This incorporates a set of beliefs, habits, dislikes, norms, and practices. Training may include information regarding health and illness, which varies from the student's background. It is essential for occupational therapy students to be trained in the recognition of cultural norms across a wide spectrum (Govender *et al.*, 2017; Sonn and Vermeulen, 2018), especially in mental health, so that 'the occupations in which the person engages and the amount of time doing the occupation, is very specific to the circumstances and culture in which the person lives' (Lesunyane 2010: 53).

Culture is all-pervasive and impacts occupational therapy practice in multiple ways. Working in different cultures can be rewarding and exciting, as well as confusing and frustrating (Sherry 2010). The occupational therapist needs to have an open mind, despite his/her own beliefs, to provide *useful* care to consumers who retain traditional beliefs (McGruder 2009; Padilla 2015). 'Models for the practice of occupational therapy, such as the Kawa and model of human occupation (Kielhofner 1985; Iwama 2007), urge occupational therapists to include culture as an integral component of the clinical reasoning process, as we consider complex interactions between the individual and the environment. Occupation refers to specific chunks of activity within the ongoing stream of human behaviour which are named in the lexicon of the culture (AOTA 2020). These authors also discuss the cultural influence on occupation stating that the personality of a client and his/her interests and personal experience are important factors, which should be taken into account by the occupational therapist.

HOW TO INCORPORATE CULTURAL RESPONSIVENESS STANDARDS INTO PRACTICE

Occupational therapy training programmes worldwide need to address cultural awareness as part of the intervention in mental health. This is not only because occupational therapists are making a determined shift by moving into the community and rural areas but also because individuals of different cultures are moving into urban areas and, thus, treatment centres.

Canadian Occupational Therapy (CAOT) Position Statement on Occupational Therapy and Cultural Safety (2011) proposes the following to increase cultural humility and sensitivity during therapeutic interactions:

- Occupational therapists embrace a best practice in occupational therapy that seeks to offer effective, client-centred, evidence-based, occupation-focused enablement for health, well-being and justice.

- Occupational therapists embrace a way of thinking that enables a social theory of change through occupational enablement.

The following considerations can also increase cultural sensitivity during interventions (Crouch 2014):

- Use open-ended questions to identify each person's unique cultural outlook.

- Re-evaluate intake and assessment documentation, as well as policies and procedures, to be more inclusive.

- Employ qualified mental health workers who are fluent in the language of the groups being served.

- Understand the cultural biases in programme design.

- Identify resources, such as natural supports, within the community that will help an individual to recover.

- Design and implement culturally sensitive treatment plans.

- Evaluate procedures and programmes for cultural sensitivity and effectiveness.

- Survey clients and workers to elicit their understanding of cultural sensitivity/competence and culturally competent practice.

It is important to acknowledge that the education of a community on mental illness, despite cultural beliefs, is vitally important. It is well recognised that some traditional approaches are successful, but when it comes to severe mental illness and the patient is self-destructive with devastating consequences for both the family and often the community, an educated and well-researched approach to treatment is needed. The development and research into psychotropic medication and the development of alternative medicines to treat mental illness are advanced. These approaches can and must be integrated into cultural dimensions for people so that they can live a life of quality despite mental illness. There is an abundance of literature to underpin this statement. Many people today have the privilege of living a 'normal' life despite having a mental illness. This cannot just be a privilege – it has to become a human rights principle.

CONCLUSION

This chapter highlights the challenging issue of the impact of culture on a person with a mental illness. The treatment of the mentally ill has advanced greatly over the last 10 years and the profession of occupational therapy has advanced even further, putting issues such as competency to the forefront. This chapter also attempts to explore mental health literacy and the differing views across cultures. Issues of stigma and the reasons why people with mental illnesses are treated differently from others and how the effect of stigma impacts them and their rights, continue to be a concern.

On a practical level, occupational therapists need to understand how culture can guide rapport building with clients, and influence assessments, setting of appropriate goals, and intervention planning. The occupational therapist working with a person with a mental illness must embody cultural awareness and sensitivity to provide appropriate support and intervention. Acquiring skills related to cultural humility and awareness is necessary for effectively responding to the clients' needs, respecting their beliefs and upholding their dignity.

CASE STUDY   Scenario 1 (African Rural Community)

Mr A is a 40-year-old highly respected teacher who has been selected to become headmaster of a school in his community. He has a wife and two children: a girl of 11 years old and a boy of 13 years old. His wife is a homemaker; she does not work but is active in the local groups (e.g. church and community projects) on the women's committee.

A month ago, Mr A appeared to have lost motivation and interest in the proposal for this new job. He appeared morose and depressed. He spent all day sitting in his office and not achieving anything. He seldom saw other staff members and went home early. He withdrew from contact with his family contact. He told his wife that he felt severe stress and depression as a result of the selection process for him to become headmaster. At his wife's request, he was visited by a family friend who approached the local healer for assistance.

Mr A has a family history of depressive illness, and his uncle committed suicide recently. The signs have been ignored or not diagnosed in the past, but Mr A's illness was recognised by a friend. She encouraged him to see the healer. As part of the district health service, a team of health professionals works in the area consisting of a doctor, a spiritual healer, a psychiatric nurse, and an occupational therapist. The local spiritual healer knew who Mr A was, gave him locally available traditional medicines, and communicated well with the nurse. The occupational therapist interviewed Mr A and asked him to visit his workplace at the school. He agreed but did not accompany her. She was familiar with the teachers at the school who welcomed her, and she was extremely careful to observe cultural norms by the way she approached them. She waited until she was invited into the school and sat in a small circle with them to discuss the daily events before telling them that she was working with Mr A to return him to work. She briefly discussed the illness of depression and gave them hope that he would recover and return to school. In the same way, she visited his wife. As culturally correct, she sat outside the house until invited in and sat on a grass mat in the house with the mother. She carefully explained the illness and how it could be treated, and what her contribution could be. The occupational therapist provided him with a balanced programme of activities. Mr A's occupational therapy programme consisted of:

- Regular exercise in the form of walking to school every day instead of using the local taxi and playing ball games with his children when they had all returned from school.

- Stress management principles, which the occupational therapist encouraged such as talking about his stresses, taking regular breaks and trying not to isolate himself from others.

- A regular diet of three meals a day.

- Encouragement to join the important men's group of the village, which was headed by the induna (headman).

- Compliance with the routine of traditional medicine given to him and regular meetings with the occupational therapist when she was in the area.

CASE STUDY — Scenario 2 (Generalized Western Traditional Culture)

J is 16 years old and comes from a middle-class Christian urban community. He comes from a strict community where the cultural norms of hard work, sobriety, loyalty, and honesty are strong principles. He has however never felt encouraged, or even noticed much by his family, until he did things wrong. Then, he began to be noticed by his teachers and other pupils. He did not make any friends and became increasingly isolated from others. He then started to smoke marijuana (dagga). After a while, J began to act peculiarly, making strange noises and carrying out mannerisms. As a result, he became ostracised by all of his classmates and also ridiculed by his parents who were unsupportive as they felt culturally that J did not fit into their social environment and ignored him even further. Eventually, the teacher decided that something must be done and after trying to talk to J realised at last that there was a problem. After discussing it with the headmaster, a psychiatrist was consulted, with J's parent's permission. He was diagnosed as Schizophrenic and admitted to a clinic where he was treated in the adolescent section. He was placed on medication. He was then referred to occupational therapy and joined a group of adolescents

from diverse cultures. He was also treated for drug use. It was made clear to him that although in some cultures, the use of marijuana was traditional, it was also very harmful and could be the cause of mental illness. The occupational therapist took a detailed history and with the initial assessment, prepared an occupational therapy home programme for J, which included a balance of sports and educational activities related to his schoolwork. J was referred after discharge to a community clinic for ongoing counselling. From a cultural point of view, treatment had to be in line with his family culture. His ongoing occupational therapy programme consisted of:

- A routine exercise schedule at the local gymnasium and encouragement to join an interest activity group such as a church group or skills group football or art. He was encouraged to join the local Narcotics Anonymous (NA) group.

- Attendance of his mother and father at a local support group for parents of children with mental illness and drug use was also encouraged.

QUESTIONS

1. It is important to take into consideration the culture of a mentally ill patient during the occupational therapy process. Discuss this statement in detail.

2. Explain how culture influences the occupational performance of a mentally ill patient.

3. Activities are generally culturally based. How does this influence occupational therapy intervention?

4. Describe cultural sensitivity and explain why it is important for occupational therapy to address this subject.

REFERENCES

American Occupational Therapy Association [AOTA] (2020) Occupational therapy practice framework: domain and process, 4th edn. *American Journal of Occupational Therapy*, **74 (Suppl. 2)**, 7412410010. https://doi.org/10.5014/ajot.2020.74S2001

Bhugra, D. Watson, C. & Wijesuriya, R. (2021) Culture and mental illness. *International Review of Psychiatry*, **33(1–2)**, 1–2. https://doi.org/10.1080/09540261.2020.1777748

Biswas, J., Gangadhar, B.N. & Keshavan, M. (2016) Cross-cultural variations in psychiatrists' perception of mental illness: a tool for teaching culture in psychiatry. *Asian Journal of Psychiatry*, **23**, 1–7. https://doi.org/10.1016/J.Ajp.2016.05.011

Canadian Occupational Therapy (CAOT) (2011) *Position statement on occupational therapy and cultural safety*. https://caot.ca/document/3701/O%20-%20OT%20and%20Client%20Saftety.pdf (accessed on 28 September 2023)

Crouch, R.B. (2014) Cultural considerations in the provision of an occupational therapy service in mental health. In: R.B. Crouch & V.M. Alers (eds), *Occupational Therapy in Psychiatry and Mental Health*. Wiley Blackwell, Hoboken, New Jersey.

Ehiemua, S. (2014) Mental disorder: mental health remains an invisible problem in Africa. *European Journal of Research and Reflection in Educational Sciences*, **2**(**4**), 11–16.

Gopalkrishnan, N. (2018) Cultural diversity and mental health: considerations for policy and practice. *Frontiers in Public Health*, **6**, 179. https://doi.org/10.3389/fpubh.2018.00179

Govender, P., Mpanza, D.M., Carey, T., Jiyane, K., Andrews, B. & Mashele, S. (2017) Exploring cultural competence amongst occupational therapy students. *Occupational Therapy International*, **2017**, 2179781.

Grandpierre, V., Milloy, V., Sikora, L. Fitzpatrick, E. Thomas, R. & Potter, B. (2018) Barriers and facilitators to cultural competence in rehabilitation services: a scoping review. *BMC Health Services Research*, **18**, 23. https://doi.org/10.1186/S12913-017-2811-1

Hechanova, R. & Waelde, L. (2017) The influence of culture on disaster mental health and psychosocial support interventions in Southeast Asia. *Mental Health, Religion & Culture*, **20**(**1**), 31–44. https://doi.org/10.1080/13674676.2017.1322048

Hocking, C. (1994) The model of interaction between objects, occupation, society and culture. *Journal of Occupational Science*, **1**(**3**), 33–44.

Hopton, K., Stoneley, H. (2006) Cultural awareness in occupational therapy: the Chinese example. *British Journal Of Occupational Therapy*, **69**(**8**), 386–389. https://doi.org/10.1177/030802260606900807

Iwama, M. (2007) Culture and occupational therapy: meeting the challenge of relevance in a global world. *Occupational Therapy International*, **14**, 183–187. https://doi.org/10.1002/Oti.234

Kielhofner, G. (1985) *A Model of Human Occupation – Theory and Application*. Williams and Wilkins, Baltimore.

Lesunyane, A. (2010) Psychiatry and mental health in Africa. The vital role of occupational therapy. In: V. Alers & R. Crouch (eds), *Occupational Therapy: An African Perspective*. Sarah Shorten Publishers, Johannesburg.

Mcgruder, J. (2009) Culture, race, and other forms of human diversity in occupational therapy. In: E.B. Crepeau, E.S. Cohn & B.A. Byt Schell (eds), *Willard & Spackman's Occupational Therapy*, 11th edn. Lippincott Williams & Wilkins, Philadelphia.

Mkize, D.L. (2003) Towards an afrocentric approach to psychiatry. *South African Journal of Psychiatry*, **9**(**1**), 4–6. https://doi.org/10.4102/Sajpsychiatry.V9i1.128

Monteiro, N.M. (2015) Addressing mental illness in Africa: global health challenges and local opportunities. *Community Psychology in Global Perspective*, **1**(**2**), 78–95. https://doi.org/10.1285/I24212113V1I2P78

Muñoz, J.P. (2007) Culturally responsive caring in occupational therapy. *Occupational Therapy International*, **14**, 256–280. Https://doi.org/10.1002/Oti.238

Musyimi, C.W., Mutiso, V.N., Nandoya, E.S. & Ndetei, D.M. (2016) *Journal of Ethnobiology and Ethnomedicine*, **12**(**4**). https://doi.org/10.1186/S13002-015-0075-6

Ngubane, N. & Makua, M. 2021 Ubuntu pedagogy – transforming educational practices in South Africa through an African philosophy: from theory to practice. *Inkanyiso, Journal of Humanities and Social Sciences*, **13**(**1**), 1–12.

Nguyen, D. & Bornheimer, L.A. (2014) Mental health service use types among Asian Americans with a psychiatric disorder: considerations of culture and need. *Journal of Behavioural Health Services Research*, **41**, 520–528. https://doi.org/10.1007/S11414-013-9383-6

Padilla, R. (2015) Environmental factors: culture. In: C. Christiansen C.M. Baum & J.D. Bass (eds), *Occupational Therapy - Performance, Participation, and Well-Being*, 4th edn. Slack Incorporated, New York.

Scaffa, M. E., Reitz, S.M. & Pizzi, A.M. (2010). *Occupational Therapy in the Promotion of Health and Wellness*. F.A. Davis Company, Philadelphia.

Shange, S. & Ross, E. (2022) "The question is not how but why things happen": South African traditional healers' explanatory model of mental illness, its diagnosis and treatment*. *Journal of Cross-Cultural Psychology*, **53**(**5**), 503–521. https://doi.org/10.1177/00220221221077361

Sherry, K. (2010) Culture and cultural competence for occupational therapists in Africa. In: V. lers & R. Crouch (eds), *Occupational Therapy: An African Perspective*. Sarah Shorten Publishers, Johannesburg.

Sonn, I. & Vermeulen, N. (2018) Occupational therapy students' experiences and perceptions of culture during fieldwork education. *South African Journal of Occupational Therapy*, **48**(**1**), 34–39. https://doi.org/10.17159/2310-3833/2017/vol48n1a7

The World Federation of Occupational Therapy (WFOT). (2010). *Diversity and culture position statement*. https://wfot.org/resources/statement-on-occupational-therapy. (accessed on 10 June 2023)

Townsend, E.A. & Polatajko, H.J. (2007) *Enabling Occupational II: Advancing and Occupational Therapy Vision of Health, Well-Being and Justice through Occupation*. Canadian Association of Occupational Therapist Publications, Ottawa.

Van Niekerk, M., Dladla, A., Gumbi, N., Monareng, L. & Thwala, W. (2014) Perceptions of the traditional health practitioner's role in the management of mental health care users and occupation: a pilot study. *South African Journal of Occupational Therapy*, **44**(**1**), 20–24.

Whiteford, G.E. & Wilcock, A.A. (2000) Cultural relativism: occupation and independence reconsidered. *Canadian Journal of Occupational Therapy*, **67**(**5**), 324–335.

World Health Organisation. (2019). *Intervention guide mental health gap action programme (mhgap) for mental, neurological and substance use disorders in non-specialized health settings*. https://www.Who.Int/Publications/I/Item/9789241549790h (accessed on 10 August 2023)

Zabow, T. 2007 Traditional healers and mental health in South Africa. *International Psychiatry*, **4**(**4**), 81–83.

CHAPTER 6

Clinical Reasoning in Psychiatric Occupational Therapy

Matty van Niekerk and Tania Rauch van der Merwe

Department of Occupational Therapy, School of Therapeutic Sciences, University of the Witwatersrand, Johannesburg, South Africa

KEY LEARNING POINTS

- Clinical reasoning encompasses clinical decision-making and clinical problem-solving.

- Clinical reasoning is a set of capabilities, both personal and professional, that an occupational therapist develops and hones over their lifetime.

- Clinical reasoning is affected by the knowledge bases and philosophy of occupational therapy, as well as one's worldview, professional knowledge and skill.

- The ability to communicate the results of one's clinical reasoning (e.g. clinical decisions) to others inside and outside of the profession (i.e. epistemic fluency) is a crucial skill.

- Critical thinking ability helps to develop clinical reasoning ability.

INTRODUCTION

Clinical reasoning (also referred to as professional reasoning) is arguably the most important critical thinking skill any healthcare practitioner must possess to accurately diagnose a client and to plan, provide/direct and reflect on appropriate, client-centred intervention (Garcia *et al.* 2021). Several personal, cognitive and psychosocial abilities underpin a practitioner's clinical reasoning ability (Alers 2014), including critical thinking, resilience and reflectivity/reflexivity, decision-making and problem solving. Clinical reasoning is also underpinned by professional knowledge and skills, such as communication (both with healthcare practitioners from various professional backgrounds, and laypersons such as clients and their families), cultural and contextual awareness, clinical judgement and evidence-based practice (Higgs *et al.* 2019). Clinical reasoning ability is not a static, once-off skill one acquires. Life experience as well as clinical experience improves a practitioner's clinical reasoning ability over the span of their career (Alers 2014).

WHAT IS CLINICAL REASONING?

Much has been written about clinical reasoning in occupational therapy literature, to such an extent that multiple systematic reviews of clinical reasoning have been possible over the last 10 years or so (Unsworth 2013; Unsworth & Baker 2016; Márquez-Álvarez *et al.* 2019). As Unsworth (2013, 2021) pointed out, conciseness is hard to achieve when trying to define clinical reasoning. Rather than producing yet another definition of clinical reasoning, this chapter will use a composition of various definitions in the literature, to highlight the elements of clinical reasoning ability.

'Clinical reasoning is a habitual and judicious process used by occupational therapists when interacting with significant others (such as the client, caregivers, family members and other members of the client's personal support system, other members of the health/multidisciplinary team), to collect information and to develop an understanding of the client's needs. This enables the occupational therapist to plan, direct, perform, and reflect on

Crouch and Alers Occupational Therapy in Psychiatry and Mental Health, Sixth Edition.
Edited by Rosemary Crouch, Tania Buys, Enos Morankoana Ramano, Matty van Niekerk and Lisa Wegner.
© 2025 John Wiley & Sons Ltd. Published 2025 by John Wiley & Sons Ltd.

client care. Clinical reasoning uses the following personal and professional attributes and skills of the occupational therapist: communication, personal and professional knowledge (including evidence underpinning practice) that may be tacit and overt, technical skills (including a combination of thinking/reasoning styles), critical thinking, worldview, (including emotions, values, beliefs, spirituality, motivation and personal style), decision-making, problem-solving, and reflection and reflexion.' (Unsworth 2013, 2021; Alers 2014; Unsworth & Baker 2016; Knis Matthews *et al.* 2017; Murphy & Stav 2018; Coviello *et al.* 2019; Higgs *et al.* 2019; Marcolino *et al.* 2019; Márquez-Álvarez *et al.* 2019; Alfaro-LeFevre 2020; Benfield & Johnston 2020; Oldenburg *et al.* 2020; Garcia *et al.* 2021; Rothacker *et al.* 2021)

As can be seen from the above definition, clinical reasoning incorporates aspects of what is already inherent to occupational therapy practice, for example the occupational therapy process, (clinical) problem-solving and clinical decision-making that are critical in assessment and intervention. Not all of these associated concepts will be reiterated in this chapter; only the crucial skills that will assist in developing and improving clinical reasoning skills will be discussed, namely worldview, critical thinking and reflectivity/reflexivity, communication, and reasoning styles. These skills, particularly, underpin a practitioner's ability to express social values, to formulate and solve problems and their ability to function in familiar and unfamiliar environments. Additionally, these skills facilitate a clinician's ability to communicate the outcomes and/or process of clinical reasoning to fellow healthcare practitioners and lay persons (including mental health care users [MHCUs] and caregivers).

This chapter will draw on capabilities theory and design thinking to present a concrete model to assist novices with making clinical reasoning and clinical problem-solving concrete and fostering a sense of self-efficacy regarding these skills.

CLINICAL REASONING CAPABILITY: CAPABILITIES THEORY AND DESIGN THINKING

CAPABILITIES

Clinical skills/competence and clinical reasoning are, in effect, a cluster of capabilities, constituted by various kinds of knowledges which, when artfully applied, enable the person to read and interpret familiar and unfamiliar context accurately, that in turn enables problem-solving, as well as ongoing learning. Capability is therefore an overarching concept that includes existent and future development of competence in a variety of areas (Cairns & Stephenson 2009; Higgs *et al.* 2019). In the previous edition, Alers reminded us that clinical reasoning demands three basic attributes, science, ethics and artistry. The science relates to the knowledge base of research that is theoretical or experiential, the ethics relates to the therapist's philosophy about human dignity, and the artistry relates to the therapist's ability to use personal skills and the ability to impartially guide decisions (Alers 2014, p. 76).

The scientific, ethical and artistic dimensions of clinical reasoning are inextricably intertwined, and each strand is needed to strengthen the line of thought leading to understanding. Without science, clinical inquiry is not systematic; without ethics, it is not responsible; without art it is not convincing. (Benner 1994, p. 104)

Capability is undergirded by four types of knowledges, also known as Aristotle's intellectual virtues (trans. 1883/1908; Higgs *et al.* 2019, p. 91):

- Scientific knowledge that is linked to the rigorous process of providing proof or evidence of what is known.

- Technical knowledge/skill also referred to as a craft, or the art in science with a clear and visible goal that is often also context-bound and pragmatic.

- Reasoning skills and judgement (cognition) interpreted as critical thinking skills that question taken-for-granted assumptions, identifying fallacies and avoiding defensive and irrational thinking patterns (Elder & Paul 2020).

- Practical wisdom is a reflective attribute based on experience, values and ethics, and results in action. This action is known as praxis, fusing theory with doing through careful thinking. Praxis is often informed by insight and empathy, driven by taking responsibility and making use of collective collaboration and partnerships to bring about change and transformation.

Although it has been said that clinical reasoning is an implicit process (Marcolino *et al.* 2019), this chapter specifically attempts to make clinical reasoning more explicit, that is overt. The more overtly clinical reasoning happens, the easier it is for novices to observe and practice. Making clinical reasoning overt also allows more experienced practitioners to guide novices (and themselves) in deliberate reflection about their practice, reasoning and clinical decision-making. One way of making clinical reasoning overt is by looking at clinical reasoning as more than just a process and a set of decisions a clinician must make, but to include the competencies of a capable 'clinical reasoner'. Capability is an important concept because it includes both a practitioner's current clinical reasoning competence and the practitioner's ability to develop increased capacity/capability in the future. Table 6.1, adapted from Cairns and Stephenson (2009, p. 16), demonstrates the three key elements of capability and the traits it encompasses. All three elements affect each of the traits; thus, the intention is not to illustrate that some traits belong to a specific element.

It is important for occupational therapy students (and clinical preceptors) to remember that ability, especially in the clinical setting, develops incrementally. As the occupational therapy student's clinical skills develop and increase, alongside increasing theoretical knowledge, so their sense of self-efficacy will develop. Initially, it is more difficult to practice in unfamiliar circumstances, especially in the psychiatric context that could also be quite unpredictable. One must therefore be attuned to which of their personal values and professional values could facilitate their ability to deal with uncertainty.

CASE STUDY

Kwandile is a second-year occupational therapy student who is placed at a residential facility for chronic psychiatric MHCUs. In the first year of study, Kwandile received theoretical knowledge on the Occupational Therapy Practice Framework (Fourth Edition), categories of occupation, and interviewing. She also practised her interviewing skills with her friends, family and classmates, specifically looking at obtaining background information about their occupational profiles. In the weeks leading up to this fieldwork block, she was taught about the Model of Human Occupation, a few standardised and non-standardised assessments and some basic information about the diagnosis of Intellectual Development Disorder (IDD). Mary, a 21-year-old resident with IDD, has agreed to work with Kwandile. This will be the first time that Kwandile has interviewed a psychiatric MHCU. While she knows how to ask questions, she is unsure of how to ask questions in a way that Mary with IDD will be able to understand. She is also not sure how long Mary will be able to work with her before becoming too tired. How can the elements of capability help Kwandile to practice in an unfamiliar setting amidst some uncertainty?

- *Ability:* Because she has practiced interviewing familiar people, she knows that she has the ability to ask questions in a systematic manner. She has had to explain and define categories of occupation in tests (and to her family who knows very little about occupational therapy); thus, she knows how to use everyday language to explain occupations and thus to ask questions about them in a simple way. Thus, she already has some abilities. She knows that she also has the ability to learn more by practicing, because her interviews have improved as she practiced with different family members and friends.

- *Self-efficacy:* She has been able to interview familiar people, so she knows that she can ask questions and formulate someone's occupational profile successfully. She has also asked some of her friends in the third year of study about their experiences with interviewing MHCUs with IDD. They all told her that although they were scared and nervous at first, they were able to interact successfully with MHCUs. Thus, based on her own experience and that of her friends (i.e. vicarious learning, which is an important aspect of self-efficacy), she thinks that she can be successful at interviewing Mary and looking out for cues that might indicate fatigue.

- *Values:* Kwandile believes that humans are occupational beings and values everyone's right to access treatment irrespective of their disability, and as such, Mary will be able to tell her about the things she does every day and has the right to have a healthcare worker engage with her to facilitate occupational performance and function. Kwandile also values learning and thus sees this as an opportunity to learn something about herself and about occupational therapy. Despite being scared, her professional value of humans as occupational beings and personal value of learning enable her to overcome the fear of uncertainty to practice in this new setting.

Table 6.1 Elements and traits of capability.

Elements of capability	Traits of capability
Ability (current and future potential) Self-efficacy (confidence in one's ability/capacity to perform tasks (successfully)) Values (in this context, it relates to professional and personal values that influence practice most often in uncertain circumstances, as well as a practitioner's ability to define and express one's values)	• Being capable of functioning in both familiar and unfamiliar circumstances. • Being creative, imaginative and innovative. • Being mindful about change and open to opportunities and uncertainties. • Being confident of one's abilities. • Being able to engage with the social values relevant to actions, in pluralistic environments. • Being a lifelong, self-directed learner • Being able to continuously formulate and solve problems.

Even if Kwandile does not remember to ask all of the questions she planned, or if she has a rocky start, using some of the traits of capability, such as being **confident in her own abilities**, being a **lifelong learner**, being **open to opportunities and uncertainties**, she will be able to perform the tasks required of her. When she reflects about her performance afterwards, she will be able to identify what she did well (i.e. what abilities she already has) and what skills she needs to practice more to improve. Reflection will also help her think about how her values and traits helped her to perform in this uncertain and new situation. Of course, as one's ability (both clinically and theoretically) increases, it becomes easier to foster the traits of capability to become more skilled at practice, as well as solving clinical problems.

Using the key elements of capability and the traits of capability, any practitioner can identify not only their current competencies, but also areas for development and thus continue to be prepared and able to deal with uncertainty and unfamiliar situations.

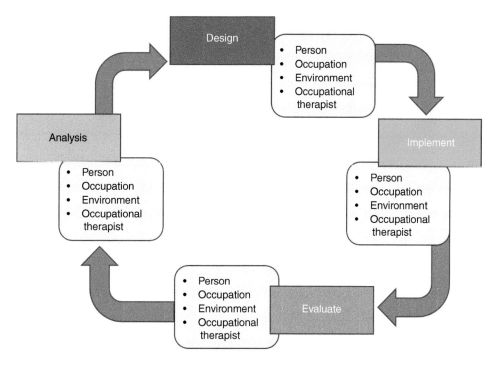

FIGURE 6.1 Design thinking as a clinical reasoning process. (Adapted from Pierce 2003, and Baum *et al.* 2015)

DESIGN THINKING

Design thinking derives from design science which originated in the early 20th century in the science engineering to address 'wicked' or very complex problems. Design thinking, as clinical reasoning, is a non-linear and iterative process. Pierce (2003) used design thinking as a theoretical and conceptual framework in her Occupation by Design Model, putting forward seven phases: motivation, investigation, definition, ideation, idea selection, implementation and evaluation. For the purposes of clarity for this chapter, the process of design thinking as clinical reasoning consists of four phases: analysis, design, implementation, and evaluation and occurs at the backdrop of the occupational therapist, the person/s receiving occupational therapy, occupation and the environment/context (Figure 6.1).

Each of the phases of design thinking as clinical reasoning involves the person (patient/client/learner), the occupation and the (student) occupational therapist (clinical reasoner) as well as the environment/context.

The **analysis phase** is undergirded by a person-centred posture by the occupational therapist of the person who is receiving occupational therapy. Thus, client-centredness will involve the complete occupational therapy assessment of their occupational profile (i.e. person and occupations) and environment/context. This environment/context includes cultural, political, geographic, historical, socio-economic, educational, demographic and ecological aspects.

In addition to a client-centred posture, accurate self-reflection is important from the outset because the (student) occupational therapist must be overtly aware of their own personal factors that may influence assessment, perception, judgement and decision-making processes. These factors include capability in knowledge, skills and thinking patterns as well as worldview – what one's expectations and beliefs are about the world, people and what constitutes a good life (see, for example Chapter 1). The analysis process may be undergirded by several modes of reasoning (see for example Table 6.3 later in this chapter) that enable one to find patterns to inform the design phase. During the analysis phase, the occupational therapy student may also start reasoning about the appropriate theoretical framework/s, occupational therapy model/s and theoretical frames of reference towards the convergent definition of the short-, medium- and long-term outcomes in the given treatment setting and practice profile.

Designing the treatment/intervention is about also designing the session plans and treatment principles. Treatment principles are the most essential scientific truths that will enable the occupational therapist and the person/s receiving occupational therapy in reaching the goal. Treatment principles are occupation-based, evidence-based theoretical guideposts that are judiciously sourced from occupational therapy theory (such as the model chosen through which to funnel one's reasoning), occupational science, theoretical frames of reference as well as the diagnosis. A treatment principle must be related to a specific goal. In the formulation of a treatment principle, the origin of the theoretical source will be evident. For example, if a therapeutic principle would state the following: 'By creating an opportunity for the person to experience a sense of mastery', it is evident that this principle's origin is in occupational science.

Part of the design phase is also the selection of, and designing the best activity requirements, activity/technique, positioning and presentation, handling and precautionary measures not only aligned with the treatment goals but also with the current context of the patient as well as future contextual considerations.

The **implementation** phase is when the intervention plan is implemented with a goodness-of-fit between time and tasks and during which the relationships between the aspects of the intervention plan are considered and critically thought through (Pierce 2003). The implementation phase occurs however not in isolation but may iterate with aspects of the analysis and design phases.

The **evaluation** phase entails the evaluation of the whole of the process from analysis to implementation. Evaluation should ideally include measuring the extent to which goals have been attained, to anchor practice as evidence (thus as a form of continuous development of new evidence for practice). Though evaluation includes reflection and reflexive practice by the clinician, also gaining feedback about the process (success and room for improvement) from all stakeholders, including the MHCU, family members/caretakers, as well as members of the multi-disciplinary team is good practice. The evaluation process should not be regarded as destructive critique but rather as a continuous opportunity for praxis and growth.

CRITICAL THINKING, WORLDVIEW AND REFLEXIVITY

Critical thinking is an important skill to develop as a clinician. It is not about destructive critique and being negative, but about thinking deeply about information and not accepting it at face value. Alfaro-LeFevre (2020) calls it 'important thinking' that is necessary for solving problems and being a lifelong learner. Critical thinking is different from just thinking, in that the latter might be as undirected as daydreaming, while critical thinking is purposeful and directed. Purposeful and directed thinking also distinguishes critical thinking from common sense, which is quite reliant on previous experience; thus, people from diverse backgrounds may have different views about what constitutes 'common' sense. Someone from New York may have a different view about using common sense to navigate streets or roads in winter than someone from Kaziikini in Botswana because their backgrounds and contexts demand different 'common sense skills'.

As can be seen from the reasoning strategies below, critical thinking skills demand thinking about factors or issues within the clinical space and outside of it, because multiple factors may play a role in the clinical decisions you make about a patient. In the clinical context, the outcome of critical thinking is to make clinical decisions and solve clinical problems about a patient, to ultimately improve your clinical judgement as a practitioner (Alfaro-LeFevre 2020).

Everybody has beliefs about the world, what is real, what is valuable, what knowledge is important and how knowledge is generated. Thus, we all have some ideas, albeit not necessarily formally situated in philosophy, about ontology (what exists in the world?), epistemology (how is knowledge created?) (Moon & Blackman 2014) and axiology (what is valuable?). These ideas are rooted in how and where we were raised and are influenced by our experiences over our life span (see Chapter 4) and contribute to our worldview. Notably, our worldview is not necessarily fixed for a lifetime. A person's worldview influences their reasoning because it colours the way in which they view situations, patients, problems and themselves, among others, as well as their expectations.

To become increasingly aware of and sensitive to how one's own worldview affects one's thinking and reasoning and to improve one's critical thinking ability, a key tool for every occupational therapist is reflectivity. Over time, practitioners must develop their reflectivity into reflexivity. Reflectivity relates to thinking about what one has learnt, and how the learning affects one's actions going forward. Reflexivity is a deeper reflective process, where one thinks about what one has learnt, and considers the implications thereof not only for oneself, but also for the broader context in which one works and even for one's profession.

Practitioners can reflect in three ways (Unsworth 2013; Alfaro-LeFevre 2020):

- Retrospectively – that is reflecting-on-action. This means thinking about what has already been done – so it comes *after* the task. You might ask yourself questions such as 'What worked well?' 'What would you change to make a treatment session or engagement with a patient better?' This kind of thinking (or reflection) is emphasised in undergraduate training, where lecturers and examiners ask students to think (reflect) about a treatment demonstration, for example, and ask these exact questions. As a clinician, it is not good enough to stop here. You must also develop competency at the next two types of reflection.

- In the situation, that is thinking-in-action: This happens *during* a task and can also be described as 'thinking on your feet'. Here you should ask yourself questions such as 'While I am learning: where does the new knowledge fit into my existing framework?' Thinking-in-action is quite difficult at first, and while lecturers expect undergraduate students to start reflecting in-action, it is a skill that builds with experience and as a practitioner gains confidence in their skills and ability to manage clinical situations.

- Prospectively, that is thinking-for-action. Here you anticipate what could possibly happen so that you can be proactive and identify what you can do to be prepared. You should ask yourself questions such as: 'What can I bring with me to help jog my memory and stay focused and energised?' For novices, thinking ahead is difficult because of their limited exposure to practical clinical situations. Therefore, novices are sometimes restricted to reading procedure manuals and textbooks. However, graduate clinicians should demonstrate the ability to think ahead.

Most importantly, reflectivity is not a once-off occurrence. All practitioners should reflect repeatedly about their practice, until this becomes an iterative process which eventually leads to reflexivity.

COMMUNICATION (EPISTEMIC FLUENCY)

> 'Imagine if we lived in a world where [occupational therapy] is globally considered as fundamental to the human rights of health and the well-being of all; a world where other disciplines such as the health sciences, political science, anthropology and economics consult the vital discipline of [occupational therapy] to inform their understanding of what humans perceive as meaningful occupation; a reality where, because of these collaborations, [occupational therapy] is in a position to actively contribute to the making of political and administrative decisions that promote occupational justice for all humans.' (Van der Merwe 2006, p. 169)

This dream expressed by Van der Merwe (2006) likely lives in every occupational therapist. Realising this dream relies on our ability to communicate our clinical reasoning and clinical decision-making confidently and clearly, as well as advocate eloquently for the rights of (among others) MHCUs. While profession-specific technical language and vocabulary are important to develop a professional identity, especially in a young profession such as occupational therapy, profession-specific technical language and vocabulary do not provide access to persons outside the profession to the body of knowledge (or episteme) used in clinical decision-making and clinical reasoning. Thus, for occupational therapy and its practitioners to be recognised as fundamental to achieving occupational justice for all human beings, we must develop epistemic fluency. As early as 1995, epistemic fluency was defined as: 'the ability to identify and use different ways of knowing, to understand their different forms of expression and evaluation, and to take the perspective of others who are operating withing a different epistemic framework' (Morrison & Collins 1995, p. 40). An epistemic framework is the way in which professional knowledge and 'ways of knowing about the world' (Markauskaite & Goodyear, 2017, p. 1) is structured or organised.

Developing epistemic fluency means that we must understand our own profession's episteme (i.e. knowledge structures and the associated philosophy and practices deriving from it, which is discussed below), as well as being able to identify that there are 'different ways of knowing' (Markauskaite & Goodyear 2017, p. 1) and that there are a variety of context-dependent and specialised knowledge (Markauskaite & Goodyear 2017; Higgs *et al.* 2019). Someone who is epistemically fluent is proficient in 'different ways of knowing about the world' (Markauskaite & Goodyear 2017, p. 1) and can flexibly move between various types of knowledge, e.g. 'abstract, contextual and situated ways of knowing' (Markauskaite & Goodyear 2017, p. 539) and are able to use 'multiple ways of knowing provided by the senses, environment and imagination'

(Markauskaite & Goodyear 2017, p. 539) to make decisions about patients and to communicate those decisions effectively within the multi-disciplinary team (Markauskaite & Goodyear 2017; Higgs *et al.* 2019).

Epistemic fluency thus, amongst others, involves using a common language with other healthcare professionals in the health and social sectors, for example using the knowledge structure of the International Classification of Function, Disability and Health (ICF) discussed below and/or the social determinants of health, discussed in Chapter 3 and to a lesser extent in Chapter 4 as part of the second generation of human rights, or in the field of psychiatry specifically, the Diagnostic and Statistical Manual of Psychiatric Disorders Fifth Edition (Text Revision) (DSM-5-TR) (American Psychiatric Association 2022).

UNDERSTANDING PROFESSIONS' KNOWLEDGE BASES TO FACILITATE COMMUNICATING CLINICAL REASONING, DECISION-MAKING AND PROBLEM-SOLVING

In Chapter 4 of this textbook, a simple definition of a profession is discussed, to distinguish professions from other occupations and actors (in the sense of doers). Building on that simple definition, Nerland and Jensen (2012, 2014) and Nerland (2016) have systematically been building an argument that professions have distinct bodies of knowledge and thus, professions are 'distinct knowledge cultures, constituted by a set of knowledge processes and practices that define expertise in the given area and serve to distinguish professional practitioners from other actors' (Nerland 2016, p. 127). It has long been known that occupational therapy has a wide knowledge base, which includes at least five broad areas, of which the first four were defined by Blom-Cooper et al. (1989):

1. 'Knowledge of the intelligence, physical strength, dexterity and personality attributes required to perform the tasks associated with the whole gamut of paid and unpaid occupations and valued leisure pursuits.

2. The professional skill to assess the potentialities and limitations of the physical and human environment to which patients have to adjust and to adjust to judge how far these environments could be modified and at what cost to meet individual needs.

3. Pedagogic skills are required, first to teach people how to acquire or restore their maximum functional capacity, and second to supervise and encourage technically trained instructors and unqualified assistants in their tasks of implementing and monitoring therapeutic recommendations.

4. The psychological knowledge and skills to deal with anxiety, depression and mood swings, which are the frequent aftermath of serious threats to health or of continuing disability, to motivate or remotivate, those with temporary or persistent disabilities to achieve their

maximum functional capacity.' (Blom-Cooper et al. 1989, pp. 15–16)

5. Occupational Science (see Chapter 3), which is a field that developed after Blom-Cooper et al. (1989) initially reflected on the knowledgebase of occupational therapy.

A profession's knowledge base does not develop in the absence of a philosophical foundation. While some professions may argue that they do not have a philosophical foundation, all professions have a disciplinary context, 'signature ways of thinking about and practicing [that] discipline' which are 'based on signature ways of thinking about and practicing [the] discipline' and follows 'accepted conceptual structures, boundaries and tribal norms and values of a discipline's community of practice' (Rahim 2015, pp. 1–2). All of these speak to the ontology, epistemology and axiology of a profession (Moon & Blackman 2014), that is its philosophical foundation. Some authors have attempted to pinpoint the philosophical foundation of occupational therapy, which includes humanism and Marxism (seeing humans as occupational beings) (Drolet 2014), and pragmatism (Ikiugu & Schultz 2006; Morrison 2016).

If occupational therapists know the diverse axiologies (values) that underpin the profession's knowledge (or epistemic) culture, they also will understand (and be better able to articulate) the 'worlds of practice' of occupational therapy and the discourses of our profession's practice knowledge: we must understand the rules for and ways in which knowledge is constructed in occupational therapy and the strategic ways in which we use our own and other professions' knowledgebases, as well as the target structures that guide occupational therapy inquiry (e.g. taxonomies and frameworks) and around which occupational therapy constructs knowledge so that we start to also understand how other professions construct knowledge (Higgs et al. 2019). If we understand knowledge bases, knowledge structures and how professions make knowledge, we can become fluent in other professions' knowledge structures (epistemes) as well, which will lead to our ability to articulate occupational therapy reasoning in ways that other professions can understand too – i.e. becoming epistemically fluent. Importantly, becoming fluent in other professions' knowledge structures should not mean that one loses one's own professional identity as an occupational therapist, but that means that at the outset, one should be well versed in the philosophy and knowledge base of occupational therapy. With secure professional knowledge as the foundation, epistemic fluency will help in not only communicating patient outcomes and clinical decisions to other members of the team involved in a patient's care, but also to better articulate the identity, value and contribution of occupational therapy to non-occupational therapists much more clearly and understandably. It should be noted that this chapter is not advocating against using occupational therapy specific language. However, it is advancing an argument, aligned to basic communication principles, that if one wants

someone else to understand a message, the onus is on the communicator (speaker) to ensure that the message is clear. Four main tools in psychiatry are available to help the occupational therapist communicate their clinical findings in such a way that other persons outside of occupational therapy can understand the message, which will be discussed briefly below.

USING COMMUNAL TOOLS SUCH AS THE ICF TO FACILITATE COMMUNICATING CLINICAL REASONING, DECISION-MAKING AND PROBLEM-SOLVING

In psychiatry and mental health, there are four main tools to facilitate epistemic fluency, namely the ICF (World Health Organization 2002), the International Classification of Diseases Eleventh Revision (ICD-11), and the International Classification of Health Interventions (ICHI) (which are all aligned) and the DSM-5-TR (American Psychiatric Association 2022).

The ICF was developed by the World Health Organisation (WHO) among others to facilitate a common language between healthcare professions and practitioners (World Health Organization 2002). It uses a model that classifies human functioning as a **dynamic interplay** between *body functions* and *body structures*, *activities* and *participation*, as well as *contextual factors*, i.e. environmental factors and personal factors (World Health Organization 2002; Escorpizo *et al.* 2015), as can be seen in Figure 6.2.

There has been some incorporation of the ICF into occupational therapy, such as the American Association of Occupational Therapy's Occupational Therapy Practice Framework (OTPF) (Boop & Cahill 2020). When some of the aspects of the ICF model are expanded, as can be seen in Figure 6.3, it becomes clear that activity corresponds well to categories of occupation as described in the OTPF (World Health Organization 2002; Boop & Cahill 2020).

Because of its adoption by many professions, there now ought to be a shared understanding among a variety of health practitioners about the dynamic interplay between the environment, the person, their affected body structures and body functions and how those impact a person's ability to participate actively in their 'Major life areas', 'community, social and civic life', 'mobility' and 'self-care' (World Health Organization 2002, p. 16). Although the way in which occupational therapy defines these areas is much more structured and refined, using the ICF terminology for activity and participation when communicating a MHCU's goals and expected outcomes of rehabilitation to other members of the multidisciplinary team, such as the psychiatrist and psychologist, will enhance teamwork and communal efforts to realising these goals and outcomes for the MHCU.

Similarly, using terminology and concepts from diagnostic frameworks, such as the ICD-11 or the DSM-5-TR, correctly will further enhance communicating clinical decisions and solutions to clinical problems. For example, when communicating about

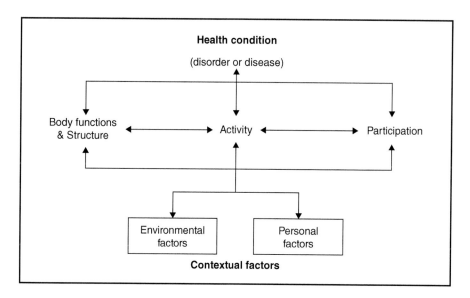

FIGURE 6.2   Model of the ICF.
Source: World Health Organization 2002/World Health Organization/Public Domain.

the prognosis of an elderly patient in the early stages of Alzheimer's disease to continue living independently, the occupational therapist should present the findings within adaptive functioning. Using the three areas of adaptive functioning (which relates to a person's ability to handle common demands in life) will help a psychiatrist to understand future planning for the patient much better than using occupational therapy jargon (see Table 6.2 for a comparison).

CASE EXAMPLE

Mrs Mnguni is a 68-year-old lady who lives in a rural community in the North of South Africa. She lives in a brick house without indoor plumbing or electricity. She is responsible for the primary care of four of her grandchildren below the age of six years, who live with her in her home. She mostly cooks in large pots on an open fire but also uses a two-plate gas cooker. Her daughter-in-law who lives 10 km away, has expressed concern about safety cooking both on the fire and on the gas stove. She recently sustained partial thickness burn injuries on her arms and torso, when she tripped on a rock and spilled boiling water on herself. She was admitted to the local district hospital, and the occupational therapist also found neuropsychiatric problems. The occupational therapist referred Mrs Mnguni for evaluation by the psychiatrist, and a diagnosis of Alzheimer's disease (mild neurocognitive disorder) was made.

One might ask, what is the difference between the two columns? Firstly, the difference lies in the way in which the information is organised, and secondly, the length of what would be a document. The left-hand column organises the information in such a way that it is already processed for the psychiatrist: there is no need for them to reorganise or interpret

the information, as it would have been necessary if the information was presented to them in the format of the right-hand column. Presenting the information in a way that places a lower demand on reinterpretation means that the psychiatrist can act more quickly on the information (i.e. make important decisions more quickly) and they understand what the occupational therapist is saying (and thus also the value and contribution of the occupational therapist in the MHCU's intervention programme).

REASONING STYLES

Unsworth (2013) described 13 modes or styles of reasoning. Some of these styles of reasoning apply professional knowledge, or patient-specific knowledge or diagnostic knowledge. Some of the styles rely on the practitioner's own context and internal processes, for example worldview. Importantly, clinicians must be aware of all these reasoning styles, but each will not necessarily be applicable to every clinical situation or clinical case, as Unsworth has shown. Nonetheless, the reflexive and skilled practitioner is able to draw on each of these reasoning styles, often in combination, to enhance clinical problem-solving and clinical decision-making. Table 6.3 attempts to group Unsworth's reasoning styles to help demonstrate how these styles may influence clinical reasoning and provides the foundation for the later discussion about how these may be used in combination to solve clinical problems and to improve one's clinical reasoning capability.

When considering this categorisation of reasoning styles, two broad approaches to clinical reasoning emerge, namely cognitive clinical reasoning processes and interactive clinical reasoning processes (Higgs *et al.* 2019). In occupational

Body	
Function:	**Structure:**
Mental Functions	Structure of the Nervous System
Sensory Functions and Pain	The Eye, Ear and Related Structures
Voice and Speech Functions	Structures Involved in Voice and Speech
Functions of the Cardiovascular, Haematological, Immunological and Respiratory Systems	Structure of the Cardiovascular, Immunological and Respiratory Systems
Functions of the Digestive, Metabolic, Endocrine Systems	Structures Related to the Digestive, Metabolic and Endocrine Systems
Genitourinary and Reproductive Functions	Structure Related to Genitourinary and Reproductive Systems
Neuromusculoskeletal and Movement-Related Functions	Structure Related to Movement
Functions of the Skin and Related Structures	Skin and Related Structures

Activities and participation
Learning and Applying Knowledge
General Tasks and Demands
Communication
Mobility
Self Care
Domestic Life
Interpersonal Interactions and Relationships
Major Life Areas
Community, Social and Civic Life

Environmental factors
Products and Technology
Nature Environment and Human-Made Changes to Environment
Support and Relationships
Attitudes
Services, Systems and Policies

FIGURE 6.3   Chapters of the ICF.

Source: World Health Organization 2002/World Health Organization/Public Domain.

therapy, specifically in the psychiatric and mental health fields of practice, a more interactive approach to clinical reasoning is necessary. Occupational therapists must actively and consciously work on improving clinical reasoning, whether using cognitive processes or an interactive approach.

HOW DOES CLINICAL REASONING DEVELOP?

Like all other occupational therapy knowledge and skills, clinical reasoning ability must be developed. Although the Dreyfus Model of Skill Acquisition (Dreyfus 2004) has been criticised, it nonetheless provides a useful set of stages, by which one can describe the development of competencies related to clinical reasoning, from novice, to advanced beginner, to competent, proficient and expert. Ideally, an occupational therapy student should move from novice to advanced beginner so that by the time they graduate, they are competent in clinical reasoning skills (Table 6.4).

Crucially, developing clinical reasoning is reliant on reflectivity and guidance; thus, collaborative reflection is especially necessary in the early stages of one's career. Competence and self-efficacy also develop as supervisors and preceptors demonstrate their own reasoning in collaborative discussions about patients.

Table 6.2 Comparing using adaptive functioning versus occupational therapy jargon to discuss independent living ability and prognosis.

Adaptive functioning	Occupational therapy jargon
Conceptual	**Client factors and performance skills**
• Mrs Mnguni is able to express herself in isiZulu, but occasionally uses circumferential language and expressions to articulate ideas.	• Poor cognition:
	• Poor memory, poor concrete and abstract decision-making, poor concrete and abstract problem-solving, poor concrete and abstract judgement.
• Her reading is slow and she no longer enjoys reading novels, preferring shorter pieces, for example short articles in the local newspaper, likely due to reduced attention span.	**Process skills**
• Her writing is slow and jittery and increasingly illegible.	• Cannot sustain performance:
• Her working arithmetic for tasks including calculating change and changing the portion sizes of recipes is no longer functional and she is at risk of financial losses related to ruined food or incorrect change.	• Does not pace during tasks such as personal care and grooming. • Does not attend during tasks such as boiling water on the stove. • Initiates tasks but often does not complete them. • Gathering, organising and restoring is of poor quality. • Adapting performance, for example notices and responds, is erratic.
• She cannot reason to solve complex problems, but simple reasoning is intact; thus, routine tasks are completed.	• Social and interaction skills are adequate:
• Her anterograde memory is poor.	• Can produce speech and speak fluently. • Sometimes does not regulate, by including excessive detail and examples that are not contextually or situationally relevant.
Social	• Adapting social interaction is increasingly difficult:
• She is able to show empathy for her grandchildren and familiar people, but is increasingly becoming egocentric.	• Does not heed the intended purpose of social interaction.
• She demonstrates adequate social judgement for simple social situations, but judgement in complex social situations resonates with her poor reasoning and egocentrism.	**Categories of occupation**
	• Personal activities of daily living
• She can communicate clearly with her grandchildren, but she avoids communication with unfamiliar people.	• Currently performs washing, dressing, toileting and grooming independently, but completion is slow. • She applies too much make-up, indicating reduced concrete judgement.
• She expects exceptions regarding adhering to rules, for example. she refuses to wear a safety belt because her arthritis makes affixing and releasing the catch difficult	• Instrumental activities of daily living
• She has become withdrawn and thus pays insufficient attention to keeping friendships. She complains of loneliness, but does not actively pursue new or existing friendships.	• Can orientate in the community using both public transport and driving herself. • When driving her sedan car, she has been involved in small accidents in the parking lot of the local shopping centre. • Has appropriate parenting skills, but quality of childcare is deteriorating. She is increasingly finding it difficult to manage all four of her grandchildren without help. She primarily looks after the one- and two-year-old children (one each), and the older children must feed and dress each other, help with washing their younger siblings/cousins and other chores such as laundry and washing the dishes. • She needs help from the two oldest grandchildren with sweeping the house, washing floors, tidying the kitchen and helping with meal preparation.
Practical	• Health management and maintenance
• She occasionally does not wash herself or change clothes. While she knows how to do this, she sometimes loses track of the routine needed to perform the tasks.	• Stops medication when she is afraid of the side effects. • Irregularly consults physician/local clinic.
• Her poor memory means that she loses track of where she has put things such as groceries and toiletries. The functional effect thereof is that she continues to buy the same things and when her daughter-in-law visits she finds goods in strange places, and also multiple duplicates of groceries.	• Rest and sleep
	• The grandchildren are helping her to maintain an appropriate sleep/wake routine, but her personal sleep preparation is taking longer. • With the grandchildren not needing to go to school, she is finding that she sleeps later in the morning and stays up later at night.
• She is increasingly using poor judgement in managing money, repeatedly complaining about not having enough money for food, firewood, gas, petrol and to pay her cell phone bill.	• Leisure/recreation
	• Most of her free time is spent with her grandchildren. • She considers some of her church activities as leisure, e.g. visiting some of the convalescent congregation members in hospitals or at their homes.
• She tries to be responsible for her grandchildren, but is increasingly relying on the two six-year-olds to take care of their younger siblings and cousins. She has difficulty keeping the house tidy and clean by herself, increasingly finding it hard to throw things like newspapers away.	• Work
	• She no longer holds a full-time job. • She has few plans for her retirement other than looking after her grandchildren. She does not know what she will do for productive activities when all her grandchildren are attending school. • She has not thought about driving cessation.

Table 6.3   Unsworth's (2021) reasoning styles categorised.

Practitioner-specific reasoning styles

Embodiment	Gathering information about a patient using one's body, e.g. sense of smell, tactile sensation when palpating muscles, etc. Sometimes broadly referred to as 'observations', but it is an emergent field of research in occupational therapy.
Worldview	How the practitioner's personal context and history influences how they see the world and thus affects clinical reasoning.
Intuition	How one's clinical experience affects a clinician's instinctive approach to a clinical situation beyond conscious reasoning.
Reflection	Iteratively performing and reviewing/examining one's performance. Most often would relate to reflection-on-action, but if that is used in conjunction with reflection-for-action and reflection-in-action (Alfaro-LeFevre 2020), reflection could become more meaningful and enhance the practitioner's ability to articulate their reasoning as well as their own development (Higgs *et al*. 2019).

Practitioner-in-interaction-with patient reasoning styles

Interactive reasoning	Focuses on the practitioner's interaction with the patient and how they adjust their clinical problem-solving and clinical decision-making based on their interaction with the patient, that is engaging the patient in occupational therapy and communicating with the client. Draws on client-centredness and therapeutic use of self.
Narrative reasoning	Using storytelling in a phenomenological way to understand the meaning of the patient's illness and illness experience.
Generalisation reasoning	When thinking about a specific concern with a patient, the clinician might reflect on general past experiences or knowledge which could relate to the situation and then apply that general past experience to one's reasoning about the patient's situation. Thus, the practitioner is making generalisations that might apply to the patient's situation.

Reasoning styles based on the health condition and its impact on ICF components of activity and participation

Diagnostic reasoning	Reasoning used to: a. Identify impairments underlying difficulties in occupational performance (i.e. activity and participation from the ICF) b. Develop interventions and solutions to address defined client-centred outcomes and goals.
Hypothetico-deductive reasoning	Also referred to as Scientific Reasoning. Generating and testing hypotheses based on clinical data and knowledge, and further data collection Often used to make a medical diagnosis, but in occupational therapy, it is also used to diagnosed occupational problems (i.e. related to the ICF component of Activity)
Conditional reasoning	Taking into account all of the following to understand what is meaningful to the patient in their lived world and to determine priorities for life going forward: • Environmental factors – social contexts • Personal factors – cultural context, personal situation/context, temporal context (patient's past, present and future)

Reasoning related to professional knowledge/issues/situations

Procedural reasoning	Using one's knowledge about the scientific or systematic components of practice such as systematic data collection, hypothesis formation and testing.
Ethical reasoning	Thinking about the ethical or moral dilemmas that one might face when dealing with a particular patient. Also, see Chapter 5 in this textbook.
Pragmatic reasoning	Also known as management reasoning, and refers to the practice and personal contexts of the occupational therapist. This includes organisational and sociopolitical environments as well as economic considerations such as resources and whether the clinician will be reimbursed for services and by whom. The clinician's personal context includes reasoning about one's own motivation, one's therapy skills and ability to interpret and understand the practice context.

Source: Adapted from Unsworth (2013, pp. 212–216).

Table 6.4   Development of clinical reasoning capabilities based on the Dreyfus Model of Skill Acquisition.

	Novice	Advanced beginner	Competent	Proficient	Expert
Clinical reasoning to interpret assessment findings	Needs rules from theory and guidance from preceptors and educators Limited and inflexible context-free application of rules	Incorporates contextual information into rule-based thinking Recognises differences between theoretical expectations and presenting problems (but unable to respond to situation quickly)	Can devise new rules specific to the situation Relating theoretical concept (condition, nature, form or function) to context Interprets data using relevant theoretical constructs	Combines different diagnostic and procedural approaches with flexibility and creativity. Putting it all together. No longer relies on guidelines to direct appropriate action for situation. Recognises assumptions	Cognitive reasoning is quick and intuitive with solutions to ill-structured problems Can predict multiple outcomes Engages global view and applies theory in a global way Recognises meaningful patterns and determines generalisations Can align thought, feeling, action into intuitive problem-recognition. Reflects in, on and for action
Decision-making	Uses rule-based procedural reasoning to guide 'actions', but does not recognise cues and therefore is not skilful in adapting rules to fit situation	Still procedural, but can recognise some patterns of behaviour or symptoms, so doesn't prioritise data well or identify what is most important	Procedural aspects more automatic and organised, so is able to prioritise problems and plan deliberately, efficiently and in response to urgency and contextual issues (including background, relationships and environment, relevant to the situation). Can see actions in terms of long-range goals.	Perceives situations as wholes, can anticipate situation and avoid irrelevant information. Prioritise issues (in HK style). Predicts multiple outcomes. Evaluates action and recognises the relationship of action and inaction. Supervisory responsibilities. Liaises with outside organisations for benefit of others	Shows confidence in own reasoning abilities Decision-making is schema-based, with automated processing. Rapid, methodical and critical evaluations of solutions. Takes nothing for granted. Meets multiple patient requests and care needs or crisis management without losing important information or missing significant needs. Prioritises quickly and efficiently. Mentors others in decision-making skills.
Judgement including reflective judgement	Unable to use discriminatory judgement	Unable to determine priorities, makes judgement based on established criteria/rules	Drawing inferences or conclusions that are supported or justified by evidence	Receptive to divergent views and sensitive to own biases	Shows confidence in own reasoning abilities. Applies judgement prudently in relevant context. Integrates feedback from others to improve practice. Insight into societal conditions generating a patient's illness.

(continued)

Table 6.4   (*Continued*)

	Novice	Advanced beginner	Competent	Proficient	Expert
	Unreflective – informed by routine. Unable to deal with unfamiliar situations	Reflective only after the event, if at all	Professional autonomy in decision-making. Conscious deliberation	Recognises ramifications of actions	Recognises ramifications and can mitigate for these through reflection-for-action
Ethics including client orientation and documentation	Recognises overt ethical issues. Defends views based on preconceptions	Begins to recognise more subtle ethical issues, judging according to established personal, professional or social rules or criteria	Recognises ethical dilemmas. Recognises individual differences. Sensitive to client's views. Capable of some contextual considerations Practices equality of practice – same rules for all	More sophisticated in recognising situational nature of ethical reasoning Able to provide options and explain possible outcomes of the options and outlines time sequences for the MHCU Can start to consider equitable practice and implement Nussbaum's principles of justice for a good life (Van Niekerk 2024)	Demonstrates clear understanding of ethical issues and practices ethically, uses practical wisdom Honest in facing personal bias Can realistically evaluate soundness of conclusions and worth of action to client and others Fully implements equitable practice an enabling a good life also for profoundly disabled MHCUs
Response to feedback	Defensive and has difficulty understanding why they have done and why they have not performed correctly	Receives feedback stoically and responds to feedback (e.g. implementing or making changes to own behaviour/ practice) erratically. Ruminates rather than reflects on feedback.	Is open to feedback, understands that feedback will result in better practice. Makes changes according to feedback. Benefits from structured or guided reflection on feedback.	Seeks feedback broadly, reflects on feedback so that the feedback also enhances the practitioner's ability to recognise their own blind spots	Seeks feedback systematically from experts, peers and subordinates. Reflexion on feedback coupled with self-reflexive practice.

Source: Adapted from Alers (2014); Higgs *et al.* (2019); Alfaro-LeFevre (2020).

CONCLUSION

Clinical reasoning is complex and develops with experience. To consciously develop one's clinical reasoning ability requires metacognition and reflection on many of the skills and abilities inherent to clinical reasoning. Using design thinking and design science, this chapter has attempted to simplify and make the process of clinical reasoning tangible and concrete. Importantly, the analysis phase includes reflection on the practitioner themselves, that is self-awareness, reflection on the MHCU and their needs, reflection on the clinical environment and the MHCU's environment and related demands, and reflection on the MHCU's priority occupations.

While experts are able to solve problems quickly, they are often unable to explain some of their reasoning to a novice because their knowledge of topics or practice areas is so deeply embedded that they practice intuitively. This chapter has attempted to elucidate some of the personal and professional skills one must possess and hone to become better at clinical reasoning, including communication and reflection.

Being able to communicate the results of one's clinical reasoning, for example the clinical decisions made, or clinical problems solved, requires that a practitioner understands their own worldview, as well as that of their profession. Communication skills demand that the occupational therapist is able to communicate in such a way that people outside the profession, such as psychiatrists, MHCUs and their caregivers or family members, are able to understand and receive the message clearly. Tools such as the DSM-5-TR and the ICF will help with interprofessional communication.

Reflection on action, reflection in action and reflection for action are important competencies to develop, in order to enhance one's clinical reasoning, clinical decision-making and clinical problem-solving.

QUESTIONS

1. Explain how reflecting on **Practitioner-specific reasoning styles** can improve one's clinical reasoning skills.

2. Explain the use of **Practitioner-in-interaction-with patient reasoning styles** in clinical reasoning.

3. Explain the use of **Reasoning styles based on the health condition and its impact on ICF components of activity and participation** in clinical reasoning.

4. Discuss the relationship between **Reasoning related to professional knowledge/issues/situations** and the profession's philosophical base.

5. Discuss the difference between reflection in action, reflection for action and reflection on action using a case from your own experience to illustrate the differences.

6. Discuss how using tools such as the ICF and the DSM-5-TR can help you to communicate your findings to the multi-disciplinary team more effectively.

7. Using the five stages of the Dreyfus Model of Skills Acquisition, write a reflection on your own self-growth regarding clinical reasoning.

ACKNOWLEDGEMENT

Thanks to Ms Kumo Sibanyoni and Ms Ryanne Foley, whose literature search as part of their final exam for the MSc OT (Applied to Psychiatric Conditions, 2022) was invaluable in updating this chapter.

REFERENCES

Alers, V. (2014) Clinical reasoning in psychiatric occupational therapy. In R. Crouch & V. Alers (eds), *Occupational Therapy in Psychiatry and Mental Health*, 5th edn, pp. 67–82. John Wiley & Sons, Ltd, West Sussex.

Alfaro-LeFevre, R. (2020) *Critical Thinking, Clinical Reasoning and Clinical Judgement: A Practical Approach*, 7th edn. Elsevier, St Louis.

American Psychiatric Association (2022) *Diagnostic and Statistical Manual of Mental Disorders (DSM-5-TR)*, 5th edn. American Psychiatric Association, Arlington. https://doi.org/10.1176/appi.books.9780890425787

Aristotle (349BC/1883/1908) *Nicomachean Ethics*. Translated by F.H. Peters. Bobbs-Merrill, New York. Made available also by Standard EBooks at https://standardebooks.org/ebooks/aristotle/nicomachean ethics/f-h-peters (accessed 13 March 2024)

Baum, C. M., Christiansen, C. H., & Bass, J. D. (2015). The Person-Environment-Occupation- Performance (PEOP) model. In C. H. Christiansen, C. M. Baum, & J. D. Bass (eds), *Occupational therapy: Performance, participation, and well-being*, 4th edn., pp. 49–56. SLACK Incorporated, Thorofare, NJ.

Benfield, A.M. & Johnston, M.V. (2020) Initial development of a measure of evidence-informed professional thinking. *Australian Occupational Therapy Journal*, **67**(4), 309–319. https://doi.org/10.1111/1440-1630.12655

Benner, P. (1994) The tradition and skill of interpretive phenomenology in studying health, illness, and caring practices. In: P. Benner (ed), *Interpretive Phenomenology: Embodiment, Caring, and Ethics in Health and Illness*, pp. 99–127. SAGE, Thousand Oaks.

Blom-Cooper, L. et al. (1989) *Occupational Therapy: An Emerging Profession in Health Care*. Duckworth, London.

Boop, C. & Cahill, S.M. (2020) Occupational therapy practice framework: domain and process fourth edition. *American Journal of Occupational Therapy*, **74** (**August**), 1–87. https://doi.org/10.5014/ajot.2020.74S2001

Cairns, L. & Stephenson, J. (2009) *Capable Workplace Learning*. Sense Publishers, Rotterdam, The Netherlands.

Coviello, J.M., Potvin, M.C. & Lockhart-Keene, L. (2019) Occupational therapy assistant students' perspectives about the development of clinical reasoning. *The Open Journal of Occupational Therapy*, **7**(2), 8. https://doi.org/10.15453/2168-6408.1533

Dreyfus, S.E. (2004) The five-stage model of adult skill acquisition. *Bulleting of Science, Technology and Society*, **24**(3), 177–181. https://doi.org/10.1177/0270467604264992

Drolet, M.J. (2014) The axiological ontology of occupational therapy: a philosophical analysis. *Scandinavian Journal of Occupational Therapy*, **21**(1), 2–10. https://doi.org/10.3109/11038128.2013.831118

Elder, L. & Paul, R. (2020) *Critical Thinking: Tools for Taking Charge of Your Learning and Your Life*, 8th edn, Foundation for Critical Thinking. Rowman & Littlefield, Maryland.

Escorpizo, R., Brage, S., Homa, D. & Stucki, G. (eds) (2015) *Handbook of Vocational Rehabilitation and Disability Evaluation Application and Implementation of the ICF*. Switzerland, Springer.

Garcia, J., Copley, J., Turpin, M. et al (2021) Evidence-based practice and clinical reasoning in occupational therapy: a cross-sectional survey in Chile. *Australian Occupational Therapy Journal*, **68**(2), 169–179. https://doi.org/10.1111/1440-1630.12713

Higgs, J., Jensen, G.M., Loftus, S. & Christensen, N. (eds) (2019) *Clinical Reasoning in the Health Professions*, 4th edn. Elsevier, Edinburgh.

Ikiugu, M.N. & Schultz, S. (2006) An argument for pragmatism as a foundational philosophy of occupational therapy. *Canadian Journal of Occupational Therapy*, **73**(2), 86–97. https://doi.org/10.2182/cjot.05.0009

Knis Matthews, L., Mulry, C.M. & Richard, L. (2017) Matthews model of clinical reasoning: a systematic approach to conceptualize evaluation and intervention. *Occupational Therapy in Mental Health*, **33**(4), 360–373. https://doi.org/10.1080/0164212X.2017.1303658

Marcolino, T.Q., Von Poellnitz, J.C., Silva, C.R. et al (2019) "And a door opens": reflections on conceptual and identity issues on clinical reasoning in occupational therapy. *Brazilian Journal of Occupational Therapy*, **27**(2), 403–411. https://doi.org/10.4322/2526-8910.ctoAO1740

Markauskaite, L. & Goodyear, P. (2017) *Epistemic Fluency and Professional Education: Innovation, Knowledgeable Action and Actionable Knowledge, Professional and Practice-based Learning*. Springer Science+Business Media, Dordrecht. https://doi.org/10.1007/978-94-007-4369-4_1

Márquez-Álvarez, L.-J., Calvo-Arenillas, J.-I., Talavera-Valverde, M.-Á., Moruno-Millares, P. et al (2019) Professional reasoning in occupational therapy: a scoping review. *Occupational Therapy International*, **2019**, 1–9. https://doi.org/10.1155/2019/6238245

Moon, K. & Blackman, D. (2014) A guide to understanding social science research for natural scientists. *Conservation Biology*, **28**(5), 1167–1177. https://doi.org/10.1111/cobi.12326

Morrison, D. & Collins, A. (1995) Epistemic fluency and constructivist learning environments. *Educational Technology*, **35**(5), 39–45.

Morrison, R. (2016) Pragmatist epistemology and Jane Addams: fundamental concepts for the social paradigm of occupational therapy. *Occupational Therapy International*, **23**(4), 295–304. https://doi.org/10.1002/oti.1430

Murphy, L.F. & Stav, W.B. (2018) The impact of online video cases on clinical reasoning in occupational therapy education: a quantitative analysis. *The Open Journal of Occupational Therapy*, **6**(3). https://doi.org/10.15453/2168-6408.1494

Nerland, M. (2016) Learning to master profession-specific knowledge practices: a prerequisite for the deliberate practitioner? F. Trede & C. McEwan (eds), *Educating the Deliberate Professional: Preparing for Future Practices*, pp. 127–139. Springer International Publishing, Switzerland.

Nerland, M. & Jensen, K. (2012) Epistemic practices and object relations in professional work. *Journal of Education and Work*, **25**(1), 101–120. https://doi.org/10.1080/13639080.2012.644909

Nerland, M. & Jensen, K. (2014) Changing cultures of knowledge and professional learning. In: S. Billett, C. Harteis, & H. Gruber (eds), *International Handbook of Research in Professional and Practice-based Learning*, pp. 611–644. Springer International Publishing, Dordrecht.

Oldenburg, H.Y., Snyder, K.L., Heinle, D.K. & Hollman, J.H. (2020) A comparison of clinical reasoning among rehabilitation students during experiential learning. *Journal of Allied Health*, **49**(4), 252–257.

Pierce, D. (2003) *Occupation by Design: Building Therapeutic Power*. F.A. Davis Company, Philadelphia.

Rahim, M.M. (2015) *Lecturing for non-law background students: assessing the cognitive load of case and legislation-based lecturing approaches.* Corporate Law Teachers Association Conference, pp. 1–21, Queensland University of Technology, Brisbane, February 2015. https://eprints.qut.edu.au/83063/

Rothacker, E., Potvin, M.-C. & Coviello, J. *et al* (2021) How I developed clinical reasoning skills during fieldwork: perspectives of OT assistant students. *The American Journal of Occupational Therapy*, **75** (**Supplement_2**), 7512505137p1. https://doi.org/10.5014/ajot.2021.75s2-rp137

Unsworth, C. (2013) The evolving theory of clinical reasoning. In: E.A.S. Duncan (ed.), *Foundations for Practice in Occupational Therapy*, 5th edn, pp. 209–232. Churchill Livingstone Elsevier, Edinburgh.

Unsworth, C. (2021) The evolving theory of clinical reasoning. In: E.A.S. Duncan (ed), *Foundations for Practice in Occupational Therapy*. 6th edn, pp. 178–197. Elsevier, Edinburgh.

Unsworth, C. & Baker, A. (2016) A systematic review of professional reasoning literature in occupational therapy. *British Journal of Occupational Therapy*, **79**(1), 5–16. https://doi.org/10.1177/0308022615599994

Van der Merwe, T. (2006) *Occupational Therapy and Ideology: A Critical Investigation*. University of the Free State. https://scholar.ufs.ac.za/bitstream/handle/11660/8742/VanderMerweT.pdf?sequence=1&isAllowed=y (accessed 15 March 2024)

Van Niekerk, M. (2024). Law, human rights and ethics in mental health-care practice. In: R. Crouch, T. Buys, E. Van Ramano, M. Niekerk, L. Wegner (eds), *Crouch and Alers' Occupational Therapy in Psychiatry and Mental Health*, 6th edn. John Wiley & Sons, Ltd., West Sussex.

World Health Organization (2002) *Towards a common language for functioning, disability and health: ICF*. Geneva. http://www.who.int/classifications/icf/training/icfbeginnersguide.pdf (accessed 14 March 2024)

Specific Issues

Occupational Therapy Groups in Mental Health

CHAPTER 7

Enos Morankoana Ramano[1] and Marianne de Beer[2]
[1]Occupational Therapy Private Practitioner, Soweto, Gauteng, South Africa
[2]Department of Occupational Therapy, University of Pretoria, Pretoria, Gauteng, South Africa

KEY LEARNING POINTS

- An understanding of occupational therapy groups.

- An application of the use of clinical reasoning in occupational therapy groups.

- The benefits of therapeutic factors during the facilitation of occupational therapy groups while following the group procedure.

- The consideration of group dynamics during occupational therapy groups.

- The therapeutic value of a group leader.

INTRODUCTION

A therapeutic group is an aggregate of people who share a common purpose that can be achieved through collaboration (Scaffa 2019, p. 539). This collaboration takes place between the group members and the group leader or facilitator with the intention to achieve a particular goal for group member satisfaction. The latter is obtained through the dynamics of group and social interaction as they share, encourage, advise, learn, empower, acquire skill and support each other to derive hope for the future and overcome their challenges.

In occupational therapy, groups are used therapeutically with a broad range of age groups and settings. The age range of individuals who can be group members includes children to older adults. Settings cover all areas of practice such as healthcare settings, schools, communities, organisations and old age homes (American Occupational Therapy Association [AOTA] 2020). Occupational therapy groups in mental health care settings often form the backbone of therapy to take care of the needs of individuals with mental illness. For this reason, groups have been employed by occupational therapists as their preferred treatment modality since the origin of the profession

(Falk-Kessler *et al.* 1990; Borg & Bruce 1991; Eklund 1997; Howe & Schwartzberg 2001; Sundsteigen *et al.* 2009; Fisher 2014).

Most mental health care facilities internationally require therapeutic groups to be part of a selection of standard forms of intervention. Some facilities encourage the inclusion of occupational therapy groups because of their therapeutic potential to provide social and emotional support and to ensure that individuals with mental illness are engaged in therapeutic activities and empowered with life skills throughout the day.

Occupational therapy groups are distinct from groups run by other healthcare professionals. This chapter will focus on occupational therapy groups that are mostly offered in mental healthcare facilities. The Position Statement on Therapeutic Group Work of the Occupational Therapy Association of South Africa (OTASA) states four criteria for the use of group work by occupational therapists: (i) a focus on occupation where social participation is emphasised, (ii) a group needs to have a clear goal, (iii) an activity (activity/task/occupation) needs to be present in the session and (iv) questions that are asked by the occupational therapist in the group need to be intentional and specific as we work on the 'here and now' of group dynamics (Occupational Therapy Association of South Africa [OTASA]

2014). This position statement reminds the occupational therapist that we are in an era of holistic, occupation-based and client-centred practice (Molineux 2004), where we need to be cognisant of the dimensions of doing, being, becoming and belonging (Hitch *et al.* 2014) and where we need to ensure that our therapeutic groups are contextualised and evidence-based.

The group size for occupational therapy groups usually ranges from 4 to 10 individuals in small groups; 10 to 15 in a mid-size group; 16 to 30 in a median-size group and 30 to 60 in a large group (Howe & Schwartzberg 2001). Groups can be classified as open groups, semi-open groups and closed groups. In open groups there is constant change of group members, which may alter the dynamics of the group. The semi-open group has stable group members and new group members join if anyone leaves. Closed groups have constant group members for the entire duration of the group; thus, they usually are able to maximise trust and cohesiveness. Both semi-open and closed groups of small to mid-sized groups foster effective interaction amongst the group members.

DESCRIPTION OF OCCUPATIONAL THERAPY GROUPS

Occupational Therapy groups are categorised as functional groups, activity-based groups, life skills groups, psychoeducational groups and expressive groups, which could be employed depending on the group members' needs (Cole 2018; Scaffa 2019; American Occupational Therapy Association [AOTA] 2020; Crouch 2021). Different categories of occupational therapy groups can be used in mental healthcare facilities to allow individuals with mental illness to explore and develop skills for participation including basic social interaction skills, tools for self-regulation, goal setting and positive choice-making (AOTA 2020, p. 62). These categories of groups are explained below:

- Functional groups focus on the therapeutic use of occupations related to activities of daily living, work, play and leisure. Examples include cooking groups, work-related skills groups and sports and game-playing groups.

- Activity-based groups focus on the process of engaging in meaningful activity with others. Examples include creative arts such as art, pottery, dance, music and creative writing; craft activities such as beadwork, making stress-balls, construction of collage, decorating gift boxes and card making.

- Life skills groups help individuals to learn new skills or coping skills to manage their life or themselves. Examples include training in relaxation methods, how to resolve interpersonal conflict and stress management strategies.

- Psycho-educational groups are used to educate individuals about their health concerns that impact their occupation and well-being. Examples include information sharing on diagnosis and medication.

- Expressive groups focus on expression of deeper emotions by using art, clay, paint and music to enable the expression of feelings and ideas and to reflect on behaviours (Cole 2018; Scaffa 2019). Other examples of methods used to stimulate reflection include reminiscence techniques, creative writing and psychodrama.

Table 7.1 summarises the types of groups that fall into categories used in occupational therapy.

Table 7.1 Categories of groups.

Functional groups Use of occupations as	Activity-based groups Engagement in activities as	Life skills groups Training and coaching in	Psycho-educational groups Didactic information on	Expressive groups Enabling introspection for personal growth through
Work-related skills (woodwork)	Expressive arts	Stress management	Diagnosis	Journaling
Pre-vocational skills training groups	Creative arts	Assertiveness skills training	Medication	Reminiscence methods
Leisure groups (sports, drumming and games)	Crafts (mosaic, material painting)	Conflict management	Discharge planning	Psychodrama methods
Activity of daily living groups (Cooking)	Music	Self-awareness	Problem-solving steps	Self-awareness techniques
Play	Dance	Vision-board	Sensory integration	Projective techniques
Sleep hygiene		Relaxation therapy	Personal recovery	
		Social skills group (role play)		
		Boundaries		
		Communication skills		
		Time management		
		Anger management		

Source: Scaffa (2019); AOTA (2020); Crouch (2021).

BENEFITS OF OCCUPATIONAL THERAPY GROUPS

The purpose and effects of occupational therapy groups have been studied for many years by different authors in the occupational therapy profession (Borg & Bruce 1991; Lund et al. 2017; Radnitz et al. 2019; Ngooi et al. 2021; Ramano et al. 2021). The evidence of occupational therapy's effectiveness in treating individuals in groups is widespread. The aim of occupational therapy groups is to help individuals with mental illness to have improved relationships, lifestyle changes and overall mental health (Lund et al. 2017).

Occupational therapy groups improve social interaction and interpersonal skills (Lund et al. 2017; Radnitz et al. 2019; Ramano & de Beer 2020; Ngooi et al. 2021). Occupational therapy group programmes with tangible activities provide opportunities for socialisation amongst individuals with mental illness in a peer group environment. The use of activities in occupational therapy groups facilitates spontaneous social interaction, encourage individuals with mental illness to experience a sense of cohesion and belonging (Ramano & de Beer 2020). Healing takes place as a result of the support provided, acceptance offered and the learning that occurs by giving each other feedback (Ramano & de Beer 2020). Importantly, a recent study found that meaningful activities used in occupational therapy groups are a catalytic means to recovery (Ramano et al. 2021).

Individuals with moderate to severe Major Depressive Disorder (MDD) who participated in a two-week occupational therapy group programme showed an improvement in the cognitive and affective functioning performance components, which are characteristically affected as a result of diagnosis (Ramano et al. 2018). The therapeutic use of tangible activities and participants' social interaction in occupational therapy groups were found to be curative and appropriate in reducing symptoms and improving functioning of individuals with MDD since it enhanced their well-being (Ramano et al. 2017). Adult inpatients with moderate to severe MDD remarked that their involvement in occupational therapy activity-based groups assisted in improving their mood (Ramano et al. 2021). However, more research is needed to corroborate these findings.

In a study by Lim et al. (2007), three-quarters of their participants found occupational therapy intervention to be helpful and most of them valued occupational therapy groups as assisting them with the improvement of concentration, daily structuring, proper planning, opportunities for socialisation, promoting their creative expression and improving their self-confidence, practicing new skills, support, relaxation and relieving boredom. Hutcheson et al. (2010) found that activities are useful to assist individuals to gain problem-solving skills, distraction from thoughts of illness and promote interaction.

By taking part in meaningful occupations, the activity group is found to stimulate spontaneity, humour, and energy and influence self-efficacy and well-being (Sundsteigen et al. 2009). Furthermore, activity encouraged continued participation in the community (Hutcheson et al. 2010).

Engagement in occupational therapy groups promotes group members' personal growth in a supportive environment, for example empowerment, sharing of ideas and learning a new skill (Crouch 2021). Personal growth is mostly enhanced through psychoeducational (didactic) groups and life skills groups. The group leader facilitates learning through imparting information and directing group interactions so that group members learn coping skills and new activity skills from each other through sharing, practice and repetition (Ramano 2017). In a study by Radnitz et al. (2019, p. 9) on occupational therapy groups as a vehicle to address interpersonal problems in social systems, the group members reported that they felt empowered and that they were able to either accept the system, change their part of the system, or leave the system. In a mixed-method study by Ramano (2017), the group members reported that they felt empowered with different skills that they learned to enable them to face life challenges and to improve their well-being. These studies show the power of occupational therapy groups to enhance the group members' ability to assist themselves (Howe & Schwartzberg 2001).

CLINICAL REASONING

Clinical reasoning is described by Rogers as the thought process that guides treatment that is offered in occupational therapy (Rogers 2004). Following this notion, various authors started to research and document their own clinical reasoning styles while planning occupational therapy interventions (Mattingly & Fleming 1994; Liu et al. 2000).

Occupational therapists working in the field of mental health guide their group intervention by using their clinical reasoning skills as discussed in Chapter 6. The style of their clinical reasoning may include, amongst others scientific, interactive, narrative, ethical, pragmatic and conditional reasoning (Scaffa 2019). Although the different styles are described separately, they are interconnected. A short description of six reasoning styles used during group work is set out below.

SCIENTIFIC REASONING

It is important for occupational therapists to use sound theory so that their reasoning is based on logical and defendable ideas, enabling them to explain how their group work intervention could have an effect on group members' well-being (Ikiugu et al. 2009). Scientific reasoning is used when occupational therapists apply 'scientifically derived' theory (Mattingly & Fleming 1994, p. 317) and evidence-based practice. It is used to understand the mental health condition affecting the group members and to decide on appropriate treatment intervention strategies, including the best type of group exposure. Scientific reasoning consists of two forms of reasoning, namely occupational diagnostic and procedural reasoning (Scaffa 2019). Each will be discussed briefly.

OCCUPATIONAL DIAGNOSTIC REASONING

According to Rogers (2004, p. 29) occupational diagnostic reasoning is the process of thinking that is used to formulate the group members' problems before they are 'summarized as occupational diagnosis'. This process consists of four components, (i) a 'descriptive component' which describes the occupational dysfunction such as difficulty in relating to others, (ii) an 'explanatory component' which describes the most likely cause of the problem for instance social anxiety, (iii) a 'cue component' that identifies signs or symptoms that can broaden the therapist's understanding of individual group members' performance component problems, for example tension headaches in social situations and withdrawal from interpersonal relationships at work, and finally (iv) a 'pathological component' that specifies the mental health disorder, for instance social anxiety disorder (Rogers 2004). According to this process, a top-down approach is followed. The functional problems are identified first, then the possible cause is explained, followed by describing the psychiatric symptoms and finally the psychiatric diagnosis that was made by a psychiatrist.

In contrast, a bottom-up approach is frequently used in the planning of occupational therapy groups, since referrals from psychiatrists indicate the provisional psychiatric diagnosis. Subsequent to these referrals, occupational therapists focus on the assessment of psychiatric signs and symptoms, as well as an evaluation of each individual group members' level of creative ability (du Toit 2009), and finally, the conclusion of the possible impact the signs and symptoms could have on their task performance and occupational functioning.

PROCEDURAL REASONING

Following the problem identification using occupational diagnostic reasoning, occupational therapists are most likely to use procedural reasoning (Cole 2018; Scaffa 2019) to the occupational therapy group intervention. In this style of reasoning, they search for appropriate theories, frames of references, approaches, including principles and techniques, as well as meaningful activities to treat the group members (Cole 2018; Scaffa 2019).

CLIENT-CENTRED APPROACH

The client-centred approach was pioneered by Carl Rogers during the 1930s (Rogers 1951). In this approach group members are seen as inherently having the ability, as well as the tendency to self-actualise unless there are obstacles in the environment that prevent them from doing so. The client-centred approach is non-directive in nature and the occupational therapist offers unconditional positive regard, empathy and genuineness (Rogers 1951; Egan 2002; Tickle-Degnen 2002). It is believed that group members have knowledge about themselves and their needs, while the occupational therapist is an expert professional who embraces partnership with the group members. Thus, occupational therapists ought to engage each group member in the decision-making process, believing in their ability to change for the better including improved occupational performance (Tickle-Degnen 2002; Maitra & Erway 2006; Casteleijn & Graham 2012).

The three conditions identified by Rogers (1951) and summarized by Vorster (2011) that could facilitate group members' growth are the following:

- **Unconditional positive regard**
  The occupational therapist should accept the group member without judgement of feelings, attitudes or behaviour.

- **Accurate empathy**
  The degree to which the occupational therapist can listen to the individual and be able to sense accurately the feelings the individual group member is experiencing.

- **Congruency**
  The degree to which the occupational therapist is genuine and transparent.

Interactive Group Approach Existentialists remind the group leader that group members are social beings and they mostly depend on interpersonal relationships for their humanness (Cole 2018). Therefore, the group leader should facilitate interaction amongst the group members and give them the opportunity to practice and form meaningful connections (Cole 2018:66). The value of occupational therapy groups includes amongst others togetherness, belonging, occupational engagement and socialising in a supportive environment (Lund *et al.* 2017). The need to belong is innate, therapeutic and healing as it allows the group members to share their inner world (Lund *et al.* 2017).

In occupational therapy groups, the group members interact with each other and the effect of their interaction might be unpredictable (Cole 2018:60). Due to the complexity of the interaction during occupational therapy groups, some scholars suggest consideration of complex system theory as a conceptual foundation for group work practice (Cole 2018).

In the widely cited work of Yalom and Leszcz (2005, p. 47), the point is made that 'psychological symptomology emanates from disturbed interpersonal relationships'. In line with this statement, Vorster (2011) also maintained that there is a correlation between a person's interpersonal relationships and degree of mental health, while Lepine and Briley (2011) point out that mental disorders are associated with problems in social interaction and close relationships. Group members with mental illness usually present with problems such as poor interpersonal skills, difficulty forming relationships, poor social skills, conflict with authority, dependency, social isolation, social exclusion, inability to express and control anger and hypersensitivity to separation (Radnitz *et al.* 2019).

The interactive approaches applied in occupational therapy groups as described by Fouche in Crouch (2021) are set out below:

- **No man is an island**
  No man is an island highlights the fact that people need people. This notion is strongly emphasized in the African Philosophy on collectivism, which maintains that 'a person is a person through other persons' (Gathogo 2008; Gade 2017). Gathogo (2008, p. 4) simply summarises the African Philosophy as 'we are meant to complement each other as I am because we are . . .' As most individuals with mental illness experience isolation, rejection, and problems with close relationships (Lepine & Briley 2011), occupational therapy groups create opportunities for social interaction, sharing of thoughts and feelings, reflection and feedback.

- **The here and now**
  The here-and-now focuses on the interaction that occurs amongst the group members in the current moment of the group. 'The here-and-now implies that the focus is on what is happening now within the group, right at this moment, here in this group' (Crouch 2021, p. 26). The group leader addresses the relationship problems between group members on what they are feeling towards other members, group leader and the group as a whole right now. The group members are able to receive feedback from each other and learn about themselves. The interaction in the occupational therapy group is triggered by the use of an activity to focus attention on particular actions and reactions. Focusing on the here and now helps the group to exert optimal influence on the group members.

- **Leading from behind**
  Leading from behind emphasises that the group leader is the facilitator of the group and should allow the group to progress at its own pace. The occupational therapist should allow the group members to express themselves so that their needs are addressed.

- **Safe, therapeutic environment: takes risks to get feedback**
  A structured, supportive social environment and setting limitations help the group members to integrate into the group (Ngooi *et al.* 2021). Groups provide a safe space to practice social skills and to strengthen relationships (Radnitz *et al.* 2019:9). The skills of group members improve within the supportive environment and group members learn to apply skills in their personal relationships, for example by learning to set firmer boundaries in some relationships and deepening connections with others (Radnitz *et al.* 2019).

- **Interaction is important**
  Fouche in Crouch (2021, p. 42) refers to interaction as 'having an effect to one another, or mutual, or reciprocal action or influence'. This highlights the fact that group members

influence each other when they connect within the group. It is assumed that once group members develop feelings of warmth, trust and care (belonging), they might feel safe enough to open up resulting in improved interpersonal relations (Ramano & de Beer 2020). The interaction allows the group members to form their own identity as they share and give each other feedback (Crouch 2021).

SOCIAL COGNITIVE THEORY

The social cognitive theory was developed by Albert Bandura and his colleagues in the 1960s (Hjelle & Ziegler 1981; Bandura 2018). This theory describes how new social behaviour can be learned by means of observational learning and the practice of desired behaviour. The practical application of this theory in occupational therapy groups is set out below.

- **Client observes desired social behaviours**
  The group leader models or demonstrates how a specific social behaviour is handled in a more effective manner, which provides for observational learning. By observing a desired social behaviour, the group members form a cognitive image of how certain behaviours are supposed to be performed. Through the observation of these behaviours and on subsequent occasions, this coded information might serve as a guide for their action.

- **Practice of desired social behaviour**
  Group members have the opportunity to practice desired social behaviour in a simulated situation where they might feel safe enough to take risks as errors have few negative consequences.

- **Individual group members to receive affirmative and or corrective feedback**
  Accurate and specific feedback might help group members to make changes in their thought patterns and behaviour. Affirmative or positive feedback should be provided as it may foster hope and encourage the group members. Corrective feedback should also be given in conjunction with suggestions or alternatives on how to improve.

- **Coaching**
  Clear instructions are necessary to facilitate the necessary adjustments to behaviour. While coaching is done in a clear and unambiguous way, instructions should also be given on what to do as well as the reason for doing so.

- **Repetition**
  It is assumed that repetition will result in increased learning. Desired social behaviour should therefore be repeated by means of brief practice trails, with immediate and frequent positive and corrective feedback.

PSYCHO-EDUCATIONAL APPROACH

During psycho-educational groups, an occupational therapist plays an educator role to enhance group learning (Cole 2018). Under the curative factor 'imparting of information' Yalom &

Leszcz (2020) referred to the application of this approach in groups where didactic instruction by the occupational therapist, or direct advice from group members is offered. Didactic groups, based on the psycho-educational approach, often form part of the occupational therapy group programme in mental health care. The psycho-educational approach provides group members the opportunity to learn information which will be of use when they leave the mental health care facility. The occupational therapist might use cognitive behavioural principles to design psycho-educational groups for skills training such as coping skills, assertiveness, social skills or stress management (Cole 2018). Furthermore, psycho-educational groups might be used for educating group members on relapse prevention, symptom management, skills for co-dependency problems and functional skills such as medication management or cooking healthy food for mental wellness.

PSYCHO-ANALYTICAL/PSYCHODYNAMIC FRAME OF REFERENCE

As indicated previously, group members are mostly treated by means of activity-based occupational therapy groups where the focus is on the group members' occupational needs and occupational performance including social interaction. Group members' socio-emotional needs however are sometimes treated by means of projective techniques, which are based on psychoanalytic or psychodynamic theory. As projective techniques frequently evoke deeper interpersonal conflicts, it is suggested that an interdisciplinary and collaborative approach be used to facilitate optimal group members' care.

The psychodynamic approach was brought into occupational therapy in the early 1960s by Fidler and Fidler (1963). They were of the opinion that the process and end product of projective activities, such as art activities, can help group members to communicate non-verbally their feelings and thoughts. The occupational therapist facilitates group interaction and allows the group to self-direct their participation in the projective activity. Projective activities serve as catalysts for introspection and offer the opportunity for emotional expression and personal growth. These techniques are not ends in themselves but rather a means to emotional expression. The occupational therapy groups that may be offered using the psychodynamic frame of reference include expressive groups such as creative drawing, sculpture, poetry, creative writing and psychodrama to express the hidden parts of self. Other activities that can be used to express emotions and communication are painting, free clay modelling, storytelling or narratives, music, movement or musical expression, journaling, and role-play techniques such as role reversal and empty chair (Cole & Tufano 2019).

ECLECTIC FRAME OF REFERENCE

A number of occupational therapists apply an eclectic/integrative frame of reference (Burnard 2005; Ikiugu et al. 2009) in their treatment of group members during occupational therapy groups. Borg and Bruce (1991) support the eclectic use of frames of reference as it allows cogent sharing of information and effective adaptation of activity. Ikiugu and Rosso (2003, p. 208) argue that occupational therapists need to focus mostly on occupation-centred practice (authentic occupational therapy) focusing on the view of humans as occupational beings, occupation as a medium of change and group leader as agents of change.

INTERACTIVE REASONING

Since occupational therapists follow a client-centred approach (described under procedural reasoning) the group members' needs, values and requests should be considered in designing the occupational therapy groups. This reasoning mode refers to the interaction between the group leader and group members. It encourages the group leader to connect with the group members as they are social beings, including the establishment of therapeutic relationships, and understanding the group members' cultural background, life story and experience of their illness (Cole 2018, p. 61). It emphasises therapist-client interaction and relationship building (Cole 2018, p. 61).

Interactive reasoning, as a continual process, aims to engage group members in their group treatment planning. The occupational therapist should therefore not only reason about what is problematic for the group member and how to fix it, but how to involve the group members in the 'fixing' process. Thus, doing with as opposed to doing to or for the group members (Mattingly & Fleming 1994, p. 179).

NARRATIVE REASONING

During the early 1990s Mattingly (1991) proposed a reasoning style that she called narrative reasoning. According to her, this reasoning style should enable occupational therapists to think about the individual group members' life stories. These 'life stories' should then reflect the group members' occupational roles and activities (Mattingly & Fleming 1994). Mattingly (1991) concluded that narrative reasoning or storytelling and story creation forms the cornerstone of clinical reasoning in occupational therapy and maintains that narrative, rather than scientific reasoning, forms the basis of clinical reasoning, thus enabling the group leader to think about the group members' life stories as it is in the here-and-now as well as helping them to visualise how the group members' life might be in the future. Narrative reasoning therefore plays an important role in the selection of (i) group objectives, (ii) topics or themes for group discussions and (iii) activities. The type of activities introduced to the group have to be meaningful and valued by group members. The group leader should consider the group members' stories, subjective experiences, gender, age groups, educational level, employment, socioeconomic status, stressors and context.

PRAGMATIC REASONING

Pragmatic reasoning is seen as another style of clinical reasoning in occupational therapy (Schell 2003), which consists of both the practice and the personal aspect of therapy. Contextual factors that facilitate or enhance treatment should be included as part of the clinical reasoning process, for example practical aspects such as treatment resources, reimbursement issues, facilities (place of group intervention), time for group intervention and trends in the profession (Unsworth 2013). High-quality facilities (indoor and outdoor) and resources that are suitable for the selected group activities such as sport equipment, games, materials and tools to create valuable and meaningful end-products should be considered. Furthermore, the objectives for the group should require careful planning that considers the duration of hospitalization or community group programme.

ETHICAL REASONING

After deciding on what would be scientifically sound, practically possible and within the group members' cultural interest and realities, the group leader should reflect on 'what ought to be done' during the occupational therapy group. Through ethical reasoning the occupational therapist proposes group interventions in relation to the ethical principles of practice. The ethical principles are the systematic exposition of the moral code that describes the group leaders' responsibilities and the fundamental principles of right and wrong action. The occupational therapy ethical codes of conduct such as beneficence, autonomy, veracity, justice and others are discussed in Chapter 4.

A Code of Ethics provides a set of principles which are based on values that guide practice and maintain high standards of professional behaviours while facilitating groups. Of outmost importance in mental health settings where unpredictable behaviours may arise, the group leader needs to be mindful of safety precautions such as team-based risk assessment and availability of security measures. The occupational therapy groups should consider occupational justice for the group members.

CONDITIONAL REASONING

Conditional reasoning is another style of clinical reasoning described by Fleming. This multi-dimensional process involves thinking across dimensions in time, past behaviour, present status and possible future outcomes. It constructs an image of the group members' possible challenges and future goals (Fleming 1991). The group leaders use conditional reasoning when they 'move beyond specific concerns about the person and places them in broader social and temporal contexts' so that meaningful experiences can be created for the group members (Mattingly & Fleming 1994, p. 133). Conditional reasoning requires a deep understanding of the group members in their totality and places the focus on

continuous adaptation of group intervention strategies (Cole 2018). Since conditional reasoning seldom happens in isolation, the group leader needs to shift between the different modes of reasoning during the group therapy process. This style of reasoning requires deep levels of insight and it is the more experienced occupational therapists who will apply this kind of reasoning (Liu *et al.* 2000; Unsworth 2013).

THERAPEUTIC FACTORS IN OCCUPATIONAL THERAPY GROUPS

One model that strongly guides occupational therapy group treatment is based on the theory and practice of group therapy as devised by Yalom and Leszcz (2020). It is assumed that individuals with mental illness may have disturbed interpersonal relationships and other functional challenges across their life, which could be addressed in occupational therapy groups. Individuals with mental illness value the relationship developed with other group members during group therapy (Joyce *et al.* 2007). Yalom and Leszcz further highlight various therapeutic factors that are facilitated during group therapies to assist with healing (Yalom & Leszcz 2020).

A therapeutic factor is 'an element occurring in group therapy that contributes to improvement in a group members' condition and is a function of the actions of a group leader, the individual or fellow group members' (Scaffa 2019). Therapeutic factors reflect those qualities that are inherent in group therapy and are valued by group members (Yalom & Leszcz 2020). Yalom and Leszcz (2020) divide the therapeutic experience into 11 primary factors facilitated as common mechanisms for change. These therapeutic factors include instillation of hope, universality, imparting information, altruism, the corrective recapitulation of the primary family group, development of socialising techniques, imitative behaviour, interpersonal learning, group cohesiveness, catharsis and existential factors (Yalom & Leszcz 2020).

Group members become interdependent on each other as a result of self-acceptance and being accepted by others (Yalom & Leszcz 2005). Universality, self-understanding and cohesiveness are viewed as important therapeutic factors (Caruso *et al.* 2013). Finlay (1993) explains that the level of trust and cohesiveness predetermines the depth of group members' involvement. In short-term therapy groups, the significance of cohesion is seen as valuable (Joyce *et al.* 2007). This allows group members to take risks as there is a sense of security which allows them to self-disclose (Vorster 2011). A supportive atmosphere creates a sense of togetherness, being accepted and valued, which leads to the experience of catharsis, lessens depression and increases life satisfaction (Chao *et al.* 2006). This benefit of group membership is also supported by Radnitz *et al.* (2019) in their study as they reported the value of support and group cohesion in the occupational therapy groups.

Occupational therapy groups are strong in cohesiveness, interpersonal learning, altruism, hope and cathartic factors and are ranked similar to psychotherapy groups (Webster &

Schwartzberg 1992). Therapeutic factors that were found to be important by the occupational therapists and group members in occupational therapy groups are cohesiveness, hope and interpersonal learning (Falk-Kessler *et al.* 1990). Both old studies by Webster and Schwartzberg (1992) and Falk-Kessler *et al.* (1990) agreed on the effectiveness of cohesiveness, hope and interpersonal learning as effective therapeutic factors in occupational therapy groups. Their results differed in terms of altruism and catharsis as they were not considered in the study of Falk-Kessler *et al.* (1990).

In the study by Lund *et al.* (2017), group cohesiveness, universality, interpersonal learning, imparting information (direct advice and didactic instructions) and altruism were found to be strong in addition to catharsis, imitative behaviour and installation of hope. Interpersonal learning, which focuses on the importance of relationships and cohesiveness in which members belong, feel valued and accepted, is viewed as powerful in group therapy (Yalom & Leszcz 2005).

The group therapeutic factors by Yalom and Leszcz were not broad enough to encompass occupational therapy groups (Eklund 1997). Furthermore, Eklund (1997) found the common therapeutic factors that are related to occupational therapy groups as relaxation, creativity, distractions, enjoyment and increasing a new skill as unique to that of Yalom and Leszcz (2005) in group psychotherapy. These are perceived as forming occupational therapy therapeutic factors (Eklund 1997). Despite the therapeutic factors, the occupational therapist uses different theoretical frameworks to guide the occupational therapy groups.

STRUCTURING OF THE GROUP

Each occupational therapy group is structured according to the size of the group, type of group, activity (tools and materials) to be used and positioning of the group members. During the opening and closing of a group session, members as a rule, sit in a circle, which promotes eye contact and interaction. The venue should be appropriate for the type of group and free of interruptions as far as possible. Moreover, the group leader should be aware of ergonomic principles in the selection of tables and chairs so that clients will be comfortable during activity participation. The positioning of group members should be determined by their conditions, level of functioning, their need for help, behaviour and the interaction required. The group leader should always face the door to be aware of the movements in the group. In the case of co-leadership, it is advisable that the co-leader sit opposite the group leader for natural non-verbal communication. Lastly, the layout often creates an atmosphere which communicates a message about what could be expected in terms of the activity that lies ahead.

GROUP PROCEDURE

A number of South African occupational therapists often follow a particular group procedure, which was developed by Beyers and Vorster (1985), Vorster and de Beer (1997), and revised by Ramano (2017) into three phases: initial phase, working phase (activity), and termination phase (reflection and discussion phase). Table 7.2 shows the summary of the revised group procedure which will be discussed below.

PHASE 1: INITIAL PHASE

Orientation

The purpose of the orientation is to create structure for the group session as the provision of external structure . . . promotes the acquisition of internal structure . . . (Yalom & Leszcz 2005). The group session starts with the group leader acknowledging and welcoming each group member. Then the group leader clearly explains the purpose of the group. This is

Table 7.2 Summary of the interactive occupational therapy group procedure.

Phase 1: Initiation phase
- Orientation
- Introduction
- Group norms/group rules
- Emotional level on arrival
- Warm-up activity
- Bridging

Phase 2: Working phase

Core group activity
- Group goals/aims/objectives
- Principles of approaches applied
- Presentation of activity
- Structuring
- Precautions
- Grading

Post-activity discussion
- Reflection on the activity
- Asking open-ended questions
- Facilitate Yalom and Leszcz therapeutic factors
- Work in the here and now

Phase 3: Termination phase
- Group members' final closing comments
- Group leaders' summary of the group session
- Reinforcement of confidentiality
- Emotional level on departure
- Affirming the group members' effort to personal recovery
- Plan of action

followed by informing the group members about the regular time of group sessions and the duration of the group session.

Introduction

It is important for the group leader to introduce him- or herself (demographic self-disclosure) first by setting the norm. By doing so, it will indicate to the group members what is required from them. Then the group leader will self-disclose something as simple as his place of birth or favourite food and request similar disclosure from the group members. These will be followed by the group members introducing themselves by name and anything else that the group leader would have used during norm-setting. Usually in the first group, the group leader at this point has to both set the norm of what is required and to lessen group members' anxiety. It is important for the group members to introduce themselves by name and something else at the beginning of each group session in order to acknowledge their presence.

Group Norms/Group Rules

As it is important to set group norms from the outset, group members and the group leader should formulate explicit group norms or rules and ethical aspects such as confidentiality, honesty, open sharing, respect for each other, giving each other a chance to talk, language preference for the group and that no one should leave the room until the group session is completed unless approved by the group members or prior arrangements with the group leader, and decided upon.

Emotional Level on Arrival

After the explicit setting of group norms, interactional norms should be created wherein each group member is met on his or her emotional level through selective self-disclosure in the here-and-now. In other words, the group leader should touch base with each group member. Group members have to reflect on their feelings within the group context, followed by an informal discussion within the group. The group leader should ensure that the mood of the group matches the goal of the group.

The reasons for meeting group members on their emotional level are twofold. Firstly, to give the group leader an idea of how the group members feel in the here-and-now and secondly, to allow the group members to recognise and identify their feelings in the here-and-now. This could be done in different ways, for instance group members could rate their feelings on a scale of 1 (sad) to 10 (happy), or relate their feelings by using colours, animals, the weather, seasons, cards with different facial expressions or informal discussion of each members' feelings.

Warm-Up Activity/Ice Breaker

The aim of the warm-up activity is to create a frame of reference for what is to follow in the main activity. It is a short activity that should last for approximately 5–10 minutes. From clinical experience, the group leader should be aware that group members who enter a group session for the first time often feel apprehensive and unsure. With this in mind, the warm-up activity has several purposes and should capture the attention of the group members.

Firstly, the warm-up activity has to lessen the group members' anxiety; secondly, social interaction has to be stimulated; thirdly, universality has to be facilitated in order to develop group cohesiveness and trust; fourthly, spontaneity has to be increased; and finally, the warm-up has to direct the group members attention towards their needs or the challenges they have to overcome in the main activity.

An example of a warm-up activity is to arrange the group members in a circle. The number of chairs in a circle needs to be one less chair than the number of members (10 members would therefore need 9 chairs) so that one member would be left standing inside the circle. The one who is standing would say something about what he or she likes and those members who like the same thing that was said, should stand up and move to the different available chair than the one they were sitting on. Once someone stood up, he or she cannot sit on the same chair. The one who remained standing would be the one who would ask the question until every member had a chance to ask a question.

Other examples of warm-up activities are musical chairs, balloon volleyball, jumping jack, parachute, tug of war, human knot game (unknotting the human knot), find someone who . . ., getting acquainted. Fouche and Crouch in Crouch (2021) highlighted some examples of warm-ups such as sending the hula hoop around the group without letting go of each-others' hand, Johari's window, blind walk, and stickers. The group leader should adapt the activity of the warm-up so that it meets the full criteria for warm-up activities and it links to the main activity.

Bridging

Bridging is mainly used to link the warm-up activity with the main activity in phase two of the group procedure. The first step in bridging from the warm-up to the main activity is what is referred to as 'problem spotting' (Fouche 2021). Once the group members are aware of the problem, they need to work on formulating the group objective and once formulated, an agreement has to be taken by all the group members to work on the problem and to participate in the main activity. This process is also referred to as verbal contract signing. Following on this step, the group members' frame of reference regarding their handling of similar challenges in the past should be obtained. An example of the steps that may need to be followed during 'bridging' are as follows.

Firstly, the group leader will ask a general question about the group members' experience of the warm-up activity; secondly the group leader will facilitate problem spotting (client should identify with the problem) "what did you think when . . .; Do you find it difficult to . . .; Do you sometimes feel . . .; What do you do when . . .; Would you like to tell us . . .?"; thirdly the group leader will formulate first (1st)-order objective of the group session (it should be formulated in such a way that it can be measured at the end of the session); fourthly, the group leader will verbally contract with all the group members individually to ensure that the group members are willing to work on the problem (facilitate agreement to participate), for example I would like to show you how to do . . . Would you like to . . .; lastly, the group leader will determine the group members existing knowledge with regard to topic at hand, for example how often do you do . . . or what method do you use . . . What have you tried . . . What do you know? in order to establish their frame of reference. Group pressure may coerce a member to agree to the verbal contract. Resistance to participation in the group process must be allowed, discussed and resolved as a normal part of group dynamics.

PHASE 2: WORKING PHASE

Core Group Activity

The use of activity as a medium of treatment is unique to occupational therapists and vital to improve group members' mental health. Occupational therapy groups are unique as activities or occupations are used as a means to achieve group members' needs and goals. Activity is a therapeutic medium used to change the group members' performance and functioning. It is important for the group leader to analyse the activity that will be used in the group and adapt it to ensure that its therapeutic potential assists in achieving the aims and objectives of the group. The group leader should take cognisance of the physical and mental capacities of the group members while selecting the activity. Engagement in an activity should take 20–30 minutes depending on the type of the group.

- **Group aims/objectives**
  The group leader should make sure that the group members' aims and objectives are established. The group leader should structure activity in a way that it addresses both individual and collective aims and objectives.

- **Focus of the group**
  Consider the therapist's focus on the group and group members. The group leader should ensure that the group is focused on its own therapeutic value and to ensure that it addresses the needs of the group members.

- **Principles of approaches applied**
  As discussed before, there are various theories, approaches and frames of references that are used in the group. The group leader should apply the principles of those approaches that are used to assist the group members. In addition, the Vona du Toit Model of Creative Ability (VdTMoCA) is often used to assist group therapists with the grouping of the MHCUs according to their functional level of creative ability. Furthermore, it helps the group leader to present activities according to the principles and techniques as stipulated in the VdTMoCA (du Toit 2009; Van der Reyden *et al.* 2019).

- **Presentation of activity**
  The activity will need to be presented according to the clients' level of creative ability (du Toit 2009; Van der Reyden *et al.* 2019). First of all, a clear and simple definition of the activity should be given before the group members engage in the activity. Therefore, the entire activity should be discussed. Then the sequence of steps and content of each step should be described. Following on this, the group leader will first start by demonstrating to the group members how the activity works so as to set the norm of what is expected. Owing to the group members' level of creative ability, ample support should be provided by the group leader to ensure that the group members participate according to the expectations of the activity. The group leader should reflect and provide feedback to group members regarding their reactions to the activity.

- **Structuring**
  A group leader will need to ensure that the environment is well organised to accommodate a group. The layout of materials and tools should be structured in a way that it will assist the group leader to achieve the aims and objectives of the group session. The seating arrangements should be according to the type of group and group leaders' objectives of the group session. The group leader should structure the materials and tools to accommodate the group members' level of creative ability, group members' interest and the appropriateness of the activity.

- **Precautions**
  The physical and mental capacity of group members should be taken into consideration and the group leader should set realistic targets. Group activities which are below the clients' capacity might lead to boredom and those activities which are beyond their capacity could cause a fear of failure and lack of self-esteem. Corrective feedback should always be constructive in nature. The group leader should count the sharp objects (scissors, knives) and dangerous chemicals (thinners, glue) and ensure that all of them are handed in at the end of the group session.

- **Grading**
  The activity should have the just right challenge to facilitate success experiences. It should be graded in terms of complexity (simple to difficult), number of steps, novelty (familiar to unfamiliar), uncertainty (predictable to unpredictable), amount of support, duration of the activity and duration of the group.

Post Activity Discussion
- **Reflection on the activity**
  The group leader should facilitate sharing and feedback from group members about their experience of the group by facilitating group interaction and emotional feedback. During phase 3, the group leader should facilitate feedback from the group members about their inter-subjective experience of the group session and also to what extent the group objective was achieved.

- **Asking open-ended questions**

  Open-ended questions such as 'how did you experience the activity' should be employed to generate discussion of feelings. Each group member should be encouraged to evaluate their effort. Retrospective, informative and positive evaluation should be encouraged. In addition, task satisfaction should be encouraged through positive feedback from other group members.

    Despite the duration of the group session, the intensity and vulnerability experienced by each group member should be kept in mind by the group leader. The impact of the group on each group member should not be underestimated.

- **First-order objectives**

  The first-order objectives are the main objectives the group leader has set for the group. During this phase, the group leader should ensure that the primary objectives (first-order objectives) of the group are met.

- **Yalom and Leszcz therapeutic factors**

  In addition, the group leader should facilitate therapeutic factors (second order objectives) as described by Yalom and Leszcz (Yalom & Leszcz 2020). During the first group, universality should be facilitated to create a feeling of safety for the group members to take interpersonal risks while enhancing cohesiveness (Yalom & Leszcz 2020). Other therapeutic factors that could be facilitated are interpersonal learning, altruism, instilling hope and the development of socialising techniques depending on the type of group and the goal of the group (Yalom & Leszcz 2020).

- **Work in the here and now**

  The group leader should facilitate interaction amongst the group members and address the relationship problems between group members on what they are feeling towards other members, therapist and the group at that moment. Furthermore, the group leader should allow the group members to give feedback to each other to enable them to learn about themselves.

PHASE 3: TERMINATION PHASE

Group Members' Final Closing Comments

Opportunity for final comments should be given to the group members so that each group member can give their opinion or a comment about what they have learned or found to be important to them throughout the group. The group leader will facilitate group members' clarification of their comments by asking open-ended questions that allow the group members to extend their comments further by explaining how they are going to apply what they have learned in their lives. Furthermore, the group members may be encouraged to give their final comments in relation to what they have learned or anything that touched them or that is meaningful to them throughout the entire group session.

Group Leaders' Summary of the Group Session

After the group leader has allowed each group member to share their experiences of the group, the group leader will highlight the key concepts or themes or important aspects highlighted by the group members. In some instances, the group members could assist the group leader to summarise the session. The group leader will continue by reinforcing what is learned or needs to be emphasised to further ensure that the goals of the group are achieved. If there are any final notes or comments or motivation that the group leader would like to share with the group members, then the group leader will do so.

Reinforcement of Confidentiality

The group leader will need to reinforce confidentiality regarding sensitive issues that may have been raised or discussed in the group.

Debriefing of the Group Members to Ensure Safety

The group leader will need to ask the group members individually to outline concerns or sensitive issues that are of concern to some of the group members. The group leader will need to debrief the group members to ensure that they feel safe and comfortable prior to leaving the group. Finally, the group leader may need to make sure that unfinished business left or unresolved in the group is followed up in subsequent sessions or through other mechanisms such as reporting to other relevant team members with informed consent of the group as a whole or with concerned individual members.

Emotional Level on Departure

Afterwards, the group leader will ask each group member to compare or rate their feelings to when they came in to join the group. The group leader may use the same rating that was used in the first phase while touching base with each group member during emotional level on arrival. During emotional level on departure, the group leader should touch base with each group member. Emotional level on departure helps the group leader to have a sense of the impact of the group session.

Affirming the Group Members' Effort to Personal Recovery

The last step is for the group leader to affirm the group members' effort and agency involved in pursuing their personal recovery through engagement during the group.

Plan of Action

The group leader will then update the group members about the group schedule and the next group session.

GROUP DYNAMICS

Group dynamics focuses on the interaction among members of a group, each of whom is dependent on the other (Yalom &

Leszcz 2020). Groups have a common goal and dynamic interaction amongst group members. The here-and-now reality orientation encourages the group members to grow and change as the group provides them with support and feedback. Group leaders need to combine theoretical evidence with unfolding narratives of group members and situations in order to provide relevant group experience (Cole 2014).

Yalom and Leszcz (2005) highlighted that group pressure changes a person's attitude and behaviour in the group. The group is capable of exerting pressure on a group member to change behaviour, but the group member influences the group when change occurs (Sadock & Sadock 2007).

Group process is the interrelationships and interaction between members, leaders and the group as a whole. The interaction operates simultaneously through member to member, leader to member and member to leader. Cole (2014:249) refers to the group process as 'social structure, symbolic meanings, transference and countertransference, communication patterns, non-verbal communication and emotional responses that often lie beneath one's conscious awareness'. These emergent process factors refer to the changing dynamics in the group.

PROBLEM GROUP BEHAVIOURS

The group leader should be aware of problem group behaviours (roles that individual members play in the group) which interfere with group functioning and integrity (Cole 2014). Problematic attention-seeking roles include the aggressor, recognition seeker, dominator, special interest pleader, and self-confessor. Members who display these behaviours divert the group to irrelevant issues and they need to be redirected by the group leader (Cole 2014, p. 251). The blocker, acting the playboy and help-seekers are self-centred (Cole 2014, p. 251). Yalom and Leszcz (2020) advise that the group leader should learn how to handle difficult group members such as the monopolist, the silent client, the boring client, the help-rejecting complainer, the schizoid client, the borderline client, the narcissistic client and the psychotic bipolar client as they may affect the group in different ways. Therapeutic guidelines on how to handle difficult group members are found in Yalom and Leszcz (2005). The group leader should be aware of these behaviours in the group and be able to manage them within the group with the group members.

GROUP LEADERSHIP

The group leader will need to screen the group members and select the group method that is best suited to the identified therapeutic needs of group members in the mental health setting at a particular point in time. The group leader will design the group session and structure the group for the group members.

The group leader needs to be aware of the group procedure and recognise that their style of leadership could influence the overall performance of a group (Molineux 2004). There are known styles of group leadership such as directive/autocratic style, democratic/facilitator style, and inactive/laissez-faire or co-leading. Usually, during first group or working with low-functioning group members, the group leader may need to use the directive leadership style, which entails a high profile from the occupational therapist as they will be expected to be actively involved in leading the group throughout its duration. The directive or autocratic leader overtly encourages the participation of the group members by directly addressing individual members to elicit their opinions.

The democratic or non-directive leader or facilitator adopts a low profile (not actively involved in leading the group) by allowing the group as a whole to make decisions, encouraging spontaneity, guiding where needed to increase cohesiveness and morale. When working with high-level group members, the group leader may need to lower their profile using a democratic style of leadership.

The inactive or laissez-faire leader allows the group members to make all the decisions of the group. The co-leader will work with the group leader as a back-up person and their roles may need to be discussed in advance with the group leader.

The style of leadership and the group leader's profile are influenced by the group members' level of functioning according to VdTMoCA (du Toit 2009; Van der Reyden *et al.* 2019), behaviour of the group members and dynamics of the group, group size, type of group and the group leaders' experience as a group facilitator. The group leader will always be a role model to set the norm so that the group members will understand what is expected from them. The group leader should be caring, offer support, facilitate emotional expression, clarification and set limits (Yalom & Leszcz 2005).

It is advisable for the group leader to be thoughtful and understanding of each group member and show respect for their values, wishes, preferences and unique culture (Cole 2018, p. 59). A group leader should also create an atmosphere that is open, accepting and supportive so that group members will feel safe enough to explore and take interpersonal risks in the group. It is important for the group leader to maximise the groups' potential for interaction, open self-disclosure and mutual support and select the appropriate activity that will address the group members' goals and occupational needs (Cole 2018). Moreover, the group leader should be able to read the group process, follow the group procedure and observe each group members' role and problems that they are experiencing and intervene appropriately (Beyers & Vorster 1985; Yalom and Leszcz 2005). The group leader is the facilitator of social interaction (Ngooi *et al.* 2021).

In occupational therapy groups, the group leader is seen as a therapeutic factor (Eklund 1997). The group leader functions as a therapeutic agent for group members' change, healing and growth (Ramano 2017). The therapeutic positioning of the leader encourages occupational presence and flow, which contributes to group members' autonomy and satisfaction through completion of the tasks, personal growth through learning, self-esteem and consideration of their lifestyle changes (Ramano 2017).

Therapeutic use of self refers to an occupational therapist's skill in forming and maintaining therapeutic relationships during occupational therapy groups (Cole 2018, p. 70). The trusting therapeutic relationship between the occupational therapist and group members is established through collaboration, communication, therapist empathy and mutual understanding (Cole 2018, p. 71). It is beneficial for the group members to feel accepted with authentic support in order to enhance their social connection and strengthen their self-esteem (Radnitz et al. 2019). The stronger social connection in the group is brought about by the group leader while ensuring the development of trust in the group. Crouch (2021) explains that trust develops when there is openness, sharing, acceptance, support and cooperative intentions amongst the group members. Ramano and de Beer (2020) found that occupational therapy groups stimulate social interaction when the interpersonal demands vary in intensity for group trust to be established. As trust develops and group members bond with each other they feel comfortable to freely express themselves and share their feelings in a group (Ramano & de Beer 2020). This is mostly facilitated by the group leader who listens, believes and values the group members (Lund et al. 2017). The group leader's leadership maintenance roles include being an encourager, harmoniser, ensuring that the group members clarify their unclear statements, consensual validation, handling different roles played in the group, reflecting, using silence, mirroring, using minimal verbal responses and summarization. These approaches to group handling assist with facilitation of interaction in the working phase (post-activity discussion) of the group procedure (Howe & Schwartzberg 2001; Scaffa 2019).

EVIDENCE-BASED PRACTICE

OUTCOMES

It is important that occupational therapists routinely measure the outcomes of the occupational therapy groups that they offer in their different settings. An occupational therapy group

intervention that is well structured and planned should provide a therapeutic effect to the group members on their physical, cognitive, emotional, motor activity, physical, psychosocial and functional independence (Borg & Bruce 1991; Lund et al. 2017; Ramano et al. 2017, 2018, Ramano & de Beer 2020; Radnitz et al. 2019; Ngooi et al. 2021; Ramano et al. 2021).

It is advisable for occupational therapists who are doing occupational therapy groups in different settings to reflect on the day-to-day running of their occupational therapy groups and to develop a routine of sharing ideas. This is supported by practicing occupational therapists to continue sharing their ideas, experiences and stories related to their groups. Furthermore, occupational therapists should attend courses as part of their continuous professional development to help them evaluate and critique their knowledge and skills.

RESEARCH

There is a critical need for evidence-based research in occupational therapy interventions including occupational therapy groups. The authors of this chapter support the international call for more evidence research on occupational therapy groups. Furthermore, more studies on evidence-based research, interactive group approach and development of group models and theories may need to be undertaken by different occupational therapists who are interested in research.

DEVELOPMENT OF AN INTERVENTION GROUP PROGRAMME

It is important for occupational therapists to develop occupational therapy group programmes that are scientific and evidence-based. The enablers for the successful development of occupational therapy group intervention programmes are relevant theoretical frameworks, clinical and professional reasoning, theory of occupation in occupational therapy, inclusion of activities for their therapeutic value in enhancing speedy recovery, therapeutic factors as put forward by Yalom and Leszcz, client centeredness, activity analysis, and following the group procedure. The occupational therapist should ensure that the topics that are included in the occupational therapy group programme are properly graded to address the objectives, aims and goals of the group. Attached is an example of a group intervention session plan that may be used for student training.

GROUP INTERVENTION SESSION PLAN

Venue: Date of session:

Facilitator: Co-facilitator:

Names of group members:

Type of group:

First order objective:

Session target:

[First order objective, is the main aim or goal of the group/theme or topic the area or skill you are addressing = e.g.

- *Overall: Health and wellness, quality of life, participation, well-being, occupational justice*

- *Occupations: Social participation, Leisure (Leisure exploration, Leisure participation)*

1. Initiation phase		
Introduce self and others		
Duration of group		
Set norms/rules for the group		
Meet on emotional level (Arrival)		
Warm-up: Ice-breaker		
Bridging Close the contract		
2. Working phase		
Type of Activity/Description		
Structure		
Materials/Equipment/Tools (Including Est Cost involved)		
Presentation according to VdTMoCA		
Therapeutic foundation used (including principles and techniques)		
Second order objectives		
Precautions: General, Activity & Clients		
Upgrading/Downgrading		
Post-activity discussion		
3. Termination phase		
Group members' final comments		
Leader's summary		
Affirming group members		

Further evaluation

Session targets met	
Choice of activity	
Critical incident (positive or negative)	
Phases of the group (group procedure)	
Occupational therapy therapeutic factors	

Impact made by the therapist (therapeutic use of self, therapist behaviour and skill/task of group leader/leadership role and skill)	
Roles played in the group	
Handling problem group members	
Aspects that should / could have been changed	
Plan for the next session	

CONCLUSION

Occupational therapy groups are an effective treatment modality for the management of individuals with mental illness in different settings. For occupational therapy groups to be effective, the group leader should ensure that the group therapy sessions are client-centred, holistic, contextualized, evidence-based, and occupation-centred. Furthermore, the group leader should focus on the here and now, apply the principles of interactive group approach and use Yalom's therapeutic factors. To ensure the flow and proper structure of the group, the group leader should follow the three phases of the group procedure.

CASE STUDY

Ms Z is a 35-year-old single woman who works for an accountant firm as a clerk. She has no children. She has no living relatives and stays with an 80-year-old woman who provides her with basic needs such as food and clean clothes. Besides reading, Ms Z has no leisure time activities and avoids social events, which leaves her feeling lonely and isolated. She has not had a boyfriend for almost five years. She reported serious financial problems and declining work performance owing to her depression.

Ms Z was admitted to a mental health care facility for two weeks. On admission, Ms Z was diagnosed with MDD-single episode by her treating psychiatrist. She was referred to occupational therapy. She presented with emotional problems (depressed mood, irritable mood, restricted affect and low self-esteem), cognitive problems (impaired concentration, forgetfulness and impaired decision-making), conation/motor activity problems (low energy levels and hypoactivity) and occupations (social withdrawal, impaired social skills, no leisure participation and poor vocational skills).

As the occupational therapist followed a client-centred approach, Ms Z was accepted unconditionally, supported and took an active role in setting up her treatment plan. It was resolved that the focus of her occupational therapy was first of all to improve her interpersonal skills and social confidence, thus altering her self-perception as a person who is unable to communicate effectively and make friends, and secondly, to explore meaningful leisure time activities. The occupational therapist used narrative reasoning to find out about Ms Z's past and present stories and helped to modify her future story in terms of activity participation and social relationships. From a scientific reasoning perspective, an interactive group approach and cognitive behavioural approach were followed to facilitate social interaction and social skills in a secure and a supportive environment. As part of her comprehensive holistic treatment plan, Ms Z was introduced to a two-week occupational therapy group programme. The group consisted of ten members including the occupational therapist. Each occupational therapy group session differed in terms of the first-order objective, activities and interpersonal demands. The group procedure remained the same for each occupational therapy group session.

On entering the first group session, Ms Z seemed emotionally distant and apprehensive. The occupational therapists' welcoming nature, warmth and support seemed to have reassured her. The group session started as everybody was welcomed by the occupational therapist followed with a request to introduce themselves by merely stating their name, and hometown. Although this request required self-exposure, Ms Z was able to do so and seemed slightly relieved. This was followed by a statement of the time and duration of each group session before group norms were set and ethical aspects such as confidentiality were also decided upon. Then, explicit norm setting, interactional norms were created wherein each group member was met on their emotional level. This gave Ms Z the opportunity to reflect on, and became aware of, her effect within the group context. The group was facilitated by means of the client-centred principles to establish cohesion development.

A warm-up activity was initiated where each group member was asked to move around and try to answer five formulated questions about five different group members. Each group member was expected to answer one question about themselves. The first-order objective of the first group session was to get acquainted on a superficial level. A card game was introduced with minimal interpersonal demands apart from sharing information about likes and dislikes. On completion of the card game, group members were asked to verbalise their experiences of the game.

As part of cohesion development and trust, it was important for the occupational therapist to facilitate the principle of universality. The process and intensity of the group experience were acknowledged by the occupational therapist as the impact of group interaction and exposure were not underestimated. Before departure from the group session, group members were asked to do a final reflection on their feelings in the here-and-now. Ms Z indicated that she felt 'emotionally fine and ok'.

On the subsequent days, group members were orientated once more by referring back to the previous groups' objectives and activities. At the beginning of each group session, actual time limits and suggested targets were stated and agreed on by group members and the occupational therapist who was the group facilitator.

Different types of groups were facilitated within the two-week group programme. Three group sessions focussed on the exploration of leisure time activities using sports and games (fingerboard, 30 seconds, adapted volleyball), which necessitated social interaction in the group context. Ms Z was also exposed to craft activities (painting jewellery boxes, beadwork – making a bracelet, collage – making a portrait of their future self, vision-board) for relaxation, creativity, learning new activity skills, enjoyment and to improve their self-confidence. As Ms Z experienced a number of successes while participating in sports, games (mainly card games), and craft activities, it appeared that she experienced flow and happiness. Engaging in meaningful activities gave her the opportunity to interact with others and to improve her self-confidence.

Ms Z attended self-management groups to assist with her coping skills, which included stress management, assertiveness, boundaries, conflict management and financial management. In groups such as assertiveness skills training, the occupational therapist used role play as a technique to improve group members' social skills. In the final group session, group members made a card for themselves in which feedback was given to one another. Ms Z received positive verbal and written feedback, whereby positive social behaviour was reinforced.

TREATMENT OUTCOMES

As Ms Z's self-confidence and feeling of accomplishment increased, she began to take the risk of self-disclosure during the group sessions. At first, her efforts were restrained and she was soft-spoken, but active listening and a willingness to focus on what she had to say helped her to develop trust and to take interpersonal risks. Treatment outcomes for Ms Z were positive as she was committed to change her past life story as she wanted to create a new story for herself. She reported that her symptoms had improved with some functional independence. Post-discharge, Ms Z returned to work. She informed the occupational therapist that she set up a monthly budget, laid down financial boundaries for herself and monitors her expenses. With regards to her leisure time, the occupational therapist assisted the client in finding a card game club in her community. The client reported that she joined a Saturday morning Bridge Training Club, which she enjoys thoroughly.

QUESTIONS

1. Name the types of groups according to the Occupational Therapy Practice Framework (Fourth edition).

2. Discuss the benefits of occupational therapy groups.

3. Explain the relevance of client centeredness in occupational therapy groups.

4. Explain the use of procedural reasoning to plan a group session.

5. How does the use of the interactive group approach assist with the success of the group?

6. Discuss the relevance of five therapeutic factors that are related to occupational therapy.

7. Discuss the relevance of Yalom's therapeutic factors in occupational therapy groups.

8. Discuss the steps of bridging in group procedure.

9. Name one warm-up activity and explain how it meets the criteria for a warm-up activity.

10. Explain how you will ascertain the impact of the group while using the group procedure.

REFERENCES

American Occupational Therapy Association (AOTA) (2020) Occupational therapy practice framework: domain and process. 4th edn. *The American Journal of Occupational Therapy*, **74** (**Supplement 2**), 1–87.

Bandura, A. (2018) Towards a psychology of human agency: pathways and reflections. *Perspectives on Psychological Science*, **13** (**2**), 130–136.

Beyers, D. & Vorster, C. (1985) Opleiding van die groepterapeut. *Psychotherapia and Psychiatry in Practice*, **40**, 26–33.

Borg, B. & Bruce, M.A. (1991) *The Group System: Therapeutic Activity Group in Occupational Therapy*. SLACK Incorporated, West Deptford.

Burnard, P. (2005) *Counselling Skills for Health Professional*, 4th edn. Nelson Thorne, Cheltenham.

Caruso, R., Grassi, L., Biancosino, B., *et al.* (2013). Exploration and experiences in therapeutic groups for patients with severe mental illness: development of the Ferrara group experiences scale (FE-GES). *BioMed Central Psychiatry*, **13**(**242**), 1–9.

Casteleijn, D. & Graham, M. (2012) Incorporating a client-centered approach in the development of occupational therapy outcome domains for mental health care settings in South Africa. *South African Journal of Occupational Therapy*, **42**(**2**), 8–13.

Chao, S.Y., Yuan-Liu, H., Yen Wu, C. *et al* (2006) The effects of group reminiscence therapy on depression, self-esteem, and life satisfaction of elderly nursing home residents. *Journal of Nursing Research,* **14**(**1**), 36–44.

Cole, M.B. (2014) Client-centred groups. In: B. Wendy, J. Fieldhouse & K. Bannigan (eds), *Creek's Occupational Therapy and Mental Health*, 5th edn, pp. 241–259. Churchill Livingstone Elsevier, China.

Cole, M.B. (2018) *Group Dynamics in Occupational Therapy: The Theoretical Basis and Practice Application of Group Intervention*, 5th edn. SLACK Incorporated, Deptford.

Cole, M.B. & Tufano, R. (2019) *Applied Theories in Occupational Therapy: A Practical Approach*, 2nd edn. SLACK publishing, Deptford; Placeholder Text

Crouch, R. (2021) *Occupational Group Therapy*. Wiley Blackwell, Oxford.

Du Toit, V. (2009) *Patient Volition and Action in Occupational Therapy*, 4th Revised edn. The Vona & Marie du Toit Foundation, Pretoria.

Egan, G. (2002) *The Skilled Helper: A Problem-Management Approach to Helping*, 7th edn. Brooks/Cole. (Wadsworth Group), London.

Eklund, M. (1997) Therapeutic factors in occupational group therapy identified by patients discharged from a psychiatric day centre and their significant others. *Occupational Therapy International*, **4**(**3**), 200–214.

Falk-Kessler, J., Momich, C. & Perel, S. (1990) Therapeutic factors in occupational therapy groups. *The American Journal Occupational Therapy*, **45**(**1**), 59–66.

Fidler, G.S. & Fidler, J.W. (1963) *Occupational Therapy: A Communication Process in Psychiatry*. Macmillan, The University of Michigan.

Finlay, L. (1993) *Groupwork in Occupational Therapy*. Chapman and Hall, London.

Fisher, A.G. (2014) Occupation-centred, occupation-based, occupation-focused: same, same or different? *The Scandinavian Journal of Occupational Therapy*, **20**, 162–173.

Fleming, M.H. (1991) The therapist with the three-track mind. *American Journal of Occupational Therapy,* **45**(**11**), 1007–1014.

Fouche, L. (2021) The Occupational Therapy Interactive Group Model (OTIGM). In: R. Crouch (ed), *Occupational Group Therapy*. Wiley Blackwell, Oxford.

Gade, C.B.N. (2017) *A Discourse on African Philosophy: A New Perspective on Ubuntu and Transitional Justice in South Africa*. The Rowman and Littlefield Publishing Group Inc, South Africa.

Gathogo, J. (2008) African philosophy as expressed in the concepts of hospitality and ubuntu. *Journal of Theology for Southern Africa*, **130**, 39–53.

Hjelle, L.A. & Ziegler, D.J. (1981) *Personality Theories: Basic Assumptions, Research and Applications,* 2nd edn. McGraw-Hill, London.

Hitch, D., Pepin, G. & Stagnitti, K. (2014) In the footsteps of Wilcock, part two: interdependent nature of doing, being, becoming and belonging. *Occupational Therapy in Health Care*, **28**(**3**), 1–7. https://doi.org/10.3109/07380577.2014.898115.

Howe, C. & Schwartzberg, S.L. (2001) *A Functional Approach to Group work in Occupational Therapy*, 3rd edn. Lippincott Williams & Wilkins, Baltimore.

Hutcheson, C., Ferguson, H., Nish, G. & Gill, L. (2010) Promoting mental wellbeing through activity in a mental health hospital. *British Journal of Occupational Therapy*, **73**(**3**), 121–128.

Ikiugu, M.N. & Rosso, H.M. (2003) Facilitating professional identity in occupational therapy students. *Occupational Therapy International*, **10**(**3**), 206–225.

Ikiugu, M.N., Smallfield, S. & Condit, C. (2009) A framework for combining theoretical conceptual practice model in occupational therapy practice. *Canadian Journal of Occupational Therapy*, **76**(**3**), 162–170.

Joyce, A.S., Piper, W.E. & Ogrodniczuk, J.S. (2007) Therapeutic alliance and cohesion variables as predictors of outcome in short-term group psychotherapy. *International Journal of Group Psychotherapy*, **57**(**3**), 269–296.

Lepine, J.P. & Briley, M. (2011) The increasing burden of depression. *Neuropsychiatric Disease and Treatment*, **7**(**1**), 3–7.

Lim, K.H., Morris, J. & Craik, C. (2007) Inpatients' perspective of occupational therapy in acute mental health. *Australian Journal of Occupational Therapy*, **54**(**1**), 22–32.

Liu, K.P., Chan, C.C. & Hui-Chan, C.W. (2000) Clinical reasoning and the occupational therapy curriculum. (W. P. Ltd, Ed.). *Occupational Therapy International*, **7**(**3**), 173–183.

Lund, K., Argentzell, E., Leufstadius, C., Tjornstrand, C. & Eklund, M. (2017) Joining, belonging, and re-valuing: a process of meaning-making through group participation in a mental health lifestyle intervention. *Scandinavian Journal of Occupational Therapy*, **26**(**1**), 56–68. https://doi.org/10.1080/11038128.2017.1409266

Maitra, K.K. & Erway, F. 2006 Perception of client-centered practice in occupational therapists and their clients. *The American Journal of Occupational Therapy*, **60**(**3**), 298–310.

Mattingly, C. (1991) The narrative nature of clinical reasoning. *The American Journal of Occupational Therapy*, **45**(**11**), 998–1005.

Mattingly, C. & Fleming, M.H. (1994) *Clinical Reasoning: Forms of Enquiry in a Therapeutic Practice*. F.A. Davis Company, Philadelphia.

Molineux, M. (2004) *Occupation for Occupational Therapists*. Blackwell Publishing, Hoboken.

Ngooi, B.X., Wong, S.R., Chen, J.D. *et al* (2021) Benefits of occupational therapy activity-based groups in Singapore acute psychiatric ward: patients perspective. *Occupational Therapy in Mental Health*, **37**(**1**), 38–55.

Occupational Therapy Association of South Africa (OTASA) (2014) Position statement on therapeutic group-work in occupational therapy. *South African Journal of Occupational Therapy,* **44**(**3**), 43–44.

Radnitz, A., Christopher, C. & Gurayah, T. (2019) Occupational therapy groups as a vehicle to address interpersonal relationship problems: mental health care users perception. *South African Journal of Occupational Therapy*, **49**(**2**), 4–10.

Ramano, E.M. (2017) *A Comparison of Two Occupational Therapy Group Programmes on the Task-Oriented Functioning of Mental Health Care Users with Major Depressive Disorders. Doctor Philosophiae*. University of Pretoria, Pretoria.

Ramano, E.M. & de Beer, M. (2020) The outcome of two occupational therapy group programs on the social functioning of individuals with major depressive disorder. *Occupational Therapy in Mental Health*, **36**(**1**), 176–187.

Ramano, E.M., de Beer, M., Roos, J.L. & Becker, P.J. (2017) A comparison of two occupational therapy group programs on the functioning of patients with major depressive disorders. *Minerva Psichiatrica,* **58**(**3**), 125–134.

Ramano, E.M., de Beer, M., Becker, P.J. & Roos, J.L. (2018) Mental health care users with major depressive disorders: initial outcomes of an occupational therapy group programme. *African Journal for Physical Activity and Health Sciences*, **24**(**3**), 60–71.

Ramano, E.M., de Beer, M. & Roos, J.L. (2021) The perceptions of adult psychiatric inpatients with major depressive disorder towards occupational therapy activity-based groups. *South African Journal of Psychiatry*, **27**(**0**), 1–8.

Rogers, C.R. (1951) *Client-centred Therapy: Its Current Practice, Implications and Theory*. The Riverside Press, Cambridge, Massachusetts.

Rogers, J.C. (2004) Occupational diagnosis. In: M. Molineux (ed), *Occupation for Occupational Therapists*, pp. 17–31. Blackwell Science, Oxford

Sadock, B.J. & Sadock, V.A. (2007) *Kaplan & Sadock's Synopsis of Psychiatry: Behavioural Sciences Clinical Psychiatry*, 10th edn. Lippincott Williams & Wilkins, Philadelphia.

Scaffa, M.E. (2019) Group process and group intervention. In: B.A.B. Schell & G. Gillen (eds), *Willard and Spackman's Occupational Therapy*, 13th edn. pp. 539–555. Wolters Kluwer, Philadelphia.

Schell, B.A. (2003) Clinical reasoning: the basis of practice. In: E.B. Crepeau, E.S. Cohn & B.A. Schell (eds), *Willard & Spackman's Occupational Therapy,* 10th edn, pp. 131–140. Lippencott Williams & Wilkens, Philadelphia.

Sundsteigen, B., Eklund, K. & Dahlin-Ivanoff, S. (2009) Patients' experience of groups in outpatient mental health services and its significance for daily occupation. *Scandinavian Journal of Occupational Therapy*, **16**, 172–180.

Tickle-Degnen, L. (2002) Client-centered practice: therapeutic relationship, and use of research evidence. *The American Journal of Occupational Therapy*, **56**(**4**), 470–474. Placeholder Text

Unsworth, C. (2013) The evolving theory of clinical reasoning. In: E.A.S. Duncan (ed), *Foundations for Practice in Occupational Therapy*, 5th edn, pp. 209–232. Churchill Livingstone Elsevier, Edinburgh.

van der Reyden, D., Casteleijn, D., Sherwood, W., de Witt, P. (2019) *VdT-MoCa The Vona du Toit Model of Creative Ability: Origins, Constructs, Principles and Application in Occupational Therapy*. Softcover published, South Africa.

Vorster, C. (2011) *Impact: The Story of Interactional Therapy*. 1st edn. Satori Publishers, Pretoria.

Vorster, C., & de Beer, M. (1997). Group activities in occupational therapy. Unpublished notes. University of Pretoria: Pretoria.

Webster, D. & Schwartzberg, S.L. (1992) Perception of curative factors and occupational therapy groups. *Occupational Therapy in Mental Health*, **12**(**1**), 3–7.

Yalom, I.D. & Leszcz, M. (2005) *The Theory and Practice of Group Psychotherapy*, 5th edn. Basic Books, Cambridge.

Yalom, I.D. & Leszcz, M. (2020) *The Theory and Practice of Group Psychotherapy*, 6th edn. Basic Books, Cambridge.

Human Ecosystems and Other Disasters

The Impact on Health, Wellness and Human Occupation

Robin Joubert and Chantal Juanita Christopher

Discipline of Occupational Therapy, University of KwaZulu-Natal, Durban, KwaZulu-Natal, South Africa

KEY LEARNING POINTS

- Expanding our understanding of human ecosystems and disasters.

- Insight into, and an appreciation of, the effects of disasters on health, wellness, human occupation and biodiversity.

- An understanding of the underlying principles that drive the occupational therapy approach and interventions to disaster management.

- Exploring the role of occupational therapists in disaster situations.

"Because of the current atrophy of an utopian imagination, apocalyptic imaginaries and narratives of cataclysmic disasters and unknown futures have colonised the spirit of our time. But what politics do visions of apocalypse and catastrophe engender, if not a politics of separation, rather than a politics of the humanity, as species coming into being?"

(Mbembe 2018, p. 1)

INTRODUCTION

Mbembe's (2018) quote forefronts the lack of '*a utopian imagination*' that thwarts humanity's action against disasters and centres this chapter's intention. We, the authors, hold similar thoughts, particularly concerning our action and inaction as a profession, in terms of meeting, preventing and mitigating the impact of these 'disasters'. The chapter aims to expand the understanding of human ecology relative to disasters, offering insights into its impact on wellness and reflections upon the occupational therapy profession's emerging role/s in the future.

Human ecology studies the interface and interrelations between human and non-human nature within their built, natural, socio-cultural and political contexts (Department of Geography, Lund University, Sweden 2022). This important understanding emphasises intersectional pressures and conditions; nevertheless in this chapter, it prompts our intentional focus on human ecology as specifically seen in terms of disasters.

A human ecosystem is an ecosystem characterised by its people and the human values they pursue both as individuals and within society, and their influence on their wider context (Moore et al. 2022, pp. 55–56). Human ecosystem disasters are natural disasters created by humans through acts which impact negatively upon the natural environment, such as pollution, deforestation, nuclear explosions and oil spills.

Crouch and Alers Occupational Therapy in Psychiatry and Mental Health, Sixth Edition.
Edited by Rosemary Crouch, Tania Buys, Enos Morankoana Ramano, Matty van Niekerk and Lisa Wegner.
© 2025 John Wiley & Sons Ltd. Published 2025 by John Wiley & Sons Ltd.

Global disasters have occurred throughout history on an annual basis in areas of hazard and as a result of diffuse causative elements; however, it appears that the incidence, widespread location and severity of disasters are reaching unprecedented levels in documented history. Disasters can be divided into either events through natural causes, for example earthquakes or as a result of human activities such as nuclear fallout. They occur predominantly as a result of natural ecological disasters, particularly weather and climate catastrophes, and others such as earthquakes, volcanoes, and tsunamis. However, they are also generated through human activities such as conflict and war and exploitation of the environment. Never before in the history of occupational therapy have we faced such a challenging future in terms of the changing face and profile of human occupation (Joubert 2020, p. 77). In 2022, The World Federation of Occupational Therapists (WFOT) acknowledged this dire situation, and produced a Disaster Preparedness and Risk Reduction Manual (WFOT 2022, pp. 1–75).

Human activities pose serious consequences for life on Earth, and these human-generated outcomes are evident in global warming, global unrest and the COVID-19 pandemic. Thus, while this chapter will focus on the impact and consequences of these disasters on occupational stability, health and wellness, it will also explore a broadening of our disaster concept and how these disasters, whatever their cause, affect all life on Earth. Leaning on Mbembes utopian imagination (2018), we posit that our acts of human occupation and creativity can either be positive or negative agents and advocates in creating, compounding or alleviating disaster effects, and therefore each one of us, individually, collectively and professionally, are responsible for creating solutions to these problems.

The United Nations International Strategy for Disaster Reduction (UN-ISDR 2017, p. 1) defines a disaster as a serious disruption of the functioning of a community or a society causing widespread human, material, economic or environmental losses which exceed the ability of the affected community or society to cope using its own resources. We would like to broaden this description as our contemporary lives intersect with disasters at different levels. We, therefore, theorise disasters to include:

- Part of an intersecting continuum of disasters or longue durée (long-term effects) that impact our lives over decades. For example global warming and the proliferation of plastics in the environment.

- Human propagated disasters of the 21st century, for example increasing stress and work-life disproportion, decreasing connection with others in real-time, individual orientated life focus versus thoughts on the collective.

- Disasters of the Other. For example, the isolation of the majority of world disasters as happening to Others/Them upholds some people's continued marginalisation with limited attempts to ameliorate conditions. Making this case is the Gini co-efficient, which tracks the difference between the rich and poor globally, and is thus an analytical tool that captures human injustice. As revealing as the Gini coefficient is, it has not promoted widespread and focused intervention in mitigation of these findings. This is evident through the same cluster of countries being at the top of the list over many years which illustrates the problem of seeing but not acting in relation to the Other.

- Fallout sequelae of individual disaster events. For example, wars or nuclear disasters that have global effects such as oceanic radioactivity following the nuclear disaster at Fukushima, Japan or lifetime losses following a house being swept away during floods.

- Disasters are overwhelmingly framed through the human species lens and must of necessity also include all living species.

- Economic disasters – these disasters include food insecurity and hoarding of essentials, profiteering on life-supporting goods, corruption and denudation of natural resources.

- Disasters of a political nature – the rise of fascism, nationalism and political agendas that prevent people from flourishing are on the rise across the planet.

This broadening of our understanding of disasters illustrates that disasters do not always occur as singular events or are linear, timebound or non-intersecting as seen at this stage in our history. The world is experiencing a series of mostly prolonged disasters that affect the entire world and their impact, in terms of damage and consequences, is thus compounded. These phenomena are now at a stage where our quality of life as well as our very existence on Earth is threatened for both humans and other species, some of which are already extinct.

Regardless of the nature, type or severity of disasters, they: threaten injury, precipitate decreased quality of life, cause death and displacement to large groups of people and animal and plant life; cause the destruction/disruption of habitat and livelihood and ways of life, and the disruption of essential resources and infrastructure. Other consequences are psychological and social as they impact the occupational processes of doing, being and belonging, disrupting social relationships and networks and related services. Ultimately, they impact not only the physical, mental and spiritual wellness and health of those affected but also the occupational potential and quality of life of large numbers of individuals (Goldmann & Galea 2014, pp. 169–183).

PUTTING THIS INTO CONTEXT

While global human population statistics are now showing a decline, the human population in 2022 was close to 8 billion people and projections for the next 30-odd years suggest an increase of anything up to 10 billion people (UN 2022, p. i). The growing impact of sustaining such huge numbers, of mostly resource-needy humans, is placing a strain on ecosystems such that it is having catastrophic effects on the biodiversity of our planet (Attenborough 2020). The emerging reality of global warming, with its climatic effects, poses an ongoing threat to the continued stability of the existence of global humanity.

Added to this, global unrest and difficult living conditions in many parts of the world are resulting in the unprecedented displacement of fleeing refugees and asylum seekers. On top of these conditions, the prolonged COVID-19 pandemic has deeply challenged the confidence of the world's health care systems, while causing human hardship and millions of deaths. In addition, and although not usually classified as a disaster, the burgeoning digital revolution, which while it has provided extraordinary technological advancement, has contributed to wide-ranging issues such as unemployment and other health-challenging side effects which are emerging, such as the effects of social media distraction and unproductivity, social anxiety and depression, cyberbullying, cyber misogyny, cybercrime and internet addiction (Huddleston 2015, pp. 3–196).

The collective consequences of these prolonged disasters are resulting in burgeoning and irreversible social and economic need, mass displacement of millions of people, in many instances with concomitant destruction of property, illness, injury, death, growing food insecurity and poverty. These conditions create unrelenting pressure upon basic resources such as energy, water and food. From a health perspective, the ultimate effects of this upon the overall quality of life, health and wellness of humanity continue to reveal themselves.

In a profession called upon to be contextually relevant and embedded within sociocultural circumstances, these contemporary conditions require occupational therapists to research and analyse these changing occupational profile/s. Specific research focused on a careful revision and transformation of the role and scope of occupational therapy is necessitated if it is to maintain its invaluable contribution to humanity's quality of life and good health. It will require a broadening of our approach and ethos to view occupation not only for its positive therapeutic effects but also for how these aforementioned disasters are impacting negatively upon human occupation, occupational choices and collective consciousness. The aforementioned conditions of disaster and the insidious creep of digital technology with their concomitant health consequences, are undermining wellness generally, and are challenging the very ethical fibre of humanity.

Because of the evolving and emerging nature of these phenomena, this chapter will attempt to briefly summarise the salient consequences of disasters as they impact health, wellness, spirituality and human occupation. To adequately face the future, we suggest that the occupational therapy profession undertakes transformative work, to acquire a novel, moral and axiologically driven approach. This would include how occupational therapists can align their interventions to contribute to improving and maintaining the quality of life of humanity through a dynamically evolving attitude. This chapter does not intend to suggest that we relinquish our existing important remedial, therapeutic and rehabilitative roles, which are directed primarily at disability, disorder and diagnosis-related interventions, but that we broaden our perspective so that it encompasses the preventive, promotive, restorative, and advocacy directed focus that is required of post-disaster interventions. Since this situation is an evolving one, the authors are not in a position to categorically stipulate the consequences on mental health, but we have attempted to allude to these throughout the chapter as they have been revealed through our literature review. Predictably, we can anticipate an incremental and debilitating impact on the mental health of humanity as and when these disasters and situations multiply, as has been anticipated in the preceding introduction.

A BROAD SUMMARY OF THE CURRENT DISASTERS IMPACTING UPON HUMAN OCCUPATION, HEALTH, WELLNESS AND EXISTENCE, PARTICULARLY IN THE AREA OF MENTAL HEALTH

To ground our thinking and future orientation as a profession, these contemporary disasters deserve to be unpacked through our professional lens. This will enable us to read the disasters from Mbembe's (2018, p. 1) atrophied utopian imagination and the opposite. The careful unpacking will serve to document, reflect and create an understanding of ways forward.

GLOBAL WARMING AND CLIMATE CHANGE

The summary of the sixth assessment report of the Intergovernmental Panel on Climate Change (IPCC 2021, p. 3) for policymakers reveals the unequivocal fact that the planet has warmed, causing widespread and rapid changes in the atmosphere, ocean, cryosphere and biosphere.

The accumulated effect of this is that the world will be increasingly exposed to severe wet and dry events such as extremely hot temperatures, freak storms and cyclones, monsoons and flooding, droughts, runaway fires and encroachment of oceans onto low-lying land. In addition, oxygen levels are dropping in the upper ocean, but temperatures are rising which, together with increased levels of carbon dioxide, are causing acidification of the surface of the ocean affecting marine life and thus also the availability of this as a food source. Climate zones are shifting poleward in both hemispheres influencing growing seasons for agriculture, which in turn will result in regional shifts in social and economic occupations and ways of life with the potential widespread displacement of humanity. All these factors will collectively affect residential security, agriculture and marine security with a concomitant effect on food security including the occupations that sustain these various securities.

GLOBAL UNREST, INSTABILITY AND DISPLACEMENT

Competition for dwindling worldly resources and related hoarding, overpopulation, nationalism coupled with territorialism and ideological differences, as well as ever-present inhumane political leaders and dictators, has resulted in increasing unrest and warfare amongst various nations (Joubert 2020, p. 78). Coupled with this is a rising decline in the levels of freedom and democracy throughout the world (Frank & Santos 2020, p. 1), the growing Gini coefficients within the majority world and a gulf of difference between these living conditions versus the Global North.

Apart from the devastating effects upon infrastructure, social disruption and human life that such unrest, invasions and wars bring, perhaps the most serious is the displacement that it causes of millions of people fleeing for their lives, into other countries. This in turn may result in an additional strain on these host country's resources, many of which are already struggling to sustain their own populations.

In their 2022 Year in Review, the United Nations Human Rights Commission reported that one hundred million people had been displaced (United Nations News Report 2022, p. 1). These displacements may occur internally, within a specific country or they mostly occur externally where displaced persons seek refuge and/or asylum in neighbouring countries or countries that they select as being a safer option or one of greater potential for a different/better life. Some of these people have been exposed to repeated displacement. Children below 18 years of age are particularly affected during these displacement crises and are estimated to constitute 43.3% of all forcibly displaced people (UNHCR 2023). This is made worse when the displacement is not quickly resolved and persists for many years. Consequences following a disaster can result in developmental delays and children may experience anxiety, fear, sadness, sleep disruption, distressing dreams, irritability, difficulty concentrating, and anger outbursts (Centre for Disease Control and Prevention [CDC] 2020).

Displacement usually results in immeasurable trauma, emotional turmoil and loss of loved ones, pets and possessions, identities, traditions and culture, with severe implications for physical, mental and spiritual health and development. It also results in the loss of livelihood, social capital and the ability to practice one's way of life. For many of those displaced, this is experienced as a lack of financial and personal security with increasing dependence related to the need for social relief and the sheltering country's largesse and accommodation for ongoing survival.

THE COVID-19 PANDEMIC AND OTHER ZOONOTIC DISEASES

Zoonotic diseases are on the rise across the world, particularly over the past decades. These diseases are a result of viruses, parasites, and bacteria jumping from one animal species to humans, e.g. monkeypox, Ebola and HIV. This increasing incidence is a direct consequence of limited food resources, overpopulation growth, urbanisation, encroachment of humans into animal territories, close animal–human interfaces, and cultural eating preferences including exotification of animal meat/parts.

Since late 2019, the COVID-19 pandemic has disrupted lives and caused the deaths and disability of millions of people across the world. At the time of writing, this pandemic is still active and research around its complex consequences is ongoing. It is, thus, too early to fully comprehend the total and emerging impact it has had upon human existence. What is a common cause is that it has had a major impact on employment, education, rethinking the workplace environment and population health (Sigahi et al. 2021). For some, it has had long-term effects which are impacting function and occupation. It also raises the real possibility that this could be the start of more frequent similar pandemics as humanity continues to encroach on other species coupled with compromised world health by global warming, overpopulation and overcrowding. The accumulated effects of COVID-19 lockdowns, the sporadic bans on intercontinental travel, disruption of cultural and religious gatherings, and separating children and adults from their schools, communities, recreational spaces and places of work have resulted in wide-scale social isolation, fractured developmental milestones, narrowing of human occupation and loss of employment and income. The World Economic Forum (WEF) estimates that 114 million people lost their jobs over the course of 2020 (WEF 2021, p. 1).

In addition, the COVID-19 pandemic has caused ill health both directly and indirectly. The sequelae of being infected are still being reported; however, long-term changes have already been documented. COVID-19 can lead to post-acute COVID syndrome, which is a multi-system disorder resulting most commonly in respiratory, cardiovascular, hematologic and neuropsychiatric symptoms either alone or in combination (Chippa et al. 2022). These effects may last weeks, months or even years and may have negative consequences for many areas of occupation. Indirectly, reduced exercise due to space and recreational limitations imposed by isolation and social distancing, coupled with fear, anxiety and depression have in turn created rising levels of mental and physical health problems and exacerbated old ones.

Of particular relevance is our belated attention as occupational therapists to pandemics and other endemic disorders. It is important to remember that in sub-Saharan Africa and particularly southern Africa, the HIV pandemic (another zoonotic disease) has continued to affect and destroy lives in much the same way as the COVID-19 pandemic. It has fallen into the background as a result of anti-retroviral efficacy; however, it continues to impact mortality and decrease general health and occupational performance and participation. Indeed, anti-retroviral access and distribution, testing and uptake were disrupted during the COVID-19 lockdowns, which demonstrates the intersecting influences of these pandemics.

THE DIGITAL REVOLUTION

While the advances in digital technology are unprecedented in their ability to enhance human existence and contribute to the health and wellness of the planet, we would be naïve not to also be alarmed by the emerging and long-term negative effects of aspects of digital technology upon the world. We need only recall how excited humanity became as the plastic revolution overwhelmed the world from the late 1800s to the present day, but we also need to heed how plastic pollution continues to seriously and adversely affect humans, wildlife, the oceans and their inhabitants.

It can be argued that automation, artificial intelligence, and a worldwide digital communications network are an empowering platform for unprecedented innovation and new job opportunities; however, they also create considerable challenges with regard to unemployment, displacement, job polarisation, career instability, ethical challenges and overall economic insecurity. The threat exists that while technology races ahead, technological skills development lags behind. Further to this, a technological divide is evident in terms of access and the ubiquitous nature of technology across the world. While the Global North streaks ahead, technology limitations in some parts of the world (for various reasons) create further conditions of marginalisation and deprivation.

Computers and robots have already replaced millions of jobs and continue to do so. The McKinsey report (2017, p. 11) on the loss and gain of jobs estimated that by 2030, 3–14% or 75–375 million of the global workforce may have to transition to new occupational categories and learn new skills. The WEF's Future of Jobs Report for the year 2020 estimated that the workforce is automating rapidly and that it will displace 85 million jobs in the next five years (Zahidi 2020, p. 26).

While digital technology may offer certain advantages to the cognitive, social and emotional development of children as well as opportunities to explore, play and learn, research and anecdotal evidence also reveals that overexposure to digital sources can have detrimental effects on creativity, language development, motor and spiritual development and social interaction (Huddleston 2016, pp. 3–61) And when used for negative purposes such as cyberbullying, cybercrime, cyberstalking or for non-reciprocated sexualisation this may have severely detrimental implications for moral and mental health. In his book *Digital Cocaine A Journey Toward iBalance* Brad Huddleston (2016, pp. 6–15) likens the current addiction of many of us to our mobile phones, the internet and social media, as demonstrating similar patterns to those of someone addicted to cocaine. Indeed, Maria Ressa, in her 2021 Nobel Peace Prize lecture, presented the metaphor that an invisible atom bomb has exploded in our information ecosystem. She pressed the urgency of the current human condition, liking it to the post-Hiroshima world, calling for us to likewise create new institutions and declarations that state our position and values such as the United Nations and the Universal Declaration of Human Rights, in order for us to monitor and stand up against humanity repeating what she refers to as an arms race in the (mis)(dis)information(sic) eco-system (The Reading List 2023, p. 25).

GLOBAL EFFECTS OF DISASTERS RELATED TO HUMAN OCCUPATION AND WELLNESS

We start by noting that any disaster, and particularly multiple disasters, impacts most seriously upon the poor and vulnerable and upon women and children. The negative effects of disasters on access to amenities and services, employment, housing, health care, education and legal protection exacerbate an already vulnerable situation creating greater risk to health, welfare, wellness and quality of life. There is growing evidence that the cumulative effects of disasters result in serious, often long-lasting mental effects such as post-traumatic stress disorder, anxiety, depression, increased substance use/abuse, suicidal tendencies, sleep problems and the exacerbation of existing psychiatric disorders (Goldmann & Galea 2014, pp. 169–183; Math *et al.* 2015, pp. 261–271; Makwana 2019, pp. 3090–3095).

The following is a summary of the impact of most if not all of these disasters.

Loss of livelihood/s and unemployment continue to be some of the most serious impacts of the global disasters and the digital revolution. New jobs are emerging through changing technology, but they are not enough to fill the gap of those jobs that are becoming obsolete or have been lost through advanced technology and disasters.

Unemployment: Global unemployment is expected to remain above pre-COVID-19 levels until at least 2023. The 2022 level of unemployment is estimated at 207 million, compared to 186 million in 2019 (International Labour Office 2022, p. 1). Unemployment appears to disproportionately affect women and the youth. These statistics do not include the impact of wars such as the Tigray War on the African continent and the Russian invasion of Ukraine. Wars displace people with the resultant livelihood disruption usually felt locally and in neighbouring countries and with that country's trading partners. These knock-on global effects are felt as a result of most cataclysmic disasters such as wars, earthquakes or nuclear disasters. Furthermore, places of livelihood are closed or suspended, and the lack of workforce and untenable work conditions disrupt supply chains and economic life. Should the disaster cause displacement of people to another region, then livelihood disruption is long term; people may not be easily absorbed into host countries and employment reshaping and re-skilling may be necessary.

Reshaping employment: Humanity continues to change the shape and nature of work and livelihoods as a result of the current conditions of the planet. While some changes have negative consequences, others are part of the human race's ongoing development and technological prowess. For example, the COVID-19 pandemic has globally disrupted restaurants and caused people's avoidance of public places. This resulted in the closure of many institutions; however, others have creatively redesigned their services to offer delivery with apps such as Uber Eats or local motorcycle delivery workers proliferating across urban cities.

Many repetitive jobs have now been made redundant by industrial advancement and digital technology and new ones are emerging as a result of new technologies. Global warming and the need for recycling have resulted in a growing recycling industry that starts from waste pickers and specialised collectors (industrial waste pickers) on dump sites and ends in recycling factories that turn used or single-use plastic, metal and glass back into reusable products. Climate change has affected traditional jobs within the agriculture and fishing industry but also created work for tree planters, vegan cuisine, fish restocking and hydroponic farms. While water remains a dwindling commodity, we predict new ventures will seek to address this, creating space for new livelihood imaginings.

Redeployment, skilling, re-skilling and upskilling: Regardless of whichever of these disasters or circumstances are the cause of unemployment, it has meant that many people have had to seek alternative employment and this in turn may require the acquisition of new skills or upgrading of existing skills. Displaced peoples need as a human right, opportunities to participate in livelihood activities as well as local assistance in transitioning more easily to the open labour market. Part of this assistance should include being offered job guidance, language courses, being taught job/related work-related policies and being carefully inducted into employment.

Alternate/intermittent employment: The COVID-19 pandemic has illustrated the dynamic nature of employment in contemporary times. According to the International Labour Office, the total working hours globally in 2022 were projected to be 2% below the pre-pandemic level, and that is equivalent to the loss of 52 million full-time jobs (ILO 2022, p. 1). Remote and hybrid workplace models are becoming part of the norm with many people working from home or distant from their normal place of work. Companies have downsized their workplaces and workplace culture has changed. The corporate world is transforming into pop-up businesses that are powered by 'gig' workers, who work on a freelance basis with limited connection to their site of business (Joubert 2020, p. 79). The concept of co-workers and workplace culture being part of a collective has also changed with less connection to, and with, others. Virtual non-face-to-face contact and online etiquette have displaced real-time face-to-face meetings and important personal human contact.

EFFECTS UPON THE QUALITY OF LIFE AND HEALTH AND WELLNESS

Our overpopulated world, complicated by this wide-scale displacement, has resulted in competition for space and resources and placed a strain upon interpersonal tolerance. The offshoot of which are unpleasant side effects such as xenophobia, violence and racism, which in turn impact negatively upon the levels of mental contentment of humanity. It is impossible to quantify the stress and grief that may accompany individuals caught up in these disasters and having to rebuild a life with very little left to build with, in often hostile and foreign contexts. This is further exacerbated if and when it becomes an everyday occurrence, which ultimately develops into the long-term conditions of dehumanisation and life stress.

The relatively short-term impact of the long periods of isolation for millions, and especially those living alone, for example during the COVID-19 pandemic and the fears related to being infected with it has resulted in loneliness, depression, anxiety and despair for many and has exacerbated existing psychological problems. Post-COVID effects include ongoing physical symptoms, neuro-psychiatric and cognitive issues while further studies continuesand will undoubtedly expand our understanding.

Effects upon mental health Emerging research on the impact of social media and virtual reality on the mental health of the world reveals that messaging and other activity on digital devices results in the release of the neurotransmitter dopamine, which is also released in large quantities when we consume drugs or engage in sexual activity, a finding that reinforces the concerns over the addictive effects of some digital devices (Huddleston 2015, pp. 6–15). With its quick and largely superficial gratification and addictive influence, it is resulting in those who are affected demonstrating symptoms such as anxiety, stress, low self-esteem, and cognitive problems that affect academic performance. Other documented problems have been related to fear of missing out (FOMO), seeking validation through social media posts, being influenced to participate in or imitate dangerous activities (the pod challenge) and the proliferation of fake news. There is increasing evidence that the internet and social media are contributing towards increasing levels of suicide-related behaviour and depression (Luxton *et al.* 2012, pp. 195–200; Luby & Kertz 2019, pp. 1–2). The worldwide ownership of smartphones is contributing to a deeply disturbing effect on interpersonal relationships in which many families and friends, while they may share social spaces together, and which were originally used for vibrant interaction, are now frequently utilised for solitary virtual interaction with their phones and disconnection with each other. As Huddleston (2015, p. 7) describes it, 'they are all together but they are not "together"'.

EFFECTS ON PHYSICAL HEALTH

Humanity's physical health is under attack from all fronts. Illnesses of lifestyle proliferate and cause mass deaths yearly (obesity, diabetes), while the increase in cancers has been linked to the state of the planet, pollution and generalised stress. Paradoxically, the world is at its most accessible and this apparent broadening of our horizons has also created the narrowing of our lives. We see this in many examples such as refugees who are confined to camps where space and opportunities for play and recreation are minimal; the quick spread of the SARS-Cov-2 virus across the world and the diverse protocols of various countries regarding border admission, or access to life-saving vaccines; the disconnection from real-time as an effect of the digital revolution and lockdowns. These conditions have resulted in people either willingly or unwillingly finding themselves in mostly sedentary situations where physical activity is limited. In these situations, adults and children alike are confined to small spaces, and/or sit for hours in front of a computer, the television or their mobile phones and playstations, where movement is confined to mostly fine manual activities rather than gross motor activities. As a result, the risk of developmental delays in children as well as lowered energy and endurance levels in especially older persons can impact negatively upon quality of life, productivity and general cardiovascular health. Anecdotal evidence from occupational therapists in paediatric practice has suggested that greater numbers of children assessed after lockdowns showed signs of reduced fine and gross motor skills compared to those assessed prior to the COVID-19 pandemic, which could be attributed to this enforced physical inertia. However, research is needed in this area.

EFFECTS ON RELIGIOUS AND SPIRITUAL HEALTH

In times when the global sustainability of humanity is threatened by disasters of apocalyptic proportions and over which we have little if any control, succour is provided through religious and spiritual activities including reflection. A common and natural response is for individuals to turn to what we consider a higher power/s or their god/s, and to prayer as a means of coping with these threats. This is often the only source of comfort and strength in what otherwise may appear to be a hopeless situation. For those who are spiritual, existential reflection may weigh heavily as the internal focus brings to bear the degree of the unfolding disaster/s. The side effects of these global disasters are disruptive in this important life domain as it may create strains in human relations and sometimes a loosening connection to religious deities who appear to be non-responsive to human suffering, which adds to the experienced stress.

Our interrelatedness and interdependence upon one another become accentuated in times of disaster. It is in such times that the compassion for those who are affected, by those who are less affected, is demonstrated through acts of care and altruism that help to sustain those who are recipients and create opportunities for meaning-making in the contributors. Ultimately, these are times when there is a rekindling of faith in humanity, *ubuntu*[1] and personal fortitude including for

those who previously did not find solace in placing their destiny in the 'hands' of a higher power. These experiences are positive in that they bring out the best in humanity and can be harnessed to deal more compassionately and humanely with the victims of disasters.

EFFECTS ON PERSONAL AND SOCIETAL VALUES, HUMANISM AND MORALITY

The cause of so-called human-facilitated disasters and circumstances discussed in this chapter is rooted in the actions of humanity and the control of resources as well as sometimes intersecting with environmental disasters. A case in point is that of marginalised people eking out life on the banks of a river and living in informal housing, who are prone to floods as a result of all or a combination of the following: the weather phenomena, poor water management, denudation of the environment, capitalistic tendencies that encourage migration and urbanisation without providing facilities to accommodate the working class, limited personal choices, and the need to be close to economic hubs. Our values, although compassionate at the time of the disaster when these homes are destroyed, may be linked to the event only, as we may be annoyed/frustrated by the pollution of the river, the destruction of the river bank as a riverine ecosystem, at the illegality of the settlement and the lack of political solutions. Our values are thus at war with each other.

Throughout a large part of the world's history, humans have been controlled and governed by socio-political forces including class and race hegemonies. World leaders have tended to place more importance on accumulating material wealth and comfort for themselves and sometimes for their countries/citizens rather than for the global health of our environment and humanity. This has driven waves of colonialism and current imperialism. The World Inequality Report (2022, p. 1) reveals that there are wide disparities in wealth distribution between, and within, countries. The richest 10% of the global population currently earn 52% of the global income, whilst the remaining 90%, including mostly the poorest half of the global population, earn just 8.5%. These statistics expose the dire humanitarian state of the world while exposing the continued situation as morally and ethically bankrupt. This greed has resulted in the exploitation of our natural and mineral resources to such an extent that it is arguable whether global warming will be reversible. Certainly, the destruction of our biodiversity through human action has resulted in the extinction of millions of valuable species of insects, flora and fauna (Attenborough 2020, pp. 3–259).

This continuing evidence of an individualistic and morally declining world strongly suggests that we support the adoption of an altruistically oriented ethos from an occupational therapist and occupational scientist perspective. This is an ethos that is already emerging in the writings and actions of progressive therapists and scientists (Whalley-Hammel 2014, pp. 39–50; Rushford & Thomas 2015, pp. 3–273;

---

[1] Ubuntu is an African philosophical concept which literally means *'I am who I am through others'*.

WFOT 2019a, pp. 4–24; WFOT 2019b, p. 1–2; WFOT 2022, pp. 1–75). This value-laden attitude should become an essential part of our ethos and how we approach our role in contributing to the global challenges of the future as they impact upon human occupation or human occupation impacts upon them.

These humanitarian disasters also link to the profession's axiological orientation and ethical systems. Is occupational therapy at the vanguard of attempts to ameliorate the effects of these disasters? Are we responsive and working strongly towards disrupting the 'disaster of the day' or are we experiencing an atrophy of the utopian imagination? Are we (for the majority) undertaking work that focuses on traditional modes of intervention with typical populations? Does our work uphold definitions of health that we take from the World Health Organisation? These questions require us as a profession to look at our contemporary values and enact our ethical responsibilities.

The authors do not offer intervention strategies, or answer where and how we work under these conditions. We rather ask you to consider the lack of practice sites for people like Adla, lack of funding as well as lack of professional and systemic support. We propose that we see our work as an ecology of practice, seeking to impact different elements within the vignette simultaneously. Practice interventions need to centre family and living in a hostile environment when they fled hostility to emphasise safe cultural expression alongside significant acculturation that may offer increased safety. Occupational therapy practice needs to include coping strategies, depression and anxiety treatment, and techniques that suit the individual from narrative work and journaling, to cognitive behavioural techniques and plans for safe evacuation and family contact in times of xenophobia.

A SUMMARY OF OCCUPATIONAL CONSEQUENCES

The cumulative effects of these disasters are likely to remain with us for many years to come. They may indeed become attenuated and decrease, but there is also the greater possibility that they will grow and be made worse by the fact that they are becoming more frequent, diverse in nature and may occur simultaneously, for example the war in Ukraine started during the COVID-19 pandemic. Further, an event such as a flood, as seen in the 2022/4 floods in KwaZulu-Natal in South Africa resulted in wastewater pipelines being disrupted, flow of sewage into water systems and the damaging of sewage treatment centres that were not maintained by municipalities. These natural and human-related elements collided to create bacterial growth in the sea off the local beaches, affecting marine life. Human occupations such as surfing, beach bathing, catching and consumption of marine life, have been disrupted, at both personal and economic levels and therefore impacted on quality of life.

The collective angst that these situations create and their impact on the mental health of entire communities and societies is currently immeasurable and, as we have tried to demonstrate in the preceding discussion, may result in generating mental illness that affects occupational capacity and well-being to such an extent that whole communities become embroiled in, and by, it. Throughout this chapter, we have summarised and alluded to the types of mental illnesses that are currently being revealed through research and those that are anticipated; however, because this is an emerging/evolving scenario, we can only predict that these described disaster situations will categorically affect mental wellness/health.

DISPLACEMENT VIGNETTE

Adla is a 43-year-old mother from the Democratic Republic of Congo (DRC). She is currently documented as a refugee in Durban, South Africa following war and conflict in her home country. Her story is marked by her experiencing repeated internal displacement within the DRC for most of her life as a result of war between different factions. Prior to undertaking the long arduous journey to southern Africa, she was based at a displacement camp near Kivu, when fresh fighting spread into the camp, which was razed and women were tortured and sexually abused. This experience prompted her to leave. She has been a resident in Durban, KwaZulu-Natal for eight years and sought help from an occupational therapist for her teenage daughter who is struggling at school. As the family case was explored, it emerged that Adla is experiencing anxiety and depression alongside post-traumatic distress as a result of her lifelong experiences as well as increasing xenophobia in South Africa.

Analysis of Adla's situation reveals disasters that are perpetrated by humans, on an ongoing basis across decades, the experience of traumatic events including violence, witnessing of killing, gang-rape and torture of women and girls, alongside fear for life and family. Once in South Africa, Adla originally felt adrift from her culture, language and way of life, exacerbated by her initial inability to negotiate life across many aspects: from where to shop, to how to apply for refugee status.

Adla is thus a symptom of a variety of human disasters that collide to make the marginalised and the vulnerable easily bullied, beset upon and 'Othered'. Adla's hypervigilance, fear and anxiety has also made her controlling and negative regarding her children's activities. She finds little meaning in her job at a local hair salon within the central business area, which is foreign-owned. She is patronised cross-culturally as she is a trained kindergarten teacher. She was unable to answer the question, *'tell me about activities that make you happy?'*

As a profession, we will have to be particularly vigilant to this and look to creative ways to counter the emergence and prevent mental illness reaching debilitating heights. We will briefly discuss these at the end of the chapter.

THE ROLE OF OCCUPATIONAL THERAPY IN MITIGATING DISASTER EFFECTS

The essence of our humanness is dependent upon our daily engagement in occupation and it is within this *'doing'* (Wilcock 1999, pp. 1–11) that we become ourselves or we become what is better described as our totality as humans. This totality, apart from consisting of our biopsychosocial being, also consists of our spiritual being, which constitutes what, and how, we become creative beings (du Toit 1962, pp. 1–19) and how we attain a sense of purpose and belonging within the communities and world in which we live. Each one of these components is essential to being holistically healthy and is largely dependent upon the context within which we live. According to Whalley Hammel (2014, pp. 35–50), the priorities for human well-being of the majority of the world's peoples are belonging, connectedness and interdependence, which echoes with the concept of totality espoused by du Toit (1962, pp. 1–19).

Because occupational therapy is based upon the belief that a human-centred focus on health and well-being is brought about by humanity's essential engagement in occupation, the primary goal should be that we can freely engage in the everyday activities that we need to, we are required to, and in which we choose to engage in. If circumstances prevail that block our ability to adequately engage in these occupations over prolonged periods, then it will negatively impact our physical and/or psychosocial and/or spiritual well-being and thus affect our health either through creating new illnesses or exacerbating existing ones. An example of this can be seen in neighbourhoods with high levels of poverty and limited resources. A child born into these conditions may struggle to thrive as a result of malnourishment or being cared for in an informal creche with little resources. The child is understimulated and presents as functionally illiterate a few years later, and may have behavioural issues.

Up until recently, the focus of occupational therapy has largely been institution-based and disability focussed, with the community focus being mostly centred on rehabilitation. In order to meet the challenges posed by the disaster scenarios sketched in this chapter, we will have to transform our current focus, which concentrates more upon individual or small group interventions, to include a greater emphasis on large group, community, organisational and societal interventions. We will have to work more as agents, advocates and sometimes even as activists in collaboration with affected communities, governmental and non-governmental organisations and specialist professions in finding solutions that will accommodate the wide-scale disruption and devastation that these disasters may have upon victims, particularly from an occupational perspective.

We will also need to adapt our current biopsychosocial focus to one which incorporates an ecological focus that is driven by environmentally healthy occupational attitudes and behaviours. In this way, occupation becomes a transformative medium in change and a socioecological process of engagement which is closely related to the protection, preservation and management of natural resources and the well-being of world populations (Rushford 2015, pp. 1–13).

Significant to the ethos of this chapter, in research on occupational therapy culture as seen through the multifocal lens (Martin *et al.* 2015, p. 86), 'Occupations are social practices' was identified as one core category and it included three subcategories: 'Occupation, health and well-being as a personal and community experience'; 'Co-occupations, collective occupations and collaborative occupations are the most important occupations'; and 'Occupation, health and well-being mutually influence each other'. The overall findings of this research indicate that to accommodate this concept, it requires taking different worldviews into account for the development of an occupational therapy culture that is useful globally and hosts diverse meanings and occupation-focused/based practices.

Occupational therapy is thus required to step up to this moment, disrupt its business-as-usual work, and enter a professional moment where we begin to revisit those hegemonic practices within the grand narrative of the profession that perpetuates the occurrence, exacerbate the impact and provide basic disaster intervention. We need to ensure that we are not the 'handmaidens' to economic and privileged systems that impact disasters and disaster tolerance. This calls for the examination and unmasking of these practices. Our reading of disasters and the future necessitates the formulation and expression of a responsive and human rights focus. This should be guided by a strong axiological/ecological rights-based focus, for it to work. These universal bonds are required in a world whose connections, although more diverse and culturally sensitive, remain in the whole disconnected and power-laden. The world of disasters and our expanded definition belies disastrous societal conditions and related constructs that nuance our work.

UNDERLYING PRINCIPLES THAT WILL DRIVE THE APPROACH AND INTERVENTIONS

- The effectiveness of disaster preparedness and risk reduction initiatives depends largely on the cultural sensitivity, political awareness, respect and critical reflexivity of the professionals involved (WFOT 2022, p. 5).

- Interventions have to work within the parameters of occupational stewardship and collaborative engagement (Rushford 2015, pp. 1–13) which is underpinned by sensitive, collaborative and responsible management of at-risk populations.

- Application of an eco-oriented approach that focuses on environmental protection, preservation and natural resource management in any relevant interventions that bring about occupational transformation (Rushford & Thomas 2015, pp. 1–2).

- Occupational therapists are concerned with human rights in pursuing occupational justice (WFOT 2019b, pp. 4–24). Thus, intervention should be in keeping with a participatory occupational justice framework (POJF) (Whiteford & Townsend 2011, pp. 65–83), which accords with the norms of stewardship and collaborative engagement and strives towards providing populations with the opportunities, resources, privilege and rights to participate in their desired occupations and achieve their potential within such occupations. The POJF also emphasises community development, population approaches and occupational participation whilst also being constantly vigilant towards abuse of power and inequity in everyday life.

- Techniques/principles need to be developed, revisited or borrowed, especially those that operationalise our axiological and justice-orientated work, particularly into disaster zones, prevention of disasters, or generally in our current perpetual state of disaster. These techniques need to create/foster opportunities to disrupt us/them and othering as a modus operandi in lieu of who is impacted the worst as a result of disasters (Christopher 2023).

- The approach supports a critical or radical practice approach which, through collaborative means, focuses on influencing and transforming regulations, policies, laws, economic and professional practices and forces that determine what people can, need or want to do.

- Linking to this is the development of processes that unravel intersectional oppressions which together form both the conditions and contexts for, and of, disasters, but also drive our inability to adequately address these obstacles. These processes should incorporate these deeper levels of analysis and understanding into the particular professional applications related to marginality, oppression and constructions (central mechanisms) that perpetuate intersectionality (Christopher 2023).

- It should raise ethical, moral, civic and philosophical questions about opposition to occupational injustice and the tensions or gaps that exist between ideals and the reality of communities or populations living daily with the iniquitous disadvantages or oppression that may be associated with the outcomes of natural disasters and avaricious societies.

- Interventional projects should be designed to contribute to the betterment of the affected individuals or populations and ecosystems; they should be sustainable and preferably provide incentives that enhance the quality of life of those concerned, for example, collective occupations.

- Due to the evolving nature of such interventions, the process requires reflective practice and constant evaluation and adaptation of, and to, these intervention processes.

- The understanding that people know best needs to be carefully mediated as a principle of practice.

EXPLORING THE ROLE OF OCCUPATIONAL THERAPISTS IN DISASTER SITUATIONS

The role and scope of occupational therapy in this evolving situation are emergent and will require extensive research and dialogue across continents as these are diversely affected and have diverse cultural and contextual dynamics. But as a start, we suggest the following as guidelines for the transforming role of occupational therapists in disaster situations:

- Working collectively and cooperatively with all relevant role players with regard to identifying, planning and implementing relevant occupational programmes and creating adequate spaces to accommodate the needs of those who are unemployed, quarantined, displaced, or confined to refugee camps.

- Working together with the various role players and professionals in identifying at-risk populations in order to create appropriate occupational spaces, interventions and opportunities for them. Such as, for example, collectively implementing a situational analysis that reveals temporary, intermediate or permanent needs of the population under threat. It would identify skills and abilities within that population and mobilise these to assist with the provision of the necessary infrastructure and resources such as housing, food security (agriculture/market gardening), educational and developmental programmes for children, recreational programmes, health maintenance and other programmes which will enhance societal upliftment and quality of life.

- Working together with relevant religious and spiritual role players to provide essential opportunities for the fulfilment, nurturement and sustainability of spiritual needs.

CONCLUSION

Historically, occupational therapy is based upon the belief in the holistic nature of humanity and its need to exist, survive and procreate through involvement in meaningful interaction with each other and through involvement in relevant occupations. If we revisit Vona du Toit's (2015) concept of human creative ability being dependent upon the integrity of the totality of the human, that is the psyche (the psychological/emotional component), soma (the physiological component) and soul (the spiritual component) as it exists within a particular contextual environment, it is integral to remember that the one component cannot exist without the others. Thus, all these components are inseparably linked and interact together to drive the person to become greater or lesser than their innate creativity, depending on their circumstances and context. The moment circumstantial disruptions such as disasters, ill health/injury and/or other destructive human-generated influences occur, they have the potential to seriously disrupt the normal interaction of these three components and thus seriously compromise the physical, mental and spiritual health of the individuals concerned. In the context of this chapter, we are referring to millions of affected people.

The reality of the current state of global disasters and disruption, and the likelihood of their sustained occurrence, requires a collaborative effort that arguably supersedes anything like it in our past. A collaborative effort that may require a whole new restructuring of our socioeconomic, and concomitantly also our occupational, ethos. In so doing, we will have to decide whether our role as occupational therapists is going to remain confined to primary, secondary and tertiary health care interventions or whether it is going to spread itself into a more intense preventive and promotive domain with an axiological foundation that requires of us as occupational therapists to be advocates, agents and, yes even activists, in turning our world into a better place to live in for all.

To give birth to this new child, we need to be liberated from the chains of adherence without losing the essential foundations that history has taught us about human occupation. We should be guided by Franz Fanon (1963, pp. 7–311), who maintains that liberation is often the substitution of the one species of humankind by another. So whatever form this liberation takes, it is still a form of colonisation of new ideas and attitudes substituting old ones. We need to be 'angelic troublemakers who will fight for a better future' (Makgoba 2023, p. 12) for our chaotic world by using our unique knowledge of occupation to take us into this future.

Finally, Professor Sandra Maria Galheigo – Assistant Professor at the University of São Paulo, in her Foreword to the WFOT Disaster Preparedness and Risk Manual (2022, p. 80), summarises the core of this chapter in a quote from Paulo Freire: 'Every tomorrow, however, what one thinks about, and which one fights for, necessarily implies dream and utopia. There is no tomorrow without a project, without a dream, without utopia, without hope, without the work of creating and developing the possibilities that make its realization viable. It is in this sense that I have said on different occasions that I am hopeful not out of stubbornness, but out of an existential imperative'.

QUESTIONS

1. Given your particular, unique geographical context, do you think occupational therapy could play a role if any of the disasters discussed in this chapter happened to occur there? And if so, briefly what would that role be?

2. If your context found itself in a situation where there was an influx of thousands of refugees due to a disaster, who were currently living in a refugee camp, reflect on some of the interventions that occupational therapy could contribute to implementing.

3. Interventions in situations as described here are too large for a single professional group to resolve on their own. List some of the role players that occupational therapists would work together with, how they would complement each other and how their various roles would differ.

4. It is suggested here that we should become more involved in advocacy promoting spaces and programmes that would contribute to greater health and wellness for affected communities. Consider how and what programmes/spaces would be appropriate.

5. It is suggested here that we should, where appropriate, even become involved as activists. Can you list some of the areas where this might be appropriate?

REFERENCES

Attenborough, D. (2020) *A Life on Our Planet: My Witness Statement and a Vision for the Future*, 1st edn. Witness Books, London.

Centre for Disease Control and Prevention (2020) *Caring for children in a disaster: your child is at risk for mental health issues after a disaster*. December 2020. https://www.cdc.gov/childrenindisasters/features/disasters-mental-health.html (accessed on August 2023)

Chippa, V., Aleem, A. & Anjum, F. (2022) *Post acute coronavirus (COVID-19) syndrome National Library of Medicine, National Center for Biotechnology Information*. February 3, 2023. https://www.ncbi.nlm.nih.gov/books/NBK570608/ (accessed on December 2022)

Christopher, C. (2023) *(Un)becoming re-creation: exploring "Coloured" women's suffocation versus rejuvenation*. Submitted in fulfilment of the requirements for the degree of Doctor of Philosophy in the School of Health Science, University of KwaZulu-Natal, Durban. January 2023. (Currently undergoing examination).

Department of Geography, Lund University, Sweden (2022) *Human ecology, people and environment*. HUMAN GEOGRAPHY | DEVELOPMENT STUDIES | HUMAN ECOLOGY https://www.keg.lu.se/en/education/subjects/human-ecology#:~:text=Human%20Ecology%20is%20the%20study,biology%2C%20economic%20history%20and%20archeology. (accessed on 8 August 2023)

Du Toit, V. (1962) Initiative in occupational therapy. In: V. du Toit (2015), *Patient Volition and Action in Occupational Therapy*, 5th edn, pp. 1–19. Vona and Marie du Toit Foundation, Pretoria.

Frank, G. & Santos, V. (2020) Occupational reconstructions: resources for social transformation in challenging times. *Cadernos Brasileiros de Terapia Ocupacional*, **28**(2) https://doi.org/10.4322/2526-8910.ctoED2802

Galheigo, D.M. (2022) *Foreword in world federation of occupational therapists (WFOT)* (2022). Disaster Preparedness and Risk Reduction Manual. www.wfot.org (accessed on 12 January 2023)

Goldmann E. & Galea S. (2014) Mental health consequences of disasters. *Annual Review of Public Health*, (**35**), 169–183. https://doi.org/10.1146/annurev-publhealth-032013-182435

Huddleston, B. (2015) *Digital Cocaine, A Journey Towards iBalance*, 1st edn. Brad Huddleston Ministries, Stuarts Draft.

Huddleston, B. (2016) *Digital Rehab: Learning to Live Again in the Real World*.

Intergovernmental Panel on Climate Change (IPCC 2021) (2021) *Summary for policymakers*. IPCC Switzerland. www.ipcc.ch (accessed 12 January 2023)

Joubert R.W.E. (2020) Occupational catastrophe! The digital revolution, global warming, unrest and pandemics: are we prepared? [Online] *South African Journal of Occupational Therapy*, **50**(**2**), 77–83. https://doi.org/10.17159/2310-3833/2020/vol50no2a10

Luby, J. & Kertz, S. (2019) *Increasing suicide rates in early adolescent girls in the United States and the equalization of sex disparity in suicide: the need to investigate the role of social media. JAMA Netw Open*, **2**(**5**), e193916. https://doi.org/10.1001/jamanetworkopen.2019.3916

Luxton D.D., June, J.D. & Fairall, J.M. (2012) Social media and suicide: a public health perspective. *Am J Public Health*, **102**(**2**), S195–S200. https://doi.org/10.2105/AJPH.2011.300608

Makgoba, T. (2023) *We need 'angelic troublemakers' who will fight for better future*. Sunday Times Newspaper. (9 April 2023).

Makwana, N. (2019) Disaster and its impact on mental health: a narrative review. *Journal of Family Medicine and Primary Care*, **8**(**10**), 3090–3095. https://doi.org/10.4103/jfmpc.jfmpc_893_19

Math S.B., Nirmala M.C, Moirangthem S. & Kumar, N.C. (2015) Disaster management: mental health perspectives. *Indian Journal of Psychological Medicine*, **37**(**3**), 261–71. https://doi.org/10.4103/0253-7176.162915

Martin I.Z., Mortos, J.A.F., Milares P.M., Bjorklund, A. (2015) Occupational therapy culture seen through the multifocal lens of fieldwork in diverse rural areas. *Scandinavian Journal of OT*, **22**, 82–94.

Mbembe A. (2018) *The idea of a borderless world* (online) https://africasacountry.com/2018/11/the-idea-of-a-borderless-world (accessed 26 April 2023)

McKinsey Report (2017) *Jobs lost, jobs gained: workforce transitions in a time of automation (December 2017)* McKinsey and Company. https://www.mckinsey.com/~/media/BAB489A30B724BECB5DEDC41E9BB9FAC.ashx (accessed 28 April 2023)

Moore, J.F., Rong K. & Zhang, R. (2022) The human ecosystem. *Journal of Digital Economy*, **1**(**1**), 53–72.

Rushford, N. (2015) Chapter 31, Occupational stewardship and collaborative engagement: a practice model. In: N. Rushford & K. Thomas (eds), *Disaster and Development: An Occupational Perspective*. pp. 236–243. WFOT, Elsevier, London

Rushford N. & Thomas K. (2015) *Disaster and Development: An Occupational Perspective*. WFOT. Elsevier, London.

Sigahi, T.F.A.C., Kawasaki, B.C., Bolis, I. & Morioka, S. (2021) A systematic review on the impacts of Covid-19 on work: contributions and a path forward from the perspectives of ergonomics and psychodynamics of work. *Human Factors and Ergonomics in Manufacturing and Service Industries*, **31**(**4**), 375–388. https://doi.org/10.1002/hfm.20889

The Reading List (2023) *Social media without the rule of law endangers democracy*. Daily Maverick 168 (05-11 August, Volume 03 Issue 42), p. 25.

United Nations (2022) *World Population Prospects 2022: summary of results*. Department of Economic and Social Affairs, Population Division. UN DESA/POP/2022/TR/NO. 3. https://www.un.org/development/desa/pd/sites/www.un.org.development.desa.pd/files/wpp2022_summary_of_results.pdf (accessed 15 December 2022)

United Nations High Commission on Refugees (UNHCR, 2023) *Global trends*. https://www.unhcr.org/refugee-statistics/ (accessed on 15 June 2023)

United Nations International Strategy for Disaster Reduction (UN-ISDR 2017) *Sendai framework terminology on disaster risk*. https://www.undrr.org/terminology/disaster (accessed on 15 December 2022)

United Nations News Report (2022) *News in Brief 16 June 2022 Global perspective, human stories*. https://news.un.org/en/audio/2022/06/1120572 (accessed on 20 December 2022)

Whalley-Hammel, K. (2014) Belonging, occupation, and human wellbeing: an exploration. *Canadian Journal of Occupational Therapy*, **81**(**1**), 39–50. https://doi.org/10.1177/0008417413520489

Whiteford G. & Townsend E. (2011) Participatory occupational justice framework (POJF): enabling participation and inclusion. In: F. Kronenberg, N. Pollard & S. Dikaios (eds), *Occupational Therapy Without Borders*, **2**, pp. 65–80. Churchill Livingstone (Elsevier)

Wilcock, A. (1999) Reflections on doing, being and becoming. *Australian Occupational Therapy Journal*, **46**(**1**), 1–11.

World Economic Forum (2021) *COVID-19 has caused a huge amount of lost working hours on Feb 4, 2021*. https://www.weforum.org/agenda/2021/02/covid-employment-global-job-loss/#:~:text=The%20COVID%2D19%20pandemic%20and,lose%20their%20jobs%20over%202020. (accessed on 28 April 2023)

World Federation of Occupational Therapists WFOT (2019a) *Resource manual: occupational therapy for displaced persons*. World Federation of Occupational Therapists, March 2019. https://wfot.org/resources/wfot-resource-manual-occupational-therapy-for-displaced-persons (accessed on 30 April 2023)

World Federation of Occupational Therapists WFOT (2019b) *Position paper: occupational therapy and human rights* [2019] file:///C:/Users/joubertr/Your%20team%20Dropbox/Robin%20Joubert/My%20PC%20(455849-OCCT)/Downloads/Occupational-Therapy-and-Human-Rights.pdf (accessed on 30 April 2023)

World Federation of Occupational Therapists (WFOT) (2022) *Disaster preparedness and risk reduction manual*. www.wfot.org (accessed on 12 January 2023)

World Inequality Report (2022) *Executive summary*. World Inequality Lab, Paris School of Economics.48 Boulevard Jourdan 75014 Paris. https://wir2022.wid.world/chapter-10/ (accessed 12 January 2023)

Zahidi S. (2020) *World economic forum, the jobs of tomorrow*. Finance & Development | December 2020. https://www.imf.org/external/pubs/ft/fandd/2020/12/pdf/WEF-future-of-jobs-report-2020-zahidi.pdf (accessed on 15 December 2022)

Occupational Therapy in Forensic Psychiatric Wards

CHAPTER 9

Nicole Rautenbach[1] and Matty van Niekerk[2]

[1]Department of Occupational Therapy, Sterkfontein Psychiatric Hospital, Mogale City, South Africa

[2]Department of Occupational Therapy, School of Therapeutic Sciences, University of the Witwatersrand, Johannesburg, South Africa

KEY LEARNING POINTS

- Understand criminal responsibility and related concepts.

- Understand the forensic process and how forensic state mental health care users (MHCUs) are admitted.

- Understand forensic report writing.

- Understand treatment for the forensic psychiatric population.

- Understand the development of a prevocational skills programme within the forensic psychiatric context.

- Understand how theory guides the development of a therapeutic programme in the forensic psychiatric context.

- Emerging fields within forensic psychiatry.

INTRODUCTION TO FORENSIC PSYCHIATRY

Forensic psychiatry is a subspeciality of psychiatry incorporating criminology. Although in some countries forensic psychiatry might involve private, or civil contexts as well, this chapter focuses on the criminal public health context.

Forensic psychiatry is complex and varies across the world, as each country has its own legislation and policies. As occupational therapists, it is important to be familiar with the legislation in one's country regarding forensic mental health and the processes involved. In addition, Snively and Dressler (2005) emphasise the importance of knowing, understanding and using criminal justice language as a means to increase credibility within the multi-disciplinary team (MDT) (i.e., epistemic fluency in the context within which one works – refer also to Chapter 6 of this book). Forensic psychiatry in the context of criminal law involves the assessment and treatment of those who committed a criminal offence, but are either deemed unfit to stand trial or deemed not criminally responsible during the commission of the offence. Both of these considerations (i.e. fitness to stand trial or criminal responsibility) require an assessment of the accused's mental capacity, but happen at different times in the process (Combrinck 2018).

A defendant's fitness to stand trial refers to the accused person's ability to instruct their attorneys, participate in and formulate their defence and follow the trial proceedings. They need to understand the trial, respond appropriately to questions and adjust their instructions to their attorneys according to how the trial unfolds (Combrinck 2018). This ultimately refers to the accused person's present state of mind. Conditions that may impact a defendant's ability to stand trial include moderate intellectual impairment, neurocognitive disorder, cognitive impairment due to a head injury, and currently experiencing a psychotic or manic state (Snively & Dressler 2005).

Generally, for a defendant to be criminally responsible for an offence, there must be proof that they committed the offence (*actus rea*) and at the time of the offence, they 'acted of

Crouch and Alers Occupational Therapy in Psychiatry and Mental Health, Sixth Edition.
Edited by Rosemary Crouch, Tania Buys, Enos Morankoana Ramano, Matty van Niekerk and Lisa Wegner.
© 2025 John Wiley & Sons Ltd. Published 2025 by John Wiley & Sons Ltd.

his or her own free will, intentionally and for rational reasons (*mens rea*)' (Allnutt *et al.* 2007). Criminal responsibility is retrospective and consists of two components: namely whether the accused person was able to distinguish between right and wrong, and if so, could act in accordance with such an appreciation. Importantly, what is assessed with these questions is the accused person's mental state at the time of the offence, making collateral information vital in this assessment (Moore 2005; Snively & Dressler 2005; South African Criminal Procedure Act no 51 of 1977). In the South African context, forensic psychiatric MHCUs are governed by both the Mental Health Care Act (MHCA) and criminal legislation such as the Child Justice Act (in the case of children) and the Criminal Procedure Act.

When there is a suspicion that a defendant is not able to stand trial, or that they were not criminally liable at the time of committing the crime, they will be sent for forensic observation at a psychiatric hospital. In the South African system, there are specific hospitals that are designated to perform this duty (e.g. Sterkfontein Hospital), but this may vary from country to country.

FORENSIC OBSERVATION PROCESS

South African criminal legislation has its roots in English law (see Chapter 4, where common law is discussed), which means that there will be many similarities with other countries that are also founded on English law. Although there may be similarities in various countries about how accused persons' criminal responsibility and ability to stand trial are determined, the legislation and processes vary between countries. It is therefore important for practitioners to be familiar with the specific legislation and processes in their country regarding the forensic observation process.

In the South African context, defendants whose ability to stand trial or criminal capacity are questioned are referred for a 30-day observation at a specialised psychiatric facility (see Figure 9.1). In her seminal chapter, Fairhead (1997) explained that an individual may be referred because they are unable to adequately communicate and instruct their defence team, they may have displayed strange behaviour within the courts or around the time of the offence, the nature of the offence may be bizarre, or there is suspicion or a history of intellectual impairment or another past psychiatric condition, or substance abuse, or a history of a head injury or epilepsy, or any other physical or medical condition which may have impacted on the accused person's criminal responsibility or trialability. In South African contexts, such accused persons who are undergoing observation are referred to as observandi (although the word is the plural form, it is used to refer both to individuals and persons being observed collectively).

During admission for a 30-day observation period, the observandi will be regularly interviewed by the forensic psychiatrist and case manager (psychiatric registrar or clinical psychologist). They are also monitored by nursing staff 24 hours per day and a multi-drug test is administered upon their admission (amongst others to distinguish intoxication from psychiatric

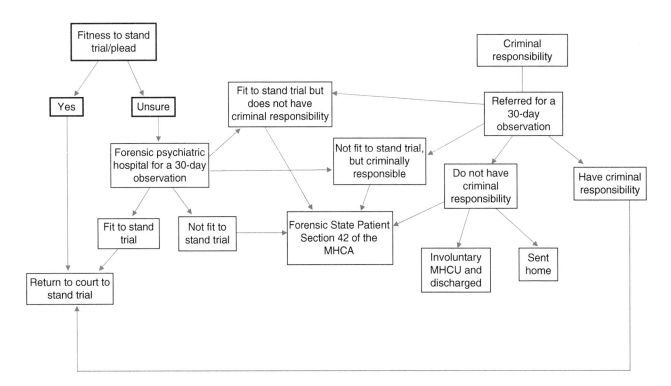

FIGURE 9.1 Figure reflecting the forensic psychiatric observation process.
Source: Adapted from Fairhead (1997, p. 385).

conditions [Bohrman *et al.* 2018] and to alert the staff to the potential for withdrawal that might have serious medical implications). The social workers will start the process of obtaining collateral information from the investigating officer, the family, victim, employer or any other sources that may be needed. In addition, the forensic psychiatrist will determine which investigations will be required during the 30 days that may include HIV testing, specific blood work, CT-brain scans etc. Personality testing or neuropsychological testing may need to be performed by clinical psychologists. One of the investigations could also be an occupational therapy functional assessment. All the investigations contribute to determining whether an observandi is fit to stand trial and whether they have criminal responsibility. What happens to the observandi after the 30-day observation period is dependent on multiple factors (see Figure 9.1), including the finding about fitness to stand trial and the finding about criminal responsibility.

It should be noted that if an observandi is not fit to stand trial, they may, depending on the severity of the charge, be admitted as a forensic state MHCU or an involuntary mental health care user with the aim of treating them and allowing them to return to court to stand trial. The reality of this though is that in certain cases, such as those not fit to stand trial due to specific conditions such as moderate intellectual impairment, significant head injuries or neurocognitive disorders, individuals may never be able to stand trial due to the nature of the diagnosis.

Criminal responsibility is complex and if an observandi cannot distinguish right from wrong, one can deduce that they could not appreciate the wrongfulness of their actions. In addition, the fact that an observandi presents with a mental illness does not automatically mean they may not have criminal responsibility. It is only if the symptoms impact the observandi's ability to understand wrong from right and act in accordance with that, they will not have criminal responsibility (Moore 2005; Snively & Dressler 2005). See Box 9.1 for an interesting variant of this question, used by courts in many countries, including the United Kingdom and the United States of America.

Where the observandi goes after their 30-day observation period is dependent on the magistrate who may, depending on the charge and considering the observandi's previous forensic history and the psychiatrist's report, either

- Send the observandi home.

- Classify them as an involuntary mental health care user to be admitted to a psychiatric hospital for treatment.

- Classify them as a forensic state MHCU to be admitted to a forensic psychiatric setting for treatment and rehabilitation.

- Stand trial.

THE SPECIFIC ROLE OF OCCUPATIONAL THERAPY IN FORENSIC OBSERVATION ASSESSMENTS

Although there has been an increase in the literature regarding the benefits of an occupational therapy programme within forensic psychiatry, there is not much research regarding the contribution and specific role of the occupational therapy profession within forensic assessment of those having committed crimes (O'Connell & Farnworth 2007). Kromm *et al.* (1982) wrote a comprehensive case study regarding how the occupational therapy assessment of a woman observandi who murdered her mother contributed to the findings for court after numerous psychological and psychiatric assessments. From their understanding, it is understood that the occupational therapy contribution is that through the use of activities, occupational therapists create a more realistic, safe and natural environment for assessment and thus it is easier to obtain a more realistic presentation of the observandi and their abilities and level of activity participation (Kromm *et al.* 1982; O'Connell & Farnworth 2007).

WHAT WOULD AN ASSESSMENT INCLUDE?

An occupational therapist approaches a forensic assessment in a similar manner in which one would approach a functional assessment, with the differences being in the interview process and report writing and setting in which the assessment occurs. The reality of the observandi's admission to a forensic hospital during the forensic observation period is that they are often not allowed to leave the unit, and thus whichever assessment one plans does need to occur within that setting. In addition, certain precautions must be adhered to, which will be discussed later in the chapter.

So how would the occupational therapist start an assessment to aid the psychiatrists in determining the observandi's criminal responsibility? The occupational therapist starts with a comprehensive, in-depth interview focussing on personal and developmental history including demographic information including home circumstances (living alone, or

---

BOX 9.1   THE 'POLICEMAN AT THE ELBOW' TEST

The test is based on the concept of 'irresistible impulse', which means that the accused knew that what they were going to do is wrong, but were unable to restrain themselves from doing it. The 'policeman at the elbow' test asks them if they still would have done it if a policeman was standing right beside them.

In jurisdictions where a plea of insanity is a defence, irresistible impulse cannot be used, because it only leads to diminished capacity, and thus is only a partial defence.

with others and who specifically), what language(s) they speak, histories, e.g. family, medical history, school history and participation (and highest level of education), work history and participation, leisure participation, personal management participation, relationships, conflict management. In addition, one must ask the observandi about the charge. It is essential to determine whether they understand the reason for referral, the nature of the charge and what they understand about the charge. For triangulation purposes, the occupational therapist will also ask the observandi about their version of offence, whether they know who works in the court and what those people's jobs entail, how they will plead and what their defence is. Question whether they understand what the implications are if they are found guilty. In addition, one can corroborate the personal history with the information obtained from the social worker and thus establish the reliability of the observandi through the interview process.

After the interview process, the occupational therapist plans the assessment which can be a combination of standardised tests and activities such as games, paper-based tasks and occupation-related tasks such as making tea or making a sandwich. It is also useful to plan the assessments at varying times of the day to aid in determining the observandi's activity participation over time.

One would comment on the observandi's performance in their various categories of occupation and the associated performance skills and patterns that impact this. In addition, plan the occupational therapy assessment to assess the observandi's specific and global mental functions along with the values, beliefs and habits (Boop *et al.* 2020). All of these factors are included in the occupational therapy report.

FORENSIC OBSERVATION REPORT

The format and outline of an occupational therapy report are generally guided by the standards and expectations of the unit and context within which the occupational therapist works. One important aspect to remember when compiling the report is that the reason for the referral is purely forensic: either to determine the capacity to stand trial, or to determine the criminal responsibility of the observandi (or both). Consequently, the report is not for therapeutic purposes and does not typically include clinical recommendations. Furthermore, it is important to write the report in 'direct, unambiguous language that avoids using technical terminology' (Kalisky 2007, p. 567). When profession-specific terminology is used, it should be defined or described adequately (Kalisky 2007), but should preferably be avoided (see also Chapter 6 about communicating occupational therapy findings to other professionals).

An example of a report format, with some guidance as to contents, appears in Figure 9.2.

It is also important to remember that reports should remain objective and comply with the referral. The report has to describe the observandi's participation within their various categories of occupation, using the Occupational Therapy Practice Framework Fourth Edition (Boop *et al.* 2020) to understand and describe how the various performance skills, performance patterns, body functions and body structures along with values and habits impact activity participation. Also discuss the observandi's basic social skills and higher-order social skills and the impact thereof on their relationships. Their work, prevocational and vocational skills, and task concept must be discussed. In addition, obtain a thorough substance use history and its impact on activity participation.

CHILDREN AND CRIMINAL CAPACITY

Children committing crimes is not an unfamiliar phenomenon (Bezuidenhout & Joubert 2003) and often there is a discussion about whether children should be held accountable for their actions and whether they truly understand the impact of their actions (Pillay & Willows 2015). Although occupational therapists may not be involved in criminal capacity evaluations of children in conflict with the law in all countries, in South Africa, it is an emerging field, with occupational therapists forming part of the MDT conducting these assessments.

Over the centuries, the views of children and their development changed from a child being viewed as an adult, with adult punishments for criminal behaviour, to the current times where it is understood that they need protection and guidance (Bezuidenhout & Joubert 2003).

The biggest changes with regards to juvenile justice came about during the 20th century with the focus of child justice moving towards restorative justice and protecting children (Bezuidenhout & Joubert 2003). Four international instruments were developed with the aim to protect the rights of children in conflict with the law and guide countries in the development of child justice policies and legislation (Gallinetti 2009):

- The Standard Minimum Rules for the Administration of Juvenile Justice (Beijing Rules [United Nations 1985]).

- The United Nations Convention on the Rights of the Child (CRC 1989).

- The United Nations Guidelines for the Prevention of Juvenile Delinquency (Riyadh Guidelines 1990).

- United Nations Rules for the Protection of Juveniles Deprived of their Liberty (JDL 1990).

It is the above instruments that shape child justice within each country. For example, in South Africa, the instruments, against the backdrop of the South African Constitution, shaped the development of the Children's Act no 38 of 2005 (2005), and eventually the South African Child Justice Act no 75 of 2008 (CJA) (South Africa 2008), with section 11 specifically dealing with the determining of criminal capacity of children (Gallinetti 2009).

When children commit criminal acts, their age plays an important role in understanding whether they have criminal capacity or not. Although the minimum age of criminal capacity is set differently for each country (Pillay & Willows 2015), in South Africa, the CJA (2008) considers children in three age bands: younger than 12 years, 12–14 years and children older than 14 years (South Africa 2008).

Children under the age of 12 years are presumed to not have criminal capacity and no charges may be laid against them. Children over the age of 14 years are assumed to have criminal capacity and are managed according to sections 77, 78 and 79 of the Criminal Procedure Act no 51 of 1977 (South Africa 1977) with criminal responsibility being managed the same as the adult population. Children between the ages of 12 and 14 years are presumed to have criminal capacity, but it is this age group where the presumption of having criminal capacity could be challenged and prosecutors need to prove

that the child possessed criminal capacity at the time of committing the crime. If a child is deemed to have criminal capacity, they will be tried in the Children's Court. If a child is deemed to not have criminal capacity, they are managed according to section 9 of the Children's Act no 75 of 2008.

The criminal capacity evaluation of children differs from the criminal responsibility evaluation of adults, since there are specific domains that must be assessed to determine a child's criminal capacity. These domains are the child's 'cognitive, moral, emotional, psychological and social development' (South Africa 2008). According to Burchell (2016), this is a subjective assessment based on the specific circumstances facing the child at the time of committing the crime, which is important, because each child develops uniquely (United Nations 1985; Pillay & Willows 2015).

NAME OF HOSPITAL

DEPARTMENT OF OCCUPATIONAL THERAPY

FORENSIC UNIT: OBSERVATIONS

FUNCTIONAL ASSESSMENT REPORT

SECTION A: PARTICULARS OF ADMISSION

Name of Observandi :

Date of Birth   :

Period of Assessment :

Charge   :

Ward   :

Date of Report   :

REFERRAL

Referred by   :

Reason for referral   :

SECTION B: ASSESSMENT FINDINGS

1. BACKGROUND INFORMATION

(Should be brief and include living situation and home context, socio-economic

information, and a brief developmental history)

2. GENERAL OBSERVATIONS

(Should include a brief description of the observandi's appearance, interaction with the

therapist and how they participated in the assessment)

3. ASSESSMENTS

   3.1. <u>COGNITIVE EVALUATION</u>

FIGURE 9.2 Report format example.

Observandi's version of the crime and understanding of the charge

Level of Consciousness

Attention and Concentration.

Thought Processes

Memory

Higher Order Cognitive Functions

3.2.   AFFECTIVE EVALUATION

3.3.   CONATIVE EVALUATION

3.4.   INTERPERSONAL RELATIONSHIPS

3.5.   OCCUPATIONALPERFORMANCE AREAS

Activities of daily living

Personal Management

Education

   Highest Level of Education:

   Grades Failed:

   School History

   Additional Qualification:

Work History

Employment at time of Arrest

Leisure Time/Recreational Activities

ASSESSMENT ACTIVITIES

SUMMARY

Compiled By:

Name: _____

Designation: _____

Signature: _____

Date: _____

FIGURE 9.2   (*Continued*)

Because of the subjectivity of the assessment, assessing a child's criminal capacity in terms of these five domains is a complex assignment. There is little guidance from international jurisdictions, since minimum ages of criminal capacity vary internationally (Pillay & Willows 2015).

Even though children's criminal capacity must be assessed based on their specific circumstances at the time, psychiatrists, clinical psychologists and social workers are most frequently involved in these assessments. Occupational therapists are rarely involved, but could play an important role from an occupational participation perspective to provide input regarding children's particular circumstances.

The process of assessing children's criminal capacity is lengthy. Even within one country, there is not necessarily uniformity. One example is the occupational therapists at Sterkfontein hospital in South Africa who are involved in conducting children's criminal capacity assessments (Pillay & Willows 2015), but this is not the case at all specialist psychiatric hospitals in the country.

How one approaches the criminal capacity evaluations of children is similar to those of the adults, but with a greater focus on school participation and the developmental history of the child. Theory related to cognitive, emotional, social, moral and psychological development plays an important role in the clinical reasoning of the occupational therapist when interpreting assessment results. It is imperative that occupational therapists who conduct criminal capacity evaluations of children are familiar with the developmental milestones of the child to understand what can realistically be expected of a child of a particular age. Other standardised assessments that can be incorporated are specific tests for visual perception as this may impact their school participation.

FORENSIC STATE MHCU

ADMISSION AND DISCHARGE

Once an MHCU has been declared a forensic state MHCU, occupational therapists must understand how MHCUs leave the hospital and the long process involved. It is also important to remember that similar to the criminal responsibility assessments, the legal processes may vary from country to country and therefore it is important to be familiar with the processes and legislation.

In South Africa, forensic state MHCUs are admitted under section 42 of the Mental Health Care Act no 18 of 2002 (South Africa 2002) and it is important to understand that these admissions are indefinite until certain expectations have been met. There are two main avenues that are available to MHCUs, which are complex and demonstrated in Figure 9.3.

The aim is for MHCUs to be granted leave of absence (LOA) from the hospital so they can reintegrate back into the community (see Case 1 and think about how the occupational

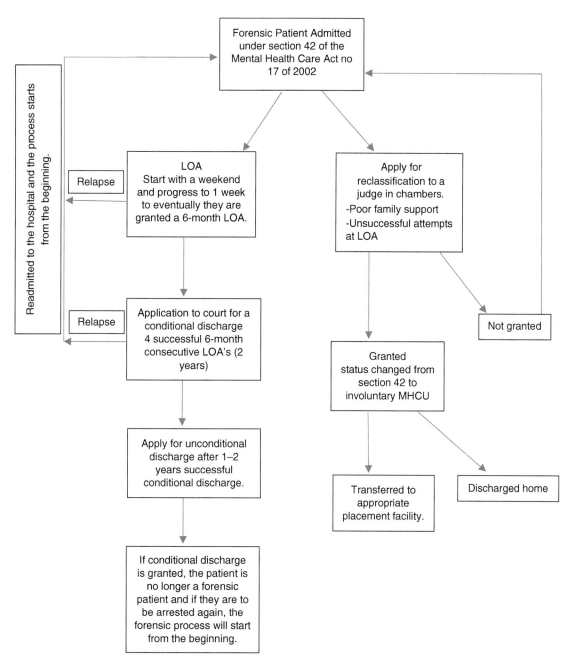

FIGURE 9.3   Process demonstrating how MHCUs leave the hospital.
Note: LOA = leave of absence.

therapist could use design thinking [see Chapter 6] to plan specific activities alongside the MHCU so that LOA is not haphazard). Cautious consideration (which could be supported by design thinking) and continuous risk assessment guide the entire process. The occupational therapist must know what the discharge plan is for the MHCU because this plan forms the basis of goal setting with the MHCU, including whether goals need to work towards reintegration back into their community and family system or towards long-term institutional psychiatric care (and of course whether the latter is available in the country).

Leave of absence usually is graded: if the first LOA was successful, subsequent leave periods increase gradually in length, depending on its continued success. The MHCU must have at least four successful six-month LOA periods in succession before the psychiatrist can apply for a conditional discharge. Ultimately, this means that although the MHCU is no longer a forensic state MHCU, the conditional discharge will be revoked and they will be readmitted as a forensic MHCU should they breach any of the conditions of their conditional discharge. If the MHCU complies with the specific conditions set out in the conditional discharge for the 1- to 2-year period, they may apply for an unconditional discharge.

Unfortunately, relapse during this process is common and occurs frequently, necessitating that the occupational therapist learns how to manage the disappointment of the MHCU and their family in a constructive manner by working together to identify the causes of the relapse. It is also important to ensure that the occupational therapists manage their own disappointment as the treating therapist.

If the MHCU either has no family, or the family is unable to provide adequate supervision or is not interested in caring for the MHCU, the MDT can apply for a reclassification for the MHCU. This is an application to the judge in chambers (i.e. the application is not heard in open court). These applications will only be considered for MHCUs who are deemed low risk, as their status will be changed from a forensic state MHCU to an involuntary mental health care user [see Chapter 4]. The purpose of a reclassification is often with the intention of placing the MHCU in a long-term mental health facility where constant care and supervision can be provided.

INTERVENTION IN OCCUPATIONAL THERAPY

Occupational therapy intervention in forensic psychiatric units is not much different from that of occupational therapy intervention in general psychiatry except for the secure setting and the emphasis on precautions (Snively & Dressler 2005).

The OTPF Fourth Edition (Boop et al. 2020) and the occupational therapy process guide how the therapist approaches assessment, treatment and the development of a ward therapeutic programme. It is important and beneficial for the programme to be comprehensive and focus on the various categories of occupation as MHCUs will often have impairment in all the areas.

Deinstitutionalisation, or at least curtailing institutionalisation as far as possible for these MHCUs who are likely to stay at the hospital for many years, is crucial, and should already be implemented in the lock-up or secure wards. Incorporating important celebratory days on the calendar, such as International Women's Day (8 March, or in South Africa on 9 August to coincide with the commemoration of an anti-Apartheid march by women to the Union Buildings), and religious celebratory days such as Divali, Hanukkah and Christmas, helps to keep MHCUs involved in the usual happenings of everyday life in the outside world. When noteworthy international events, such as sporting world cup events, take place, these could also be incorporated into the treatment programme to stimulate the forensic MCHUs' interest in the outside world. Making decorations could be included in the therapeutic activities. Consideration should be given to making an event of a decoration day, considering MHCUs' level of Creative Ability (according to the Vona du Toit Model of Creative Ability (VdTMoCa) [see Chapter 2], their energy levels, and sensory processing and ability to handle stimuli. Involving them in making decorations for the ward not only reinforces the approaching events but also spreads the workload of decorating the ward and provides opportunity for MCHUs to give and receive positive feedback on their efforts. Where possible or feasible, also include MHCUs' birthdays.

Forensic MHCUs often have difficulty with social participation; thus, social events should be included in occupational therapy intervention programmes. Examples of these activities include large-group sports events and calendar-related large-group events where MHCUs are invited to recite poems, sing songs, etc. These are effective in not only facilitating physical health, but also in encouraging social interaction. Another consideration is to celebrate MHCUs' birthdays, as a way of making MHCUs aware of each other (which is important on levels of Creative Ability at Self-presentation and lower) [see Chapter 2] and thus increasing social interaction. Necessarily, care should be taken to consider different cultural and religious views about these celebrations (considering, e.g. Jehovah's Witnesses who do not celebrate events such as Christmas and personal birthdays).

Most occupational therapy interventions in state forensic facilities are likely to be in the form of large-group and creative group interventions, depending on MHCUs' level of Creative Ability [Chapter 2].

Prevocational skills/work programmes are extremely effective in developing not only work skills, but also social skills and skills related to self-care. Consider Jubilee's experience in Case 1.

CONTEXT

The forensic psychiatric unit looks different for each hospital. MHCUs can be divided into wards based on their risk and where they are in their rehabilitation process. These would be open-wards, pre-open wards, moderate-security wards and

CASE 1   Jubilee Motsamai

My name is Jubilee Motsamai. I am 44 years old and a mother of two children (ages 13 and 15). I was born in a remote rural village in Botswana, but grew up in an agricultural town in the East of the country. I was diagnosed with Bipolar Disorder Type 1 roughly 18 years ago. At the time, I was a medical student at a coastal university in South Africa. I presented with increased energy, singing loudly and doing a lot of things at once, which was consistent with the characteristics of a manic episode. I have been on treatment ever since. I was so embarrassed by my behaviour at the time, that I dropped out of university and did not complete my studies.

About seven years ago, I slept at a Bed-and-Breakfast establishment in Francistown, one of the bigger cities in Botswana. I left without paying. A criminal case was opened and I was found unfit to stand trial. After a lengthy procedure, I was declared a State Forensic MHCU two years later and after more delays, was admitted to a forensic unit in the capital city two years later. This was five years ago.

Being in a forensic unit, I have received treatment and support from different people/professionals. This includes the medical doctors, social worker, psychologist and nurses. Although there are very few occupational therapists in my country, I was lucky enough that my unit did have an occupational therapist who was also included in my care, treatment and rehabilitation. Our unit was fortunate to have sensitive and well-trained security guards and also had regular visits from spiritual counsellors such as pastors, which are facilitated by the occupational therapist. My condition has brought me closer to God and I am a born-again Christian. My religion and spirituality give me a strong sense of identity and efficacy; thus, I place great value in it. Having opportunities to attend fellowship here in the forensic unit, which was made possible by the occupational therapist, has been very helpful. I am mostly stable, with fewer relapses compared to when I was first admitted.

I am lucky to have been involved in the occupational therapy projects such as beading, batik, gardening, sewing, library and vetkoek* making. These activities have helped to give structure to my days in the forensic unit. They keep me busy and occupied, which prevents me from having negative thoughts. I have also learnt different skills that I can practice when I go back home. I have been able to generate a little money through being part of

the various projects. Currently, I am in the Praise-and-Worship group, sewing, vetkoek and bread-making projects.

Through my involvement in occupational therapy projects, I have started a small business of baking vetkoek and artisanal bread and selling it at the Tuckshop to staff and fellow MHCUs. I have been able to get an income from selling bread that I can use to help myself in addition to what I get from the sewing projects in which I am involved. I plan to continue with the baking business upon discharge.

I have recently been included in the pre-discharge programme of the forensic unit. I will be here (hopefully) for one year. Because I have indicated that I want to continue with my artisanal bread and vetkoek, I have been supported with business planning and management information. Together with the occupational therapist, I have planned my first LOA to gather information about the need for artisanal bread and vetkoek in various areas, and investigating suitable and affordable places from which to bake and/or sell my bread.

Considerations and Questions:

1. Can you surmise Jubilee's level of Creative Ability (yes, there is not a lot of information directly pointing to a level of Creative Ability, but think about indicators such as initiative and prevocational skills) [see Chapter 2]?

2. Did you notice that in the programme in which Jubilee was involved, the occupational therapist appears not to have used low-cost activities (or activities using recycled material/waste)? One possible reason is that Jubilee is likely to be involved in an independent living wing of the forensic ward, and that she and her cohorts are likely to be involved in an extended pre-discharge plan. How would you design the programme for the pre-discharge wing of a forensic ward, incorporating higher-level prevocational (and vocational) skills?

* A vetkoek is a small, deep-fried ball of dough, like a donut without a hole. It is made from yeasted (bread) dough. It is an Afrikaans word, but it could probably be traced back to the Dutch 'oliekoek' and thus could have found its way into Southern African cooking via the Dutch East India Company. Historically, it was made from leftover white bread dough, but nowadays making vetkoek is the objective. Once they have cooled down, they are cut open and filled with savoury and sweet fillings.

high-security wards (Fairhead 1997; Moore 2005). Another way to place MHCUs in units is through establishing wards for MHCUs of various levels of functioning. The occupational therapy programme is based on the level of functioning of the patients in the specific ward context. When MHCUs are placed in wards based on their level of functioning, the VdTMoCA [Chapter 2] can be beneficial in aiding to place the MHCUs in the correct wards. This will also ensure that most MHCUs in the ward would benefit from the same programme as the

other MHCUs in the ward and that group planning would be aimed at the MHCU's specific level of functioning.

Wards for MHCUs on the Levels of Creative Ability Below Self-Presentation/High-Security Wards

MHCUs in these wards are often diagnosed with moderate to severe intellectual development disorder or schizophrenia with prominent negative symptoms and cognitive decline. Within high-security wards, these would often be recently admitted forensic MHCUs or those who are problematic in other wards or those who relapsed while they were on an LOA. Often MHCUs require much support and supervision with regards to the execution of their personal and instrumental activities of daily living.

Usually, when it is a high-security ward, these MHCUs are not allowed to leave the ward, but when it is a ward for low-functioning forensic MHCUs who are lower-risk, they may be allowed to leave the ward with supervision/escorting. Both these sets of wards remain categorised as high-security wards.

The focus of occupational therapy intervention for high-security wards is often to stimulate basic social skills, stimulate task concept, stimulating leisure engagement, stimulating engagement in activities of daily living and sensory stimulation. Behavioural programmes can be very beneficial in these wards to encourage desirable behaviour. MHCUs are often involved in small gardening groups and when they are involved in projects, it is often tasks/activities that require 1–3 step tasks that are not complex. Physical activities such as volleyball, cricket or soccer are an effective way to channel energy and frustration in a constructive manner (Fairhead 1997; Moore 2005).

Medium-Functioning Wards/Moderate-Security Wards

These wards admit MHCUs who still require supervision when executing personal management and instrumental personal management tasks, but need less supervision than high-security wards. The MHCUs are more independent in participating in leisure activities in the ward and display better basic social skills. They may be allowed to leave the wards with escorts to attend occupational therapy at the occupational therapy department. The focus remains on developing social skills and stimulating leisure participation. There is also a focus on task-based groups to help develop task concept and games such as morabaraba/mlabalaba (which is an indigenous African strategic game of which the spelling differs according to language; here we use Northern and Southern Sotho), ludo, card games and checkers are effective. Groups focusing on physical activity, gardening and creative tasks are enjoyed as they allow the MHCUs the opportunity to explore and present themselves to others (Fairhead 1997; Moore 2005). When MHCUs are transitioning to Self-presentation (patient-directed or transitional level), they should be involved in prevocational programmes such as carwash and coffee shop programmes (where MHCUs serve as 'chefs'/cooks and waitrons in a coffee shop for staff and other MHCUs who are paying customers, executing simple tasks under relatively close supervision).

High-Functioning Wards/Low Security

These are often open wards and MHCUs are independent in activities of daily living and instrumental activities of daily living (thus at the least on Self-presentation, patient-directed, but with less active symptomatology than the previous group).

They generally display better basic social skills and present themselves more effectively to others. These are often MHCUs that require involvement in life skill groups, substance use groups and psychoeducation groups, although the latter should be used sparingly [see Chapter 7]. They are more independent in routinely engaging in leisure, and leisure aims will focus on independent engagement in leisure activities and expanding leisure interests. Additionally, there is a focus on improving higher-order social skills, and a greater focus on developing work skills. The MHCUs should be able to leave the wards to participate in the therapeutic programme independently, which is likely to include similar prevocational skills as the previous level, but with increased social demands (such as serving as waitrons to fellow patients at first and later to staff in the coffee shop programme).

Prevocational/Work Programmes

A prevocational skills project is extremely beneficial in developing work skills but also practical skills which can be used for self-employment or to obtain a job. In order to set up a successful prevocational skills programme aimed at meeting the needs of the MHCUs, the occupational therapist must understand the challenges MHCUs face and the environment from which they come because this is the environment to which they will return. This is no easy feat for either the occupational therapist designing the programme or the MHCU who has to return to a community.

In South Africa, many MHCUs are from low socio-economic environments, which are high risk due to poverty, prevalence of substance use and often the presence of violence. These are often areas where people experience occupational imbalance, alienation, and deprivation. These MHCUs' reality is a lack of access to further education or training opportunities, which further limit their employment opportunities. They often have severe financial constraints, compounded by limited levels of education (usually because financial constraints meant that they needed to start generating an income as early as possible – usually 15 years old, but frequently even earlier although it is illegal to work before the age of 15 years).

Consequently, these MCHUs come from backgrounds with limited resources, and often home instability. Stigma attached to having a mental illness further complicates their lives, and they are often ostracised by the community and even their own family, more so when they committed an offence and if the crime was against a family member. After they are admitted the reality of the hospital is an environment that perpetuates occupational alienation and imbalance due to the physical environment, and in certain contexts, lack of staff and general resources. Despite this, it is vital to think out of the box to provide the best rehabilitative care possible for the MHCUs with a focus on deinstitutionalisation and reintegration into the community and family. Necessarily, the occupational therapist has to be creative in designing a prevocational skills programme, as well as a pre-discharge programme that incorporates well-structured and designed leaves of absence.

Occupational therapists know and understand the importance of work for MHCUs. Research has indicated that experiencing meaningful engagement in work forms an essential part of life, socio-economic contribution and independence, and contributes to shaping personal identity (Bank *et al.* 2015). Research further emphasises that psychiatric MHCUs benefit from a means of employment, yet they are often excluded from both formal and informal employment due to their experience of functional difficulties and the stigma towards psychiatric MHCUs, especially forensic psychiatric MHCUs (Swart 2005; Bank *et al.* 2015). Furthermore, research has proven the benefits of engagement of individuals with disability involved in protected workshops and supported employment (Swart 2005; Bank *et al.* 2015). Being aware of this knowledge and understanding MHCUs' needs guides the setting up of a programme that allows for skill development while providing intervention in the domains of social, work, ADLs and IADLs.

It is important to plan and set up a prevocational skills programme that is most suited to the context and MHCU needs, and guided by theory to develop a successful prevocational skills programme.

A prevocational skills programme should aim to facilitate choice and individuality for the MHCUs to combat institutionalisation. To further encourage this, the prevocational skills programme can incorporate events mentioned earlier (including birthdays and celebratory calendar events), selecting a 'worker of the month', allowing sick leave while in the programme, selecting MHCUs to be team leaders for specific projects to provide more responsibility and to participate in caring for the work environment through aiding in organising the area and washing of uniforms. As the forensic units are generally extremely structured, a well-planned prevocational programme can facilitate independence within a very structured environment.

MHCUs should have the opportunity to present their work to others such as the MDT, which can be achieved through consumer-related events such as the coffee shop and market days to sell end-products. There must be disciplinary procedures as the prevocational skills programme aims to create a more realistic environment and there should be consequences for undesirable behaviours (Jolivette & Nelson 2010). Disciplinary procedures however should also be graded according to the projects and the MHCU's level of creative ability and functioning. Behaviour such as smoking during work hours or not following the rules despite reminders result in warnings issued and with enough warnings, the MHCU can be suspended. More concerning behaviour such as aggression, theft, attempting to escape, or using substances results in immediate dismissal due to the risk these behaviours hold towards other MHCUs and staff. MHCUs can re-enter the projects again, but only after involvement within in-ward occupational therapy. Behavioural frames of references may be used to guide disciplinary procedures.

Outcomes measures such as the APOM (Casteleijn & Graham 2012) are useful in tracking MHCUs' participation and progress. It is important that occupational therapists working in forensic psychiatric hospitals select outcome measures that best suit their needs and the needs of the context. The APOM allows for multiple assessments to occur and thus it aids not only in tracking change but also in when a referral is needed to a different project, which would better benefit the MHCU's needs.

When initiating a prevocational skill project, it is extremely important to continue to evaluate the success of the programme. It is important to consider whether (i) the projects are relevant to the MHCUs, (ii) it equips the MHCUs with the necessary skills they may need, (iii) the programme is effective and (iv) MHCUs benefit from the programme.

Precautions

Due to the nature of the context and the nature of the MHCU and their admission, there are very specific precautions to be aware of when either working in the forensic assessment unit or the forensic psychiatric MHCU unit to ensure the safety of all staff and other MHCUs. Generally, the units will have very specific expectations for staff to adhere to such as ensuring all doors are always locked, emergency alarms and security cameras are operational, and higher staff: MHCU ratios are implemented. Other precautions that the occupational therapist must consider are:

- Awareness of the tools and materials taken into a unit or used in sessions and the risk they may pose. Certain tools and materials can be used as weapons (e.g. scissors) or as substances (e.g. vaporous or volatile substances such as glue and methylated spirits).

- Ensuring that all tools are accounted for at the start and the end of the session and that specifically high-risk tools are used under the supervision of the occupational therapist.

- Secure storage of tools in a safe and lockable area/cupboard.

- Being alert and aware of any changes that happen within the MHCUs' behaviour and affect (i.e. emotional expression) and how this may impact the session. If a MHCU does become aggressive, it is important to remain calm, not to turn your back on the MHCU and to attempt to de-escalate the situation. Certain facilities provide calming and restraining training for their staff, which are useful skills to possess to ensure the safety of the MHCU and the occupational therapy staff.

- Communicating with the nursing staff, carers, cleaners, security staff and others about the occupational therapist's movements in the unit and alert them of her whereabouts. It is important to *habitually* greet and chat for a couple of seconds with all the staff encountered on the way to and from the therapy area in the ward, so that multiple people are aware that there is an occupational therapist in the ward and can raise alarm if necessary.

- Conducting constant risk assessments when having sessions with MHCUs. When an MHCU is particularly agitated prior to a session due to a specific reason, evaluate the decision to include them in the therapy sessions on that specific day.

- Never make promises to MHCUs that cannot be guaranteed, as this can not only lead to mistrust within the therapeutic relationship, but it can also agitate MHCUs.

- Plan and be aware of the physical structuring of the session, that is, where is the occupational therapist positioned in relation to the MCHU, the exit/door and any obstructions to an exit.

- Occupational therapists should be cognisant of the clothing they wear. Ideally, professional and modest clothing should be worn (Snively & Dressler 2005).

CASE 2 — Considering the Importance of Programmes

Hospital X is a specialised, public health psychiatric facility in South Africa catering for 500–600 mental health care users, most of which are forensic psychiatric MHCUs. Due to resource limitations, the ward MDT programme is often limited with MHCUs experiencing high rates of idleness, boredom, occupational imbalance, occupational deprivation and occupational alienation. This has been linked to increase in adverse events and risk-taking behaviour within MHCUs and high rates of institutionalisation observed amongst MHCUs.

The formal prevocational skills programme was initially developed in 2014 and it has continued to evolve over the years and has been found to be extremely effective in providing quality treatment for large groups of MHCUs. The prevocational skills foundations are the VdTMoCA (Chapter 2), but also incorporates principles from frames of references such as the client-centred and behavioural frames of reference (Chapter 1; Duncan 2011). The programme has further incorporated the APOM (Casteleijn & Graham 2012), which is used to track changes as the MHCUs progress through therapeutic programme. Projects are graded and divided to cater to various levels of functioning and needs of the MHCUs with the aims differing in each level of project, building on each other as the MHCU progresses through the prevocational program. Everything from supervision provided, responsibilities placed on MHCUs, and complexity of duties given to the MHCU is graded.

The projects selected for the programme are relevant to the client population and thus it is important to be familiar with their needs. Due to the MHCU population described earlier, the projects focus on developing skills around being self-sustaining and self-employment and thus projects included in this programme include various gardens catering to different levels of MHCU on creative ability. Other projects include recycling, car wash, shoe repair, making bath products, sewing, thrift shop, basic woodwork, cable clip project, peanut project, decorations and the coffee shop.

How each project operates is dependent on the MHCU's level of Creative Ability (see Chapter 2). Projects range from taking place in two to four 90-minute sessions per week, to seven 2-hour sessions in a 4-day week. This allows for the building of endurance. In addition, the sizes of the groups also vary from the MHCUs catering to those on a lower level of Creative Ability (usually below Self-presentation) comprising 6–12 MHCUs per session to the projects catering to MHCUs on a higher level of Creative Ability (around Passive Participation) accommodating up to 25 MHCUs per session. There are usually one to two occupational therapists managing the MHCUs.

The aims of the various projects vary in the focus of prevocational skills, ranging from basic personal presentation skills such as quality of execution of activities of daily living and focusing on basic social skills and work habits, to focusing on higher social skills, social presentation, more complex problem solving and planning and more complex work skills (see Chapter 2).

When selecting projects to include in a prevocational skills programme, activity analysis is essential to determine the projects and products to include, as well as the client factors and performance skills (Boop et al. 2020) required of the MHCUs to enable them to function optimally in that specific project.

Any MHCU who is referred to the prevocational skills programme must be involved in ward occupational therapy, where they would have gained much of the enabling skills such as conflict management, assertiveness and social skills, to perform well in the prevocational skills programme. The MHCUs who participate in the prevocational skills projects must practice these skills in a more realistic environment. If an MHCU successfully participates in the in-ward occupational therapy groups, they can be referred to one of the projects in the prevocational skills programmes that will meet their needs and interests, provided they are low risk and the MDT has agreed (thus also showing the graded nature of the intervention programmes in the hospital).

Questions:

Compare Jubilee's experience of a pre-discharge and vocational skills intervention programme in Case 1 with the prevocational skills programme described in Case 2.

a. Which of the two programmes would best prepare a MHCU to live independently outside of the hospital?

b. What are the implications for skills development of the occupational therapist, or occupational therapy technicians, or employing/contracting skilled artisans to teach patients skills such as artisanal baking and being a barista?

c. Could the programme at Jubilee's hospital be presented to all pre-discharge patients, considering that some MHCUs with chronic conditions such as severe Intellectual Development Disorder may be eligible for discharge? Patients on which level of Creative Ability should be included in a vocational skills programme such as the artisanal baking programme?

Although being aware of precautions is necessary, it is extremely important to not let fear dominate interaction with and views of MHCUs. They are human beings who deserve kindness, respect and proper rehabilitative care just like any other person. Approaching and interacting with them with fear will impede the therapeutic relationship.

RISK ASSESSMENT

Cordingley and Ryan (2009, p. 532) defined risk assessment as 'making a prediction, based on an evaluation of the potential of an individual carrying out risk behaviours'. Kalisky (2007) discusses how discharges are based on the perceived risk of an individual, which is usually based on the MDT members' judgment rather than quantitative measures. Furthermore, there is an understanding that risk is a dynamic process that changes depending on the MHCUs, their emotional and psychiatric state, and changes over contexts and situations (Cordingley & Ryan 2009).

Although occupational therapists do not perform formal risk assessments to the same level as psychiatrists and clinical psychologists, the feedback provided by the occupational therapist to the MDT contributes to the risk assessment. In addition, informal risk assessments are continuously occurring during the intervention process. Constant, honest and effective communication between the therapist and the MDT is vital in this process (Snively & Dressler 2005; Kalisky 2007). The occupational therapist considers the MHCU's ability to follow instructions and comply with norms, manage emotions and impulses, interaction with others, the level of supervision and structure required and their level of insight regarding the charge against them, evidence of mental illness and general behaviour.

PRISON POPULATION

Occupational therapists do not only work in forensic psychiatric wards in hospitals. The level of involvement of occupational therapists within the prison population varies across the world with some countries incorporating occupational therapists as well-established members of the team while other countries do not employ occupational therapists in the prison system at all. Notably, community reintegration for the prison population upon release is not only challenging, but is also the largest predicting factor for recidivism (Bradbury 2015). Occupational therapy is key to tackling the occupational injustice and occupational risk factors experienced by the prison population (Bradbury 2015), by offering a comprehensive therapeutic programme addressing the various categories of occupations and the occupational risk factors, for example, occupational deprivation, to ensure successful reintegration into the community.

ETHICS IN FORENSICS

Health professions ethics and professionalism (see Chapter 4) are inherent to forensic psychiatry, but are nonetheless complex and difficult to navigate. There is limited confidentiality in the occupational therapy (and other) assessment because occupational therapy reports will be seen by the psychiatrist and potentially the court. Once the observandi becomes a forensic state patient, confidentiality must be ensured, with the only exception that keeping a confidence does not threaten someone else's safety. Transparent feedback to the MDT is important for continuity of care, but a careful balance must be struck between effective care and confidentiality.

Clinical ethics in treatment is also a challenging topic because of forensic state patients' limited ability to refuse care treatment and rehabilitation (see Chapter 4), due to being mandated by the court to receive care, treatment and rehabilitation. Occupational therapists must consider the impact that being unable to refuse treatment may have on MHCUs' interest and motivation to engage in the therapeutic programme.

CONCLUSION

Forensic psychiatry is complex, broad and multi-faceted. Working with this particular MHCU population is challenging, but it can be truly rewarding, for both the occupational therapist and the MHCU. Consider these words from a patient who had been admitted to a public health forensic ward in a Southern African country:

> 'I would like to put it out there that occupational therapy projects are contributing to the social, occupational and psychological wellbeing of us as patients in the Forensic Unit. Even though we were diagnosed with mental illness, through occupational therapy, we have been able to do what other people can do. We are learning valuable skills that can help us when we are discharged. We are therefore grateful to have occupational therapy services here, and I would recommend occupational therapy for other patients as well.'
>
> Ms X, forensic MHCU.

It is vital for occupational therapists working in this field to be *au fait* with the processes involved in their country's legislation and forensic mental health system, in order to grasp the needs of the MHCU population.

Occupational therapists must understand the various types of wards and implement appropriate intervention programmes for each group. LOA should be well-designed to ensure that the MHCUs benefit optimally from the experience and that those who are capable of independent living, such as Jubilee in Case 1, are able to achieve it successfully.

QUESTIONS

1. Critically evaluate from an ethics perspective, whether the craft and artisanal products produced by forensic MHCUs should be sold at cost or at market value.

2. Critically evaluate how MHCUs should be remunerated/rewarded for their contribution to the end-products.

REFERENCES

Allnutt, S., Samuels, A. & Driscoll, C.O. (2007) The insanity defence: from wild beasts to M'Naghten. *Australasion Psychiatry*, **15**(**4**), 292–298. https://doi.org/10.1080/10398560701352181

Bank A.A., Harries P. & Reynolds F.2015) Without occupation you don't exist: occupational engagement and mental illness. *Journal of Occupational Science*, **22**(**2**), 197–207. https://doi.org/10.1080/14427591.2014.882250

Bezuidenhout, C. & Joubert, S. (eds) (2003). *Child and Youth Misbehaviour in South Africa: A Holistic View*. (Illustrate). Van Schaik Publishers, Cape Town.

Bohrman, C., Blank Wilson, A., Watson, A. et al (2018). How police officers assess for mental illnesses. *Victim Offender*, **13**, 1077–1092.

Boop, C., Cahill, S.M., Davis, C. et al (2020). Occupational therapy practice framework: domain and process fourth edition. *American Journal of Occupational Therapy*, **74** (**Supplement_2**), 7412410010p1–7412410010p87. https://doi.org/10.5014/ajot.2020.74S2001

Bradbury, R. (2015) *The role of occupational therapy in corrections settings*, 153. https://core.ac.uk/download/pdf/217288237.pdf (accessed 12 March 2024).

Burchell, J.M. (2016) *Principles of Criminal Law*, 5th edn. Juta, Mar Cape Town.

Casteleijn, D. & Graham, M. (2012) Domains for occupational therapy outcomes in mental health practices. *South African Journal of Occupational Therapy*, **42**(**1**), 26–34.

Combrinck, H. (2018) Rather bad than mad? A reconsideration of criminal incapacity and psychosocial disability in South African Law in light of the convention on the rights of persons with disabilities. *African Disability Rights Yearbook*, **6**, 3–26. https://doi.org/10.29053/2413-7138/2018/v6a1

Cordingley, K. & Ryan, S. (2009) Occupational therapy risk assessment in forensic mental health practice: an exploration. *British Journal of Occupational Therapy*, **72** (December), 531–538. https://doi.org/10.4276/030802209X12601857794736

Duncan, E.A.S. (ed) (2011) *Foundations for Practice in Occupational Therapy*, 5th edn. Churchill Livingstone Elsevier, Edinburgh.

Fairhead, D. (1997) Occupational therapy as applied to forensic psychiatry. In: R.B. Crouch & V.M. Alers (eds), *Occupational Therapy in Psychiatry and Mental Health*, 3rd edn, pp. 382–397. Maskew Miller Longman, Cape Town.

Gallinetti, J. (2009) *Getting to Know the Child Justice Act*, Child Justice Alliance, Bellville.

Jolivette, K. & Nelson, C.M. (2010) Adapting positive behavioural intervention and supports for secure juvenile justice settings: improving facility-wide behaviour. *Behavioural Disorders*, **36**(**1**), 28–42.

Kalisky, S. (2007) Legal aspects of psychiatric practice. In: S.E. Baumann (ed), *Primary Health Care Psychiatry: A Practical Guide for South Africa*, pp. 560–568. Juta, Cape Town.

Kromm, J., Vasile, R.D. & Gutheil, T.G. (1982) Occupational therapy in the assessment of a woman accused of murder. *Psychiatric Quarterly*, **54**(**2**), 85–96.

Moore, M. (2005) Forensic psychiatry and occupational therapy. In: R. Crouch & V. Alers (eds), *Occupational Therapy in Psychiatry and Mental Health*, 4th edn, pp. 250–263. Whurr Publishers Ltd, London.

O'Connell, M. & Farnworth, L. (2007) Occupational therapy in forensic psychiatry: a review of the literature and a call for a united and international response. *British Journal of Occupational Therapy*, **70**(**5**), 184–191.

Pillay, A.L. & Willows, C. (2015) Assessing the criminal capacity of children: a challenge to the capacity of mental health professionals. *Journal of Child and Adolescent Mental Health*, **27**(**2**), 91–101. https://doi.org/10.2989/17280583.2015.1040412

Snively, F. & Dressler, J. (2005) Occupational therapy in the criminal justice system. In: E. Cara & A. MacRae (eds), *Psychosocial Occupational Therapy: A Clinical Practice*, 2nd edn, pp. 567–590. Thompson Delmar Learning, New York.

South Africa (1977) *Criminal Procedure Act 51 of 1977*. www.justice.gov.za/legislation/acts/1977-051.pdf (accessed on 17 April 2018)

South Africa (2002) *Mental Health Care Act 17 of 2002*. https://www.gov.za/sites/default/files/gcis_document/201409/a17-02.pdf (accessed on 19 September 2023)

South Africa (2005) *Children's Act 38 of 2005*. https://www.justice.gov.za/legislation/acts/2005-038%20childrensact.pdf (accessed on 19 September 2023)

South Africa (2008) *Child Justice Act No. 75 of 2008*. www.justice.gov.za/legislation/acts/2008-075_childjustice.pdf (accessed on 17 April 2018)

Swart, L. (2005) Vocational rehabilitation in psychiatry and mental health. In R. Crouch & V. Alers (eds), *Occupational Therapy in Psychiatry and Mental Health*, 4th edn, pp. 208–229. Whurr Publishers Ltd, London.

United Nations (1985) *United Nations standard minimum rules for the administration of juvenile justice ("The Beijing Rules")*. http://www.ohchr.org/Documents/ProfessionalInterest/beijingrules.pdf (accessed on 17 April 2018)

United Nations (1989) *Convention on the rights of the child*. www.ohchr.org/Documents/ProfessionalInterest/crc.pdf (accessed on 17 April 2018)

United Nations (1990) *United Nations guidelines for the prevention of juvenile delinquency (Riyadh guidelines)*. https://www.crin.org/en/docs/resources/publications/hrbap/IHCRC/UnitedNationsGuidelinesforthePreventionofJuvenileDelinquency.pdf (accessed on 17 April 2018)

Occupational Therapy Assessments and Interventions

Priorities in Acute Mental Health

Annah Lesunyane[1], Lebogang Lefine[2], Rosemary Crouch[3] and Catherine Shorten[4]

[1]Occupational Therapy Department, Sefako Makgatho Health Sciences University, Pretoria, Gauteng Province, South Africa

[2]Occupational Therapy Department, Sefako Makgatho Health Sciences University, Pretoria, Gauteng Province, South Africa

[3]School of Therapeutic Sciences, Faculty of Health Sciences, University of Witwatersrand, Johannesburg, South Africa

[4]Occupational Therapy, Gauteng, South Africa

KEY LEARNING POINTS

- Assessment and intervention with the acutely ill mental health care user.

- Techniques and activities appropriate for intervention.

- Occupational therapy within the mental health care team.

- Discharge planning, relapse prevention and follow-up care.

INTRODUCTION

This chapter focuses on the contribution of occupational therapy in assessment and intervention planning in an acute care mental health care setting. The unique role of occupational therapy within a multidisciplinary mental health care team and the importance of early discharge planning in relapse prevention are discussed. Engagement in meaningful occupations and proper support are central features to recovery and resumptions of important roles for persons suffering from mental disorders. Occupational therapy contributes to recovery as it reflects goals of health and well-being regarding participation in meaningful occupations (American Occupational Therapy Association [AOTA] 2020; Ngooi et al. 2021).

Acute mental health care services in many countries are provided under the provisions of legislation guiding mental health service delivery. The World Health Organisation guidelines (2020), as well as country-specific legislation, for example the Mental Health Care Act of South Africa (2002), ensure that services for acute mental health are prioritised for efficient service delivery. Services rendered in acute mental health care settings are a critical part of the mental health service system (Johnson et al. 2022). Acutely ill psychiatric patients are a vulnerable population and the provision of care poses a challenge to the mental health care team. These patients often present with severe symptoms of mental illness, rendering them to be at risk of harming themselves or others. The dilemma facing the team is that an acutely ill patient with a severe psychiatric illness is not in a position to fully understand the need and implications for treatment at this stage. According to Sims (2014), the acute symptoms are distressing and may affect a person's cognition, beliefs, perceptions and behaviour. Diagnoses include schizophrenia spectrum disorders, depressive disorders, bipolar and related disorders, and substance-related disorders.

Crouch and Alers Occupational Therapy in Psychiatry and Mental Health, Sixth Edition.
Edited by Rosemary Crouch, Tania Buys, Enos Morankoana Ramano, Matty van Niekerk and Lisa Wegner.
© 2025 John Wiley & Sons Ltd. Published 2025 by John Wiley & Sons Ltd.

The staff members in in-patient settings are obligated to exercise ethical responsibility towards the care of the patients in keeping them safe and maintaining their dignity. Safeguarding the well-being of people with mental health conditions is essential to alleviate the stigma, low self-esteem, withdrawal and social isolation.

Acute care settings are highly structured environments and provide intensive treatment (Sims 2014; Syed 2020). The highly structured environment aids in managing the severe symptoms of acute illness. The environmental structure of the acute mental health care setting contributes to ensuring the safety of the mental health care users for the promotion of personal, occupational, and social functioning and well-being (Bowers *et al.* 2009). Thus, mental health care users' symptoms are closely monitored and improvement can be noted (Skaltsi *et al.* 2021).

The emphasis in acute care is on the admission being for as short a time as possible, with early discharge and community support being implemented (Lloyd & Williams 2010; Fitzgerald 2016). The legal length of stay for acute mental health mandated by human rights instruments is necessary to ensure that the users receive intervention promptly and are referred to the appropriate mental health service for continued care (refer to Chapter 4). The length of admission in an acute psychiatric ward is often less than 21 days depending on the context (public/private sector). There are many reasons for this, the main reason being financial. Costs incurred in the treatment of acutely ill patients frequently result in a short hospital stay and early discharge.

Acute care settings are also shifting attitudes about hospitalisation and are now focused on reducing the duration of stay in hospitals and moving to continued supportive care offered by the development of community mental health services. Rössler (2006) stresses the importance of a shift away from a focus on an illness model towards a model of functional disability in psychosocial rehabilitation. This empowers people living with mental illness by enabling them to live normal lives in the community. Shorten and Crouch (2014) point out that the approach to treatment in an acute setting is not curative but rather the initiation of the rehabilitation process, highlighting the importance of assessment, control of psychiatric symptoms, and discharge planning using occupational therapy interventions.

Psychiatric rehabilitation aims to help individuals with mental illness to develop the skills needed to live in the community with minimal professional support regarding social relationships, work, and leisure as well as the quality of life and family (Liberman *et al.* 2001). This implies that continued care is necessary for the maintenance of functioning and recovery with emphasis on correct assessment and aftercare planning.

Rössler (2006) explains the overall philosophy of psychiatric rehabilitation as comprising both individual-centred and ecological strategies. The individual-centred approach aims at developing the patient's skills in interacting with environmental demands, and the ecological strategy is directed towards the development of environmental resources to reduce potential pressures and stressors. The environmental resources in this context would be the appropriate physical settings for the intervention of mental health care users and the tools and equipment used in the acute mental health care setting.

Available literature indicates that the historical developments of the contribution of occupational therapy are grounded within mental health settings and studies have reported on the efficacy of specific occupational therapy interventions in acute psychiatry (Peters 2011; Paterson 2014; Fitzgerald 2016). Occupational therapy involvement is therefore important in the acute care of psychiatric patients (Sims 2014).

The occupational therapist is most likely to encounter the acutely ill psychiatric patient in an in-patient hospital, clinic or treatment centre. To make a meaningful contribution to the management of acutely ill psychiatric patients, an occupational therapist requires both expert knowledge of psychiatric conditions and a clear strategy of occupational therapy intervention with short-term dynamic goals. High patient turnover and rapid discharge of patients affect the implementation of the occupational therapy process. Despite these challenges, occupational therapists are experts in the assessment and remediation of functional performance and are skilled to provide quality and consistent care to deliver service outcomes (Fitzgerald 2016). Sims (2014) explains that the process of providing occupational therapy services follows a specific protocol intended to meet individual needs and goals completed within a very short time period. Occupational therapy provides the first steps on an often-long road to recovery for the patient, who is at a very vulnerable time of recovery. The overall objective is recovery, stabilisation on the medication and continued recovery after discharge. The aim is to reach the ultimate goal of improved quality of life (Shorten & Crouch 2014).

The Occupational Therapy Practice Framework (OTPF) (AOTA 2020) outlines the process of occupational therapy in providing services to their clients. This three-part process forms the basis for understanding the contribution of the occupational therapist in acute health care (Syed 2020; Skaltsi *et al.* 2021) and encompasses:

- Evaluation
- Intervention
- Outcomes

OCCUPATIONAL THERAPY ASSESSMENT

The primary role of the occupational therapist during the evaluation or assessment is to determine 'the relationship between health, illness, and occupational functioning' (Sims 2014). The occupational therapist must assess the patient's occupational performance in ascertaining how able the patient is to complete the activities presented and the activities that form part of his/her role after discharge (Rogers & Holm 2016). This assessment must be non-threatening and socio-culturally acceptable. The level of creative ability must be assessed so that activities suggested for the patient are relevant and realistic, enabling them to succeed at completing the activities (Shorten & Crouch 2014). Assessment of the level of creative ability focuses on assessment of the client's performance as well as an environmental analysis (De Witt & Sherwood 2019). This focus assists the occupational therapist to apply clinical reasoning in understanding how motivation, performance abilities and problems/difficulties/challenges in different environments influence the client's health and well-being (De Witt & Sherwood 2019).

It is important to engage the client in assessment and formulate appropriate goals, which can be challenging during the acute phase of an illness (Steede & Gough 2022). Occupational therapy assessment in an acute setting is characterised by the rapid changes in the mental health care user (d'Oliveira 2020). This means that the occupational therapist needs to select the appropriate assessment methods to understand the client (WFOT 2019). It is not always easy to engage an acutely ill patient in the occupational therapy programme, and obviously, no force or coercion may take place. The occupational therapist requires good insight into the methods of assessment for these mental health care users as their symptoms can influence the outcome of assessment greatly.

Standardised occupational therapy assessments can be difficult to administer especially because the tests require the mental health care user to have some knowledge and awareness around their symptoms. Assessments such as the Canadian Occupational Performance Measure (COPM) (Law *et al.* 1990) or the Hospital Anxiety and Depression Scale (HADS) (Zigmond & Snaith 1983) are client-centred and therefore an acutely psychotic or severely depressed and anxious patient may not be able to complete them successfully. Non-standardised assessments such as clinical observations and generic ADL assessments are useful in this acute phase of illness (Manee *et al.* 2020). The power of clinical observation, therefore, is the best method of assessment. Different training programmes have various observation recording methods, but they all result in the same evaluation of the patient.

To facilitate observation, the skilful use of activity is essential. It is here where the occupational therapist can engage with the mental health care user in a structured assessment environment, however, not making use of formal standardised assessment tools yet. The use of clinical reasoning becomes important for the occupational therapist to conclude what and how the user presents. The use of activity is key, as it is through the means of activity participation that the occupational therapist can ascertain the primary symptoms affecting the functioning of the user (Bryant *et al.* 2014). Activity selection is dependent on the clinical reasoning of the occupational therapist to inform their understanding of the client's health condition and related dysfunctions, assessment, intervention planning, activity analysis, and synthesis (Cole 2018). It is therefore vital that the occupational therapist selects activities that are purposeful and relate to the context of the mental health care user. These activities may be introduced individually or in occupational group therapy.

In some countries such as the United States, the United Kingdom, some East African countries, and South Africa,

occupational therapy technicians (OTTs) or occupational therapy assistants (OTAs) are trained and available to provide and implement the activities for the daily programme in the occupational therapy department. It is here that the important assessment and observation of acutely ill patients take place. These mid-level health workers in occupational therapy are invaluable and must be well trained particularly in the handling and understanding of psychiatric patients and their illnesses, in order to work in this particular field.

During the assessment, the occupational therapist must also ascertain whether there are any external contributing factors to the patient's illness. It is important to note that in South Africa and other countries, a high percentage of persons with acute psychiatric conditions have a co-morbid diagnosis such as HIV/AIDS and substance use or abuse. This is often a complicating factor, either as a precipitator of the illness or in the illness itself, and therefore impacts negatively on the quality of life of the client (Lefine & Lesunyane 2022).

In the case of drug addiction or alcoholism, it is often part of a person's attempt to cope with a psychiatric condition. It is therefore imperative that the occupational therapist is aware of the possibility of this problem, which will require attention within the total intervention. This co-morbidity is often overlooked.

INDIVIDUAL OCCUPATIONAL THERAPY INTERVENTION

The intervention process follows an in-depth assessment of the mental health care user, which has been completed. The intervention process consists of therapeutic activities that are provided by occupational therapists to enhance the engagement in occupation for the improvement of well-being (AOTA 2020). The invention process requires planning, implementation, and review to occur to keep abreast of the progress of the client. Occupational therapists draw from theories, practice models, frames of reference, and research to inform their intervention with clients (AOTA 2020).

In an acute setting, the use of individual intervention is important, as clients are severely ill and may not be suitable for group intervention. Therefore, individual intervention offers the opportunity to address challenges such as anxiety and poor interpersonal functioning in occupational role engagement (Lloyd & Williams 2010). Occupational therapy facilitates participation in activities by creating an environment that is conducive to mental health where the creativity and performance of mental health care users are stimulated. Individual engagement in activities provides alleviation of symptoms that are present when the client is not engaged in activities (Steede & Gough 2022). Control and supervision of the patient are required so that ongoing assessment and observation can take place during intervention. The OTT/OTA's general observations in individual and group intervention provide valuable feedback in terms of the symptoms present in therapy and therefore assist the occupational therapist in evaluating the progress of the mental health care user (van der Reyden 2014).

Activities that can be used at an individual level as well as in small groups include activities of daily living (ADL) and creative activities and therapeutic groups.

ACTIVITIES OF DAILY LIVING (ADL)

The occupational therapist's intervention in this regard is important, as occupational therapists can pay specific attention to the performance of these activities and therefore ascertain the level of independence in performing them. ADL is often, one of the first indications of poor occupational performance that can be noted in the lack of personal hygiene and grooming of a mentally ill person (Edemekong *et al.* 2022). As a result of their illness, ADL is often neglected. A recently admitted patient into an acute psychiatric ward will often be dirty, smelly, unshaven, and wearing dirty clothes. ADL is therefore intended to empower the client in their recovery by ensuring that they acquire the skills of paying attention to their self-care for them to confidently engage in other occupations (Lean *et al.* 2019) and can be useful to help orientate the client to reality and engaging their senses. The occupational therapist, therefore, has to prioritise ADL as this forms the foundation of the mental health care user taking responsibility for their self-presentation. At this stage, the OTA/OTT can record information regarding the mental health care users' hygiene and grooming skills.

Personal ADL activities can be graded to suit the level of functioning of the client and therefore create an opportunity for the client to practice self-care skills before discharge and reintegration into the community. Self-care activities encourage patients to take pride in themselves and their appearance; therefore, activities such as bathing, showering, shaving, dental hygiene and toileting are appropriate. Grooming activities include hair care, nail care, make-up and care of clothing such as washing and ironing. A study undertaken by Gibson *et al.* (2011) found that ADL was effective in the intervention of acutely ill clients. Instrumental ADL (IADL) activities include activities such as meal preparation and clean-up, home establishment and management, financial management, and shopping. The occupational therapist aligns these activities with the roles that the client has in their home set-up. It is therefore important for the occupational therapist to take serious consideration of the cultural and spiritual background of the client, as this can influence the kind of activities expected of a client. The socio-economic status, level of creative ability, and symptoms of the illness are to be considered during the selection and analysis of these activities.

Holmqvist & Holmefur's study (2019) provides an adapted version of the ADL taxonomy for persons with mental disorders. Their study reports on the effectiveness of the ADL taxonomy as a tool for the assessment and checking of progress in the intervention of ADL. ADL occupations are vital in the initial stages of intervention for acutely ill mental health care users as they can promote participation in other occupations like work, education and leisure (AOTA 2020).

CREATIVE ACTIVITIES

Creative activities have therapeutic value in the intervention of mental health care users (Hansen *et al.* 2021). Creative activities such as arts and crafts engage the mind and body, and allow for creative processes, development of skills and enhancing occupational performance. As a result of a short hospital stay and often the disturbed cognition and behaviour of the acute patient, the craft projects chosen for a patient should require only a few steps to complete. The completion of a craft project allows the client to experience meaning in the task and enhances their occupational performance, eliciting a sense of pride. All activities must promote the constructive use of free time and must build self-esteem and confidence. These activities aim to develop new skills and revive or maintain old skills. They should be both process- and end-product focused, thus allowing the client to go through the entire process (all the steps) of creating an end product, as well as emphasising the value and importance of a good quality end product. Creative activities are reported by Griffiths and Corr (2007) to pose an inherent nature to meet specific needs and aid in achieving diverse objectives in individual and group situations. The occupational therapist has to have an understanding of the potential of creative activities to bring about relaxation, stimulate self-expression and reduce levels of stress for the client (Martin *et al.* 2018). It is therefore vital for the occupational therapist to work towards a good end product of which the client will be proud. This will aid in achieving the aims of alleviating hopelessness and promoting self-esteem.

Because many occupational therapy department budgets are not generous, much thought needs to go into what materials will be used for craft projects. Many acceptable end products can be made from low-cost materials; however, this will depend on the economic resources of the facility. Craft projects need to be specifically chosen for the patient according to his/her level of creative ability (refer to Chapter 2). It is sometimes tempting to be apathetic and give a patient an easy craft, as he/she will be discharged soon and probably not be seen again, which undermines the just-right challenge.

Using creative activities and ADL activities will depend greatly on the culture and socio-economic status of the patient. Crafts must be meaningful and appropriate for the patient. If a patient operates a jackhammer in a mine, a birthday card is not appropriate for him to make; however, making a man's stamped leather belt would be much more acceptable. A chief executive officer of a company would be best involved in an administrative activity such as collating documents or attempting a crossword puzzle, perhaps even a ceramic painting activity like decorating a coffee mug.

Patients need to be encouraged to start a craft project and to complete it. Comments such as 'I'm not creative or artistic' should be ignored, and gentle guidance and help offered. Be warned not to complete the project for the patient; this would not be therapeutically beneficial as the patient would not feel proud of an end product completed by the therapist.

In fact, this could even increase feelings of incompetence as the patient would not take ownership of the product and not experience task satisfaction. The environment where creative activities occur has to therefore stimulate the creativity of a client. A welcoming environment that is warm and comfortable, a place where the clients love to be in will assist the therapist in ensuring productivity in this environment.

The analysis of the activities must take into consideration the physical and psychological demands of the activity. Craft projects should not require fine motor coordination, as an acute psychiatric patient would become frustrated and possibly angry and give up or fail at the task. Activities using large arm movements will help to productively channel hyperactivity and aggression, and the added physical exercise will be therapeutic. Therefore, specific consideration needs to be made for the level of the creative ability of the client to ensure the just right challenge is given to him/her. Examples include painting on paper, on the wall, or the floor with large brushes; kneading clay or dough; cutting out shapes in biscuit dough; stamping leather; painting using stencils with sponges and paint; digging in the department's vegetable garden (if available); sanding a tray or wooden breadboard, hammering in nails and sawing wood. Examples of other one-step activities that can be used are:

- Printing on paper or fabric using a stamping tool
- Simple marbling, where the patient is only involved in placing the paper on the water
- Decorating bought candles by dipping them in different coloured waxes (be mindful of the hot wax with disturbed patients)
- Making simple cookies with melted marshmallows and Rice Krispies (cereal)
- Making sandwiches
- Making simple pizzas by adding different toppings to a ready-made (or pre-prepared) pizza base

Important aspects of using creative activities in the occupational therapy department must be noted:

- As OTAs and OTTs are usually responsible for all materials, they must ensure that equipment and materials, such as paints and paintbrushes, are kept in good condition. Paint bottles, jars, or tubes need to be cleaned, and the lids firmly replaced after every session. Paintbrushes need to be cleaned properly to prolong their life. Looking after equipment and material also saves money as there is less wastage. Occupational therapy students should be made aware of this as well, to prevent them inadvertently wasting precious departmental resources.

- Ensure that there are adequate materials in stock to complete craft projects. There is nothing more frustrating or disappointing than if one cannot complete a task because the paint or glue is finished and there is no replacement. Stocks need to be regularly checked, and any material that is finished or soon to be finished needs to be purchased and replaced. Occupational therapy students can also be included in stock-taking, which contributes to their broader understanding of managing a department, as well as the value/cost of tools and materials.

- As the occupational therapy department is in an acute psychiatric setting, great care needs to be taken to ensure the patient's safety. Sharp tools, such as scissors, craft knives, and scalpels, and toxic substances, such as turpentine, methylated spirits, lacquer thinners, leather dye, and glues, need to be locked away in a storage cupboard. These items can only be used under supervision. Safety in an occupational therapy department is an ethical issue, both for the patient and the occupational therapy staff. Harm or injury to a patient due to negligence in an occupational therapy department may become a legal issue.

- Physical exercise: Exercise must be graded by the occupational therapist and OTA/OTT. It is an important activity as it promotes physical and psychological well-being and is also an excellent way to channelise hyperactivity and aggression constructively. However, very psychotic and disturbed patients may injure themselves or others during exercise activities, and therefore, it is important that the exercise is chosen carefully and graded according to the patient's physical and mental fitness. Gentle stretching exercises to music may be appropriate, and music must be culturally appropriate.

- Leisure and recreation activities include tabletop games, such as Checkers, Monopoly and South African Morabaraba. Intellectual games would include games such as Trivial Pursuit, crossword puzzles, and card games. Games should be country- and culture-specific. These activities provide fun and encourage social interaction; they also lessen feelings of isolation and relieve stress and anxiety.

- Gardening is a very beneficial activity. It provides exercise outside in the fresh air and sunshine and results in a good end product. Gardening, if encouraged after discharge, will provide the patient with a fulfilling hobby, fresh vegetables, and flowers and possibly also new skills such as propagating plants from cuttings. This activity will depend on the length of hospital stay and available facilities.

OCCUPATIONAL GROUP THERAPY

The use of therapeutic groups is a core part of occupational therapy practice in the acute mental health setting (Cole 2018). Recent studies affirm the value of occupational therapy groups in achieving beneficial treatment goals/outcomes (Ramano & De Beer 2020; Ngooi et al. 2021). Group work provides focus in therapeutic intervention with one aim being to facilitate an environment where the client feels accepted and has a great sense of belonging (Crouch 2021). Occupational group therapy encompasses a whole spectrum of group work (Finlay 2002). A model for classification of groups in occupational therapy describes the transition from the task and socially centred groups to the expressive and explorative groups (Finlay 2002). Patients should also be carefully chosen for any occupational group therapy according to their level of creative ability (de Witt & Sherwood 2019). It is very important to note that all group work in occupational therapy is therapeutic from table-top games to life skills training and psychodrama.

In the acute psychiatric setting, the use of creative activity-based group work is beneficial at this stage of the illness. This is a result of the clients not being clinically ready for more medium and intense groups. Creative activity-based groups are valuable in acute settings as the focus of the group is on the experience of the process of the activity as clients can gain skills (Crouch 2021). The occupational therapist in the acute psychiatric setting has to have good knowledge and understanding of the group process to facilitate effective groups for these kinds of clients. In many parts of the world, including South Africa, acute psychiatric admission is characterised by short stays; therefore, there is very little time to form an authentically cohesive group, hence adapting to constant change is vital. The choice of group to run is therefore also important for the occupational therapist. Educational groups, ADL groups, and creative craft groups are all appropriate for the acute setting (Ngooi *et al.* 2021; Cole 2018). Lifestyle management groups are also presented by the occupational therapist to promote a balanced lifestyle including balancing work/productive activities, leisure activities, and sleep and restorative activities. In addition, these groups could be used to educate the patients about life skills such as budgeting and home management, all of which are important coping skills to be used once the patient has been discharged.

There is often no time to develop cohesiveness in higher intensity groups because once the patient is stabilised on their medication, they usually are discharged. However, where possible, it is valuable to introduce groups on stress management, anger control and anxiety management. It should be noted that certain occupational therapy groups are beneficial in acutely psychotic or depressed and hypomanic patients; however, severity of the condition needs to be considered (Rocamora-Montenegro *et al.* 2021). Patients should be carefully chosen for occupational group therapy according to their level of creative ability (Crouch 2021).

EVALUATION OF OUTCOMES

Evaluation of outcomes in hospital-based settings is challenging because of the shortened length of stay, the acuity of illness, and the high turnover in the patient population. Creating an evaluation protocol and choosing specific assessments requires sound clinical reasoning based on a theoretical practice model. This selection guides the process of choosing appropriate assessments, allows the therapist to explain the

rationales for their choices to members of the treatment team, and supports the production of outcomes evidence (Mahaffey & Holmquist 2011). 'Outcomes emerge from the occupational therapy process and describe the results clients can achieve through occupational therapy intervention. Outcomes should be measured with the same methods used at evaluation and determined through comparison of the client's status at evaluation with the client's status at discharge or transition' (AOTA 2020, p. 26).

The rapid discharge of clients from an acute setting has a significant impact on the full occupational therapy process being completed satisfactorily; therefore, the occupational therapist has to prioritise assessment methods, the intervention aims and outcomes to be established before discharge and recommendations for post-discharge and follow-up (Syed 2020). In occupational therapy, outcomes are considered right from the beginning of the process, but they can also be modified during the intervention part of the process. With the end in mind, health, well-being, and participation in life through engagement in the occupation are facilitated through occupational therapy (AOTA 2020).

ROLE OF OCCUPATIONAL THERAPY WITHIN A COMPREHENSIVE MENTAL HEALTH CARE TEAM

Comprehensive intervention planning is important for continuity of care and support in the provision of mental health care services. The goals of psychiatric hospitalisation include symptom relief and coordination of care to promote recovery. The stabilisation of clients living with mental illness starts with the initiation of the psychosocial rehabilitation process in an acute setting. Psychosocial rehabilitation requires a multidisciplinary approach as many competencies are required for its implementation to promote recovery and reintegration in the community (Liberman *et al.* 2001).

Teamwork should expand beyond hospitalisation to include assessment of risk and ongoing contact with friends, family and relevant professionals, to develop continuing support plans in preparation for discharge. The composition of the treatment team depends on context and the philosophy of the setting. Each team will vary in its skill mix and level of staffing, depending on the size of the unit, the needs of the people, and the funding provided. A multidisciplinary team of health professionals typically includes psychiatrists, psychiatric nurses, psychologists, occupational therapists and psychiatric social workers. Other team members can include recreational or activity therapists, and expressive therapists (such as art, music, and dance or movement). In addition, facilities employ staff members to provide structure to the unit, and help with meals and daily scheduled activities (Brown *et al.* 2011). Social workers or licensed counsellors provide family intervention, process group therapy, and provide placement and referral support. Therapy services in acute settings are provided by a team that could include support staff, activity coordinators, other therapy staff and teachers, technicians, and volunteers.

The occupational therapist has a significant contribution to make within the multidisciplinary team. This includes having an occupational focus that identifies strengths, as well as areas needing development. Occupational therapists can contribute a unique perspective on a person's occupational functioning in domains such as self-care, productivity, and leisure (Bryant et al. 2014) and provide insight into the impact of illness on a person's ability to carry out meaningful occupations. In addition, the occupational therapist's knowledge of cognitive and sensory needs can help the team determine the best approach to treatment as well as the best discharge environment.

DISCHARGE PLANNING, RELAPSE PREVENTION AND FOLLOW-UP CARE

An individual's stay in an acute care setting is typically very brief, but it is often the beginning of a person's recovery. The short admission periods and uncertain impending discharge of clients pose challenges to occupational therapy treatment planning and implementation. Discharge planning is therefore a priority in the occupational therapy process in the acute psychiatric setting. Collaboration with community occupational therapists is a resource for continued care to prevent relapse. From the moment a person comes into the hospital, the focus must be on discharge and the follow-up care that will help the individual continue their recovery. Discharge planning needs to begin at the time of admission. Sims (2014) advises that early discharge is encouraged once a person has recovered from an acute phase and is no longer a risk to themselves or others.

As acute psychiatric patients are often only afforded a short hospital stay, a large part of their recovery will take place after discharge. It is therefore imperative to source outpatient services to which the patients will be referred. The follow-up care of the patient should be provided in the community setting (Fitzgerald 2016). The occupational therapist must have a sound knowledge of the availability of outpatient services, community services such as recreation centres, community-based occupational therapy services, and recovery groups so that the patient can be referred correctly. It is very important not only to inform the patient of these details but the patient's relatives, caregivers, or whoever will be caring for the patient after discharge.

An important part of discharge planning is to enable patients to be reintroduced to the roles they played before being admitted to the hospital (Lesunyane 2010). Patients must also be able to utilise the interventions learned from their occupational therapy treatment to continue the recovery process after discharge. To this end, the occupational therapist should communicate effectively with the key people and facilities in the environment to which the patient will be referred

or discharged. This will depend on the severity of the illness, co-morbid diagnosis, forensic details, response to treatment, and environmental factors. It will also depend on the mental health facilities available in the community and the supportive environment into which the patient will be discharged. The planning of a programme of daily activities for use after discharge is essential as it will promote the constructive use of spare time and the benefits of living a balanced lifestyle. When planning leisure pursuits after discharge, consideration must be paid to the availability and affordability of items or materials needed for such pursuits.

If referring to another registered health professional, details regarding diagnosis, medication, abilities, disabilities, preferences and goals can be revealed only if permission is given by the patient. It will enable the encouragement of ongoing treatment and build on the goals already accomplished, which will continue to enhance the patient's recovery. Follow-up is recommended but will depend on available services. Occupational therapists have distinctive expertise in linking service users to community support resources and/or facilitating discharge to more appropriate placements (Simpson et al. 2005; Fitzgerald 2016)

Relapse prevention is an important element of recovery and aims to put support in place to prevent another acute episode. It is important to explore relapse prevention options, support people in their discharge and reduce or prevent future admissions (Sims 2014).

CONCLUSION

Occupational therapy provides the acutely ill patient with the first steps on an often-long road to recovery and is responsible for providing well-managed, relevant evaluation and intervention, and supporting ongoing recovery after discharge. Acute mental health interventions in occupational therapy focus on the use of meaningful activities and occupations that help patients recover, develop and maintain positive behaviours as well as prevent relapses (Skaltsi et al. 2021). The specialised use of observation, assessment and activities either in individual or group intervention provides therapeutic, relevant, dynamic short-term interventions for the acutely ill psychiatric patients. The unique contribution of the occupational therapist in the mental health care team is that it promotes optimal occupational well-being for the patient. As a result, occupational deprivation is minimised.

In many countries, readmission rates are high due to environmental factors such as a lack of health support facilities, poor housing and poverty. The responsibility is profound for the mental health care team in the effective treatment of acutely mentally ill patients. The value of the multidisciplinary mental health care team lies in the recognition, use and integration of the expertise of the different professionals, with a combined focus and the shared goal to enable the patient to meet their personal life goals and roles.

CASE STUDY

OCCUPATIONAL PROFILE

Nthabiseng (name changed) is a 43-year-old Setswana-speaking South African woman. She was brought to the hospital by her family, who complained that she had begun isolating herself from her family, always sleeping and talking to herself. They started to worry when they noticed that she was neglecting herself (refusing to eat, wash, dress and care for her household). She was recently widowed. On admission to an acute unit in a general psychiatric hospital, Nthabiseng was diagnosed with Major Depressive Disorder with complicated grief after the loss of her husband. She was found to be psychotic with suicidal thoughts and presented with severe weight loss. It was suspected that she was also immunocompromised.

ANALYSIS OF OCCUPATIONAL PERFORMANCE

Upon occupational therapy assessment, Nthabiseng presented with severe deficits in a primary area of occupation: BADL, in which she was disinterested. Her ability to perform personal hygiene and grooming lacked refinement resulting in an overall unkempt appearance. Her deficits in IADL indicated an inability to achieve independence and affected her role performance. She did not comply with medication and therapy (occupational therapy and psychotherapy) routines as she believed that this was part of her grief for her husband and therefore in the cultural context, she felt the need to isolate. Client factor deficits included deluded content of thought, depressed mood, and poor motivation. Her mood affected her functioning tremendously and everything she did depended on how she was feeling emotionally. The ADL and IADL functioning affected her ability to fulfil the tasks of her role as a mother, as she was too depressed to offer the emotional support her children required.

INTERVENTION PLAN

Nthabiseng displayed significant acute symptoms, which had to be addressed. The main objective is to manage the symptoms by organising thought processes and alleviating her depressed mood to activate purposeful action. These SMART (specific, measurable, attainable, realistic and time-bound) objectives were upgraded to incorporate life skills training during the later stages of therapy.

The initial occupational therapy intervention approach selected was the restoration of impaired skills and abilities, later followed by maintenance to ensure sustainable performance after intensive rehabilitation. Therapeutic services would be delivered as inpatient rehabilitation five times a week, and upon discharge as outpatient follow-up appointments once every month. For therapy to be most effective, activity demands were carefully considered to facilitate reality-bound interactions with her.

INTERVENTION IMPLEMENTATION

Implementing the intervention plan required the use of BADL, IADL and craft activities, which fell within Nthabiseng's roles and interests. These activities were considered purposeful as they were able to alleviate her depressed mood and improve her performance in her role as mother. Before discharge, the consultation process was followed whereby Nthabiseng's family was advised on health management, supported role resumption and skills maintenance to prevent relapse.

INTERVENTION REVIEW

The intervention plan was reviewed 3 weeks after the commencement of therapy. Nthabiseng's condition, having complied with the medication routine and occupational therapy, was stable. Acute symptoms appeared to be managed, and the plan was modified to incorporate life skills, discharge planning sessions and follow-up support.

SUPPORTING HEALTH AND PARTICIPATION THROUGH ENGAGEMENT IN OCCUPATION

The outcomes set for Nthabiseng were that of achieving improvement in occupational performance as well as achieving a state of physical, mental, and social well-being in terms of health. She was able to fulfil the role of mother particularly in IADL, where with the help of social services and psychology, these objectives were achieved. Overall, Nthabiseng's quality of life was improved, engagement in all spheres of occupational performance was once again possible and she was able to fulfil her roles.

QUESTIONS

1. What is the relevance of intervention by the occupational therapist with the acutely ill psychiatric patient?

2. Describe the main roles of the occupational therapist in the field of acute psychiatry.

3. Describe the structuring of the treatment environment for an acutely ill psychiatric patient.

4. What difficulties confront the occupational therapist in the acute psychiatric setting?

5. Discuss the role of the OTT or OTA in this treatment setting to support the objectives/roles of occupational therapy intervention.

6. Discuss the use of creative activities in this treatment setting.

7. Explain why the use of ADL is so important in the acute phase of illness.

8. Explain why the discharge programme is important in this field.

9. Describe the role of the occupational therapist within a multidisciplinary team as part of planning the discharge of an acutely ill psychiatric patient.

REFERENCES

American Occupational Therapy Association (AOTA) (2020) Occupational therapy practice framework, 3rd edn. *The American Journal of Occupational Therapy*, **74** (**Supplement_2**), 7412410010p1–7412410010p87. https://doi.org/10.5014/ajot.2020.74S2001

Bowers, L., Alexander, J., Grange, A. & Warren, J. (2009) The nature and purpose of acute psychiatric wards: the Tompkins Acute Ward Study. *Journal of Mental Health*, **14**(**6**), 625–635. https://doi.org/10.1080/09638230500389105

Brown, J., Lewis, L., Ellis, K., Stewart, M., Freeman, T.R. & Kasperski, M.J. (2011) Conflict on interprofessional primary health care teams can it be resolved? *Journal of Interprofessional Care*, **25**(**1**), 4–10. https://doi.org/10.3109/13561820.2010.497750

Bryant, W., Fieldhouse, J. & Bannigan, K. (eds) (2014) *Creek's Occupational Therapy and Mental Health*. Elsevier Health Sciences.

Cole, M.B. (2018) *Group Dynamics in Occupational Therapy. The Theoretical Basis and Practice Application of Group Intervention*, 5th edn. Slack Incorporated, Thorofare, New Jersey.

Crouch, R.B. & Shorten, C. (2014) Acute psychiatry and the dynamic short-term intervention of the occupational therapist. In: R.B. Crouch & V.M. Alers (eds), *Occupational Therapy in Psychiatry and Mental Health*. Wiley Blackwell, Hoboken, New Jersey.

Crouch, R.B. (2021) *Occupational Group Therapy*. Wiley Blackwell, Hoboken, New Jersey.

de Witt, P. & Sherwood, W. (2019) Assessment of creative ability. In: D. van der Reyden, D. Casteleijn, W. Sherwood & P. de Witt (eds), The Vona du Toit Model of Creative Ability: Origins, constructs, principles and application in Occupational Therapy. Vona & Marie du Toit Foundation, Pretoria.

d'Oliveira, J. (2020) *Occupation-centred practice: perspectives of occupational therapists working in acute mental health care*. Dissertation from the University of Pretoria. Available from: https://repository.up.ac.za/bitstream/handle/2263/78424/D%27Oliveira_Occupation_2020.pdf (accessed 17 August 2023)

Edemekong, P.F., Bomgaars, D.L., Sukumaran, S. & Schoo, C. (2022) *Activities of daily living*. In: StatPearls [Internet]. Treasure Island (FL): StatPearls Publishing. https://www.ncbi.nlm.nih.gov/books/NBK470404/ (accessed 17 August 2023)

Finlay, L. (2002) Groupwork. In: J. Creek (ed), *Occupational Therapy and Mental Health*, pp. 245–265. Churchill Livingstone, Edinburgh.

Fitzgerald, M. (2016) The potential role of the occupational therapist in acute psychiatric services: a comparative evaluation. *International Journal of Therapy and Rehabilitation*, **23**(**11**), 514–518.

Gibson, R.W., D'Amico, M., Jaffe, L. and Arbesman, M. (2011) Occupational therapy interventions for recovery in the areas of community integration and normative life roles for adults with serious mental illness: a systematic review. *The American Journal of Occupational Therapy*, **65**(**3**), 247–256.

Griffiths, S. & Corr, S. (2007) The use of creative activities with people with mental health problems: a survey of occupational therapists. *British Journal of Occupational Therapy*, **70**(**3**), 107–114. https://doi.org/10.1177/030802260707000303.

Hansen, B.W., Erlandsson, L.K. & Leufstadius, C. (2021) A concept analysis of creative activities as intervention in occupational therapy. *Scandinavian Journal of Occupational Therapy*, **28**(**1**), 63–77. https://doi.org/10.1080/11038128.2020.1775884

Holmqvist, K.L. & Holmefur, M. (2019) The ADL taxonomy for persons with mental disorders - adaptation and evaluation. *Scandinavian Journal of Occupational Therapy*, **26**(**7**), 524–534. https://doi.org/10.1080/11038128.2018.1469667

Johnson, S., Dalton-Locke, C., Baker, J. *et al* (2022) Acute psychiatric care: approaches to increasing the range of services and improving access and quality of care. *World Psychiatry*, **21**(**2**), 220–236

Law, M., Baptiste, S., McColl, M., Opzoomer, A., Polatajko, H., & Pollock, N. (1990) The Canadian occupational performance measure: an outcome measure for occupational therapy. *Canadian Journal of Occupational Therapy. Revue canadienne d'ergotherapie*, **57**(**2**), 82–87. https://doi.org/10.1177/000841749005700207

Lean, M., Fornells-Ambrojo, M., Milton, A. *et al* (2019) Self-management interventions for people with severe mental illness: systematic review and meta-analysis. *British Journal of Psychiatry*, **214**(**5**), 260–268. https://doi.org/10.1192/bjp.2019.54

Lefine, M.L. & Lesunyane, R.A. (2022) Enablers and inhibitors to quality of life as experienced by substance abusers discharged from a rehabilitation centre in Gauteng, South Africa. *South African Journal of Occupational Therapy*, **52**(**3**), 62–72. https://doi.org/10.17159/2310-3833/2022/vol52n3a8

Lesunyane, A. (2010) Psychiatry and mental health in South Africa: the vital role of occupational therapy. In: V. Alers & R. Crouch (eds), *Occupational Therapy: An African Perspective*, pp. 286–304. Sarah Shorten Publishers, Johannesburg.

Liberman, R.P., Hilty, D.M., Drake, R.E. & Tsang, H.W. (2001) Requirements for multidisciplinary teamwork in psychiatric rehabilitation. *Psychiatric Services*, **52**(**10**), 1331–1342. https://doi.org/10.1176/appi.ps.52.10.1331

Lloyd, C. & Williams, P.L. (2010) Occupational therapy in the modern adult acute mental health setting: a review of current practice. *International Journal of Therapy and Rehabilitation*, **17**(**9**), 436–442.

Mahaffey, C.L. & Holmquist, B. (2011) Hospital-based mental health. In: C. Brown, V.C. Stoffel & J.P. Muñoz (eds), *Occupational Therapy in Mental Health: A Vision for Participation*. 5th edn. FA Davis, Philadelphia.

Manee, F.S., Nadar, M.S., Alotaibi, N.M. & Rassafiani, M. (2020) Cognitive assessments used in occupational therapy practice: a global perspective. *Occupational Therapy International*, **2020**, 8914372. https://doi.org/10.1155/2020/8914372

Martin, L., Oepen, R., Bauer, K. *et al* (2018) Creative arts interventions for stress management and prevention - a systematic review. *Behavioral Sciences (Basel, Switzerland)*, **8**(**2**), 28. https://doi.org/10.3390/bs8020028

Mental Health Care Act of South Africa (2002). Mental Health Care Act No 17 of 2002. https://www.gov.za/sites/default/files/gcis_document/201409/a17-02.pdf (accessed 17 August 2023)

Ngooi, B.X., Wong, S.R. Chen, J. D. *et al* (2021) Benefits of occupational therapy activity-based groups in a Singapore acute psychiatric ward: participants' perspectives. *Occupational Therapy in Mental Health*, **37**(**1**), 38–55.

Paterson, C.F. (2014) A short history of occupational therapy in mental health. In: W. Brown, J. Fieldhouse & K. Bannigan (eds), *Creek's Occupational Therapy and Mental Health*. Churchill Livingstone (Elsevier), Edinburgh.

Peters, C. (2011) History of mental health: perspectives of consumers and practitioners. In: C. Brown, V.C. Stoffel & J.P. Muñoz (eds). *Occupational Therapy in Mental Health A Vision for Participation*. FA Davis, Philadelphia.

Ramano, E.M. & de Beer, M. (2020) The outcome of two occupational therapy group programs on the social functioning of individuals with major depressive disorder. *Occupational Therapy in Mental Health*, **36**(**1**), 29–54. https://doi.org/10.1080/0164212X.2019.1663336

Rogers, J.C. & Holm, M.B. (2016) Functional assessment in mental health: lessons from occupational therapy. *Dialogues in Clinical Neuroscience*, **18**(**2**), 145–154. https://doi.org/10.31887/DCNS.2016.18.2/jrogers

Rocamora-Montenegro, M., Compañ-Gabucio, L.M. & Garcia de la Hera, M. (2021) Occupational therapy interventions for adults with severe mental illness: a scoping review. *BMJ Open*, **11**(**10**), e047467. https://doi.org/10.1136/bmjopen-2020-047467

Rössler, W. (2006) Psychiatric rehabilitation today: an overview. *World Psychiatry: Official Journal of the World Psychiatric Association (WPA)*, **5**(**3**), 151–157.

Shorten, C. & Crouch, R.B. (2014) Acute psychiatry and the dynamic short term intervention of the occupational therapist. In: R.B. Crouch & V.M. Alers (eds), *Occupational Therapy in Psychiatry and Mental Health*, 5th edn. Willey Blackwell, Oxford.

Skaltsi, P., Konstantinou, G., Papagathangelou, M., Angelopoulos, E. and Papageorgiou, C. (2021) The role of occupational therapy within an acute mental health setting: a naturalistic cohort study. *Psychiatric Annals*, **51**(**3**), 131–139. https://doi.org/10.3928/00485713-20210207-01

Steede, K. and Gough, R. (2022) Service user experiences of occupational therapy in acute mental health settings: a qualitative evidence synthesis. *Occupational Therapy in Mental Health*, **38**(**4**), 364–382, https://doi.org/10.1080/0164212X.2022.2064031

Syed, Z. (2020) Occupational therapy: the process in acute psychiatry. *African Journal of Health Professions Education*, **12**(**1**), 9–11.

Sims, K.L. (2014) The acute setting. In: W. Brown, J. Fieldhouse & K. Bannigan (eds), *Creek's Occupational Therapy and Mental Health*. Churchill Livingstone (Elsevier), Edinburgh.

Simpson, A., Bowers, L., Alexander, J., Ridley, C. & Warren, J. (2005) Occupational therapy and multidisciplinary working on acute psychiatric wards: the Tompkins Acute Ward Study. *The British Journal of Occupational Therapy,* **68**(**12**), 545–552.

van der Reyden, D. (2014) Auxiliary staff in mental health care: requirements, functions and supervision. In: R.B. Crouch & V.M. Alers (eds), *Occupational Therapy in Psychiatry and Mental Health*, 5th edn. Willey Blackwell, Oxford.

World Federation of Occupational Therapy (2019) *WFOT position statement: occupational therapy and mental health.* https://wfot.org/resources/occupational-therapy-and-mental-health. (accessed on February 2023)

World Health Organisation (2020) *Mental health atlas 2020.* https://www.who.int/publications/i/item/9789240036703 (accessed 17 August 2023)

Zigmond, A.S. & Snaith, R.P. (1983) The hospital anxiety and depression scale. *Acta Psychiatrica Scandinavica*, **67**(**6**), 361–370. https://doi.org/10.1111/j.1600-0447.1983.tb09716.x

Improving Health and Access to Health Services through Community-Based Rehabilitation

CHAPTER 11

Stephanie Homer[1] and Olindah Silaule[2]

[1]Department of Occupational Therapy, University of the Witwatersrand, Johannesburg, South Africa

[2]Division of Occupational Therapy, Department of Rehabilitation Sciences, University of Cape Town, Cape Town, South Africa

KEY LEARNING POINTS

- Direct intervention within the Health Sector: Preparing for discharge and occupational therapy in the home.

- Community-based rehabilitation (CBR) service delivery: Occupational Therapy and inter-sectoral approaches to care, the community context, establishing district services and advocacy for mental health.

- Barriers to integration into the family or community.

- Factors affecting CBR service provision.

- Recognising when people with disability are empowered.

INTRODUCTION: WHY WORK IN THE COMMUNITY?

Internationally there is a shift towards Universal Health Care (UHC), for people with disabilities, at the primary level of a public health system based on the philosophy of Primary Health Care (PHC) (World Health Organisation [WHO] 2022). UHC refers to the shift towards primary-level care and means that it is more likely that people with mental illness will be living with, and accessing, mental health services in the community rather than in secondary- and tertiary-level hospitals. The moderate or severe mental health disorders for which rehabilitation is the primary intervention are seen in Table 11.1 (Cieza et al. 2020). The need for occupational therapy in the community will increase, due to a number of factors related to these disorders:

people living with serious mental illness and co-morbidities have lifelong impairment in function as measured by years lived with disability (YLD), the population of people with mental illness is increasing commensurate with the birth rate, HIV survival post–anti-retroviral treatment is associated with enduring common mental disorders (Gouda et al. 2019) and recognition that people with chronic physical illness or disability are at risk of depression (WHO 2022). However, there is a large gap in service delivery and up to 70% of those with severe disorders do not have access to mental health treatment (WHO 2020). Moderate and severe chronic disorders require greater health resources and time and may remain on the occupational therapy caseload for several months or years; therefore, community-based rehabilitation (CBR) is both appropriate and effective (Asher et al. 2016; Department of Health 2023).

Crouch and Alers Occupational Therapy in Psychiatry and Mental Health, Sixth Edition.
Edited by Rosemary Crouch, Tania Buys, Enos Morankoana Ramano, Matty van Niekerk and Lisa Wegner.
© 2025 John Wiley & Sons Ltd. Published 2025 by John Wiley & Sons Ltd.

Table 11.1 International mental disability trends 1990–2019.

	Prevalence (millions)	Increase since 1990	Years lived with disability	Increase since 1990
Alzheimer's and dementia	52.0 (44.0–59.0)	161% (156–166)[†]	7.4 (5.2–10.0)	165% (159–171)[†]
Developmental intellectual disability	137.0 (97.0–177.0)	37% (32–46)[†]	10.0 (6.1–14.0)	44% (37–54)[†]
Schizophrenia	24.0 (20.0–27.0)	66% (63–69)	15.0 (11.0–19.0)	65% (62–69)[†]
Autism	28.0 (24.0–34.0)	39% (39–40)	4.3 (2.8–6.2)	39% (38–40)[†]

Source: Cieza et al. (2020)/Elsevier.
[†]Statistically significant using 95% uncertainty interval (UI). Increases are largely due to population growth.

The term mental health care user (MHCU) is used in this chapter to cover the population associated with these disorders that require community-based mental health services.

The term rehabilitation midlevel worker (MLW) has been used to encompass occupational therapy assistants and community rehabilitation workers that are primarily employed by the Department of Health as well as care workers, peer supporters and parent facilitators primarily trained or employed by NGOs involved in rehabilitation.

PREPARING FOR HOSPITAL DISCHARGE

Mental health care users at a district hospital are usually discharged to the community after short hospital stays of a few days (Thomas et al. 2015). However, after discharge, despite substantial improvement in activity participation from self-differentiation to self-presentation levels of Creative Ability (see Chapter 2) in the hospital, the decline in activity participation can be noticed within three months (Silaule & Casteleijn 2021). Additionally, the readmission rates of MHCUs with schizophrenia are very high (Tomita & Moodley 2016), and MHCUs with substance abuse-related psychoses are readmitted within a few months of discharge (Thomas et al. 2015). Possible reasons are twofold. Firstly, short-stay hospital admissions mean MHCUs are discharged on the constructive explorative action level of Creative Ability before they are medically and functionally stable and therefore need assistance to cope in the community. Secondly, MHCUs are discharged with poor health literacy regarding their illness and medication (Silaule & Casteleijn 2021). Early discharge from hospital leads to incomplete rehabilitation which, combined with poor medication adherence, results in a 'revolving door' phenomenon (Thomas et al. 2015).

Due to poor resources in low- and middle-income countries (LMICs), families are expected to become the main caregivers post-discharge (Silaule & Casteleijn 2021), so the discharge programme must include health literacy to improve insight, for both MHCUs and their caregivers about

- *Their mental condition*: Signs and symptoms, the reasons for admission, medicine adherence and the common side

effects of medication. Ensuring they understand the instructions for taking medicine even when feeling well (Mokwena & Ndlovu 2021).

- *Awareness of activities and stressors that make the illness worse:* These may include family celebrations, alcohol and drug taking, topics of conversation, unexpected occurrences, e.g. a visitor, and the effects of the family's attitude and behaviour towards MHCUs. Identify those stressors to be avoided and enable them to predict and prevent the effects of unavoidable stressors.

- *Occupation routine*: A structured time use routine is particularly relevant in cultures that believe illness or disability means one does not have to participate in premorbid daily activities. Building an occupational routine is important for maintaining health and change in occupations may be early signs of relapse.

- *Options for continued medical care and rehabilitation*: Information on resources such as a district hospital outpatient clinic, the multidisciplinary team (MDT) clinic outreach service to MHCUs' homes or referral to another service provider is helpful. Most commonly, the psychiatric outpatient clinic is offered at district hospitals (WHO 2020) but research indicates up to 75% of MHCUs living in the community do not access these services (Seedat et al. 2009). It is important to check if the MHCU will (i) remain in the area or move to where they have a better support system or fewer stressors (such as moving from an urban area to a rural area); (ii) use the alternative points of care. Provide them with written information place and days/dates on which rehabilitation service delivery will take place.

- *Recognising the start of relapse:* Knowing the steps to follow when a change in mental state is noticed (either by self or by household members) may serve as an early prevention strategy for readmission.

This learning opportunity increases caregivers' acceptance of the MHCU and reduces the likelihood of the MHCU blaming the family for an admission, resulting in an easier adaptation to living with their family again. A more detailed description follows in the 'Intervention in the Home' and 'Health Promotion' sections.

OUTREACH REHABILITATION AT THE CLINIC OR IN THE HOME

The local clinic may be a good point of contact with MHCU, as they usually attend monthly for chronic medication. If there is no dedicated occupational therapy service at the clinic, a district hospital rehabilitation outreach team could provide a service. To ensure referrals to the rehabilitation team, inform the PHC nurse about the service offered and who can benefit (Cieza et al. 2020). Groups, rather than individual intervention, are cost-effective at the clinic level, and PRIME has developed an excellent Support Group Programme for MHCU and caregivers (PRIME 2014).

Nonetheless, access to clinics can be problematic. Most MHCUs in LMIC have difficulty attending clinics (Modiba *et al.* 2000). They have to walk to the clinic, may not be in the area on the day of appointment (e.g. at a traditional healer or visiting relatives), they went to the clinic/hospital for another complaint, e.g. flu that month and did not realise they still needed to have their regular appointment, there was no one to assist them to the clinic, or they have no money for transport (Mokwena & Ndlovu 2021) (see Vignette 1). Therefore, the outreach team should consider whether their service is at times that suit the MHSU or times that suit the therapist. Even if the MHCU goes to the clinic there is no guarantee that psychotropic medication will be available (Docrat *et al.* 2019) or that the team has transport to get to the clinic, reducing the chance of MHCU adherence to a rehabilitation schedule. For these reasons, home visits should be considered, especially for those who have problems attending a clinic.

VIGNETTE 1: HOW TO FAIL DESPITE GOOD INTENTIONS

In a situational analysis of the health service in a rural farming area (Homer 2014), the following questions were asked of the clinic manager:

'When do the therapists come to do outreach?',

'On Wednesdays, but it is hard to get people to come and there is often no one for them to see',

'So is there a day when you see a lot of people with chronic problems?'

'Yes most people with MHCU, strokes, and diabetes come on Thursdays'.

In a deinstitutionalised mental health system, with limited access to community mental health services, families and relatives play a unique role in the care and management of MHCUs making them responsible for the MHCUs' recovery. Home visits are essential for the therapist to understand the facilitators and barriers for successful rehabilitation. In resource-poor areas, try at least two visits to revise the pre-discharge mental health literacy and assess whether occupational function has been retained and whether the MHCU has been reintegrated into family life. Further intervention includes structuring an occupational performance routine appropriate to their level of creative participation and advising family on handling behaviour. In areas where a rehabilitation MLW is available the therapist and MLW should discuss whether they will work together or if the MLW will be the main person carrying out the intervention, and how the MLW will be supported.

PLANNED MENTAL HEALTH LITERACY

Checking how much of the pre-discharge health education the MHCU and the caregiver can recall is important. Insight is demonstrated if people can describe in their own words, medical terminology is not obligatory. Reinforce what they do know and re-educate if necessary. Knowledge alone may not change medical adherence (Sibeko *et al.* 2017) and medicine routines need to be established.

To assess medicine adherence, check the number of tablets left against the number of days since collecting medication

with the MHCU and the caregiver. It is important to include the caregiver, because Masilela and MacLoed (1998) report that only 12.55% of caregivers supervise taking medication. Counting tablets introduces a discussion on adherence with the MHCU and their caregiver, which should include

- The importance of lifelong medication for controlling the symptoms and preventing relapse.

- Signs of under- or over-medicating, e.g. increased aggression, drowsiness and extrapyramidal rigidity which affects motor functioning.

- Establishing that both MHCU and the caregiver understand how to take the medication correctly.

- Storage places for medicine must be safe (away from children), but easy to see, e.g. with their toothbrush, to establish a medication routine.

- 'Alarms' for medication times and 'calendars' for clinic or home visit dates.

- Short message system (SMS) reminders about clinic attendance or home visits.

- Reporting side effects of medication to the clinic nurse or doctor.

- An adult family member attends the clinic with the MHCU to report on the illness; as people with poor memory, judgement or insight may report that they are well when they are getting worse.

Poor medication compliance will affect family relationships as the MHCU's behaviour deteriorates. See Vignette 2.

VIGNETTE 2: WHEN THERE IS NO MEDICINE

One night we received a phone call from a colleague. Her cleaner's son was a MHCU. His behaviour had deteriorated over a few days and he had gone to the local hospital where he sat all day in 'outpatients' waiting for a consultation, only to be told the doctor was not seeing any more patients. He returned the next day, again without getting help. He became psychotic – hitting his mother. His mother was now locked inside the house, and he was outside threatening her.

System failures created a family in fear, a son and family who would have to cope with the trauma of the police coming to collect him and forcibly take him to hospital and a family that would find bridges hard to mend when the son returned from hospital.

HEALTH MAINTENANCE: OCCUPATIONAL PERFORMANCE

A routine may be difficult because MHCUs are forgetful, have low energy or low motivation, or poor planning; or they perceive themselves as needing less assistance than the caregivers actually give them (Masilela & MacLoed 1998). Many MHCUs suffer from nutritional deficits due to poor appetite or eating habits, e.g. they may go for several days without eating or they may only eat one type of food or eat excessively or wastefully.

Changing routines requires personal assistance on a daily basis by the caregiver or home-based care (HBC) workers. First discuss the perception of assistance of 'caring for' or 'changing occupational performance'. In order to task-shift rehabilitation to these carers, discuss their goals; frequently these are daily washing, wearing clean clothes, making beds and cleaning the room or helping in the yard, and may precede changing social interaction. Start simply and be knowledgeable of the local and family activity norms. Facilitate the selection of one of these occupations that conforms to the MHCU's interests and level of Creative Ability. Model practical ways such as shaping behaviour and using rewarding language to deal with problematic behaviours, e.g. not dressing, and then observe them practising these. Depending on the MHCU's level of Creative Ability, the family may

- Tell the MHCU what to do, watch him and give appropriate encouragement.
- Share the task with the MHCU.
- Divide the task into steps and supervise the MHCU doing one part of it.

Grade from a single daily activity to several activities, and finally a full day of structured activities. Social activities may start simply: sharing a meal, listening to the radio or TV together, sitting in the same room or going for a walk. Grade to having visitors: family, neighbours and friends, but to begin with the MHCU may be a spectator rather than a participant. Social roles and activities in the community include widening the social circle by visiting nearby family or friends; and attending community events. In impoverished communities, the variety of social and recreational activities may be limited: attending church, playing football/netball, being in a choir and the local bar or shebeen (informal tavern serving traditional beer). If work and home roles are not resumed, it is easy to return to alcohol or drug habits as a means of 'filling the day'.

A structured day of personal care, home chores and leisure activities, e.g. watching TV, develops skills and prevents the MHCU from ruminating on their disorder. In rural areas, a structured day may include assisting the household with fuel gathering, fetching water, cultivating crops and herding livestock. By improving independence skills, the burden of care is reduced and can change the attitude of both the MHCU and family members, creating hope for the future.

EXTENDING REHABILITATION AT HOME USING PRINCIPLES OF CBR

Developing a *comprehensive rehabilitation home programme* requires an understanding of factors that may affect the success of rehabilitation in the home, including the family in intervention. By completing a situational analysis of the available resources, family life, their needs (as self-expressed), and their beliefs, the occupational therapist and/or CRW will contextualise the MHCU within their social and physical environment and understand how the family can contribute to the rehabilitation programme. This approach should be explained to the family, as standard health services are based on a medical model rather than a social model (the former is health care practitioner/facility-centric, whereas the latter is more inclusive of the MHCU's wider support system including family). Explaining the approach is the first step in family participation, establishing the relationship between the therapist/CRW and the family and moving rehabilitation from a therapist-directed approach to a patient/family-directed approach to the recovery journey.

Participatory Rural Appraisal (PRA) has useful facilitating tools that enable caregivers and family members to identify problems and needs and discuss issues through doing tasks:

- Drawing a timeline may show the effects of illness on the MHCU and family, e.g. initial episode interrupted schooling, and non-medical intervention used, e.g. traditional or alternative medicine and health practices.

- Making a map (plan) of the home and yard may identify physical problems with which they deal daily, and whether the MHCU is in the main part of the home or segregated from the family.

- Creating a Venn diagram of the social relationships with the MHCU may show who should be the main caregiver or that the MHCU has little social support within the family. They can also be used to get the family to identify and prioritise problems and needs.

- A transect walk through the neighbourhood with the MHCU will show their awareness of local resources and a map of the distance and costs (transport and time) to clinics and hospitals will illustrate the ease (or not) of access to those services.

The expressed needs of MHCU and family should be prioritised for intervention. Mental health care users frequently express the need for acceptance within the family and the need to work. Children with intellectual disability identified organised leisure, school, caring for family and participating in family meals (Huus *et al.* 2021).

WORKING WITH FAMILIES

FACTORS AFFECTING FAMILY PARTICIPATION IN REHABILITATION

Social Context

Families may be reticent about sharing, or show little interest in rehabilitation, requiring several visits to get accurate information. This may be understood in the context of their society, experience and burden of care.

Mental disability is identified as behaviour outside acceptable *social* behavioural norms and therefore reflects local culture and knowledge of health. Traditional African beliefs link mental illness (and co-morbid neurological conditions such as epilepsy) with witchcraft (often associated with beliefs that someone is jealous of you), the wrath of the ancestors (because you have done something wrong or immoral), or a calling to become a healer. These beliefs result in stigma, even within a family (Kimotho 2018). Even health-literate people may 'blame' genetic inheritance, and this may affect family relationships. Therefore, protecting the family's reputation from strangers may be culturally appropriate, and many cultures believe that discussing mental illness or interacting with MHCU spreads the illness.

Various strategies may be tried before the family accepts that the disability persists despite intervention. Hallucinations may be interpreted as the ancestors calling the person to become a traditional healer, or a church prophet as they are possessed by a holy spirit. In Africa, treatment is usually by a traditional healer (Van Niekerk *et al.* 2014) who is an expert in herbal medicine, interpreting the spirits of the ancestors, or the will of the gods/God. Use of herbalists, spiritual healers and consultation with the ancestral family is not confined to African cultures. People in developed countries seek help from revivalist churches, alternative therapies (herbal remedies, vitamin supplements and acupuncture), mystics and fortune tellers.

Past experience of medical care may lead to expectations of a cure as people with epilepsy are 'cured' with anti-epileptics and those with psychosis may have their violent behaviour and hallucinations controlled by anti-psychotics. However, occupational performance impairments due to changes in cognitive abilities, energy levels and motivation remain. Families realise no matter what they try nothing works – a cycle of learned helplessness ensues. Why should they believe a therapist or rehabilitation MLW (relatively unknown types of health workers) who says that things will get better? If the family agrees to intervention, they may expect quick change as with medicine, whereas the rehabilitation MLW expect change and recovery over an extended period of time. Their expectation is that the rehabilitation MLW will be the agent of change, just as the traditional healer, clinic nurse or doctor provides a cure. The CBR approach expects that the family and the MHCU will continue with therapy and recovery-orientated strategies without the occupational therapist. While this dichotomy can lead to misunderstanding and frustration it can be addressed through longitudinal support from rehabilitation MLWs that are, in turn, supported by an occupational therapist. For successful CBR, select the first goal together with the family and MHCU to ensure interest, success and commitment to the longitudinal recovery process.

Burden of Care

The role of caregiving in mental health is determined by the state of relationships and social responsibility that the carer has towards the MHCU and tends to be obligatory in nature (Olagundoye & Alugo 2016). Most families and relatives occupy this role of caregiving without any knowledge and skills required to handle its demands (Chadda 2014). Families may not cope with the stress of this additional burden nor have the time and energy to carry out intervention, especially if the burden of care is coupled with the burden of poverty (Marimbe *et al.* 2016). High levels of burden (Akbari *et al.* 2018) are composed of

- Objective burden related to the impact of caregiving: financial strain, prolonged time spent on caregiving, disrupted family routines, disruption or conflict in family relationships, restrictions on the family's occupational performance, loss of social support in the community due to beliefs about the cause and spread of mental disability, as well as problems caused by the behaviour of the person with mental illness and lack of access to community mental health services (Masilela & MacLeod 1998; Chadda 2014; Egbe *et al.* 2014; Kimotho 2018; Ndlovu & Mokwena 2023). In general, those with severe disability live in households with less income and the direct costs of extra care at home and accessing monthly chronic medication, traditional healer or rehabilitation services; result in high out-of-pocket expenditure (Hanass-Hancock *et al.* 2017; Addo *et al.* 2018) and indirect costs (Addo *et al.* 2018). Further direct costs include additional household costs such as food (due to increased appetite or wastage) and habits such as smoking and drinking used to reduce anxiety and improve mood. Indirect costs include loss of productivity which is associated with loss of income because of losing a job to take on caregiving responsibilities and increased role responsibility for the primary caregiver, as well as loss of income and roles of the MHCU (Chadda 2014; Addo *et al.* 2018). Mental disability exacerbates the poverty cycle leading to poor diet and low energy levels, yet in LMIC hours of heavy labour are required to provide water, food and fuel energy, leaving little energy for rehabilitation.

- Subjective burden related to the mental and emotional impact of caregiving: feelings of loss, guilt, shame, anger, grief, frustration and resentment (Chadda 2014). This burden is influenced by patient, caregiver and material resource factors (Yerriah *et al.* 2021).

- The patient factors are related to the characteristics of the MHCU such as the chronic nature of a mental disorder, violent behaviour, roaming the streets, not heeding family advice, recurrent relapses, poor treatment compliance, duration of a mental disorder, deficits in occupational performance skills and routines that changes in occupational profile and routines of the caregiver and lower level of education of an MHCU (Yesufu-Udechuku *et al.* 2015; Caqueo-Urízar *et al.* 2016; Yerriah *et al.* 2021).

- Caregiver factors are the age of the caregiver (for older caregivers, the role may be too demanding), the gender (female caregivers may have difficulty balancing multiple roles they are expected to occupy such as being a mother, worker, house maintainer and key emotional supporter), lower level of education and strained relationships with the MHCU (Adeosun 2013; Flyckt *et al.* 2015; Lippi 2016; Yerriah *et al.* 2021).

- Material resource factors are limited access to mental health services which has to do with the lack of information on mental disorders and decreased social support that is closely linked to the community stigma experienced by the caregiver and the MHCUs.

Healthy families are essential if MHCUs are to live in the community. If the health status of family and caregivers is neglected, they have no chance to express their concerns and needs, and use trial and error to develop coping strategies (Chadda 2014; Akbari *et al.* 2018). Expressed needs include information about mental illness, its treatment and cure; skills to handle behaviour and training of the MHCU in occupational performance, financial support (such as social grants) or work, reducing stigma by changing attitudes in the community, access to appropriate services and support from the community, e.g. religious organisations and local government; prioritisation of access to housing; and 'empowerment' (Chen *et al.* 2019; Kumar *et al.* 2019). Sadly, only 10% of caregivers reported that they got help coping from health personnel; they were more likely to receive advice from community members (Homer 2014).

SUPPORT FOR THE CAREGIVER

The burden among families and relatives can be alleviated by integrating caregiver assessments into routine mental health care and providing support strategies for the families and relatives in the community.

Integrating Caregiver Assessments in Routine Mental Health Care

Early identification of the burden of care in the caregivers of the MHCUs (Chadda 2014; Silaule *et al.* 2023) is essential for planning and strengthening the MHCU's support systems. Assessment methods include

- Screening during the initial interviews with the MHCU and their families: aiming questions that directly identify the caregiver's ability to cope with the demands of caregiving, the need for and availability of support, and contextual factors such as stigma.

- Observation for warning signs of depression or compassion fatigue: irritability towards a MHCU, feelings of being overwhelmed, feelings of fatigue, expression of hopelessness and helplessness in dealing with the MHCU's condition.

- Occupation-based assessment to establish the impact of caregiving on the ability of the caregiver to engage in and balance occupations.

Burden measures such as the Caregiver Burden Inventory (Novak & Guest 1989) and Caregiver Self-Assessment Questionnaire (American Medical Association 2015) can be used to establish the level of the burden experienced by the families and relatives of the MHCUs. They also serve as a reference point for discussion about caregiver well-being. The utility and contextual relevance of these and other non-standardised tools may be increased by translating them into local vernacular.

Assessment should lead to the occupational therapist's spoken recognition of the burden of care and the establishment of a caregiver well-being care plan (Chadda 2014).

Support Strategies for the Families and Relatives in the Community

Prolonged time in caregiving and inability to engage in all occupations as expected becomes the main concern for many caregivers. Caregiver education and occupation-based interventions are two strategies for supporting caregivers. These should be tailored to meet their expressed needs (Chadda 2014; Rosas-Santiago *et al.* 2017; Zeng *et al.* 2017; Chen *et al.* 2019; Seshadri *et al.* 2019; Yu *et al.* 2020):

- Health literacy on the mental illness, practical handling and management of problem behaviours and ability to structure engagement of the MHCUs in daily occupations were discussed earlier.

- Orientation to available community mental health services for the MHCU (clinic services, ward-based outreach teams, community health workers with CBR competences and any day centres) and informal support organisations, such as peer-led support groups, for themselves.

- Looking after your own health, and a balanced engagement in daily occupations.

- Using burden and coping strategies, e.g. appropriate anxiety and stress management techniques.

- Temporary relief of burden: time to engage in activities of their choice such as social and leisure activities and sharing roles and duties with other members of the family may relieve stress (Souza *et al.* 2017). In cases where there is no family to assist, community workers such as rehabilitation MLWs, community health workers and HBCs could be involved in respite care.

EXTENDING THE DEFINITION OF REHABILITATION FOR THE INDIVIDUAL

For most occupational therapists, rehabilitation as a direct intervention may be the only service they offer but the WHO recognises that other factors influence health and well-being, and the important role of other sectors in mental health (WHO 2021). This multi-sectoral approach to disability-inclusive development is embodied in the definition of CBR and has recently been applied directly to WHO's Quality

Rights Programme materials for training, guidance and transformation (2019). CBR is:

> '*A strategy within general community development for the rehabilitation, reduction of poverty, equalisation of opportunities, and social inclusion of all people with disabilities through the combined efforts of people with disabilities themselves, their families, organisations and communities and relevant government and non-government health, education, vocational, social and other services*' (Joint Position Paper 2004).

Initially seen as needed for an overarching societal change, the components of the WHO CBR Matrix extends rehabilitation by ensuring that the MHCU has access to available resources across different sectors.

Figure 11.1 describes the WHO CBR matrix (WHO 2010a), which covers all components of life.

In well-resourced communities, all components may be present and working together but in LMIC resources are limited. In areas where occupational therapy is a scarce resource knowledge of the MHCU, family and local role players and services they offer should result in

- Identification of life goals for the MHCU

- A coordinated inter-sectoral care and recovery pathway plan

- Referral to existing community organisations to extend the period of rehabilitation

- Task shifting rehabilitation activities to carers and rehabilitation MLWs, or to other health professionals and mid-level health workers such as CRWs and relevant community organisations

LIFE GOALS

Onset of MHCU early in life means their entire adult life is affected: friendships, schooling, work, marriage and having their own house and family become impossible dreams for many. Those who have a later onset of problems may face the stresses of losing friends, jobs, homes, marriage partner and children. All have to face the death of relatives, especially family members who support them. They may not be able to hold down a job or complete regular tasks within the home, their behaviour may be erratic and socially inappropriate, and this may result in them being ostracised by the community or their family. Despite this, many MHCU still have dreams to earn money, have a loving relationship with a life partner, have children and a positive relationship with them and live away from their parents' home. To do this, they need to be as healthy as possible, learn, have options for employment, a support system and access to local social, recreational and cultural activities.

HEALTH

- In LMIC, clinic services are dependent on the PHC nurse. PHC nurses may have limited mental health literacy (Korhonen *et al.* 2022) and fear people with MHCU due to cultural beliefs and their experience of a confused, aggressive or violent MHCU refusing help (Homer 2014). These nurses may avoid extended contact with MHCUs (Gerber 2018) and limit the care they offer. Care at the PHC primary level involves identifying cases and referring, issuing medicine, monitoring for deterioration and some basic 'healthy lifestyle' advice (Robertson *et al.* 2018). Extended

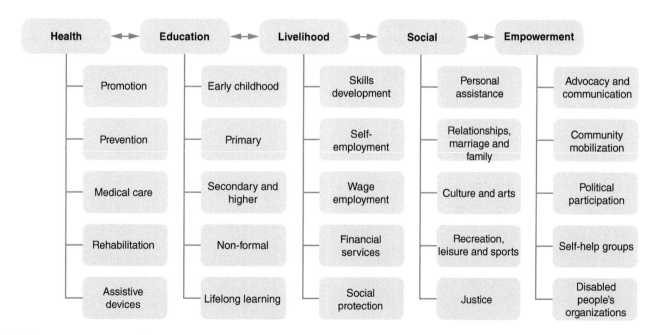

Health	Education	Livelihood	Social	Empowerment
Promotion	Early childhood	Skills development	Personal assistance	Advocacy and communication
Prevention	Primary	Self-employment	Relationships, marriage and family	Community mobilization
Medical care	Secondary and higher	Wage employment	Culture and arts	Political participation
Rehabilitation	Non-formal	Financial services	Recreation, leisure and sports	Self-help groups
Assistive devices	Lifelong learning	Social protection	Justice	Disabled people's organizations

FIGURE 11.1   Components of community-based rehabilitation.

Source: Adapted from Components of community-based rehabilitation: The WHO CBR Matrix (WHO 2010a, p. 71).

mental health care may be offered by District Mental Health Teams that include mental health nurses and occupational therapists. These professionals are an important source of mentorship for all health workers as well as having a vital role in monitoring the health of people with MHCU in their district. However, there may be a gap between policy rhetoric and what is available (RHAP *et al.* 2015) and this gap may be filled by non-government organisations (NGOs):

- Lay counsellors such as the PRIME programme and the Zimbabwean Friendship Bench scheme are successful in reducing symptoms of emotional distress (WHO 2021).

- Traditional healers may use occupation as part of their intervention and evaluation of progress, so therapists need to collaborate with them more (Van Niekerk *et al.* 2014).

- MHCU-based Disabled People's Organisations (DPOs) offer support services in the field of mental health. DPOs provide leaflets and talks about mental health and the work of the organisation, interventions such as home care, counselling and support groups for MHCU or caregivers. Their contribution may extend to the livelihood and empowerment components with work opportunities through sheltered workshops, self-help groups and work placement.

EDUCATION

Although education is a right for all children in many areas, if there is no support offered for MHCU at school and the pressure of education work may be too stressful for MHCUs returning after hospital admission. School teachers may be fearful and unaware of available educational support or how to access it, resulting in low enrolment and leaving parents to cope with children with epilepsy, autism, behavioural disorders and intellectual impairment at home. The resultant gaps in education have a long-term impact on employability (WHO 2021).

Discussions with the Department of Education should be around accommodations for learning, e.g. resources for the classroom, how to handle seizure or how to handle a child who does not concentrate. District Education Teams may include occupational therapists who are equipped to advise on disability-inclusive universal design or adaptations for learning in the classroom, playground and home. They advise and educate teachers, and channel referrals to special schools, although these may be far away and have long admission waiting lists. Formal and informal childcare facilities should be encouraged to accept children with mental disabilities, but they require education and training on managing these children.

A SUSTAINABLE LIVELIHOOD: OVERCOMING POVERTY

The unemployment rate for MHCU is high (WHO 2021). It is important to liaise with the Department of Labour and the social worker about unfair dismissal from employment, and difficulties obtaining unemployment benefits. Those hoping to return to work may not cope with their previous role and work pressure. Employers may not cope with relapses. In these cases, a company 'medical pension' may be an option. Without formal employment opportunities, work retraining, alternative employment, social protection, and food security become necessary.

An occupation-based CBR programme may improve work skills (Lui *et al.* 2023) and local municipalities and the Department of Labour may offer skills training for microenterprise projects such as making kitchen units, small bread-making projects and creative handwork such as batiks. Community self-help groups may do income-generating activities, e.g. baking, sewing and woodwork. Their set-up may be supported by the Department of Social Development (DSD) community development officers, who also support DPOs establishing protective workshops.

Social grants may be available and occupational therapists have an important role in grant education as those applying for grants for mental health problems may not be recognised as debilitating (Hanass-Hancock *et al.* 2017). People living on farms or in rural areas do not have easy access to grants (Modiba *et al.* 2000). Grants may cause family problems, e.g. the grant is spent on alcohol or drugs, or given away by the grant holder, or the family has control of the grant and uses it for themselves and not the grant holder. The occupational therapist, social worker or rehabilitation MLW should discuss control of money and budgeting with MHCU and carers.

Even with grants food security is vital as there are links between household food insufficiency and short-term and lifelong mental health problems (Sorsdahl *et al.* 2011). Food gardening is rarely perceived as a leisure activity in a poor rural area, as it is considered a survival or work occupation. The Department of Agriculture may support community garden development and in some countries, municipalities may have an 'allotment scheme'. A food garden at home may create food security and decrease food expenditure. Gardening may promote correct energy expenditure, build physical fitness, improve self-esteem by having an end product (even digging a patch of ground over can be satisfying) and by being involved in an activity recognised and valued by the family and community. Food gardening may increase motivation to participate in other activities and bring the family together. If enough food is produced, it can be sold to create income.

Saving clubs such as Christmas clubs and stokvels (a South African invitation-only community-based savings group where members contribute a fixed amount at an agreed-upon frequency, with the payout going to members on a rotational basis) are common throughout southern African communities.

SOCIAL

Illness may have a negative effect on family relationships (Brooke-Sumner *et al.* 2014). Social interaction is avoided or discouraged or the MHCU's attempts are ridiculed. Families may neglect, isolate or abuse the MHCU. MHCUs may avoid interaction because it is always stressful. If conflict remains even with occupational therapy or rehabilitation MLW intervention, or the MHCU has no family and needs support to care for their own needs, then refer to the DSD as community social workers help resolve family conflicts and assist with grant applications for financial relief. In South Africa, the DSD subsidises residential care for adults with mental disabilities who need personal assistance, though since the Life Esidemeni debacle the Department of Health is responsible for the quality of care at the centres (Department of Health 2018). Care centres for children with disabilities may come under the Social or Education sector.

Studies show that stable housing is important for MHCU, some of whom are homeless because of their illness and others who wish to be independent of their family. There are a variety of working international models for shared or independent living (WHO Guidance on Community Mental Health Services 2021) In South Africa, the Department of Housing's low-cost housing scheme allows new houses to be built in existing family homesteads, thereby eliminating the stress of relocating to a new area and losing social support systems.

The Department of Sport and Recreation is involved in promoting recreational activities at pre-schools and primary schools, building facilities such as playgrounds, as well as supporting sports and drama for adolescents and adults. The occupational therapist's role in collaboration with Rehabilitation MLWs is mainly to enhance access to these resources and ensure those with disability are included.

Community social groups form around sport, religion, music and dance, drama, funerals, celebrations, self-improvement, making food and earning or saving money. Meeting savings club members on a monthly basis is also a way to socialise. Informal social support providers include a good listener that people go to talk about their problems with, the local priest, a village elder or someone with social standing in the community (often a person with a higher level of education).

By ensuring access to a range of community resources, the occupational therapist in collaboration with Rehabilitation MLW enables the MHCU to live a richer and more productive life. However, to find these resources may require an understanding of the resources in a district and not just the local area.

BEYOND THE INDIVIDUAL – CBR DISTRICT SERVICE DEVELOPMENT

CBR is more than therapeutic, rehabilitative and recovery-orientated intervention under the health component; it is a means of changing the place in society of people with disabilities as reflected by the United Nations (UN) Disability Inclusive Sustainable Development Goals for 2030 (UN General Assembly 2015):

- Reduce premature mortality through improved health and livelihood.
- End poverty and hunger through improved social protection and livelihood.
- Ensure dignity and equality through empowerment component.
- Foster peaceful, just and inclusive societies through the social and empowerment component.
- Ensure prosperity and living with nature.
- Implement strategies with partners working within each component.

Such development goals need the existing health services and community to work together to build awareness of mental health and illness to ensure a 'full range of services and supports to enable people to live independently and be included in the community (including rehabilitation services, social services, educational, vocational and employment opportunities, housing services and supports, etc.)' (WHO 2020). Whilst few OTs may work at the district level, many of these principles and activities can be done in the local hospital service area.

To ensure UHC, a situational analysis of existing services and community needs is essential for planning and budgeting services. Analysis includes resources that are available within the community as well as understanding whether people with disability have 'equal access' to these resources or if stigma is a barrier to achieving the best possible assistance in rehabilitation, health, wealth, education, employment, adequate living conditions, transport and protection against violence (WHO 2022).

Situational analysis is followed by

- A 'gap analysis' of services and disability advocacy that needs to be developed.
- Awareness raising of service availability and equal access to existing services.
- Transferring knowledge and skills of occupational performance to people with MHCU and their families so they cope better and reduce their poverty.
- CBR policy development.
- Raising awareness about disability acceptance and inclusion in the community and supporting families affected by MHCU.
- Advocacy development for MHCU and carers and community organisations and inclusion of them in service development.
- Training new rehabilitation MLW to deliver CBR services.

SITUATIONAL ANALYSIS

Existing Services

The minimum analysis should cover MHCU prevalence and the local health and community resources for inter-sectoral referrals identified above. Not everyone with a mental health problem accesses health services so the hospital register is not enough. Depression, alcoholism, or dementia, and stress and depression masked by physical symptoms may not be perceived as illnesses by the community. Depression is associated with chronic illness and physical disability, the long-term effects of COVID-19 are not yet understood and those with psychosis may not seek any service for up to 35 weeks from onset (Burns *et al.* 2010). They also default treatment. If district prevalence is unknown, national or international prevalence found in the Global Burden of Disease project can be used as a proxy, see Figure 11.2 (Dattani *et al.* 2023).

Local Health Resources Analysis   This includes service coverage, human resources, funding, and what services are used or rejected by the MHCUs. Mental disorders rank third in the South African National Burden of Disease (Seedat *et al.* 2009) yet rank low in resource allocation with only 1.53 OTs:100 000

uninsured population (Docrat *et al.* 2019). Such scarce resources result in inequitable distribution over provinces (Ned *et al.* 2020) and lower numbers of occupational therapists in rural areas.

District hospital occupational therapy services in LMIC may depend on a single district post held by expatriate therapists working a fixed-time contract (voluntary service model) or by newly qualified therapists doing a year of community service (South African model) so it is unlikely that an occupational therapist will offer dedicated mental health service. Personnel rotate frequently and re-advertised posts may not be filled immediately, quickly leading to each therapist starting new projects that collapse when they leave, or 'reinventing the wheel'. Rapid bed turnover and limited human resources create an environment for CBR as an appropriate strategy for increasing access to rehabilitation and determining the best role for the OT.

Inter-sectoral Resources Analysis

An inter-sectoral approach enhances the sustainability of CBR services and is 'best use of available resources'. Communities are rich in resources that may help and support the MHCU and their families. OTs need to identify other service

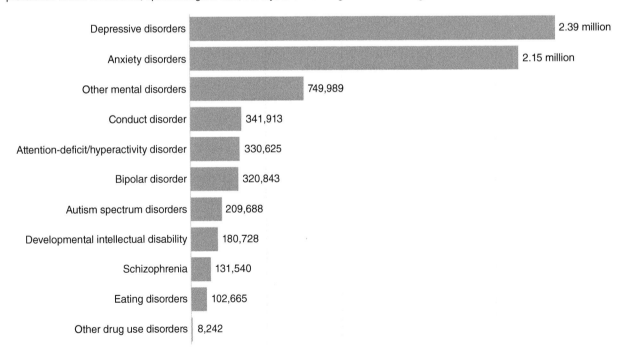

Number with a mental or neurodevelopmental disorder by type, South Africa, 2019

Our World in Data

Substance use disorders are not included. Figures attempt to provide a true estimate (going beyond reported diagnosis) of prevalence based on medical, epidemiological data, surveys and meta-regression modelling.

Disorder	Number
Depressive disorders	2.39 million
Anxiety disorders	2.15 million
Other mental disorders	749,989
Conduct disorder	341,913
Attention-deficit/hyperactivity disorder	330,625
Bipolar disorder	320,843
Autism spectrum disorders	209,688
Developmental intellectual disability	180,728
Schizophrenia	131,540
Eating disorders	102,665
Other drug use disorders	8,242

Data source: IHME, Global Burden of Disease (2019)

FIGURE 11.2   Prevalence of mental health care users South Africa 2019.
Source: Dattani *et al.* (2023) / Oxford University Press / Public domain.

providers, and then compare all existing services to determine if there is duplication of services, equal access to CBR services, and the local barriers/facilitators to access and service gaps. DPOs and NPOs can be identified using 'disability directories' and the online NPO register run by the DSD.

IDENTIFYING MHCUS TO CREATE AWARENESS AND INCREASING ACCESS TO REHABILITATION

To find MHCU and those outside the health system use:

- Local clinic list of MHCU on chronic medication.

- Referrals from the District Hospital.

- A 'Meet and Greet' session over the radio (make sure an easy to remember day and venue are chosen).

- A Household Survey (this may be the most inclusive way to find people, but it is expensive and time-consuming).

- Mapping. See Figure 11.3 Low-cost and high-tech mapping of the same area.

Mapping is an enjoyable PRA tool (Shields-Zeeman *et al.* 2017) that can be used to map MHCU and non-users in local areas as well as local resources. Most people in rural communities know someone with MHCU (Masilela & MacLeod 1998): a youth group may know those with alcohol/drug problems or school-related stress, Ante Natal Clinics attendees may recognise mothers with postpartum disorders and young children with learning or developmental problems. Mapping the community may be the beginning of the occupational therapist's understanding of the community and initiating relationships with community members. Involving community leaders such as councillors or local tribal offices can create political support for the future CBR service.

Follow-up mapping with a home visit or a community meeting to ensure MHCUs and their families are aware of their rights, have information about the CBR services, and you, ideally in collaboration with rehabilitation MLWs or CHWs, can begin to identify specific MHCU and family needs. Unfortunately, few MHCUs know local support options so the therapist and/or rehabilitation MLW should increase awareness and access to these organisations ensuring that referral is

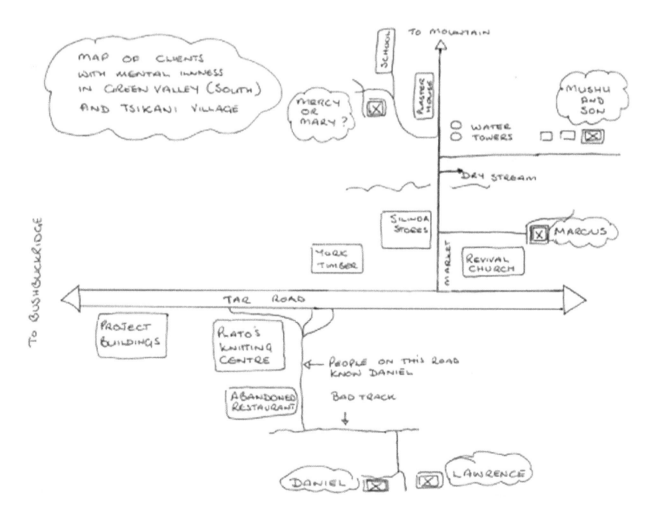

FIGURE 11.3   Low-cost and high-tech mapping of the same area.

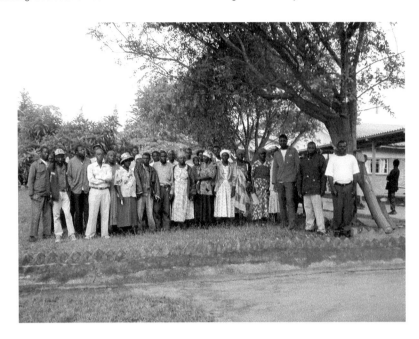

FIGURE 11.4 Sizanani Mental Health Support Group. (Author's photograph)

to a locally accessible group appropriate to the MHCUs culture and socioeconomic level.

Local Mental Health Needs and Mental Health Advocacy – The Bigger Picture

A resource analysis is not enough; people have mental health needs and expectations. OTs should not assume they know the needs of the MHCUs. A simple PRA exercise described by Petrick, Homer and Evans (Homer 2014) showed that therapists and young adults with disability prioritised different needs, did not speak the same 'language' (leading to misunderstanding about priorities) and therapists ignored their expressed needs. These needs underpin mental health and rehabilitation advocacy.

MHCUs and Community Needs Analysis Common needs can be identified through quantitative research, but qualitative research such as focus group discussions and PRA tools (Venn diagrams and matrix ranking) can provide rich information. Throughout the analysis process, MHCUs, organisations, community members and health service staff will develop expectations about the CBR service. The priority *need* of the MHCU may be the love and understanding of their family, with the expectation the therapist will align with them against the family. The family's priority *need* may be for the MHCU to contribute to the productivity of the family by looking after the home, so that others can go to work. Their expectation is the therapist ensures that the MHCU works. Communities have to deal with inappropriate behaviour at community gatherings, damage to property, aggression and assault (Homer 2014) and community leaders are concerned with protecting the community and *need* to confine people with mental disabilities

so that they do not endanger property and the health of others and they expect better access to mental health centres and care centres. The therapist may *expect* that education to MHCU, family and community on causes of MHCU and treatment will increase compliance with treatment and acceptance by the community.

The completed analysis should become part of the community profile document maintained within the occupational therapy department; and service providers, MHCUs and community should be informed of the results.

Use the Situational Analysis to create discussion and possible activities around:

- CBR Programme Goals to integrate those with MHCU into the community, based on existing inter-sectoral service delivery.
- Service gaps identified by the needs and barriers.
- Attitudes and prejudices.
- Collaborators in the programmes.
- The timeline of the programme to monitor and evaluate it (WHO 2010b).

Care should be taken to ensure that everybody understands needs will be prioritised, that not all needs will be met in the short term, and that solutions should be realistic in terms of personnel, technology and funds.

ADVOCACY FOR BETTER MENTAL HEALTH AND EMPOWERMENT FOR PEOPLE WITH DISABILITY

First steps in developing CBR may be to have the needs of those with MHCU recognised and some basic services offered at the community level may need priority attention. The outcome of a good advocacy programme is for mental health to be valued by all and 'recognised as a requirement for community development' (WHO 2010b, p. 5), to ensure the rights of people with disability are known, and MHCUs are accepted and included into family and community life and have equal rights to community resources. Mental health advocacy is built on raising awareness and mobilising change in the community.

Awareness of Mental Health and Prevention of Mental Health Conditions Within the Community

As for the family health, literacy is often the first step to develop insight into disability within the community. Raising awareness in community groups, e.g. teachers at a school or a local sewing group, should create a learning cascade as they pass on knowledge gained to friends, family and neighbours. However, professional knowledge has to be translated so it is easily understood by lay people, and should provide healthy lifestyle skills so they become responsible for their own well-being, can help others in stressful situations or help the early detection and referral of those who are ill to prevent further loss of function (WHO 2010b). In areas of low literacy, talk shows on the local radio, at public events or in clinics and schools are a better option than leaflet distribution. Plan sessions that facilitate active participation, e.g. short role plays on a stressful situation, followed by a discussion of what everyone can do to help themselves or nearby families in stressful situations, as well as helping MHCU. Ordinary people may offer solutions, e.g. social, emotional and donations of goods to families affected by MHCU (Modiba *et al.* 2000; Homer 2014).

Few people are aware of the importance of occupations, performance patterns and the need to balance areas of occupation to reduce stress and live healthily. Important aspects are timetabling daily routines or weekly goals, inducing restful sleep, using relaxation techniques and avoiding extra responsibilities when you are already burdened by disability or caring. Teenage pregnancy, truancy, alcohol and drug use are common in poverty-stricken areas with limited choices for recreation. Alcohol and drugs are linked to an increase in head injuries due to violence and traffic accidents, and, if taken during pregnancy, increased risk of cognitive problems in the child. Therapists need to work with families, schools, churches, the municipality, and youth groups to develop healthy replacement activities such as sport and recreation.

Mental health is dependent on good nutrition. Nutrient deficits during pregnancy and early childhood are associated with poor mental health and learning. Boosting the diet may prevent congenital cognitive disabilities and counteract the effects of malnutrition on learning in school-aged children, a Vitamin B-rich diet may prevent illness (particularly depression) due to stress in adolescents and adults. Even with poverty restrictions using a different starch, protein, fruit or vegetable each week creates an overall balanced diet (Sathyanarayana

Rao *et al.* 2008). Therapists may teach healthy eating if there is no dietician, but our focus on activity participation is what differentiates our health education from other health professionals: healthy eating habits and a balanced diet to prevent weight loss and improve mental function, planning healthy meals, meal preparation, budgeting to buy healthy food, growing food gardens, keeping chickens and harvesting food in the countryside.

Rehabilitation in someone's home provides the opportunity to ensure the family is protected from preventable diseases that can cause neuropsychological deficits in children and adults. When in the home check the Road to Health charts to see if children have been immunised or have risk factors and educate on the Expanded Programme on Immunisation. Know the HIV status of the MHCU and encourage people with signs of HIV to be tested and treated. Monitor families affected by HIV for stress and mental health problems (Joubert & Bradshaw 2005, p. 206). Promote the use of mosquito nets, chemical sprays or traditional methods such as burning dung or citronella to prevent malaria-related neurological conditions.

Mental health prevention and promotion school-based programmes are the most commonly reported community health programmes (WHO 2020) and ensure the equitable distribution of knowledge needed to build mental health resilience within the community (Department of Health 2023). Key topics are as follows:

- The importance of a healthy lifestyle and the dangers of drug and alcohol use.

- How to recognise signs of stress related to school, home life, stigma and traumatic events.

- How to tell if someone they know has a mental health problem.

- Contact details for help, e.g. Child Line, social workers and nurses.

Working with the Community to Bring About Change

The importance of inter-sectoral collaboration is highlighted for a comprehensive mental health care plan (WHO 2020; Department of Health 2023) and awareness raising is needed in a variety of community stakeholders to reduce stigma and discrimination towards MHCU (WHO 2010b, pp. 5 and 210). A stakeholder analysis (WHO 2010a, p. 47) to identify the government and societal groups identified earlier and other stakeholders such as the traditional leader and political parties is indicated. These stakeholders drive community projects, provide access to funds and bestow recognition or support for health projects, or for an individual health worker. Whilst mapping may tell the occupational therapist what stakeholders are present and where they meet, Venn diagrams and matrix ranking can be used to find out more about the activities, power and influence of these structures. Stakeholders can help the occupational therapist understand the local community and it may be essential to contact local leaders to gain permission to work in the community and some guarantee of safety. From this information, the occupational therapist can determine the stakeholders that could make large changes within the community if they are more aware of mental health issues and how they can contribute to changing public perceptions of MHCU and help MHCU to access existing community resources or providing resources for MHCU.

The stigma of mental illness creates many problems for the MHCU and their families (Monnapula-Mazabane & Petersen 2021). Mental health advocacy is needed to overcome community violence and sexual abuse against MHCU, which for females is 4–10 times more likely than national averages (Swartz & Bhattacharya 2017). Women with disabled children are more likely to be victims of physical or social abuse by both family members and the community. Communities with little education, or opportunity to develop leadership skills, simply may not know what to do to improve the health of their community. They may have limited expectations of what the CBR service can provide – particularly if they have seen projects started but not finished – and change can be time-consuming and frustrating. Awareness raising for these stakeholders would include education on disability rights, understanding disability, acceptable health services and integration into schools, places of work and community activities (Duncan 2016). Identify practical contributions stakeholders can make to the CBR programme such as promoting mental health and the prevention of MHCU within their own family or organisation, resource support (such as a building or piece of land that can be used by a support group) or social support by including MHCU in organisations and events. Stakeholders are usually interested in having services provided, e.g. a care centre or support group, but expect the therapist, as the expert paid to deal with mental health, to initiate them. Their role can be extended by using innovative programmes such as WHO Guidance on Community Mental Health Services (2021) and WHO's Preventing Suicide: A Community Engagement Toolkit (2017) that give practical guidance on developing community-led action plans to recognise mental illness and stigma and reduce risk of illness, violence and suicide at the local level.

Developing Support Resources

People at the creative ability level of participation may be accepted within an existing group, e.g. a choir, but those at lower levels of creative ability are less likely to be accepted or able to make a valued contribution to the group without assistance. MHCU may be socially isolated as they are suspicious of people, very anxious in social situations, and have poor conversation skills. Due to stigma, they may have little opportunity to practice social skills with family, friends and the community. As social support groups occur naturally in all communities, the concept of disability support groups is usually accepted by MHCUs and carers (Brooke-Sumner et al. 2014). Groups may

be established by nurses, social workers, community developers, DPOs, as well as occupational therapists. Whilst a MHCU support group may be more appropriate (Ghosh 2005), a general disability support group may be practical in low-resource settings. Groups create the opportunity to gain acceptance, learn about MHCU and coping and develop friendships. The starting point for developing a group may be a very simple level before the participants are ready to see themselves as part of a group with a purpose. Activities such as introducing themselves to the others attending the clinic, saying something about themselves, the problems they are having and ways in which they try to cope, whilst sharing light refreshments is how the Sizanani Mental Health Support Group started, see Figure 11.4 (Homer 2014). Caregiver support groups centre on sharing the problems of caring, learning about how others cope and ways to reduce stress. Successful support models include the Hong Kong Clubhouse Model, the Nairobi Mind Empowerment Peer Support Group (WHO 2021) and the PRIME (2014) Psychosocial Rehabilitation Support Groups for MHCU and carers.

The practicalities of organising these groups and developing their independence can be lengthy due to the inherent problems of mental disability: problems with memory and task completion mean they may not remember the dates or place of the meeting or may get sidetracked when making their way to the meeting. Low motivation and energy or the burden of care may also affect attendance.

A successful small sustainable CBR programme is better than a grand idea that raises expectations within the community but fails to deliver.

Establishing a Small Core of People Who Will Act as Champions for Mental Health

The need to task shift from health professionals to non-specialised health workers and informal health practitioners has long been recognised in South Africa, particularly in rural areas, as they are more likely to offer culturally relevant education and intervention (Vergunst 2018). Current international practice in LMIC consists of community workers, e.g. the caregiver, HBC worker or local DPO involved in the day-to-day intervention, with rehabilitation MLWs supporting and monitoring their work; and a therapist acting as programme manager developing overall service plans and managing the CBR programme. Research indicates that this model ensures better compliance with medical, occupational and social intervention resulting in improvements in mental health (Asher et al. 2018; Chen et al. 2021). This conceptual model has been trialled in South Africa (Luruli et al. 2016); however, despite the need, it is not a national model and still needs adjusting to reduce barriers to participation (Ned et al. 2020).

Therapists may be instrumental in establishing disability advocacy and rehabilitation training for:

- HBC workers to help individual MHCUs in their care.

- Centres for people with disability started by a local person with big heart but no training.

- Well-established DPOs offering care rather than rehabilitation, or

- Training programmes for formal rehabilitation MLWs, e.g. occupational therapy assistants or community rehabilitation workers (Rule *et al.* 2006).

Training varies according to the level and need, but all should comply with national policy and standards, or guidelines from the WHO; otherwise, it may lead to unrealistic expectations from the service provider and those trained. Local mental health champions may be trained in early detection and referral (Shields-Zeeman *et al.* 2017). Practical advice on handling specific behaviours as related to their job is appreciated; it is hoped improving the knowledge of people working in the informal health services will improve the service they render.

National DPOs do lobby for better services, and the Western Cape Forum for Intellectual Disability successfully lobbied for more education centres for children with intellectual impairment (Western Cape High Court 2010). Health activist groups such as the Rural Doctors Association of Southern Africa and Rural Rehab SA lobby for better rural service delivery and worked with stakeholders on the Rural Mental Health Campaign (RHAP *et al.* 2015) highlighting the plight of rural MHCU (see Vignette 3).

VIGNETTE 3: DO YOU HAVE ANY POWER TO CHANGE POLICY?

Concerned by the lack of mental health services in rural areas of South Africa, two occupational therapists from Rural Rehab SA (a small volunteer advocacy group) worked together with the psychiatric occupational therapists special interest group to plan an occupational therapy workshop to provide guidance on service provision. From this workshop, it was clear that a multi-sectoral approach was needed and invites went out for a pre-conference event at the Rural Health Conference in 2014. Here the full extent of the problem was described but there was no evidence in the literature and without evidence we could not ask for change. From those attending a small group of an occupational therapist from Rural Rehab SA, the national director of SA Mental Health Federation, the chair from SADAG who is a MHCU, a psychologist, and a health activist from the Rural Health Advocacy Project (RHAP) volunteered to develop a research plan and questionnaire which the two DPOs would use to find out the problems the rural MHCU had. This collection of stories was so powerful that RHAP used some of its funds to design and publish it as a report. The report was circulated to some of the health activist media groups who used it to take the government to task. The team was invited to the World Psychiatric Conference, the Minister of Health's Advisory Committee and eventually to the South African Human Rights Commission to present their findings and lobby for better resources. This report results in the monitoring of psychotropic medicine stock-outs and is a

reference document for the National Mental Health Policy Framework and Strategic Plan 2023–2030.

News media in South Africa such as Spotlight, Daily Maverick and Bhekisisa are interested in Disability Rights, publishing articles on local communities achieving their rights and using information provided by health activist groups such as Section 27+ to create awareness of problems.

Empowerment

Knowledge of the rights of disabled people and how to access services such as medicine, rehabilitation, grants, housing, appropriate schools and support agencies is not enough; it is only by using these services independently that they show they are empowered. See Figure 11.5. The empowerment process may be fostered by these services, e.g. therapist facilitates the MHCU and family to set and prioritise personal rehabilitation goals, help implement the activities into a routine and evaluate if the goal was achieved. Caregivers are empowered when they continue rehabilitation activities when the therapist is not present: stimulating early development for young children or including the MHCU in participation in family and community life (Narayan & Reddy 2008).

Whilst therapists do advocate on behalf of people with disability, the CBR principle is to empower people to be their own advocates. Sunkel (2017 p. 45), a MHCU and activist says, 'A system that does not recognise the "voice" of persons with Severe Mental Disability (SMD) or acknowledges their views and opinions becomes an enforcer of disempowerment. Persons with SMD must be acknowledged as the key partners in scaling up mental health care services and reducing stigma. They must be empowered to a level where they can be actively involved in policy development, implementation and monitoring of health systems'.

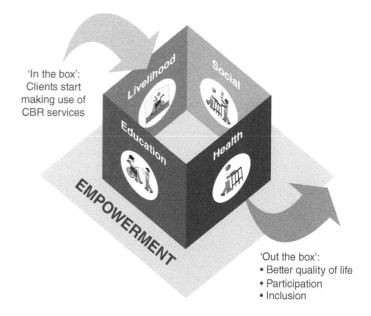

FIGURE 11.5   CBR as a simplified three-dimensional construct (Cornielje 2016).

Empowerment is seen when MHCU and carers, singly or together, raise awareness in the community, e.g. by participating in World Mental Health Day (10 October) campaigns; lobby for disability inclusive services for MHCU, and actively contribute to the planning, monitoring and evaluation of services (WHO 2020). They should sit on local CBR or clinic health committees to be involved in planning, standard setting and monitoring of rehabilitation services, even if this is just at an annual workshop. If committees do not exist, then the first step is to ensure the District or Local Municipality is aware of the mental health issues in their community and get them to facilitate local committee development, such as a Mental Health or Disability Forum. Occupational therapists could support these fora by providing training for MHCUs on leadership, how to run meetings, and how to do strategic plans. A useful resource for capacity building is the WHO (2019) Mental Health Quality Rights guidance and training tools, but it may take years for MCHUs, caregivers, grassroots DPOs and municipal fora to grow into groups active in mental health rights.

Using Policy to Advocate for Disability and Rehabilitation Services

Service delivery is dependent on health funding based on national policy and the prevalence and distribution of health problems throughout the district. However, only 21% of WHO Member States have a mental health policy or plan (WHO 2020), resulting in inefficient health programmes. These countries could be guided by the WHO Guidance on Community Mental Health Services, Chapter 5 Policy and strategy for mental health (WHO 2021).

In South Africa, 'Mental Illness' and 'Disability' are identified as priority national health programmes and the development of community mental health services is a specific goal (Department of Health 2023). There are the Mental Health Care Act 2002 and a District Health Package that includes norms and standards for mental health care in the hospital and community (Department of Health 2002). These are translated into living documents on Essential Medication and Standard Treatment Guidelines for District Hospitals and Essential Medication and Standard Treatment Guidelines for Primary Health Care (Department of Health 2020) that include rehabilitation for MHCU at the hospital and clinic levels, as well as mental health policy and plans that include occupational therapists and psychologists in the District Specialist Mental Health Team (DSMHT) (Department of Health 2023). Large districts in rural areas mean the DSMHT role is mainly advocacy and training for existing service providers.

Inclusion of CBR services is in the PHC package, but the implementation of this remains haphazard (Law 2008) and therapists usually decide independently what they will offer. Small wonder then that occupational therapy mental health services are difficult to establish at the primary level. It is vital to establish a CBR guideline within the district, based on the needs analysis, follow national policy and incorporate the principles of equity, appropriate technology, community participation, and multi-sectoral interaction. By aligning occupational therapy protocols and guidelines to these national health documents, there is an increased chance of funding. This guideline can then drive the programme development to ensure the priority needs and service gaps are met. Being aware of professional standards, policies, technology appropriate for the primary care level and cost-effective service delivery means that you have an armoury with which to lobbying for better service delivery. WHO (2023) identifies there is strong evidence for OT intervention to improve function with programmes that focus on health literacy, family intervention, Cognitive Behavioural Therapy, supported employment programmes and peer-to-peer support; and variable evidence for activities of daily living, supported housing, caring for carers and building support networks.

WHAT WILL I LEAVE BEHIND?

All therapists should do a regular 'CBR check' to monitor the CBR programme. Monitoring and evaluation tools should be established in the early stages. Monitoring tells you what is happening, e.g. are support groups established and do they meet every month? Evaluation establishes whether the programme is successful – judged on its 'relevance, effectiveness, sustainability and impact' (WHO 2010a, p. 62). In terms of *relevance*, MHCUs must speak for themselves and be active participants in the development of the service whether at an individual or programme level. For example, should a programme focus on function or financial status of the MHCU? *Effective* programmes are based on sound research so keep up to date once graduated. Programmes should comply with the principles of *equality and efficiency* and answer the questions: 'Where should the service points be to provide the easiest access for the MHCUs?', 'Is the service equal throughout the district?' and 'Is this the *most* efficient way?' For example, if an outreach service identifies people who need rehabilitation but expects them to travel to the hospital for the service, are you really providing an accessible service? Is it better to work with individual cases or develop groups? Are midlevel staff as effective as therapists at providing social groups for people with MHCU? Indicators of *impact* are the levels of inclusion of people with disability in school, work and social activities, changes in income, work or educational status and changes in attitudes in the person, their family or the community. *Sustainability* is about what one person, or one project can realistically achieve, e.g. should you work only with those who have mental health problems, or should you work on preventing mental health problems in the community by starting an activity centre for the youth? When starting in a new area identify what you want to achieve and what you will leave behind, that will continue to benefit the community. Activities should be selected on their relevance to the common mental health needs of the community and if they are affordable. Both the referral system and access to social grants should be developed enough that they would run without the direct intervention of the occupational therapists. The other area to develop is that of champions for CBR. If you are the first occupational therapist in an area, then much of your work may be taken up with networking and establishing priorities and systems rather than individual MHCU intervention. This can be a difficult transition from clinician to service developer. It is easy to feel overwhelmed by the needs of the community and over-commit to projects or committees and consequently do not fulfil the roles adequately or burn out trying to do so. By using an intersectoral approach, the occupational therapist endeavours to increase the chances of sustainability for the programme and reduce burnout in themselves.

CONCLUSION

This chapter described how to build up a community service based on the needs of the people in a particular community to ensure that people with disabilities are given 'maximum opportunity to become an equal and active member of the community'. CBR services therefore need careful planning to ensure that the needs of people with disability are met despite turnover in staff and to ensure that the succession of occupational therapists can

adapt quickly to their new role, and work stresses are minimised, which in turn should encourage occupational therapists to remain in that community. It is hoped that innovative postgraduate CBR programmes will produce a generation of committed *experienced occupational therapists* skilled in community work.

QUESTIONS

1. What *barriers* exist for people with MHCU living in the community?

2. What can you do to develop *awareness* of mental health and mental disabilities within a community, in order to reduce stigma and discrimination?

3. How can you *involve* people with MHCU and their carers in CBR programmes?

4. What can you do to ensure that people with mental health problems can *access* health, social and economic services within the community?

5. What *support* do families living with MHCU need?

6. How can you *empower* people with MHCU and their family to participate in family and community life?

REFERENCES

Addo, R., Agyemang, S.A., Tozan, Y. & Nonvignon, J. (2018) Economic burden of caregiving for persons with severe mental illness in sub-Saharan Africa: a systematic review. *PLOS ONE*, **13**(8), e0199830. https://doi.org/10.1371/journal.pone.0199830

Adeosun, I.I. (2013) Correlates of caregiver burden among family members of patients with schizophrenia in Lagos, Nigeria. *Schizophrenia Research and Treatment*, **2013**, 1–7. https://doi.org/10.1155/2013/353809

Akbari, M., Alavi, M., Irajpour, A. & Maghsoudi, J. (2018) Challenges of family caregivers of patients with mental disorders in Iran: a narrative review. *Iranian Journal of Nursing and Midwifery Research*, **23**(5), 329–337. https://doi.org/10.4103/ijnmr.IJNMR_122_17

American Medical Association (2015) *Caregiver self-assessment questionnaire.* https://www.healthinaging.org/tools-and-tips/caregiver-self-assessment-questionnaire

Asher, L., De Silva, M., Hanlon, C. *et al* (2016) Community-based rehabilitation intervention for people with schizophrenia in Ethiopia (RISE): study protocol for a cluster randomised controlled trial. *Trials*, **17**(1), 1–14. https://doi.org/10.1186/s13063-016-1427-9

Asher, L., Hanlon, C., Birhane, R. *et al* (2018) Community-based rehabilitation intervention for people with schizophrenia in Ethiopia (RISE): a 12 month mixed methods pilot study. *BMC Psychiatry*, **18**(1), 250. https://doi.org/10.1186/s12888-018-1818-4

Brooke-Sumner, C., Lund, C. & Petersen, I. (2014) Perceptions of psychosocial disability amongst psychiatric service users and caregivers in South Africa. *African Journal of Disability*, **3**(1), 146. http://dx.doi.org/10.4102/ajod.v3i1.146

Burns, J.K., Jhazbhay, K. & Emsley, R. (2010) Cannabis use predicts shorter duration of untreated psychosis and lower levels of negative symptoms in first-episode psychosis: a South African study. *African Journal of Psychiatry*, **13**(5), 395–399. https://doi.org/10.4314/ajpsy.v13i5.63106

Caqueo-Urízar, A., Urzúa, A., Jamett, P.R. & Irarrazaval, M. (2016) Objective and subjective burden in relatives of patients with schizophrenia and its influence on care relationships in Chile. *Psychiatry Research*, **237**, 361–365. https://doi.org/10.1016/j.psychres.2016.01.013

Chadda, R.K. (2014) Caring for the family caregivers of persons with mental illness. *Indian Journal of Psychiatry*, **56**(3), 221–227. https://doi.org/10.4103/0019-5545.140616

Chen, L., Zhao, Y., Tang, J. *et al* (2019) The burden, support and needs of primary family caregivers of people experiencing schizophrenia in Beijing communities: a qualitative study. *BMC Psychiatry*, **19**(1), 1–10. https://doi.org/10.1186/s12888-019-2052-4

Chen, Y., Lam, C.S., Deng, H., Yau, E. & Ko, K.Y. (2021) The effectiveness of a community psychiatric rehabilitation program led by laypeople in China: a randomized controlled pilot study. *Frontiers in Psychiatry*, **12** (**November**), 1–9. https://doi.org/10.3389/fpsyt.2021.671217

Cieza, A., Causey, K., Kamenov, K., Hanson, S.W., Chatterji, S. & Vos, T. (2020) Global estimates of the need for rehabilitation based on the Global Burden of Disease Study 2019: a systematic analysis for the Global Burden of Disease Study 2019. *Lancet (London, England)*, **396**(10267), 2006–2017. https://doi.org/10.1016/S0140-6736(20)32340-0

Cornielje, H. (2016) The potential of a new understanding of CBR for the field of leprosy. In: D.M. Scollard & T.P. Gillis (eds), *International Textbook of Leprosy*, pp. 1–19. American Leprosy Missions, Greenville, South Carolina. https://doi.org/10.1489/itl.4.4

Dattani S., Rodés-Guirao L., Ritchie H. & Roser M. (2023) *Mental health.* OurWorldInData.org. https://ourworldindata.org/mental-health

Department of Health (2002) *A district hospital service package for South Africa. A set of norms and standard.* Pretoria, South Africa. http:// www.kznhealth.gov.za/norms.pdf (accessed on 30 March 2011)

Department of Health (2018) *National Health Care Act 2003: policy guidelines for the licensing of residential and/or day care facilities for persons with mental illness and/or severe or profound intellectual disability.* Government Gazette, 16 March, pp. 15–20.

Department of Health (2020) *Essential medication and standard treatment guidelines for primary health care.* https://knowledgehub.health.gov .za/elibrary/primary-healthcare-phc-standard-treatment-guidelines-stgs-and-essential-medicines-list-eml (accessed 1 October 2020)

Department of Health (2023) *National mental health policy framework and strategic plan 2023–2030.* Pretoria. https://www.spotlightnsp .co.za/wp-content/uploads/2023/04/NMHP-FINAL-APPROVED-ON-30.04.2023.pdf (accessed 31 August 2023)

Docrat, S., Besada, D., Cleary, S., Daviaud, E. & Lund, C. (2019) Mental health system costs, resources and constraints in South Africa: a national survey. *Health Policy & Planning*, **34**, 706–719. https://doi .org/10.1093/heapol/czz085(accessed 21 March 2023)

Duncan M. (2016) Development reasoning in community practice. In: M. Cole & J. Creek (eds), *Global Perspectives in Professional Reasoning*, pp. 1–19. SLACK Inc., Thorofare, New Jersey.

Egbe, C.O., Brooke-Sumner, C., Kathree, T., Selohilwe, O., Thornicroft, G. & Petersen, I. (2014) Psychiatric stigma and discrimination in South Africa: perspectives from key stakeholders. *BMC Psychiatry*, **14**(1), 1–14. https://doi.org/10.1186/1471-244X-14-191/TABLES/3

Flyckt, L., Fatouros-Bergman, H. & Koernig, T. (2015) Determinants of subjective and objective burden of informal caregiving of patients with psychotic disorders, **61**(7), 684–692. https://doi.org/10.1177/ 0020764015573088

Gerber, O. (2018) Practitioners' experience of the integration of mental health into primary health care in the West Rand District, South Africa. *Journal of Mental Health*, **27**(2), 135–141. https://doi.org/ 10.1080/09638237.2017.1340604

Ghosh A. (2005) *Reaching the Unreached Persons with Mental Disability through Community based Rehabilatition.* Shondana Consultancy Pvt Ltd., India. http://www.shodhana.org/shodhana/papers/National%20 Conference.pdf (accessed on 18 June 2012)

Gouda, H.N., Charlson, F., Sorsdahl, K., *et al* (2019) Burden of non-communicable diseases in sub-Saharan Africa, 1990–2017: results from the Global Burden of Disease Study 2017. *The Lancet Global Health*, **7**(10), e1375–e1387. https://doi.org/10.1016/S2214-109X(19)30374-2

Hanass-Hancock, J., Nene, S., Deghaye, N. & Pillay, S. (2017) "These are not luxuries, it is essential for access to life": disability related out-of-pocket costs as a driver of economic vulnerability in South Africa. *African Journal of Disability* **6**, a280. https://doi.org/10.4102/ajod.v6i0.280

Homer, S.L. (2014) Improving health and access to health services through community based rehabilitation. In: R. Crouch & V. Alers (eds), *Occupational Therapy in Psychiatry and Mental Health*, 5th edn, pp. 126–147, Chapter 6. Wiley, Chichester, UK

Huus, K., Morwane, R., Ramaahlo, M. *et al* (2021) Voices of children with intellectual disabilities on participation in daily activities. *African Journal of Disability*. **10**, a792. https://doi.org/10.4102/ajod.v10i0.792

International Labour Organisation, United Nations Educational, Scientific and Cultural Organisation, and World Health Organisation (2004) *CBR: a strategy for rehabilitation, equalization of opportunities, poverty reduction and social inclusion of people with disabilities* (Joint Position Paper). http://www.ilo.org/public/english/region/asro/bangkok/ ability/download/otherpubl_cbr.pdf (accessed on 16 February 2011)

Joubert, A. & Bradshaw D. (2005) *Population ageing and health challenges in South Africa chapter 15 in chronic diseases of lifestyle in South Africa since 1995-2005.* http://www.mrc.ac.za/chronic/cdlchapter15.pdf (accessed on 27 March 2013)

Kimotho, S.G. (2018) Understanding the nature of stigma communication associated with mental illness in Africa: a focus on cultural beliefs and stereotypes. In: B. Canfield & H. Cunningham (eds), *Deconstructing Stigma in Mental Health*, pp. 20–41. IGI Global, Hershey, PA. https:// doi.org/10.4018/978-1-5225-3808-0.CH002

Korhonen K., Axelin A., Stein D.J. *et al* (2022) Mental health literacy among primary healthcare workers in South Africa and Zambia. *Brain and Behavior*, **12**, e2807. https://doi.org/10.1002/brb3.2807

Kumar G., Sood M., Verma R., Mahapatra A. & Chadda R.K. (2019) Family caregivers' needs of young patients with first episode psychosis: a qualitative study. *International Journal of Social Psychiatry*, **65**(5), 435–442. https://doi.org/10.1177/0020764019852650

Law F.B. (2008) *Developing a policy analysis framework to establish level of access and equity embedded in South African health polices for people with disabilities.* Masters Thesis, University of Stellenbosch, South Africa. http:// scholar.sun.ac.za/handle/10019.1/2565 (accessed on 27 March 2013)

Lippi, G. (2016) Schizophrenia in a member of the family: burden, expressed emotion and addressing the needs of the whole family. *South African Journal of Psychiatry*, **22**(1), 922. https://doi.org/10.4102/ SAJPSYCHIATRY.V22I1.922

Liu, Y.-C., Yang, Y.K., Lee, Y.-C. *et al* (2023) Occupational evaluation of community-based psychiatric rehabilitation outcomes in individuals with severe mental illnesses: a ten-year retrospective study. *Asian Journal of Psychiatry*, **81**, 103450. https://doi.org/10.1016/j.ajp.2023.103450

Luruli R.E., Netshandama V.O. & Francis J. (2016) An improved model for provision of rural community-based health rehabilitation services in Vhembe District, Limpopo Province of South Africa. *African Journal of Primary Health Care & Family Medicine*, **8**(2), a980. https://doi .org/10.4102/phcfm.v8i2.980 (accessed on 2 June 2022)

Marimbe, B.D., Cowan, F., Kajawu, L., Muchirahondo, F. & Lund, C. (2016) Perceived burden of care and reported coping strategies and needs for family caregivers of people with mental disorders in Zimbabwe. *African Journal of Disability*, **5**(1), a209. https://doi.org/10.4102/ajod .v5i1.209

Masilela, T.C. & MacLoed C. (1998) Social support. Its implications in the development of a community based mental health programme. *South African Journal of Occupational Therapy*, **27**(2), P11–P16.

Modiba P., Porteus K., Schneider H. & Gunnarsson V. (2000) *Community Mental Health Service Needs: A Study of Service Users, Their Families and Community Leaders in the Moretele District, North West Province.* Centre for Health Policy, University of the Witwatersrand, South Africa.

Mokwena, K.E. & Ndlovu, J. (2021) Why do patients with mental disorders default treatment? A qualitative enquiry in rural Kwazulu-Natal. *South Africa Healthcare*, **9**(4), 461. https://doi.org/10.3390/ healthcare9040461 (accessed 21 on March 2023)

Monnapula-Mazabane P. & Petersen I. (2021) Mental health stigma experiences among caregivers and service users in South Africa: a qualitative investigation. *Current Psychology*, **42**, 9427–9439. https://doi.org/10.1007/s12144-021-02236-y (accessed on 21 March 2023)

Narayan J. & Reddy P.S. (2008) *Training for trainers (TOT) programmes on intellectual disability for CBR workers* http://www.dinf.ne.jp/doc/english/asia/resource/apdrj/vol19_2008/tot_intellectual_disability.html (accessed on 17 June 2012)

Ned L., Tiwari R., Buchanan H., Van Niekerk L., Sherry K. & Chikte U. (2020) Changing demographic trends among South African occupational therapists: 2002 to 2018. *Human Resources for Health*, **18**, 22.

Ndlovu, J.T. & Mokwena, K.E. (2023) Burden of care of family caregivers for people diagnosed with serious mental disorders in a rural health district in Kwa-Zulu-Natal, South Africa. *Healthcare*, **11**, 2686. https://doi.org/10.20944/preprints202308.0762.v1

Novak, M. & Guest, C. (1989) Caregiver Burden Inventory (CBI). *The Gerontologist*, **29(Cb I)**, 798–803.

Olagundoye, O. & Alugo, M. (2016) *Caregiving and the Family*, p. 13. Intech, London. https://doi.org/10.5772/intechopen.72627

PRIME (2014) *Psychosocial rehabilitation (PSR) support groups facilitator's guide.* PRIME University of Cape Town. https://webcms.uct.ac.za/sites/default/files/image_tool/images/446/Manuals/PRM015%20schizophrenia%20facilitators%20manual%202014%20FA%20PRINTERS.pdf (accessed on 29 March 2023)

RHAP, RuDASA, RuReSA, SAFMH and PACASA (2015) *The Rural Mental Health Campaign Report 2015.* https://www.ruresa.org.za/200347899763983f28e0d2b/rural-mental-health-campaign.html (accessed 13 October 2015)

Robertson L., Chiliza B., Janse van Rensburg A. & Talatala M. (2018) Chapter 11: Towards universal health coverage for people living with mental illness in South Africa. In: L.C. Rispel & A. Padarath (eds), *South African Health Review 2018*, pp. 1–2. Health Systems Trust, Durban.

Rosas-Santiago, F.J., Marván, M.L. & Lagunes-Córdoba, R. (2017) Adaptation of a scale to measure coping strategies in informal primary caregivers of psychiatric patients. *Journal of Psychiatric and Mental Health Nursing*, **24**, 563. https://doi.org/10.1111/jpm.12403

Rule S., Lorenzo T. & Wolmarens M. (2006) Chapter 20. Community-based rehabilitation: new challenges. In: B. Watermeyer, L. Swartz, T. Lorenzo, M. Schneider & M. Priestley (eds), *Disability and Social Change. A South African Agenda*, pp. 273–290. HSRC Press, Cape Town. https://www.afri-can.org/CBR%20Information/CBR%20New%20Challanges.pdf

Sathyanarayana Rao T.S., Asha M.R., Ramesh B.N. & Jagannatha Rao K.S. (2008) Understanding nutrition, depression and mental illnesses. *Indian Journal of Psychiatry*, **50(2)**, 77–82. http://www.ncbi.nlm.nih.gov/pmc/articles/PMC2738337/ (accessed on 12 July 2012)

Seedat S., Williams D.R., Herman A.A. *et al* (2009) Mental health service use among South Africans for mood, anxiety and substance use disorders. *South African Medical Journal*, **99(5)**, 346–352. http://www.scielo.org.za/pdf/samj/v99n5/a23v99n5.pdf (accessed on 18 June 2012)

Seshadri, K., Sivakumar, T. & Jagannathan, A. (2019) The family support movement and schizophrenia in India. *Current Psychiatry Reports*, **21(10)**, 95. https://doi.org/10.1007/s11920-019-1081-5

Shields-Zeeman L., Pathare S., Hipple W. B., Kapadia-Kundu N. & Joag K. (2017) Promoting wellbeing and improving access to mental health care

through community champions in rural India: the Atmiyata intervention approach. *International Journal of Mental Health Systems*, **11**, 6.

Sibeko G., Temmingh H., Mall S. *et al* (2017) Improving adherence in mental health service users with severe mental illness in South Africa: a pilot randomized controlled trial of a treatment partner and text message intervention vs. treatment as usual. *BMC Research Notes*, **10**, 584. https://doi.org/10.1186/s13104-017-2915-z

Silaule, O. & Casteleijn, D. (2021) Measuring change in activity participation of mental health care users attending an occupational therapy programme in rural South Africa. *South African Journal of Occupational Therapy*, **51(3)**, 63–73. http://dx.doi.org/10.17159/2310-3833/2021/vol51n3a8

Silaule, O., Nkosi, N.G. & Adams, F. (2023) Extent of caregiver burden among informal caregivers of persons with severe mental disorders in rural South Africa. *Rural and Remote Health*, **23(2)**, 7509. https://doi.org/10.22605/RRH7509

Sorsdahl, K., Slopen, N., Siefert, K., Seedat, S., Stein, D.J. & Williams, D.R. (2011) Household food insufficiency and mental health in South Africa. *Journal of Epidemiology and Community Health*, **65(5)**, 426–431. https://doi.org/10.1136/jech.2009.091462 (accessed on 27 March 2013)

Souza, A.L.R., Guimarães, R.A., De Araújo Vilela, D. *et al* (2017) Factors associated with the burden of family caregivers of patients with mental disorders: a cross-sectional study. *BMC Psychiatry*, **17(1)**, 353. https://doi.org/10.1186/s12888-017-1501-1

Sunkel C. (2017) A service user's perspective. *World Psychiatry*, **16**, 44–45. https://doi.org/10.1002/wps.20378 (accessed on 1 August 2023)

Swartz, M. & Bhattacharya, S. (2017) The limitations and future of violence risk assessment. *World Psychiatry*, **16(1)**, 25–26. https://doi.org/10.1002/wps.20394 (accessed on 1 August 2023)

Thomas, E., Cloete, K.J., Kidd, M. & Lategan, H. (2015) A decentralised model of psychiatric care: profile, length of stay and outcome of mental healthcare users admitted to a district-level public hospital in the Western Cape. *South African Journal of Psychiatry*, **21(1)**, 8. https://doi.org/10.7196/sajp.538 (accessed on 21 March 2023)

Tomita A. & Moodley Y. (2016) The revolving door of mental, neurological, and substance use disorders re-hospitalization in rural KwaZulu-Natal Province, South Africa. *African Health Sciences*, **16(3)**, 817–821. http://dx.doi.org/10.4314/ahs.v16i3.23

UN General Assembly (2015) *Transforming our world: the 2030 agenda for sustainable development 21 October 2015.* A/RES/70/1. https://www.refworld.org/docid/57b6e3e44.html (accessed on 31 August 2023)

Van Niekerk M., Dladla A., Gumbi N., Monareng L. & Thwala W. (2014) Perceptions of the traditional health practitioner's role in the management of mental health care users and occupation: a pilot study. *South African Journal of Occupational Therapy*, **44(1)**, 20–24.

Vergunst R. (2018) From global-to-local: rural mental health in South Africa. *Global Health Action*, **11**, 1. https://doi.org/10.1080/16549716.2017.1413916

Western Cape High Court (2010) *Western cape forum for intellectual disability v. Government of the Republic of South Africa and another case: 18678/2007 (11 November 2010).* https://wcfid.co.za/wp-content/uploads/2021/12/WCFID_Right-to-Education-_Court-Case-1.pdf (accessed on 23 March 2023)

World Health Organisation (2010a) *Community-based Rehabilitation: CBR Guidelines.* WHO Press, Geneva. https://apps.who.int/iris/bitstream/handle/10665/44405/9789241548052_introductory_eng.pdf?sequence=9&isAllowed=y (accessed on 16 February 2011)

World Health Organisation (2010b) *Community-based Rehabilitation: CBR Guidelines. Supplementary Booklet.* WHO Press, Geneva. https://apps.who.int/iris/bitstream/handle/10665/44405/9789241548052_supplement_eng.pdf?sequence=1&isAllowed=y (accessed on 16 February 2011)

World Health Organisation (2019) *Mental health QualityRights guidance and training tools.* https://www.who.int/publications/i/item/who-qualityrights-guidance-and-training-tools (accessed on 16 August 2023)

World Health Organisation (2020) *Mental Health Atlas 2020* https://www.who.int/publications-detail-redirect/9789240036703 (accessed on 16 August 2023)

World Health Organisation (2021) *Guidance on Community Mental Health Services. Promoting Person-centred and Rights-based Approaches.* WHO Press, Geneva.

World Health Organisation (2022) *Global report on health equity for persons with disabilities.* Geneva. Licence: CC BY-NC-SA 3.0 IGO. https://www.who.int/publications-detail-redirect/9789240063600 (accessed 2 December 2022)

World Health Organisation (2023) *Package of interventions for rehabilitation. Module 8. Mental health conditions.* Geneva. Licence: CC BY-NC-SA 3.0 IGO. https://www.who.int/publications/i/item/9789240071308 (accessed 31 August 2023)

Yerriah, J., Tomita, A. & Paruk, S. (2021) Surviving but not thriving: burden of care and quality of life for caregivers of patients with schizophrenia spectrum disorders and comorbid substance use in South Africa early intervention in psychiatry. *Early Intervention in Psychiatry*, **16**(2), 153–161. https://doi.org/10.1111/EIP.13141

Yesufu-Udechuku, A., Harrison, B., Mayo-Wilson, E. *et al* (2015) Interventions to improve the experience of caring for people with severe mental illness: systematic review and meta-analysis. *British Journal of Psychiatry*, **206**(4), 268–274. https://doi.org/10.1192/bjp.bp.114.147561

Yu Y., Li T., Xi S. *et al* (2020) Assessing a WeChat-Based Integrative Family Intervention (WIFI) for schizophrenia: protocol for a stepped-wedge cluster randomized trial. *JMIR Research Protocol*, **9**(8), e18538. https://doi.org/10.2196/18538

Zeng, Y., Zhou, Y. & Lin, J. (2017) Perceived burden and quality of life in Chinese caregivers of people with serious mental illness: a comparison cross-sectional survey. *Perspectives in Psychiatric Care*, **53**(3), 183–189. https://doi.org/10.1111/ppc.12151

KEY CBR DOCUMENTS

Coleridge, A. & Hartley, S. (2012) *CBR stories from Africa: what can they teach us?* University of East Anglia. http://www.afri-can.org/CBR%20Information/CBR%20Stories%20from%20Africa.pdf (accessed on 18 June 2012)

Food and Agriculture Organisation of the United Nations (2014) *A Vegetable Garden for All*, 5th edn. E-ISBN 978-92-5-108106-8 (PDF) (accessed 12 January 2021)

Heinicke-Motsch, K. (2010) *CBM CBR policy paper 2010.* Cristian Blinden Mission.

International Labour Organisation, United Nations Educational, Scientific and Cultural Organisation, and World Health Organisation (2004) *CBR: a strategy for rehabilitation, equalization of opportunities, poverty reduction and social inclusion of people with disabilities* (Joint Position Paper).

World Federation of Occupational Therapists (2004) *Position paper on CBR.* http://www.wfot.org/ResourceCentre/tabid/132/cid/16/Default.aspx (accessed on 16 February 2011)

World Health Organisation (1994) *Community-based Rehabilitation and Health Care Referral Services. A Guide for Programme Managers.* WHO Press, Geneva. (accessed on 10 June 2013)

World Health Organisation (2010a). *Community-based Rehabilitation: CBR Guidelines.* WHO Press, Geneva.

World Health Organisation (2010b). *Community-based Rehabilitation: CBR Guidelines. Supplementary Booklet.* WHO Press, Geneva.

World Health Organisation (2018) *Preventing Suicide: A Community Engagement Toolkit.* World Health Organization, Geneva. ISBN 978-92-4-151379-1.

READING TO UNDERSTAND THE REALITY OF MHCU IN LMIC

Malan, M. (2014, May 30) *The people told me they are coming to take me away tonight.* https://bhekisisa.org/article/2014-05-30-desperate-search-for-answers-to-schizophrenia-puzzle/ (accessed on 3 October 2022)

RHAP, RuDASA, RuReSA, SAFMH and PACASA (2015) *The rural mental health campaign report 2015.* https://www.ruresa.org.za/200347899763983f28e0d2b/rural-mental-health-campaign.html

The Model of Occupational Self-Efficacy

CHAPTER 12

A Contemporary Model to Return Individuals with Mild-to-Moderate Brain Injury to Work

Mogammad Shaheed Soeker

Occupational Therapy Department, University of the Western Cape, Cape Town, South Africa

KEY LEARNING POINTS

- The Model of Occupational Self Efficacy can be used in order to enhance the work skills of individuals diagnosed with a mild-to-moderate brain injury.

- Individuals who sustained a traumatic brain injury may require holistic intervention in order to address the functional limitations that they may experience post-injury.

- The Model of Occupational Self-Efficacy advocates for the use of a supported employment framework and ongoing support in order to facilitate the successful return to work of individuals who sustained a brain injury.

INTRODUCTION

Traumatic brain injury (TBI) is a burden to the global public health system. In countries such as the United States of America, 70 000–90 000 individuals experience resultant functional impairment that is long term in nature (Wehman et al. 2003). In South Africa, the TBI mortality is six times higher and individuals with TBI often have less access to health care resources (Soeker & Darries 2019). Internationally, there is a void in research related to brain injury rehabilitation, with research mainly couched in the medical model of disability (Soeker & Ganie 2019). The medical model often advocates that persons with disability require medical intervention or treatment in order to remedy them, with minimal focus on viewing the person with disability as a complete individual. Of significance is a focus on understanding how

the TBI affects the worker role of the individual with TBI. There is not a great focus on understanding the challenges individuals with TBI face when reintegrating to their communities. Having the individual with TBI involved in planning their own goals during rehabilitation is important as this helps enhance their motivation to engage in rehabilitation programmes (Seigert & Taylor 2004). Research has proved that the unemployment rate for persons with disability is as high as 88% often causing socio-economic challenges to these individuals (Soeker 2012). It could therefore be argued that there is a need to manage the individual with TBI's condition holistically and not just from a medical perspective. Current rehabilitation interventions do not clearly enable clinicians and clients to link what they have achieved in rehabilitation to what is needed when they resume their worker roles or return to their communities.

Crouch and Alers Occupational Therapy in Psychiatry and Mental Health, Sixth Edition.
Edited by Rosemary Crouch, Tania Buys, Enos Morankoana Ramano, Matty van Niekerk and Lisa Wegner.
© 2025 John Wiley & Sons Ltd. Published 2025 by John Wiley & Sons Ltd.

LITERATURE REVIEW

EPIDEMIOLOGY

A review of TBI reported the annual incidence of TBI injuries as being between 27 and 69 million globally (GBD 2019). The general description of a TBI is that it is an injury that occurs to the head and brain (Ahmed et al. 2017) that results in physical and psychosocial limitations. Such injuries could result in impaired physical, cognitive, emotional and behavioural functioning. Research conducted at a large South African teaching hospital in 2009 revealed that 82% of head trauma was experienced by young men (Webster et al. 2015). The treatment costs of this type of injuries are high and, as a result, many TBI survivors struggle to return to full-time employment (Hyder et al. 2007). The process followed after a TBI could be viewed as a process that is lifelong (Scholten et al. 2014). In South Africa, the prevalence of disability is estimated to be 5% of the population. This in turn contributes to the national burden on health services and further facilitates the diminished ability of individuals with TBI to return to work in South Africa (Webster et al. 2015).

RETURN TO WORK

A study conducted in South Africa indicated that 40% of individuals with TBI struggle to return to work in formal employment one to two years post-injury (Ptyushkin et al. 2010). However, internationally, between 50% and 100% of individuals with TBI engage with work two years post-injury (Cancelliere et al. 2014). Research also indicates that 70% of individuals who sustained a moderate brain injury and 20% of individuals who sustained a mild brain injury struggle to return to work (Vuadens et al. 2006). Ten percent of these individuals may get dismissed from their work and a further 2% are only employed for a brief period of time (Vuadens et al. 2006). The above therefore indicates that many individuals with TBI struggle to find and maintain employment.

ENABLERS THAT ASSIST THE WORKER ROLE OF INDIVIDUALS WITH BRAIN INJURY

In a study conducted by Dawson et al. (2007), the severity of the brain injury and the degree of psychosocial limitations were associated with the ability to transition to the worker role. The authors further indicated that when a rehabilitative programme addresses challenges such as pain, depression and coping, there are better outcomes related to return to work. According to Lefebvre et al. (2005), other facilitators include the early involvement of the family of the individual with TBI in the rehabilitation process, as the early involvement of the family greatly enhances the co-operation between the family and the rehabilitation team, thus enhancing the ability of the individual with TBI to return to work. Thus, rehabilitation in

the home environment may reduce the transport costs to rehabilitation centres and consequently reduce financial impact on brain injury survivors. Soeker and Pape (2019) concurred with the above authors, as they identified that financial challenges and travelling for services were major challenges that need to be addressed during rehabilitation. Including a client-centred approach was seen as a very important facilitator, in that it enables clients to become self-sufficient and take ownership of the rehabilitation process (Abbas & Soeker 2020).

BARRIERS TO THE WORKER ROLE OF INDIVIDUALS WITH BRAIN INJURY

Typical barriers or challenges that influence TBI survivors are education, severity of the injury, pre-injury income, marital status and social support among others (Waljas et al. 2014). Poor administration procedures and communication with the individual with TBI were seen as common health system-related challenges. Poor administration procedures are specifically related to the long waiting lists that affected the individual with TBI particularly when the patient/client is trying to be referred to an appropriate health professional in order to access rehabilitation programmes and apply for a disability grant. Additional barriers that are commonly reported include the side effects of medication that affect the individual's work performance (Soeker et al. 2012).

GENERAL PRINCIPLES WHEN WORKING WITH INDIVIDUALS WITH TBI

PRECAUTIONARY PRINCIPLES

It is important to remember that the occupational therapist should always take the following TBI characteristics into consideration:

- Changes in levels of consciousness.
- Memory disturbances.
- Confusion associated with deficits in orientation.
- Neurological signs, such as brain injury observable on neuroimaging, new onset or worsening of seizure disorder, visual field deficits and hemiparesis.

HANDLING PRINCIPLES

The following handling principles should be applied when managing individuals with TBI in rehabilitation programmes:

- Build a therapeutic relationship with the client based on trust. The client with TBI may look as if they do not require help or they may feel as if they do not have a problem. However, the occupational therapist may need to facilitate the process of improving the client's insight.

- Show the client empathy by listening to what they have to say.

- Give the client an opportunity to express their feelings.

- An indirect approach may be necessary especially for clients with TBI who may have low motivation. Do not force them to participate in the programme, rather casually involve them.

- When praise is given, it should be genuine praise given for their effort.

- It is important to create a positive rapport between the therapist, client, employer and the client's family.

REHABILITATION MODELS AND THE MODEL OF OCCUPATIONAL SELF-EFFICACY

Many rehabilitation models have been proposed to assist the integration of individuals with TBI and disability in general to transition to the workplace. Some of these rehabilitation models could be costly; however, the cost-benefits in terms of securing paid employment outweigh the cost of vocational intervention for the individual with TBI (Van Niekerk et al. 2011). Supported employment (SE) is an effective strategy to promote the inclusion of persons with disability in the workplace (Van Niekerk et al. 2011). Supported employment assumes that, when the right types and intensity of support are provided, the persons with disabilities can (and should) be integrated into competitive employment (Soeker 2012, 2016). The latter strategy can be associated with the Model of Occupational Self-Efficacy (MOOSE) that aims to enhance the skills of sick or injured individuals to become competent employees who have the skills to return to, and maintain, employment. In the following section, MOOSE as a contemporary work integrative strategy will be described in detail.

THE MODEL OF OCCUPATIONAL SELF-EFFICACY

The MOOSE, developed by Soeker (2012), focuses on enhancing an individual's or client's belief in succeeding in their worker role. The model consists of four stages, namely Stage 1: A strong belief in functional ability; Stage 2: Use of self; Stage 3: Creation of competency through occupational engagement and Stage 4: A capable individual. The aim of each stage of the model is to produce goal-orientated steps that motivate the client towards achieving, and maintaining, their independent worker role. Using this model as a guide for a vocational rehabilitation programme allows the therapist to engage in client-centred intervention, and it allows self-reflection and improved insight into the TBI survivor's work potential.

The model is spiral in structure which indicates that the stages of the model are interrelated (see Figure 12.1). The individual can fluctuate between the various stages of the

model due to their level of occupational self-efficacy. In between the stages of the model is the environment that will influence the individual's performance in the four stages of the model (Soeker 2014). The environment consists of various stakeholders such as the family, medical systems, work system and insurance system. Throughout the process of developing occupational self-efficacy, there are critical contacts that serve as enablers for the individual to complete rehabilitation (Soeker 2014). These contacts include the contact with the occupational therapist or therapist that facilitates the first stage of the model. Other forms of contacts may include the person themselves, family members, health care team, other brain-injured individuals who had completed rehabilitation and work colleagues (Soeker 2014).

Stage One: A Strong Belief in Functional Ability

In this stage of the model, the individual with brain injury would be seen as an outpatient in a hospital setting, a client that is receiving home-based therapy in the community, or a client that has already resumed employment (Soeker 2014). This stage of the model could consist of two- to four-hour sessions (the number of sessions will depend on the client's response to intervention). Their cognitive status should be classified on level VIII of the Ranchos Los Amigos cognitive scale. Level VIII is described as an individual who is alert and orientated, capable of recalling and integrating past and recent events and responsive to their culture (Tipton-Burton et al. 2006). During this stage, the client is expected to follow a process of introspection and reflection. This will enable them to develop new insight and cope with their environment. The process will enable the client to develop inner strength and a sense of efficacy (Soeker 2014). The six steps of the Gibbs' reflective cycle (1988) are used by the occupational therapist to facilitate introspection with the client.

Step One: Description of the Event or What Happened These steps are defined by the client providing a detailed description of the traumatic event that they experienced or the challenge that they are experiencing. This challenge may be related to feelings regarding the acceptance of the brain injury, barriers related to the roles and community participation (Soeker 2014).

Step Two: Feelings The occupational therapist will enable the client to explore their thinking related to the critical incident. The client will explore their feelings regarding the actual event or stressors. There may be an exploration pertaining to how the incident or outcome of the event made them feel (Soeker, 2014).

Step Three: Evaluation of the Circumstances In this step, the client is expected to make a judgement and evaluate the critical incident and to consider what was good or bad about the critical incident. During this step, the client will be requested to evaluate their circumstances or make a judgement about

Occupational self efficacy

An occupational therapy practice model
for the return of the brain injured individual to work

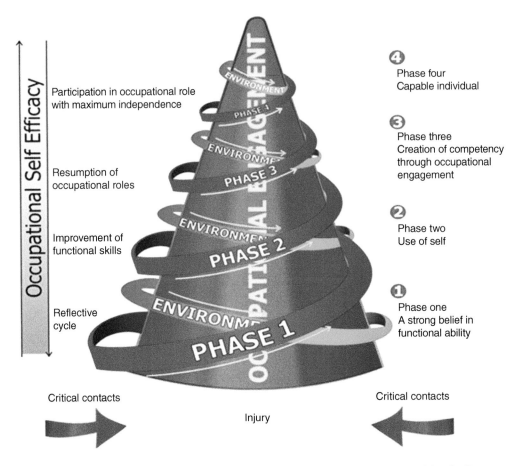

FIGURE 12.1   A graphical description of occupational self-efficacy: an occupational therapy practice model to facilitate returning to work after a brain injury.
Source: Soeker (2014) / IntechOpen /Public Domain.

their experience. For example, if the client was reflecting about a problem in carrying objects in the workplace, the occupational therapist may ask them to reflect on what is required to do the tasks (Soeker 2014).

Step Four: Situational Analysis of the Problem In this step, the occupational therapist will encourage the client to visualise the problem that they are experiencing. The occupational therapist will try to obtain clarity of the concern highlighted by the client by asking various questions. In this process, the client will gain insight into stakeholders such as doctors, family or employers who may be able to assist them with their specific problem. For example, the client may need to seek further training in order to improve their skills or adapt their work routine (Soeker 2014).

Step Five: Conclusion In this step, the client reflects on the challenge that they identified and analyses various solutions

to solve their problem. At this stage, the client has developed insight and would be able to select a solution for their problem. The client is encouraged to be as open and honest about their reflection as possible, as sometimes they may feel embarrassed about the functional limitations that they have; for example, the individual may struggle to focus while reading (Soeker 2014).

Step Six: Action Plan In this step, the client will be asked to reflect on their challenge and imagine that they need to actively develop an action plan. They need to then determine the best solution to the problem. During the above process, the client could be on their own or a family member could be present during the reflection and goal setting process. Stage one mainly focuses on introspection and reflection – once the client successfully masters the reflection process, then they will be able to move to the next stage of the model (Soeker 2014).

Stage Two: Use of Self

As the client has completed the process of introspection, they would have identified their own strength particularly in completing their various occupations. Stage two of the model could consist of two- to four-hour sessions (and the number of sessions will depend on the client's response to intervention). The occupational therapist will function in the capacity as a facilitator/case manager and will merely guide the client in overcoming the challenges that they are experiencing. The client may focus on improving their range of motion, muscle strength, tone, coordination and balance. They may also require continued cognitive behavioural therapy whereby the client's cognitive function is improved. A transdisciplinary approach will be followed as this approach will enable all stakeholders (health-related practitioner, employer and family) to be aware of the client's occupational goals. For example, should the client want to return to work, then all stakeholders should be made aware of this goal. This means that even if the physiotherapist focuses on mobility and the speech therapist focuses on communication skills, then the underlying goal of these health professionals would be to return the client to his worker role (Soeker 2014).

Stage Three: Creation of Competency Through Occupational Engagement

The establishment of competency is the main outcome of stage three of the model. There is a specific focus on the client's worker role. Should the client not have engaged with their worker role as yet, then they will gradually be introduced to this role. This stage of the model could consist of two- to four-hour sessions (the number of sessions will depend on the client's response to intervention). They now have the functional skills to resume their occupational roles. The occupational therapist will continue working as a facilitator/case manager. The utilisation of social relations by the client will be encouraged, and the client will initiate contact with various stakeholders (i.e. health professional, employer and family). The reflective process will be encouraged as a method to solve problems. For example, a client who had worked as a receptionist and may have a problem in coping with difficult customers may be assisted by the occupational therapist to brainstorm various coping strategies that they think could be used to solve the problem. The client will reflect on the reasons why they are struggling to cope with customers, for example, they may have an increase in anxiety when speaking to difficult customers (Soeker 2014).

During this stage, a work test placement will be arranged, the occupational therapist will then arrange that the client initiates training either in the workplace or the rehabilitation centre in order to practice the coping skill required during challenging work-related situations. The client performs the actual duties of his job under the guidance of the occupational therapist (in this stage, the occupational therapist could also be viewed as a job coach). The employer or line manager could be present to also observe the client's work performance. The occupational therapist could make use of a work schedule in order to observe the client's work hours, work behaviour and productivity. The latter work-related activity could take place over a period of time, for example, 1–3 days, until the client has mastered the skill. The reflection cycle could be used again in order to assist the client in identifying ways of making his job easier, for example, the use of assistive devices or adjustments to their work routine or work environment. The client can then choose to continue working in his current job or may decide to find an alternate job (Soeker 2014).

Stage Four: A Capable Individual

In this stage, the client will continue to reflect on their performance in the previous three stages of the model. They will specifically focus on how they could engage with work-related tasks. This stage of the model could consist of two- to four-hour sessions (the number of sessions will depend on the client's response to intervention). In this stage, the occupational therapist will have a discussion with the client specifically re-inforcing the work-related skills obtained in the previous stages with the hope of having the client internalise these skills and ultimately developing a strong sense of occupational self-efficacy. The outcome of this stage is that the client would be able to overcome the various challenges they experienced related to finding and maintaining employment. Due to the integrated and dynamic nature of the model, the client could revert back to one of the previous stages of the model based on their ability to overcome the barriers or challenges that they experienced. During this stage, the client would be involved in real work for a prolonged period of time. They will ultimately view themselves as capable individuals engaging in their worker role with maximum independence. The support and/or guidance given by the occupational therapist are gradually withdrawn.

GUIDELINES FOR THE UTILISATION OF THE MODEL OF OCCUPATIONAL SELF-EFFICACY

The occupational therapist can utilise the following guidelines to achieve each of the objectives below.

TO FACILITATE A STRONG PERSONAL BELIEF (SOEKER 2014)

- The occupational therapist should have knowledge of the individual's social, cultural and community context and related dynamics.

- The occupational therapist should have knowledge with regard to the medical management of the brain injury, workplace analysis and workplace ergonomics.

- The occupational therapist should be able to understand who the stakeholders are that interact with the client. The occupational therapist needs to understand how to facilitate the Gibbs' reflective cycle with the client.

TO ENCOURAGE THE CLIENT'S USE OF SELF (SOEKER 2014)

- The occupational therapist enables the client to engage in self-care tasks, as well as transport-related and vocational activities.

- The occupational therapist should have good communication skills, problem-solving skills, negotiation skills, empathy and be transparent. They need to role model the appropriate behaviour to the individual with brain injury.

- The occupational therapist would act in the capacity of a case manager and job coach. They will provide the client with choices with regard to rehabilitation and participation in work-related tasks.

- The occupational therapist will utilise a client-centred approach to the rehabilitation process.

TO ENHANCE COMPETENCY THROUGH OCCUPATIONAL ENGAGEMENT (SOEKER 2014)

- Client-centred practice allows the client to achieve competency in their various roles. This ultimately will improve life skills such as coping skills and assertiveness skills.

- The occupational therapist continues to act in the capacity as a case manager and/or job coach. The case manager and job coach will help the client to identify resources and the necessary stakeholder (health sector, family members etc.) that will assist with their worker role.

- The client should engage in work test placements either with their previous employer or in a simulated environment. This will enable the client to practice their skills in a real-life setting. Information obtained in this setting will enable the occupational therapist, employer and client to identify whether reasonable accommodation will be required.

TO DEVELOP A CAPABLE INDIVIDUAL (SOEKER 2014)

- The occupational therapist will encourage the client to focus on self-reflection in order to improve their performance in work-related tasks.

- Engagement in the role as a worker should be emphasised and good co-operation between the various stakeholders (client, employer and family) and the environment should be maintained.

- Ultimately, the client will be transformed into a capable person, who would be able to engage in their worker role with complete independence.

CASE STUDY 1

SD is a 40-year-old male who sustained a moderate brain injury after a driver lost control of their mini bus and drove into his car. SD is currently six months post TBI. He has a Grade 12 level of education and has been working as a storeman at a beverage factory. SD lives with his wife and three children in a low socio-economic area, his wife is unemployed and the family is dependent on his salary. As SD was injured in a motor vehicle accident, he qualified to have compensation from the South African Road Accident Fund. This compensation was +/− R15000 (equivalent to +/− U$550) per month.

Outcome: Individual is currently employed for eight months as a general assistant at a beverage factory.

NB: The stages of the MOOSE are applied to the case study.

Stage 1: A strong personal belief

- Ranchos Los Amigos scale VIII (Level of cognitive function)

- **Introspection**, Gibbs' (1998) reflective cycle – Initially, it was very difficult to get SD to trust the therapist as he was of the opinion that there was no problem with his functional ability post TBI. The therapist had to arrange intervention sessions with SD at his home as well as at the beverage factory where he was going to work. It was difficult to get SD to attend the sessions on his own initially as he did not feel competent in using transport and driving independently. The type of questions asked included: (i) Describe the incident, (ii) Practically, how has the incident changed your life/circumstances? (iii) Emotionally, do you think that your ability to do tasks is different when compared to your ability to do tasks before the accident?

- SD slowly responded to the questions and really had to introspect and accept what had happened to him and focus on improving his work skills. SD decided that he would want to work in the food retail industry. He initially wanted to return to his previous job but he indicated that he would struggle with the fast-paced nature of the work.

Stage 2: To encourage the client's therapeutic use of self

- *Introspection continued*: During stage two, the occupational therapist focused on work skills such as mathematical skills and reading skills. The client (SD) continued to experience endurance- and memory-related concerns due to TBI. The occupational therapist had to assess whether SD's memory concerns were going to affect his ability to initiate tasks such as stock taking and comprehension type of activities. At this stage, it was felt that no further rehabilitation would improve his memory-related challenges and that compensatory measures had to be used by the client. These compensatory measures included the use of memorisation/visualisation techniques, whereby SD had to remind himself about the tasks that he had to complete for the day. He had to visualise travelling routes, the structural barriers such as steps in the workplace, distances between restaurant tables, danger of certain equipment example shelves and containers as well as the distance of transportation pick-up points.

- The occupational therapist worked in the capacity as facilitator and **case manager** for continued **rehabilitation** (increased muscle strength and cognitive rehabilitation). The aim of this stage of the model was for the client to take responsibility for his own rehabilitation.

Stage 3: To enhance competency through occupational engagement

- Focus of this stage is on the occupational area of work. The main priority of the occupational therapist together with SD is on improving his life skills such as coping skills, decision-making skills, transport management and managing their finances. Furthermore, there was a focus on improving SDs' computer literacy by allowing him to draft his own CV and improve general work skills such as work habits (personal presentation), work endurance (ability to work an eight-hour work shift) and quality of work performed. The client is once again encouraged to self-reflect on previous goals such as to maintain employment in the beverage manufacturing industry. The occupational therapist and SD identified the job description of a general worker in a beverage factory. The occupational therapist conducted a job site analysis, whereby the physical environment, working hours, equipment used, social aspects of the job and workplace hazards were identified. The employer agreed with the occupational therapist by allowing SD to gradually return to work, that is, SD worked for four hours initially in order to determine how he will cope in the new work environment. Thereafter, a meeting was set up with the manager of the beverage factory, SD and his family and the occupational therapist. The occupational therapist focused on the number of hours that the client could work as well as their work duties. The occupational therapist also arranged a climate meeting with employees of the beverage factory in order to allow them to address any concerns that the co-workers may have in working with SD. The above process served as a climate meeting with co-workers in order to reduce any stigma that may exist with regard to working with individuals with TBI.

- The client was given the opportunity to role play different workplace situations that he deemed as problematic. The occupational therapist assisted with the provision of advice regarding the correct worker behaviours. The role plays ultimately enhance SD's life skills and work abilities. The modified work schedule provided the client with a view of how his work skills have improved (see Appendix). In this stage, the client worked a minimum of five hours per day that was gradually increased to eight hours per day. The client's work-related tasks were also increased – initially, he performed administration tasks; however, with time, physical type of work tasks were added. As the client's confidence increased so did his number of work hours and he was allowed to do night shift work as well. Furthermore, the supervision that was provided by the occupational therapist or job coach was decreased from weekly supervision to supervision on a monthly basis.

Stage 4: To develop a capable individual

- In this stage of the model, the client was encouraged to continue to self-reflect on the stages 1–3. This process allowed the client to gain confidence in his skills. The occupational therapist asked the client questions related to how their work ability and self-efficacy beliefs improved. SD indicated that he was able to independently use transport, he was able to work any shift in the beverage manufacturing factory where he worked. He could use novel problem-solving processes, that is, follow a step-by-step process to write down a problem, determine solutions to the problem and evaluate which solution is best suited to solve the problem. The supervision by the occupational therapist was further reduced from supervision once a month to supervision every second month either face to face to telephonically.

CASE STUDY 2

MD is a 19-year-old female who sustained a severe brain injury at the age of 17 due to her involvement in a sport-related accident. She has a Grade 12 level of education and was going to study at a local university. Due to the extent of her injuries, she decided not to continue her studies in order to recover and find employment. After participating in rehabilitation, namely, physiotherapy and occupational therapy, MD unsuccessfully tried to find work. MD struggled to find employment as she struggled with comprehension and numeracy skills. These skills are essential for work that required communication and clerical skills. MD was dependent on a disability grant of R2000, which is equivalent to U$120. MD reported that she had never worked before her injury but would occasionally assist her father with the delivery of flowers to customers as her father owned a florist's.

(continued)

CASE STUDY 2　　*(Continued)*

Outcome: MD is employed for 10 months at a local fast-food restaurant.

Stage 1: A strong personal belief

- Ranchos Los Amigos scale VIII (Level of cognitive function)

- **Introspection**, Gibbs' reflective cycle – MD indicated that she wanted to improve her work skills by enhancing her level of education. She was of the opinion that good paying jobs require a university degree. The results of an occupational therapy work assessment procedure revealed that she struggled with. The questions asked during this stage included: Describe the incident, (i) Practically, how has the incident changed your life/circumstances? (ii) Emotionally, do you think that your ability to do tasks is different when compared to your ability to do tasks before the accident?

- MD's response to the questions revealed that she wanted to find employment in the formal work sector. MD was particularly interested in doing SETA (Sector Education Training Authority) clerical programmes. The SETA programmes are government programmes that provide sponsored training to unemployed individuals. MD was provided with a monthly stipend of (R2000, equivalent to $120). The above sessions were initiated in the rehabilitation centre.

Stage 2: To encourage the client's therapeutic use of themselves

- Introspection continued: In this stage, MD was encouraged to continue with introspection. MD was given the information about the various short courses that would assist her. As part of the process of becoming autonomous, MD was requested to contact the skills provider about the course and was encouraged to ask questions about the course. She engaged in work preparatory tasks such as drafting her curriculum vitae, engaging with simulated clerical tasks (e.g. doing filing, basic office management type of tasks and inventory type of tasks). The simulated tasks that she was involved in focused on checking the quantity and quality of products on shelves as well as packing and unpacking shelves. The short course with the SETA programme offered by the government was successfully completed by MD over a 12-month period. Some of the questions asked to MD during this stage of the programme included: (i) How did you find the rehabilitation experience so far? (ii) What in your opinion was beneficial and not relevant about the experience? (iii) How do you think you could use what you were taught practically in a work experience or at home? (iv) Do you think you have improved as a worker?

Stage 3: To enhance competency through occupational engagement

- In this stage, the programme focuses on the individual's worker role and the occupational area of work. In this stage of the model, the occupational therapist emphasises the provision of a real work experience for MD in the formal labour market. A local insurance company indicated that they were willing to provide her with this work experience over a period of 6–12 months. The occupational therapist arranged a meeting between the employees and human resource professional of the company. The purpose of integrating MD into the workplace was explained and there was a discussion that focused on the fears that staff had in working with individuals who were diagnosed with a brain injury. This initial discussion with staff members was fruitful, in that the discussion improved insight of staff members regarding the strengths and limitations of individuals with brain injury.

Her work tasks included keeping the office filing in alphabetical order and ensuring that all invoices are filled in the correct files. She had to answer telephone queries and take minutes in some staff meetings. She also had to keep a schedule of the amount and type of office stationery that was received from suppliers as well as the amount of stationery that have been distributed to staff. The occupational therapist regularly contacted the line manager in order to monitor MD's work performance. Her work performance was measured according to the company's work performance chart. As she performed at the same level as her colleagues, this enhanced the confidence of MD as she could measure her own work standards to the standards required in the formal labour market (competitive employment). In terms of the work shifts, MD was required to work from 9 a.m. to 2 p.m. initially, thereafter her working hours were increased to work from 9 a.m. to 5 p.m. She was also required to work three days a week while she was training initially, thereafter her work week increased to five days per week. The client was provided with weekly supervision initially thereafter, the supervision was decreased to once monthly.

Stage 4: To develop a capable individual

- In this final stage of the model, the focus continues to be introspection and reflection on the previous stages of the model. MD could now reflect on the work skills that she gained and reflect on skills that she would like to obtain in the future. MD could now use transport on her own and successfully complete the SETA clerical course. She was able to work from 9 a.m. to 5 p.m., doing day shift work. She could solve work-related problems independently and used compensatory techniques such as the use of a cell phone to store important dates and a reflective diary to capture important work tasks that she needs to complete. The supervision by the occupational therapist was further reduced from supervision once a month to supervision every second month either face to face to telephonically. MD achieved her work-related goal, in that she could secure a one-year contract doing clerical work at a local property management company.

CONCLUSION

Research has proven that the MOOSE is a useful model to facilitate the reintegration of individuals with TBI to their worker role. The model advocates for client-centred practice and enables the occupational therapist to work as both a case manager and a job coach working with all stakeholders related to the individual who sustained a TBI. The treatment techniques used by occupational therapists included muscle strength training, cognitive retraining and life skill enhancement. The latter should be used in conjunction with the various stages of the model. In conclusion, the MOOSE enables the individual who sustained a TBI to overcome challenges related to engaging in work-related tasks and serves as a link between rehabilitation and the workplace. The model provides a good platform for the individual with TBI to engage in a supported process for developing occupational self-efficacy and meet work-related goals.

QUESTIONS

1. Describe the functional impairments that may affect the work skills of individuals who sustained a TBI.

2. Name three precautions and handling principles that must be taken into consideration when treating individuals who sustained a TBI.

3. What are the advantages of using supported employment as a work skills training model?

4. What are the four main stages of the MOOSE?

5. How can the MOOSE be implemented in practice?

WORK ABILITY SCREENING TOOL

Key:

1-Incapable   2-Weak

3-Below average   4-Average

5-Above average   6-Exceptional

WORK HABITS

Personal presentation	Remarks (if any)
Date	
Attendance	
Punctuality	
Self-discipline	
Helpfulness	
Attitude	

SOCIAL PRESENTATION

Date	Remarks
Ability to work with supervisors	
Ability to work with co-workers	
Need for strict limit setting	
Ability to handle criticism	
General social interaction with co-workers and supervisors in the unit	
Co-operation	
Ability to fulfil a supervisor role	

WORK COMPETENCY AND SKILLS

Date	Remarks
Ability to follow verbal instructions	
Demonstrated	
Written	
Illustrated	
Ability to follow and execute instructions 1–3 steps	
Ability to follow and execute instructions 1–6 steps	

INSTRUCTION RETENTION

Date	Remarks
Ability to listen	
Comprehension	
Interpretation	
Accurate execution of instructions with minimal or no prompts of the assessor	

TASK PLANNING AND EXECUTION

Date	Remarks
Orientation to work area	
Planning of work area in relation to structuring	
Efficiency	
Ergonomics	
Practical planning of the work task in relation to steps of activity	

TASK COMPLETION

Date	Remarks
Ability to start the task	
Tolerance to maintain task	
Ability to complete task	
Ability to retain task	
Ability to recognise errors	
Ability to correct errors	

SAFETY

Date	Remarks
Knowledge of equipment and tools needed for task	
Ability to handle tools and materials safely	
Knowledge of where to collect equipment	
Knowledge and implementation of storing equipment safely and clean after use	
Implementation of basic precautions of own safety in the area	
Awareness and implementation of safety precautions of tools	

WORK TOLERANCE

Date	Remarks
Physical endurance in extended sitting posture	
Physical endurance in prolonged sitting	
Physical endurance in repetitive mobilisation from station to station	
Psychological endurance (mood)	
Psychological endurance (ability to work under pressure)	

Ability to sustain work effort

Number of rest periods

Reasons for rests

Prompt return to work after rests

MOTIVATION

Date	Remarks
Intrinsic motivation	
Extrinsic motivation	
Derives satisfaction from being productive	

PERFORMANCE

Date	Remarks
Quality of repetitious tasks	
Assembly-line operations	
Packing-assembly-inspecting	
Physical/manual labour tasks	
Quantity produced	
Hours lapsed to reach above quantity	
Speed	

General comments (if any): _____

_____

_____

REFERENCES

Abbas, I. & Soeker, M.S. (2020) The model of occupational self efficacy, a model to enhance self-efficacy and identity in individuals diagnosed with schizophrenia. *South African Journal of Occupational Therapy,* **50**(**3**), 22–29.

Ahmed, S., Venigalla, H., Mekala, H.M., Dar, S., Hassan, M. & Ayub, S. (2017) Traumatic brain injury and neuropsychiatric complications. *Indian Journal of Psychology Medicine,* **39**(**2**), 114–121. https://doi .org/10.4103/0253-7176.203129

Cancelliere, C., Kristman, V.L., Cassidy, J., *et al* (2014) Systematic review of return to work after mild traumatic brain injury: results of the international collaboration on mild traumatic brain injury prognosis. *Archives of Physical Medical and Rehabilitation,* **95**(**3**), 201–209.

Dawson, D.R., Swartz, M.L, Wineoccure, G. & Struss, D.T. (2007) Return to work following traumatic brain injury: cognitive, psychological, physical, spiritual and environmental correlates. *Disability and Rehabilitation* **29**(**4**), 301–313.

GBD (2019) Traumatic brain injury and spinal cord injury collaborators. Global, regional, and national burden of traumatic brain injury and spinal cord injury, 1990-2016: a systematic analysis for the Global Burden of Disease Study 2016. *The Lancet Neurology,* **18**(**1**), 56–87.

Gibbs, G. (1998) *Learning by Doing: A Guide to Teaching and Learning.* Further Educational Unit, London.

Hyder, A.A., Wunderlich, C.A., Puvanachandra, P., Gururaj, G. & Kobusingye, O.C. (2007) The impact of traumatic brain injuries: a global perspective. *Neurorehabilitation,* **22**(**5**), 314–353.

Lefebvre, H., Pelchat, D., Swaine, B., Gelinas, I. & Levert, M.J. (2005) The experiences of individuals with a traumatic brain injury, families, physicians and health professionals regarding care provided throughout the continuum. *Brain Injury,* **19**(**58**), 55–97.

Ptyushkin, P., Vidmar, G., Burger, H. & Marincek, C.R.T. (2010) Use of the International Classification of Functioning, Disability and Health (ICF) in patients with traumatic brain injury. *Brain Injury,* **24**(**13–14**), 1519–1527.

Scholten, A.C., Haagsma, J.A., Panneman, M.J.M, van Beeck, E.F. & Polinder, S. (2014) Traumatic brain injury in the Netherlands: incidence, costs and disability-adjusted life years. *PLoSOne.* **9**(**10**), e110905. https://doi.org/10.1371/journal.pone.0110905

Seigert, R.J. & Taylor W.J. (2004) Theoretical aspects of goal setting and motivation in rehabilitation. *Disability and Rehabilitation,* **26**, 1–8.

Soeker M.S. (2012) The development of the model of occupational self efficacy. *Work,* **43**(**03**), 313–322.

Soeker, M.S. (2014) Returning individuals with mild to moderate brain injury back to work: a systematic client centered approach. In: T. Quinn & F. Sadaka (eds), *Traumatic Brain Injury,* pp. 373–394. In Tech Publishers, Croatia.

Soeker M.S. (2016) A pilot study on the operationalisation of the model of occupational self efficacy: a model for the reintegration of persons with brain injuries to their worker roles. *Work,* **53**, 523–534.

Soeker, M.S. & Ganie, Z. (2019) The experiences of employers and care givers of individuals returning to work through the use of the model of occupational self efficacy for returning brain injured individual to work. *Work,* **64**, 355–370.

Soeker, M.S. & Darries, Z. (2019) Challenges women with traumatic brain injury experience in their work environment after vocational rehabilitation. *Work,* **64**, 477–486.

Soeker, M.S. & Pape C. (2019) The use of the model of occupational self-efficacy for work retraining: a multiple case study. *Occupational Therapy International,* **2019**, 1–8 https://doi.org/10.1155/2019/3867816.

Soeker, M.S., Van Rensburg, V. & Travill, A. (2012) Are our rehabilitation programmes enabling our clients to return to work? Return to work perspectives of mild to moderate brain injured individuals in South Africa. *Work,* **43**(**02**), 171–182.

Tipton-Burton, M. McLaughlin, R. & Englander, J. (2006) Traumatic brain injury. In: H.M. Pendleton & W. Schultz- Krohn (eds), *Pedretti's Occupational Therapy: Practise Skills for Physical Dysfunction,* 6th edn, Elsevier Mosby, Philadelphia.

Van Niekerk, L., Coetzee, Z., Engelbrecht, M. *et al* (2011) Supported employment: recommendations for successful implementation in South Africa. *South African Journal of Occupational Therapy,* **41**(**3**), 85–90.

Vuadens, P., Arnold, P. & Bellmann, A. (2006) *Return to Work After a Traumatic Brain Injury.* Vocational Rehabilitation. Springer, Paris.

Waljas, M., Iverson, G., Lange, R. *et al* (2014) Return to work following mild traumatic brain injury. *Journal of Head Trauma Rehabilitation,* **29**(**5**), 443–450.

Webster, J., Taylor, A. & Balchin, R. (2015) Traumatic brain injury, the hidden pandemic: a focused response to family and patient experiences and needs. *South African Medical Journal,* **105**(**3**), 195–198

Wehman, P., Kregel, J., Keyser-Marcus, L. *et al* (2003) Supported employment for persons with traumatic brain injury: a preliminary investigation of long term follow-up cost and program–efficiency. *Archives of Physical Medicine and Rehabilitation,* **84**(**2**), 192–196.

Work and Mental Health – Facilitating and Sustaining Work Engagement

CHAPTER 13

Lyndsey Swart[1], Tania Buys[1] and Carol-lynn Andreitchenko[2]

[1]Occupational Therapy Department, School of Health Care Sciences, Faculty of Health Care Sciences, University of Pretoria, South Africa

[2]Ascent Rehabilitation, Canberra, Australia

KEY LEARNING POINTS

- The value and contribution of work to a person's health and well-being.

- Factors which contribute to mental health problems in the workplace.

- The effects of mental illness on a person's work performance.

- Barriers and facilitators to work engagement faced by people living with mental illness.

- Occupational therapy and the process of facilitating work engagement or re-engagement for people living with mental illness.

- Stay-at-work and return-to-work intervention strategies for people living with mental illness.

INTRODUCTION

This chapter shares the collective experiences of the authors in work rehabilitation with a specific emphasis on adults living with mental health challenges or mental illness. While attempting to use a universally relevant approach, the authors recognise that terminology and legislation may differ between countries. For the purposes of this chapter, we use the term 'vocational rehabilitation'.

Work is an essential part of life. Not only do we spend spend a large proportion of our waking hours engaged in work activities, but work is a means to earn a livelihood. It also provides us with a sense of personal identity and social contribution. Recent literature indicates that work improves health outcomes and increases the quality of life (Figueredo *et al.* 2020; Van Niekerk *et al.* 2020). However, the landscape of work is changing. According to The World Health Organization (WHO) Guidelines on Mental Health at Work (WHO 2022a), the way people work and the places in which they work are being redefined by numerous factors such as technological advancements, globalisation, demographic changes, climate change, socio-political developments and economic determinants. In particular, the COVID-19 pandemic disrupted employment settings and accelerated this pace of change. Some jobs are losing their relevance while new ones are emerging. For many workers, this ongoing barrage of unprecedented change has led to chronic levels of stress and anxiety, with negative consequences for mental health. A global increase in the prevalence of mental health disorders in the workplace is evident (Memish *et al.* 2017; Coduti *et al.* 2018; Thompson *et al.* 2021). The World Mental Health Report (WHO 2022b) estimates that 15% of working-age adults experienced a mental disorder in 2019, with 12 billion working days lost to depression and anxiety at a cost of US$ 1 trillion in lost productivity. These disturbing statistics raise two important issues: firstly, the right of persons with mental illness to perform remunerative employment and secondly, the need to manage mental health in the workplace.

THE RIGHT OF PERSONS WITH MENTAL ILLNESS TO ENGAGE IN REMUNERATIVE EMPLOYMENT

The right to work is recognised by several international human rights treaties and conventions (UDHR 1948; ILO 1958; ICESCR 1967). Additionally, legislation in many countries includes provisions for promoting the right to work and prohibiting discrimination against people with disabilities. Despite these protections, employment rates for persons with mental illness remain dismally low (Memish et al. 2017; Figueredo et al. 2020; Gühne et al. 2021). According to the WHO Mental Health Atlas 2020, individuals with mental illness worldwide are much less likely to be employed compared to those without mental illness (WHO, 2021; https://www.health.org.uk/publications/long-reads/unemployment-and-mental-health#:~:text=In%20January%202021%2C%2043%25%20of,were%20on%20furlough%20(34%25)). This issue is more pronounced in developing and low-income countries, where high unemployment rates impact the entire population (https://www.health.org.uk/publications/long-reads/unemployment-and-mental-health#:~:text=In%20January%202021%2C%2043%25%20of,were%20on%20furlough%20(34%25)).

Compelling evidence, however, indicates that people with mental illness can and should work. A growing body of research reveals that with appropriate interventions and support, most people with mental illness are able to function in various levels of competitive employment (Fukuura & Shigematsu 2021). Successful employment is associated with reduced symptoms, reduced hospital admissions, improved social skills, refined self-esteem, greater personal independence and improved quality of life (Drake & Wallach 2020; Fukuura & Shigematsu 2021; Gühne et al. 2021; Arena et al. 2022; Gühne et al. 2022). The importance of work for persons with mental illness is perhaps best encapsulated in the aphorism 'One does not get better in order to work but one works in order to get better'.

THE EFFECTS OF MENTAL ILLNESS ON WORK PERFORMANCE

Typical challenges associated with mental illness that may interfere with a person's ability to perform work safely and productively include difficulties with interpersonal relationships, the episodic and fluctuating nature of many mental disorders, medication side effects, emotional dysregulation,

cognitive dysfunction, low motivation and increased risk of substance abuse. These extent of these difficulties may vary greatly between individuals and are further influenced by social and environmental factors. In the following section, we examine each of these challenges.

Difficulties with Interpersonal Relationships

People with mental illness frequently face difficulties with interpersonal relationships in the workplace (King-Casas & Chiu 2012) for a variety of reasons, including:

* Stigma, discrimination and lack of understanding of mental illness by management, supervisors or co-workers can make it difficult for an individual to form and maintain adequate relationships at work (Hampson et al. 2020). This can lead to social isolation and exclusion as well as a reluctance to disclose their mental health status in order to receive assistance and reasonable accommodation.

* Symptoms of mental illness or side effects of psychotropic medication (Haime et al. 2021) can result in difficulties responding appropriately to social cues, leading to awkward or uncomfortable social interactions.

* High levels of depression, stress or anxiety can result in maladaptive behaviours such as avoidance, withdrawal or conflict (Sun et al. 2022), which may negatively affect the individual's ability to form and maintain healthy relationships.

* Interpersonal and behavioural problems can lead to strained relationships with colleagues and managers, challenges working in a team and difficulty dealing with conflict and feedback on work performance.

The Episodic and Fluctuating Nature of Mental Illness

Mental illness can present with periods of debilitating symptoms, or relapses, followed by periods of remission or improvement (Waghorn & Lloyd 2005). Relapses can vary in duration and intensity and can be triggered by a variety of factors such as stress, trauma, medication change or substance use. This can make it difficult to predict how an individual will respond over time, even with optimal treatment. A severe relapse can seriously impact the individual's ability to work. Work attendance, work performance and interpersonal communications are commonly disrupted. Relapses may also undermine the individual's self-confidence and motivation to work (van Niekerk 2009). It is thus imperative that the individual's mental health status and medication use be properly monitored by a qualified healthcare professional.

Medication Side Effects

The Anatomical Therapeutic Chemical Classification categorises psychotropic drugs into five classes (WHO 2023), namely anti-anxiety agents, antidepressants, antipsychotics, mood stabilisers and hypnotics. Each of these has its own specific uses, benefits and side effects including but not limited to fatigue, drowsiness, blurred vision, sleep disturbance, anxiety, nausea, weight gain, gastrointestinal problems, tremors and cognitive impairment. It is important that individuals with mental illness understand the interactions and possible side effects of their medications, as this may affect their performance and/or safety at work. Persons performing safety-sensitive occupations such as police officers, emergency responders, pilots, commercial drivers and construction workers need to be monitored with particular care.

Emotional Dysregulation

Emotional dysregulation is a common symptom of mental illness (Copeland *et al.* 2014). It refers to difficulties in managing and expressing emotions in ways that are socially and culturally appropriate. Persons with emotional dysregulation may experience intense emotional reactions, have difficulty controlling their emotions and may tend to react impulsively. In the workplace, emotional dysregulation may manifest as difficulty coping with stress, catastrophising, frequent mood swings, unpredictable behaviour and interpersonal conflict. It can also impact decision-making ability, leading to impulsive or irrational choices. A decline in an individual's ability to regulate their emotions may indicate the onset of a mental health relapse and should be referred for prompt medical assessment and support.

Cognitive Dysfunction

A recent study by Abramovitch *et al.* (2021) found that most types of mental disorders are associated with underperformance across various cognitive domains, including memory, attention, visuospatial function, processing speed and executive function (including task shifting, response inhibition, working memory, fluency and planning). People with mental health conditions thus commonly experience cognitive challenges which can affect their productivity and performance at work, particularly during times of stress or symptom relapse.

Low Motivation

Fluctuations in motivation are normal. However, when low motivation becomes pervasive or starts interfering with an individual's ability to perform their normal everyday activities, this can result in occupational dysfunction. Avolition is the term to describe a significant or severe lack of motivation or a pronounced inability to complete purposeful tasks. Avolition is a common symptom in several mental health disorders (Griffiths 2017) including bipolar disorder, depression, post-traumatic stress disorder, premenstrual dysphoric disorder, schizophrenia, traumatic brain injury and Alzheimer's disease. In the work setting, clinical avolition or low motivation is frequently misunderstood, and the individual may be labelled as lazy or as having a poor atti-

tude. It is thus important that any significant change in motivation is properly assessed and managed by mental health professionals. Occupational therapists are skilled in evaluating and intervening in motivation as it affects occupational performance. One of the occupational therapy models which provides guidelines is the Vona du Toit Model of Creative Ability (VdTMoCA) discussed in Chapter 1.

Increased Risk of Substance Abuse

Many individuals who develop substance use disorders are also diagnosed with mental illness, and vice versa (NIDA 2021). Common substances of abuse include alcohol, nicotine (cigarettes, chewing tobacco, snuff), prescription drugs (e.g. benzodiazepines, sedatives, codeine, sleeping tablets and some pain medications), cannabis, illegal drugs (e.g. cocaine, heroin, methamphetamine and LSD) and inhalants (e.g. hydrocarbons, solvents, gasoline, paints and thinners). Depending on the substance used, a variety of functional impairments may occur, including poor judgement, confusion, slowed reflexes, drowsiness, dizziness, inattentiveness, impaired concentration, impaired memory, slurred speech, loss of balance, agitation, anxiety, motor weakness, visual impairment and difficulty breathing. These impairments typically lead to low productivity, increased error rate, poor engagement in work tasks and excessive absenteeism and can have serious safety consequences in safety-sensitive occupations. Other work-related problems associated with substance abuse include drug dealing and drug use in the workplace as well as theft of controlled substances for abuse. Work-related factors that may aggravate substance abuse in the workplace include high job stress, low job satisfaction, low job agency, work-related fatigue, repetitive duties, isolation, long hours, irregular shifts, long periods of inactivity or boredom, lack of opportunity for promotion, inadequate supervision, poor job clarity and easy access to substances in the workplace.

While many countries have laws and regulations that support the accommodation of individuals with disabilities in the workforce, this right is not without limitations. In situations where absenteeism, poor work performance or behavioural issues create an unreasonable burden on the employer, employment legislation typically allows for disciplinary action and even dismissal. Prevention of symptoms, early intervention and effective management of sick leave are thus important considerations when managing employees with mental illness.

SOCIAL AND ENVIRONMENTAL BARRIERS TO EMPLOYMENT

Global data indicate that people with mental disabilities face disproportionate social and environmental barriers to employment when compared with the general population and even with those with other disabilities (Memish *et al.* 2017;

ILO 2022; Gühne *et al.* 2021). Ebuenyi *et al.* (2019) describe four main barriers to employment affecting people with mental illness, including social exclusion and stigma, work identity crisis, non-accommodative socio-political environment and socio-economic status.

Social Exclusion and Stigma

Social exclusion and stigma are major barriers to employment for people with mental illness (American Psychiatric Association 2020; Brouwers 2020; Nirmala *et al.* 2020). Misunderstandings about the nature and causes of mental illness, along with biases about the capabilities of people living with mental health impairment, often lead to reactions of fear, disdain and avoidance (Angermeyer *et al.* 2010). The American Psychiatric Association (2020) identifies three main types of stigma experienced by people with mental illness:

- Public stigma, which involves the negative or discriminatory attitudes that others have about mental illness.

- Self-stigma, which refers to the negative attitudes, including internalised shame, that people with mental illness harbour about their own condition.

- Institutional stigma, which is more systemic and involves policies of government and private organisations that intentionally or unintentionally limit opportunities for people with mental illness. Examples include lower funding for mental illness research or fewer mental health services relative to other healthcare interventions.

For the individual living with mental illness, all three types of stigma can contribute to the worsening of their condition and reduce the likelihood that they will seek treatment. This negative cycle becomes a formidable barrier to any form of employment. A 2020 systematic review by Figueredo *et al.* (2020) found that high psychosocial stress is positively linked to a greater risk of sickness absence, less job satisfaction and a deterioration in the quality of the work experience.

Work Identity Crisis

Related to, and perpetuating the barrier of social exclusion and stigma, is the prevalent perception that people with mental illness are not fit or able to work. This myth is propagated not only by society at large but also by some individuals with mental illness themselves, leading to self-doubt and low confidence in their ability to work. When an individual struggles to identify themselves in the worker role and those around them doubt their ability to work, the chances of them becoming gainfully employed are substantially reduced.

Non-accommodative Socio-political Environment

Workplace accommodation is positively associated with a reduction in symptoms and increased job tenure in persons with mental illness (Zafar *et al.* 2019). However, those with mental illness are less likely to receive workplace accommodation than individuals with other disabilities (Sevak & Khan 2017; Ebuenyi *et al.* 2019). Employers appear to be more willing to provide the physical and structural modifications typically required by persons with physical disabilities than the organisational modifications (Zafar *et al.* 2019) typically required by persons with mental health impairments. Examples of organisational modifications include flexible work hours, supportive supervision, the opportunity to work from home, and adapted communication methods. Ebuenyi *et al.* (2019) found that people with mental disabilities were unlikely to receive adequate accommodation across various social structures including education, health insurance and employment, leading to lower levels of education, inability to access adequate treatment and difficulty securing and retaining employment.

Socio-economic Status

The socio-economic status of persons with mental illness is a major determinant of their ability to prepare for and participate in meaningful employment (Ebuenyi *et al.* 2019), particularly in developing and low-income countries. Adequate management of symptoms depends upon access to appropriate healthcare, medication and an adequate diet. Those who can afford therapy and special support are also more likely to complete their education and occupational training. Access to insurance benefits which promote rehabilitation and return to work often determines which individuals can continue working. However, incapacity and disability insurance does not always promote employment. This typically occurs when disability benefits make no provision for rehabilitation or return to work, and it becomes easier for the individual to live off insurance funds than to take on the challenge of rehabilitation and return to work. It is thus essential that occupational therapists understand what social and insured benefits are available to their clients and how these might affect the individual's ability and motivation to participate in the work engagement process.

FACILITATORS OF EMPLOYMENT FOR PEOPLE WITH MENTAL ILLNESS

The literature identifies several factors that may facilitate job acquisition and retention in persons with mental illness. These include:

- Stability or reduced severity of mental illness symptoms (Ebuenyi *et al.* 2018; Rössler *et al.* 2019; Gühne *et al.* 2022).

- Improved self-awareness, self-esteem and self-acceptance (van Niekerk 2016; Ebuenyi *et al.* 2018).

- The provision of workplace accommodations (Sevak & Khan 2017; Ebuenyi *et al.* 2018; Zafar *et al.* 2019).

- Reduction in social barriers and stigma (Ebuenyi *et al.* 2018; Brouwers 2020).

- Alternative employment models such as sheltered employment, supported employment and cooperative income-generating groups (van Niekerk *et al.* 2015; Zhang *et al.* 2017; Ebuenyi *et al.* 2018).

THE ROLE OF THE OCCUPATIONAL THERAPIST IN FACILITATING WORK ENGAGEMENT

The foundational principles and practices of occupational therapy lend themselves well to the prevention and management of mental illness and the promotion of mental health and well-being in the workplace. Work is one of the nine categories of occupation described in the Occupational Therapy Practice Framework and is thus embedded both in occupational therapy and in occupational science (AOTA 2020). This field of practice has variously become known as vocational rehabilitation, occupational rehabilitation, work practice, work-related practice, vocational practice and others. Vocational rehabilitation, using the description provided by Escorpizo *et al.* (2011), which indicates a multi-professional, client-centred approach to 'optimise work participation' (Escorpizo *et al.* 2011, p. 130) is the term used in this chapter. With the growth of the field of vocational rehabilitation, occupational therapists have cultivated specialised skills, and many countries have formulated position statements to provide guidance for these practitioners. This has contributed to a perception of vocational rehabilitation as a distinct speciality within the profession. This has, somewhat lamentably, resulted in many occupational therapists hesitating to intervene in the client's occupation of work.

THE WORK ENGAGEMENT PROCESS

Returning to work, and continuing to work, for people living with mental health limitations is essential, yet fraught with numerous challenges inherent to the person, the type of work they perform, the environment in which the work is performed as well as the relationship between these three factors, the intersection of which indicates successful work performance. Occupational therapists have an undeniably valuable role to play in facilitating work engagement as well as in preventing mental health-related limitations and promoting employee well-being in the workplace. It is crucial for occupational therapists, particularly those who are new to the field, to understand that when working within a vocational rehabilitation framework, the core process remains the same as that of occupational therapy. This process involves evaluation, intervention and the attainment of specified outcomes (AOTA 2020). Work is one of the nine categories of occupation (AOTA 2020) and the connectivity to the other categories of occupation such as ADL, IADL, health management and leisure should not be neglected by occupational therapists working in vocational rehabilitation. Figure 13.1 illustrates a cyclical work engagement process model proposed by the authors. This model has five phases, namely

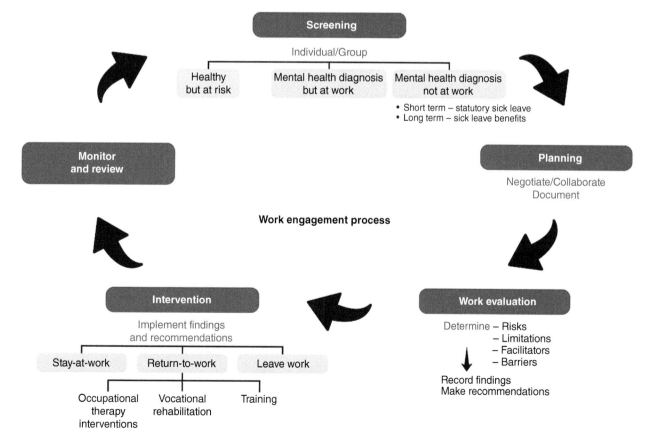

FIGURE 13.1   Work engagement process.

screening, planning, work evaluation, intervention and monitor/review. These phases, whilst generally following the process mentioned above, are often iterative and fluid, and the client may move backwards and forwards between them as the process and outcomes are adapted to meet the specific needs of the client and the external influences of the job and the work environment. The work engagement process model embraces promotive, preventive and rehabilitative interventions. Each phase is discussed in more detail.

An 'occupation-centred' (Fisher 2014, p. 163) and 'occupation-focussed' (Fisher 2014, p. 166) approach can be adopted when addressing clients' work. This requires the occupational therapist to place work at the centre of the evaluation and intervention process (Fisher 2014). Various theoretical frameworks can be applied to clients with mental illness during the work engagement process. These include the Model of Human Occupation (Kielhofner 2008), the Biopsychosocial Model (Ross 2007), the International Classification of Functioning, Disability and Health (WHO 2001), the Person–Environment–Occupation Model (Strong *et al.* 1999) and the VdTMoCA (Casteleijn & de Vos 2007). These models all describe the interaction and relationship between the person, the working environment (context) and the specific occupation (work). Occupational therapists may use these models individually or in combination.

PHASE 1: SCREENING

All referrals for vocational rehabilitation should be thoroughly screened before commencing with evaluation and intervention. The purpose of screening is to gain a clear understanding of the referral source's needs and expectations. Screening helps the occupational therapist determine the type of service required and whether they can provide it. Vague or ambiguous referrals should be immediately clarified with the referral source. Referral sources are varied and could include the treating healthcare provider, employer, employee wellness practitioner, occupational health practitioner, insurer, case manager or the client themselves. Clients for vocational rehabilitation services commonly fall into three categories: (i) those who are healthy but at risk, (ii) those with a mental health condition who are working and (iii) those with a mental health condition who are not working, either short term (statutory sick leave) or long term (insured benefits or unpaid leave). Table 13.1 summarises common risk factors for work engagement in each of these three categories using the Person-Environment-Occupation model (Law *et al.* 1996) as a thematic framework. Appropriate occupational therapy interventions are proposed.

The following screening process is suggested for vocational rehabilitation referrals, after carefully reviewing all received documentation:

1. Analyse the referral:
   - Who is the referral source and what is their interest in the requested intervention?

   - Is some form of authorisation necessary to perform the requested intervention? Some institutions may require prior approval or registration of service providers.
   - How are occupational therapy services remunerated? Are there any billing requirements or procedures that you need to be aware of?
   - What intervention has been requested? Do you have the necessary skills, experience and resources to provide the intervention?
   - To whom will you report? What should be included in the written report? Special consideration must be given to the client's privacy and confidentiality.
   - What background information is required to plan the intervention? This typically includes medical and health-care reports, job descriptions and work performance reviews, if available.
   - What types of informed consent should be obtained from the client?

2. Accept the referral in writing:
   - Provide the appointment details.
   - Provide any information the client will need to prepare for the appointment, for example, what to wear (this may include job-specific attire such as safety boots and jackets) and what to bring (medical documentation, medication, spectacles, curriculum vitae, job description, assistive devices etc.).
   - Request relevant background information. Ensure the client has provided written consent for their information to be released to the occupational therapist.

PHASE 2: PLANNING

Planning is an essential part of the work engagement process as this is when the occupational therapist, the client and other stakeholders (medical and non-medical) collectively develop a client-centred plan for the work engagement process. During this phase, it is important that the occupational therapist understands and respects the interests of all stakeholders, including the client, the employer and the funder, so that a workable and practical plan can be developed. Planning is incorporated into all phases of the work engagement process. It typically begins after screening, and is adapted throughout. Planning ordinarily involves the following four steps: evaluation, collaboration, goal setting and intervention, which may overlap with other phases in the work engagement process:

- *Evaluation*: A thorough evaluation of the client's ability to work is conducted.

- *Collaboration*: Communication and collaboration between all stakeholders are important to the success of any vocational rehabilitation initiative. The client's participation in this process is essential. Stakeholders could include the occupational health practitioner, the client's supervisor, a

Table 13.1 Risk factors associated with work engagement.

Client category	Risk factors to work engagement	Proposed interventions
Healthy but at risk	Worker characteristics that may increase the risk of mental health disorders include previous history of mental health disorder, family history of mental health disorder, poor social support, immigrants/foreigners (Di Napoli et al. 2021) and racial, ethnic (Wallace et al. 2016) and gender minorities (Lee et al. 2016). Job/environment risk factors typically include workplace stressors that increase the risk of mental health disorders (Harvey et al. 2017), include atypical work hours, high job demands combined with low job control, job insecurity, organisational change, effort-reward imbalance, workplace conflict/bullying and lack of occupational social support. Certain occupations may also increase the risk of mental health disorders (Wilhelm et al. 2004), such as those that expose the worker to danger and crisis and those that involve caring for others.	Examples of preventive interventions targeting at-risk employees include: • Education and awareness about mental health conditions. • Stress management techniques. • Monitoring of workplace culture, conflict and support mechanisms. • Work–life balance guidance and recommendations. • Supportive work environment: this could include peer support networks, manager training, improved communication channels and regular check-ins with employees. • Resilience building interventions. • Promotion of physical health and well-being. • Provision of mental health resources and benefits, for example, access to professional resources, mental health days, insurance cover for mental health interventions.
Mental health condition – working	Worker risk factors The nature and severity of client's mental health condition, inadequate treatment or poor compliance with treatment, inadequate personal support structure, poor self-confidence, social withdrawal/poor social skills, cognitive impairments, fear of disclosure of disability, reduced motivation and/or drive, substance abuse, unrealistic expectations, reduced mental and/or physical endurance, poor emotional regulation. Job/environment risk factors High levels of job stressors, including excessive workload, tight deadlines, lack of autonomy, lack of flexibility, atypical work hours, organisational change, effort-reward imbalance, workplace conflict/bullying/discrimination, lack of awareness and support by managers and/or colleagues, lack of access to mental health resources, inadequate or no accommodations, compromised privacy/confidentiality, inadequate workplace mental health/disability policies. Job insecurity or fear of job-loss	Both preventive and rehabilitative interventions may be appropriate, depending on the phase of mental illness. Examples of preventive interventions are listed under the 'healthy but at risk' column above. Examples of rehabilitative interventions include: • Case management. • Reasonable accommodation. • Employer education and awareness about mental health conditions. • Workplace monitoring (individual or group). • Upskilling or reskilling.
Mental health condition – not working	All risk factors for working clients with a mental health condition may apply with the following additional considerations: Worker risk factors Length of time out of the workplace (deterioration in work habits), insured disability benefits which form a disincentive to return to work, outdated work skills. Job/environment risk factors Changes in the workplace since last work engagement, high levels of job stressors, inadequate disability policy, job insecurity/redundant position.	Interventions will be primarily rehabilitative, but may include some preventative strategies: • Pre-vocational interventions. • Work hardening. • Work conditioning. • Graded return to work.

human resources representative, an insurance representative, a safety officer and others. The occupational therapist is well positioned to facilitate this process.

- *Goal setting*: Clear and measurable goals are established in collaboration with the client and appropriate stakeholders. These goals should be realistic, achievable and tailored to the client's specific circumstances while respecting the operational and safety requirements of the employer.

- *Intervention planning*: Based on the evaluation and established goals, a detailed plan is developed. This plan outlines the specific interventions, techniques, strategies, timelines, responsible persons and review processes that will be employed to achieve the work (re) engagement goals. It is a good idea to put this plan in writing and to share it with all stakeholders so that everyone is clear on the agreed process.

PHASE 3: EVALUATION

The terms evaluation and assessment are sometimes used interchangeably by occupational therapists, but evaluation is suggested here, as this is a broader term and encompasses a number of assessment strategies (AOTA 2020) to establish whether the worker or potential worker meets the requirements of a job. Irrespective of the term used, three components are evaluated. These are the person, the work or job or employment type that the client was or will be performing, and the work environment or context in which the job is performed. The evaluation of these three components should establish the strengths and limitations of the client, the barriers and enablers of the environment as well as the work tasks which the client can and cannot currently perform.

Work evaluation is on going process that occurs throughout vocational rehabilitation. Ongoing evaluation is particularly important for individuals with mental illness, as their work performance may fluctuate significantly due to the effects of medication, environmental influences or changes in their mental condition. An effective vocational rehabilitation programme should closely monitor these factors and identify any work-related issues that may trigger symptoms.

Preparation for the Work Evaluation

The referral instruction should clearly indicate the purpose and scope of the evaluation and/or further intervention. All accompanying documentation must be carefully reviewed, and its relevance to the process noted. As part of preparation, it is essential that the occupational therapist understands the mental health condition, its progress, prognostic indicators for employment and potential interventions. This will inform the evaluation process. For example, if a client presents with fatigue, it may be appropriate to schedule an early morning appointment to assess the client's strengths as well as a later appointment to determine the effects of fatigue on work performance. Evaluation over two or more sessions often

proves helpful where time and funding resources allow. This enables the occupational therapist to observe the client at different times and in different contexts. Should a client's documentation reveal anxiety, it may be appropriate to first build a therapeutic relationship with the client before the assessment commences to manage anxiety. In this regard, an informal interview prior to the work evaluation may be appropriate. Any accommodations made during the assessment must be carefully noted, as these will need to be carried through to the employment situation. In confirming the appointment, the client should be informed of what is expected of them and requested to bring their medication to the evaluation. This is important to confirm medication use and compliance. It is also useful to request the client to bring their curriculum vitae detailing their work history as well as their current job description and any available medical documentation.

Preparation is concluded by creating an evaluation plan that documents the assessment strategies and their sequence of administration. A typical evaluation plan might include the following assessment strategies: a semi-structured interview, self-report questionnaires, functional and cognitive tests, work simulation tasks and clinical observations throughout, preferably in both structured and unstructured settings. A customised but flexible approach allows the therapist to assess all aspects of interest while adapting to any unforeseen challenges that may occur. Whilst familiarising oneself with the referral documentation before the evaluation, occupational therapists need to guard against bias or stereotyping of the client. The occupational therapist must have a comprehensive understanding of various methods of assessments, sources of information, statistical interpretation of standardised tests as well as the value each method will contribute towards understanding the client's strengths and limitations in terms of work performance. Both qualitative (observations) and quantitative data (test results) are of value. A good evaluation plan needs to be both comprehensive and flexible within the requirements of referral requests. Evaluation provides a 'snapshot' of the client's function at a specific time, and it is, therefore, essential to plan well and to use multiple and focused assessment strategies in order to obtain a comprehensive view of the client's work abilities and occupational profile.

Selecting an Appropriate Venue for the Work Evaluation

This could be a clinic, hospital, rehabilitation setting, the client's home, or the client's place of employment. An important aspect to consider is the availability of appropriate assessment strategies and other requirements. Although the client's home may provide an important source of collateral information, the occupational therapist will miss out on appropriate work-context information, unless the client normally works from home. Evaluation conducted at the place of work, on the other hand, may draw unnecessary attention to the client but will allow the occupational therapist to directly observe the client's job and work environment demands and engage with relevant persons such as the employer, the line manager and co-workers. Irrespective of the location, the occupational therapist must ensure that the evaluation can take place without distractions and that client confidentiality is ensured. Family members and employer representatives should not be permitted to sit in on the evaluation unless formal approval and consent have been obtained from all parties.

Obtaining Informed Consent

Before commencing the vocational rehabilitation process, it is essential to obtain written informed consent in compliance with local legislation and ethical standards. The informed consent process entails a comprehensive discussion, during which the occupational therapist provides the client with all necessary information in a clear and understandable manner, addresses any questions or concerns and allows the client ample time to make a voluntary and informed decision regarding the proposed intervention.

Informed consent should encompass various aspects, including the purpose of the referral, a detailed description of the process, proposed treatments or procedures, potential risks and benefits, alternative options, expected outcomes, the names of individuals receiving feedback and/or reports as well as the client's rights throughout the process. It serves as confirmation that the client has made an informed and voluntary choice concerning the proposed assessments or interventions. When obtaining informed consent, consideration should be given to the client's level of understanding and functioning, and reliable interpreters should be employed when language barriers exist. It is also advisable to seek consent to collaborate with the client's treating healthcare practitioners, family members and other appropriate stakeholders during the informed consent process.

Initial Interview

During the initial interview, the occupational therapist collects all relevant information related to the purpose of the work evaluation and should be mindful that the initial interview is not primarily therapeutic in nature. Skilful interviewing, good communication skills and establishing rapport with the client are important. The use of an interview guide with a semi-structured format is recommended. The interview guide is developed before interviewing commences and typically includes the following information: the client's education/training background, psychiatric history, reported symptoms and functional impact, other relevant medical history, current treatment and compliance thereto, as well as current activity profile (including that of activities of daily living, sleep and leisure participation), support structures, coping mechanisms/styles, habits, functioning in the interpersonal and behavioural domains, motivation and readiness to change. The occupational therapist should consider the client's work history, whether this has been stable, whether the client is still

working, and if out of work, for how long. It is important to establish psychosocial job demands, the client's reported/perceived difficulties at work, perceived supports/facilitators, patterns of strained interpersonal relationships, history of performance management, poor time keeping etc. or if there has perhaps been a change in job demands at work, in reporting line etc. precipitating difficulty. Occupational therapists need to establish predisposing, precipitating and perpetuating factors. Therefore, the use of performance appraisals, work attendance records and collateral information are often useful. A mental status examination is recommended. Throughout the initial interview, the occupational therapist should be making qualitative observations regarding verbal and non-verbal behaviour, communication, insight, cognition and affect. In the author's experience, it works well to note observations on a timeline as this can also indicate endurance and changes in performance over time. The initial interview may include administration of self-report questionnaires on mood, emotional regulation, anxiety, sensory profile, stress tolerance, self-efficacy and resilience, to name but a few.

Physical Screening

Although the focus of the evaluation is on the functional effects of the mental illness, it is necessary to conduct a physical screening to determine any physical side effects of the medication as well as the presence of any physical and/or neurological disease. The client might also have been away from the work environment for an extended period, potentially resulting in physical deconditioning and reduced endurance, which could hinder their ability to sustain a full and productive workday. Additionally, the client may have gained weight, because of a limited activity profile or medication side effects. Measurement of heart rate, body mass index and the presence of oedema in the extremities should, therefore, be considered.

Testing

The occupational therapist should carefully select assessment strategies to adequately meet the purpose of the evaluation. Consideration should be given to the use of norm- and criterion-referenced tests (Laver-Fawcett 2007). Criterion-referenced tests, which measure the client's performance against the criteria of the work, are preferred over norm-referenced testing, which compares the performance of the test-taker to a norming group. Therefore, work samples such as the Valpar Component Work Samples and others, with well-defined time standards, based on predetermined criteria and not on specific population norms could be considered. Work simulation involves placing the person into a realistic work situation where environmental, interpersonal, task, tool and other such demands are simulated to represent the work situation as closely as possible. On-the-job evaluation involves assessing the client at the place of his/her potential or current employment. All the criteria of the job and the work environment are therefore taken into consideration. Performance standards and behavioural norms should be evaluated in accordance with the culture, standards and norms of the employer or industry. It is recommended that the occupational therapist involve company employees with appropriate expertise to assist in the evaluation, particularly when the job is of a skilled nature. On-the-job evaluation is usually appropriate towards the end of the vocational rehabilitation process when the client displays a high level of work readiness.

The client's presentation and the psychosocial demands of the job will affect the use of assessment strategies. These could encompass cognition, including executive function, work samples, work simulation/performance-based assessments, for example, a manager putting together a mock presentation of year-end sales results to present at a high-level meeting, an admin worker populating a spreadsheet to required speed and competency levels whilst answering the phone as she would normally do at work; a sales representative cold calling clients as well as role plays of potentially provocative situations to evaluate interpersonal and relational skills. The testing environment should simulate the work environment as accurately as possible, for example, if a client works in an open plan noisy environment, this needs to be included in aspects of testing. Clinical observations of the client's behaviour and task engagement throughout testing are a critical part of the work evaluation.

Obtaining Collateral Information

Obtaining collateral information from relevant people in the client's life is an essential aspect of the vocational assessment process as this will contribute towards understanding the client's background contexts, strengths, limitations and motivations. Understanding the client's functioning prior to and after the development of a mental illness can give an indication of a possible prognosis. Information from a spouse or partner can indicate the client's functioning in the home environment as well as their daily activity profile. Information provided by the employer can indicate problems with work performance such as reduced productivity levels, absenteeism, ability to work in a team, ability to handle conflict and criticism, as well as how the employer has managed these problems in the past. Early contact with the employer can foster early collaboration required for return-to-work planning as well as highlight potential barriers. Collateral information from the client's attending mental health practitioners is important to supplement information gained, assist with treatment formulation and foster interdisciplinary collaboration and common treatment goals. Collateral information must be obtained with the consent of the client. While both written and verbal forms of consent are often acceptable, written consent provides a clear and tangible record of the patient's agreement to a specific intervention, which can be critical in legal and ethical situations. It is important that the occupational therapist notes the date, time and content of any verbal agreements with the client.

Evaluation of the Workplace: Job Analysis and Work Visit

Conducting a workplace visit, meeting with people in the workplace and performing a job analysis of the client's current or potential work is important both during the vocational assessment and as part of placement or returning to work. Understanding work-related factors such as environmental factors, interpersonal relationships, work stressors, the pace of work and potential psychosocial hazards and risk factors, for example, lack of role clarity, low job control and poor workplace relationships, are important in formulating an intervention plan with the focus on work participation. It is also important to establish whether specific policies and procedures for employees with mental health conditions are in place and what these encompass and to get a sense of the workplace culture, and level of psychological safety. Visiting the workplace further facilitates an understanding of potential reasonable accommodation and realignment positions. Obtaining company job descriptions is often useful.

Analysis, Interpretation and Planning

The occupational therapist consolidates, critically reviews and triangulates. All the information gathered during the evaluation to inform the intervention approach. This involves applying clinical reasoning to understand the client's strengths and limitations and the way forward in terms of facilitating optimum work engagement. The purpose of the evaluation must be answered with a consolidated report that clearly and succinctly communicates the results of the work evaluation with a clear and realistic plan of action based on the client assessment and collaboration with all relevant stakeholders.

PHASE 4: INTERVENTION

Intervention strategies for engaging with work – whether it involves getting, maintaining, returning to, or leaving a job due to mental illness – are shaped by various factors. These include the individual's health history and factors that predispose, precipitate, or perpetuate illness; comorbid conditions; and the functional impact of their mental health issues. Additional influences include the individual's recovery stage, their unique biopsychosocial context including both barriers and supports, their educational and employment backgrounds, resource availability and accessibility, employment status, the nature of their job and work environment (if applicable), their personal goals, and the outcome of their work evaluation.

Given the well-documented rise in mental health disorders and the significant direct and indirect costs associated with these conditions, occupational therapists must take a proactive role. As part of a multisectorial, multi-stakeholder team, they need to advocate for integrated and comprehensive intervention strategies. These strategies should focus on pre-vention, actively promote and protect mental wellbeing in the workplace, and ensure early identification of issues. Coupled with targeted interventions, these efforts are crucial to foster-ing optimal mental health and promoting job retention. Healthy but struggling at-risk employees can be identified early through proactive absenteeism and presenteeism management. They can be equipped with skills to potentially combat a disability trajectory, develop a more disruptive health condition/conditions, promote and foster recovery and prevent undue work absence. In addition, critical life events, for example, the loss of a loved one, being diagnosed with a chronic medical condition, financial losses etc., could be flagged for proactive mental wellness support. Employees living with mental health conditions who have disclosed to their employer could be assisted with putting strategies in place that timeously identify relapse symptoms for early management thereof, including access to additional support in times of change or crises.

Ideally, for optimal impact occupational therapists in vocational rehabilitation need to be dual-focused, namely strategic-organisational, coupled with operational-employee interventions. Occupational therapists are ideally positioned to understand the complexities and multifactorial influences on workers given their holistic biopsychosocial approach and their grounding in the person, environment and occupa-tion model.

Strategically and organizationally, occupational thera-pists can contribute to the development of occupational health and safety-integrated, work-specific mental health policies and procedures. These include identifying and mitigating psy-chosocial risk factors related to work, environment, and occu-pation, fostering psychologically healthy workplaces, training managers to recognise and support workers with mental health conditions, and educating workers to increase aware-ness of stigmatising attitudes and improve health literacy. They can facilitate team resilience, ensure resources are read-ily available and accessible, and advocate for comprehensive management plans. Such plans should encompass early identification and support for remaining at work to prevent premature work cessation while receiving early intervention (Howell *et al.* 2022). Occupational therapists should also facil-itate a timely return to work, if necessary, as research indi-cates that prolonged absence from work can have detrimental effects on multiple levels. Should work absence be indicated, ideally, this should be coupled with vocational rehabilitation, a return-to-work coordinator and a return-to-work plan craft-ed at the outset. A disability leave plan is noted as one of the key best practice components (Dewa *et al.* 2016). Occupa-tional therapists can champion reasonable workplace accommodations/modifications and in-work support. Pol-icies need to include post-return-to-work support to foster retention, recovery, career progression and well-being.

Tailored individual–employee interventions are best determined where possible in an interdisciplinary team

setting with multi-stakeholder collaboration and where feasi-ble offered in the workplace. Ideally, the occupational thera-pist works collaboratively with involved stakeholders which could comprise the employee's mental health practitioners, employee wellness, occupational health and safety, as well as management/human resource practitioners towards common goals. This collaborative approach has its origin in the evalua-tion stage and ensures that all role players are aligned. The employee is regarded as a critical stakeholder and a person-led approach to intervention is supported.

Individual interventions could include those provided in Table 13.2.

Interventions for clients with mental illness who are transitioning gradually into retirement due to normal ageing or due to their mental illness should also be considered. This aspect of vocational rehabilitation is frequently overlooked and can exacerbate the impact of mental illness. Occupational therapists can play a crucial role in facilitating the development of new occupations, lifestyle modifications, adjustments in living accommodations, stress management and strengthen-ing of family dynamics.

Vocational Case Management

A service delivery approach utilised in vocational rehabilita-tion, for stay-at and return-to-work, is that of vocational case management defined by Ross as 'counselling and encourage-ment, referral to services, coordination of service provision, and support to and facilitation into work' (Ross 2007, p. 201). This encompasses a focus on early intervention, an individu-alised strategically planned/tailor-made approach for the employee, sourcing and referral services, coordination of all treatment; liaison with all members of the interdisciplinary team and all stakeholders including the line manager/human resource practitioners, managing expectations of all stake-holders, supporting both the employee and the employer, mitigating risks and can include recommendations for and crafting of a graded return to work plan in collaboration with all stakeholders. Results of a systematic review showed strong evidence of reduced work absence duration and higher return-to-work rates with face-to-face contact with a return-to-work coordinator (Dol *et al.* 2021).

Digital Health/Technologies

The COVID-19 pandemic necessitated a rapid pivot, acceleration of technology use, and reimagining the way we delivered traditional vocational rehabilitation in mental health from the in-person, to telehealth and hybrid/blended service delivery models. According to the World Federation of Occupational Therapists (WFOT), 'Telehealth is the use of information and communication technologies to deliver health-related services when the provider and client are in dif-ferent physical locations' (WFOT 2021, p. 1). Video conferenc-ing, telephonic engagement, remote monitoring and the use of digital apps are examples of synchronous (real-time)

Table 13.2 Individual interventions.

Interventions: stay at work

- Determining which specific barriers/stressors/triggers for an individual (individual and work-organisational level, e.g. high work volumes, time sensitive deliverables and poorly defined outputs) are modifiable and non-modifiable, and collaboratively determining strategies to address them.

- Empowering the employee with supportive self-management strategies through psychoeducation.

- Sensitisation and awareness training, for example, equipping a supervisor with the skills to recognise early warning signs of a relapse; the signs of a panic attack and how to respond appropriately etc.

- Facilitating effective communication strategies for the employee's manager/supervisor.

- Evidence-based skills/strategy-based interventions such as mindfulness, resilience-facilitation, sleep hygiene, practical stress and anxiety management, time management, work–life balance, facilitation of a more engaged-varied-constructive activity profile, problem-solving skills, facilitation/strengthening of more effective adaptive coping strategies, distress tolerance, emotional regulation, interpersonal effectiveness including assertiveness, conflict resolution and dealing with criticism. These can be offered individually or in group settings. Intervention should include practical application in life and at work to facilitate efficacy. Role play can be utilised, for example, dealing with a manager with whom the employee has a strained relationship.

- Facilitation of self-efficacy.

- Cognitive rehabilitation.

- Job coaching.

- Recommendations for upskilling, for example, an employee with a promotion that includes people management might benefit from upskilling and attending in-house training.

- Facilitating discussions around poor job–person fit/match (e.g. an employee who has been promoted without the required skill set) and person environment occupation fit (e.g. facilitating an employee's insight and understanding around his/her sensory profile to identify environmental needs and triggers) and practical solutions/strategies to self-regulate/manage this through for, for example, environmental changes/sensory ergonomics – relocating their workstation away from high-traffic areas; providing natural lighting, decluttering a desk/desktop background etc.

- Should co-morbid health conditions be present their functional impact would need to be addressed.

- Facilitation of/referral to community support structures.

- Lifestyle management.

- Addressing disclosure and requests for reasonable accommodations/modifications or adjustments/adaptations. Numerous resources are available to assist employees and occupational therapists with tailor-made reasonable workplace accommodations and disability employment issues such as The Job Accommodation Network (JAN) (JAN 2023) and Workplace Strategies for Mental Health (Life 2023) offer resources and tools for workplace mental health and psychological safety. Workplace accommodation can be temporary or permanent. Examples of accommodations include:
    - Scheduling – flexible work arrangements, flexible scheduling, completion of critical tasks with high risk at specific times when the employee's mental alertness is best, modified break schedules, use of a task checklist/to-do list and/or use of planning/scheduling software; regular reminders of, for example, upcoming deadlines; time off work to attend with healthcare practitioners etc.
    - Environment – designated safe work space for an individual to retreat to during a panic attack, remote work etc.
    - Job description – removal of marginal/non-essential functions etc.
    - Supervisory methods – weekly touch bases with line manager or supervisor to discuss daily/weekly tasks and progress with goal orientated management methods etc.
    - Communication – outlining clear and measurable expectations for respect in the workplace for all employees; provision of all instructions and assignments in writing with clear, specific and measurable expectations for all tasks etc.

Interventions: return to work

In addition to the strategies outlined above this could include:

- Facilitation of maintained contact between the employer and employee as research has highlighted this as a critical factor.

- Assisting with the practical/logistical aspects of return to work, for example, organising child care should they have taken on the role since being off work.

- Collaborative crafting of a return-to-work plan with clear responsibilities of all role players.

- They might require a period of work preparation/pre-vocational skills training which could include facilitation of an activity profile more compatible with work resumption including regular morning waking routines to promote conditioning. Work tasks from their jobs can be utilised for cognitive hardening.

Table 13.2 (*Continued*)

- The period of work preparation can be dovetailed with a graded return to work (if indicated) which could include gradual increase of work hours, exposure to work tasks – situations, volume/load etc. concurrent to supportive Occupational Therapy to allow real-time problem-solving of work-related difficulties (as they arise). The graded return to work can facilitate work hardening in situ/in vivo and to allow for opportunity to implement and practice skills taught in therapy, in the workplace, to promote work self-efficacy/self-confidence with gradual weaning of support. This process needs to be time limited.

- Longer term support/follow-up might be indicated to sustain/retain employment. This could include attendance of groups which could be peer led by individuals with lived experience.

- Ensuring that a relapse plan is in place.

- Empowering the employee with supportive self-management strategies and facilitating access to mental health resources to sustain employment and promote career progression.

Interventions: get-to-work/job seeker

- Assistance to compile a curriculum vitae.

- Advocacy around applicable disability legislation.

- Advocacy around disclosure of disability and requesting work accommodations/modifications.

- Interview role plays to assist with guidance in dealing with 'difficult' issues, such as gaps in their employment history due to hospitalisation and psychiatric treatment, as well as disclosing their illness and requesting reasonable accommodations.

- Referral for job-seeking support and where indicated, working collaboratively with occupational therapists with supported employment experience.

- Where applicable, use of volunteer work for pre-vocational skills facilitation.

- Self-employment – entrepreneurial ventures.

telehealth, with video logs, photographs and emails examples of asynchronous telehealth (offline/store and forward transmission of data). Telehealth can encompass evaluation, intervention, consulting, supervision and remote monitoring (Dahl-Popolizio *et al.* 2020). This ensured service and care continuity more notably at the height of the pandemic when stringent lockdown measures were in place. Anecdotally perceived benefits/value add of Telehealth with specific reference to video conferencing include cost/time/travel savings, greater flexibility, increased accessibility, increased convenience and comfort, value add/richness of information (e.g. employee able to log on from work or home), continuity of care and enhanced professional collaboration (easier for all members of the team to schedule an online meeting in their diaries; easier to engage with managers, supervisors etc.).

Research furthermore supports efficacy with patients providing positive feedback and high satisfaction levels, and occupational therapists experiencing it as a satisfactory and effective service delivery model (Dahl-Popolizio *et al.* 2020), with a similar therapeutic relationship between online therapy and face-to-face therapies documented (Henson *et al.* 2019).

Anecdotally some challenges identified at the outset included technical issues (e.g. availability of/access to resources, tech savviness of both the therapist and clients etc.), availability of resources, for example, online assessments and treatments and an inability to replicate certain assessments and treatment online. Rapid innovation has however led to numerous online assessments and treatment modalities becoming available. In addition, challenges with establishing/maintaining rapport, lack of personal contact, client engagement, clinical observations, richness of information, gauging body language

and subtle nonverbal cues, containment and language diversity were identified.

Post-pandemic telehealth and hybrid/blended approaches remain valuable service delivery models for appropriately selected clients.

A plethora of mobile mental health apps/digital tools/technologies are commercially available and can be utilised to augment, as an 'add-in' to treatment. The efficacy of apps are enhanced when used in combination with traditional face-to-face interventions (Torous *et al.* 2020). Functionality is broad and can range from novelty or single intervention apps (e.g. deep breathing) to diagnostic and multiple therapeutic treatments. The National Institute of Mental Health groups mental health apps into six categories according to functionality viz. self-management, cognition improvement, skills training, social support, symptom tracking and passive data collection (Chandrashekar 2018). These apps can be used in vocational rehabilitation to assist with aspects such as time management, organisation, prioritising and planning, for example, calendars and checklists etc. The advantages of incorporating apps with traditional service offerings are multiple including increased accessibility, reach and engagement outside of/and in between the in-person sessions or following discharge, the introduction of novelty and alignment with digitalisation trends as well as richness of information gathering. Anonymity has also been cited as an advantage. App selection is individualised and informed by amongst others, diagnosis/diagnoses (e.g. an employee suffering anxiety with comorbid persistent pain would benefit from a transdiagnostic app), the therapeutic goal as well as our clients' needs and preferences. App selection should be guided further by information pertaining to safety, privacy and data security, proven effectiveness, efficacy, quality and published research in terms of evidence, the latter is more onerous for diagnostic and multiple therapeutic treatment apps. There are resources available to assist with this, for example, The American Psychiatric Associations app evaluation framework, which includes five hierarchical levels for consideration viz. accessibility and background, privacy and security, clinical foundation, engagement style and therapeutic goal (Lagan *et al.* 2021), with numerous government bodies/organisations publishing guidelines for digital health technology safety and evaluation.

In the area of vocational rehabilitation, virtual reality can also be leveraged as a therapeutic tool by creating immersive and interactive environments for practising of amongst others social skills strategies, for example, job interview scenarios, dealing with criticism, conflict handling etc.

PHASE 5: MONITOR AND REVIEW

Monitoring and reviewing is an essential component of ensuring quality of care, yet guidelines for occupational therapists are often lacking (Robinson & Botha 2013). Ensuring and monitoring the quality of care especially in mental health service delivery poses 'unique challenges' (Kilbourne *et al.* 2018, p. 32) as a result of a number of factors including those related to the condition itself as well as the stigma associated with mental health (Kilbourne *et al.* 2018). The purpose of implementing monitoring and reviewing during the work engagement process determines whether the purpose of the referral has been achieved, planned outcomes have been reached and recommendations are implemented by the relevant stakeholders. In essence, the occupational therapist needs to follow up with the client – the actual patient, the employer as well as a referral agent to establish whether there are problems and to

rapidly respond and problem-solve where appropriate. This should be done in a flexible, yet scheduled manner considering the needs of the client and the context. Standardised tools can be used (Robertson 2021) including questionnaires, interviews, structured observations, visits and self-assessment (Lukersmith *et al.* 2013; Robertson 2021). Gathering standardised data will contribute towards evidence-based practice, as gaps and strengths in the work engagement process are identified. When commencing the work engagement process, this process should be clarified with all stakeholders with a plan of how and when monitoring and review will be conducted.

Once outcomes have been achieved, the occupational therapist must close the case and communicate this to both the client and other stakeholders.

CONCLUSION

Practising in work and vocational rehabilitation offers an exciting and rewarding field of practice for occupational therapists in the field of psychiatry and mental health. The aim of vocational rehabilitation is to optimally (re)integrate the individual with a disability into society and, wherever possible, into remunerative employment. Because vocational rehabilitation spans the corporate/industrial sector as well as the medical/rehabilitative sector, occupational therapists can work with a wide variety of stakeholders and professions. To do this successfully, they need to acquire new skills and expertise in vocational rehabilitation. The challenge for many schools of occupational therapy is to develop appropriate undergraduate and postgraduate training programmes that empower their graduates to move out of the clinics and into the workplace. After all, it is in the workplace and in society that true integration of people with mental disabilities can really occur.

CASE STUDY

Mark, a single 35-year-old senior accountant, was referred for a work evaluation by a psychiatrist who had recently diagnosed him with depression and anxiety. Medical management at the time of referral included pharmacotherapy to which he noted good adherence. Mark had been booked off work for a month prior to the evaluation. Mark had self-disclosed his diagnosis to his HR manager.

Mark arrived late for his evaluation and appeared somewhat unkempt. He reported a low mood confirmed on self-report questionnaires. The evaluation highlighted impaired sleep patterns, a disengaged activity profile with late inconsistent waking times and sleeping during the day, poor cognition, poor endurance and coping mechanisms as well as low reported resilience, self-efficacy and stress tolerance. Mark had withdrawn from his usual social engagements.

Leading up to treatment seeking there had been an uncharacteristic trend of absenteeism, poor time keeping and productivity–competency difficulties over a few weeks. This had been flagged by Mark's manager. Predating this Mark reported a stable and successful career with a long tenure at his current employer. There was no previous history of psychosocial difficulties. Mark identified several recent stressors including the death of a close relative, a new reporting line that had a different management style, as well as restructuring in the business which had led to staff losses with the resultant uptake of a new unfamiliar portfolio and increased workload/volume. Given the latter, he had been working longer hours and had not been able to pursue his regular off-road cycling hobby.

Mark described a good support system outside of work. Mark's goal was to resume work.

A case management approach was adopted and multilevel–concurrent intervention was implemented that included:

- Establishing a return-to-work plan in collaboration with all stakeholders with whom a relationship had already been fostered during collateral information gathering in the assessment phase. Information gathered from an organisational perspective included specific mental health policies in place which supported early return to work and workplace accommodations/modifications. Mark was to be engaged in a work preparation process for two to four weeks dovetailed with a supported reintegration into work for a further approximately six to eight weeks.

- Referral for treatment to an occupational therapist with a special interest in depression and anxiety for amongst others practical stress and anxiety management skill acquisition; sleep hygiene, facilitation of more functional coping mechanisms, work–life balance including incorporation of his previous exercise regime, facilitation of an activity profile more compatible with work, cognitive rehabilitation, time management and interpersonal effectiveness skills including assertiveness, dealing with conflict and handling of criticism. Treatment content had a strong work focus and included role play of various situations (specifically past encounters with his manager) and attendance of groups. A hybrid program was crafted with both in-person and telehealth. Cognitive rehabilitation was supplemented with an app, and he was also exposed to various apps from which he could choose if he was interested providing tools and resources to support self-practice.

- Mark attended occupational therapy during the work preparation period and during the reintegration to allow for real-time problem-solving and engagement over issues, practising of skills taught to allow for efficacy and strengthening of self-management.

- Some telehealth sessions were utilised during the reintegration so that the occupational therapist could have sight of (with consent) his desktop/daily/weekly requirements and practically reinforce time management strategies taught in therapy.

- A relapse plan was put in place.

- Mark was assisted in accessing employee wellness for supportive counselling and grief counselling.

- An interdisciplinary approach with liaison amongst his treating healthcare practitioners was fostered.

- Engagement with his employer:
  - Regarding the organisational policies and procedures in place for employees experiencing psychosocial health difficulties. The beginning of a conversation was held around the existing policies and prevention, promotion, protection and early identification and intervention.
  - It was noted that they were in the process of recruiting to replace the lost staff member, so the increased workload was only temporary.
  - His employer was amenable to Mark attending a course for upskilling to assist with the new portfolio he had acquired.
  - Clear expectations of requirements for the new portfolio.

- Workplace accommodations/adjustment recommendations included:
  - Weekly touch bases with his line manager for goal setting and assistance with planning and prioritisation.
  - Use of an electronic organiser and calendar/planners.
  - Time off work to attend to his healthcare practitioners.
  - Removal of marginal/non-essential functions.

QUESTIONS

1. Describe the ways in which mental illness can limit a person's ability to function in competitive employment.

2. Discuss employment barriers and facilitators for people living with mental illness.

3. Describe the work engagement process.

4. Discuss work evaluation as applied to people living with mental illness.

5. Discuss work intervention strategies.

6. Discuss the role of the occupational therapist in the workplace.

REFERENCES

Abramovitch, A., Short, T. & Schweiger, A. (2021) The C factor: cognitive dysfunction as a transdiagnostic dimension in psychopathology. *Clinical Psychology Review*, **86**, 102007. https://doi.org/10.1016/j.cpr.2021.102007

American Psychiatric Association (2020) *Stigma, prejudice and discrimination against people with mental illness*. https://www.psychiatry.org/patients-families/stigma-and-discrimination (accessed 08 March 2024)

Angermeyer, M.C., Holzinger, A. & Matschinger, H. (2010) Emotional reactions to people with mental illness. *Epidemiology and Pyschiatric Sciences*, **19(1)**, 26–32. https://doi.org/10.1017/s1121189x00001573

AOTA (2020) Occupational therapy practice framework: domain and process 4th edn. *The American Journal of Occupational Therapy*, **74 (Suppl 2)**, 1–87. https://doi.org/10.5014/ajot.2020.74S2001

Arena, A.F., Harris, M., Mobbs, S., Nicolopoulos, A., Harvey, S.B. & Deady, M. (2022) Exploring the lived experience of mental health and coping during unemployment. *BMC Public Health*, **22(1)**, 2451. https://doi.org/10.1186/s12889-022-14858-3

Brouwers, E.P.M. (2020) Social stigma is an underestimated contributing factor to unemployment in people with mental illness or mental health issues: position paper and future directions. *BMC Psychology*, **8(1)**, 36. https://doi.org/10.1186/s40359-020-00399-0

Casteleijn, D. & de Vos, H. (2007) The model of creative ability in vocational rehabilitation. *Work*, **29**(1), 55–61. https://pubmed.ncbi.nlm.nih.gov/17627077/

Chandrashekar, P. (2018) Do mental health mobile apps work: evidence and recommendations for designing high-efficacy mental health mobile apps. *Mhealth*, **4**, 6. https://doi.org/10.21037/mhealth.2018.03.02

Coduti, W.A., Eissenstat, S.J. & Conyers, L.M. (2018) Linking hope factors, barriers to employment and health outcomes for individuals living with human immunodeficiency virus (HIV). *Work*, **61**(2), 225–236. https://doi.org/10.3233/wor-182794

Copeland, W.E., Shanahan, L., Egger, H., Angold, A. & Costello, E.J. (2014) Adult diagnostic and functional outcomes of DSM-5 disruptive mood dysregulation disorder. *American Journal of Psychiatry*, **171**(6), 668–674. https://doi.org/10.1176/appi.ajp.2014.13091213

Dahl-Popolizio, S., Carpenter, H., Coronado, M., Popolizio, N.J. & Swanson, C. (2020) Telehealth for the provision of occupational therapy: reflections on experiences during the COVID-19 pandemic. *International Journal of Telerehabilitation*, **12**(2), 77–92. https://doi.org/10.5195/ijt.2020.6328

Dewa, C.S., Trojanowski, L., Joosen, M.C. & Bonato, S. (2016) Employer best practice guidelines for the return to work of workers on mental disorder-related disability leave: a systematic review. *Canadian Journal of Psychiatry*, **61**(3), 176–185. https://doi.org/10.1177/0706743716632515

Di Napoli, A., Rossi, A., Baralla, F. *et al* (2021) Self-perceived workplace discrimination and mental health among immigrant workers in Italy: a cross-sectional study. *BMC Psychiatry*, **21**(1), 85. https://doi.org/10.1186/s12888-021-03077-6

Dol, M., Varatharajan, S., Neiterman, E. *et al* (2021) Systematic review of the impact on return to work of return-to-work coordinators. *Journal of Occupational Rehabilitation*, **31**(4), 675–698. https://doi.org/10.1007/s10926-021-09975-6

Drake, R.E. & Wallach, M.A. (2020) Employment is a critical mental health intervention. *Epidemiology and Psychiatric Sciences*, **29**, e178. https://doi.org/10.1017/s2045796020000906

Ebuenyi, I.D., Guxens, M., Ombati, E., Bunders-Aelen, J.F.G. & Regeer, B.J. (2019) Employability of persons with mental disability: understanding lived experiences in Kenya. *Frontiers in Psychiatry*, **10**, 539. https://doi.org/10.3389/fpsyt.2019.00539

Ebuenyi, I.D., Syurina, E.V., Bunders, J.F.G. & Regeer, B.J. (2018) Barriers to and facilitators of employment for people with psychiatric disabilities in Africa: a scoping review. *Glob Health Action*, **11**(1), 1463658. https://doi.org/10.1080/16549716.2018.1463658

Escorpizo, R., Reneman, M.F., Ekholm, J. *et al* (2011) A conceptual definition of vocational rehabilitation based on the ICF: building a shared global model. *Journal of Occupational Rehabilitation*, **21**(2), 126–133. https://doi.org/10.1007/s10926-011-9292-6

Figueredo, J.-M., García-Ael, C., Gragnano, A. & Topa, G. (2020) Well-being at work after return to work (RTW): a systematic review. *International Journal of Environmental Research and Public Health*, **17**(20), 7490. https://doi.org/10.3390/ijerph17207490

Fisher, A.G. (2014) Occupation-centred, occupation-based, occupation-focused: same, same or different? Previously published in *Scandinavian Journal of Occupational Therapy* 2013; 20: 162–173. *Scandinavian Journal of Occupational Therapy*, **21**, 96–107. https://doi.org/10.3109/11038128.2012.754492

Fukuura, Y. & Shigematsu, Y. (2021) The work ability of people with mental illnesses: a conceptual analysis. *International Journal of Environmental Research and Public Health*, **18**(19), 10172. https://doi.org/10.3390/ijerph181910172

Griffiths, C.A. (2017) Determinates of mental illness severity. *International Journal of Psychosocial Rehabilitation*, **21**(2), 32–36.

Gühne, U., Pabst, A., Kösters, M. *et al* (2022) Predictors of competitive employment in individuals with severe mental illness: results from an observational, cross-sectional study in Germany. *Journal of Occupational Medicine and Toxicology*, **17**(1), 3. https://doi.org/10.1186/s12995-022-00345-3

Gühne, U., Pabst, A., Löbner, M. *et al* (2021) Employment status and desire for work in severe mental illness: results from an observational, cross-sectional study. *Social Psychiatry and Psychiatric Epidemiology*, **56**(9), 1657–1667. https://doi.org/10.1007/s00127-021-02088-8

Haime, Z., Watson, A.J., Crellin, N., Marston, L., Joyce, E. & Moncrieff, J. (2021) A systematic review of the effects of psychiatric medications on social cognition. *BMC Psychiatry*, **21**(1), 597. https://doi.org/10.1186/s12888-021-03545-z

Hampson, M.E., Watt, B.D. & Hicks, R.E. (2020) Impacts of stigma and discrimination in the workplace on people living with psychosis. *BMC Psychiatry*, **20**(1), 288. https://doi.org/10.1186/s12888-020-02614-z

Harvey, S.B., Modini, M., Joyce, S. *et al* (2017) Can work make you mentally ill? A systematic meta-review of work-related risk factors for common mental health problems. *Occupational and Environmental Medicine*, **74**(4), 301–310. https://doi.org/10.1136/oemed-2016-104015

Henson, P., Wisniewski, H., Hollis, C., Keshavan, M. & Torous, J. (2019) Digital mental health apps and the therapeutic alliance: initial review. *BJPsych Open*, **5**(1), e15. https://doi.org/10.1192/bjo.2018.86

Howell, K.-L., Govender, P. & Naidoo, D. (2022) Factors influencing prevention and early intervention within the disability claims management process: South African insurer's perspective. *South African Journal of Occupational Therapy*, **52**(2), 16–25. https://doi.org/10.17159/2310-3833/2022/vol52n2a3

ICESCR (1967) *The international covenant on economic, social and cultural rights (article 6) and the right to form and join trade unions (article 8)*. https://treaties.un.org/doc/treaties/1976/01/19760103%2009-57%20pm/ch_iv_03.pdf (accessed 08 March 2024)

ILO (1958) *C111 - Discrimination (Employment and Occupation) Convention, 1958 (No. 111)*. https://www.ilo.org/dyn/normlex/en/f?p=NORMLEXPUB:12100:0::NO::P12100_Ilo_Code:C111 (accessed 08 March 2024)

ILO (2022). https://ilostat.ilo.org/new-ilo-database-highlights-labour-market-challenges-of-persons-with-disabilities/ (accessed 19 March 2024)

JAN (2023) *Job accommodation network*. https://askjan.org/index-old.cfm (accessed 08 March 2024)

Kielhofner, G. (2008) *Model of Human Occupation. Theory and Application*, 4th edn. Wolters Kluwer. Lippincott Williams & Wilkins, Baltimore.

Kilbourne, A.M., Beck, K., Spaeth-Rublee, B. *et al* (2018) Measuring and improving the quality of mental health care: a global perspective. *World Psychiatry*, **17**(1), 30–38. https://doi.org/10.1002/wps.20482

King-Casas, B. & Chiu, P.H. (2012) Understanding interpersonal function in psychiatric illness through multiplayer economic games. *Biological Psychiatry*, **72**(2), 119–125. https://doi.org/10.1016/j.biopsych.2012.03.033

Lagan, S., Emerson, M.R., King, D. *et al* (2021) Mental health app evaluation: updating the American Psychiatric Association's framework through a stakeholder-engaged workshop. *Psychiatric Services*, **72**(9), 1095–1098. https://doi.org/10.1176/appi.ps.202000663

Laver-Fawcett, A. (2007) *Principles of Assessment and Outcome Measurement for Occupational Therapists and Physiotherapists. Theory, Skills and Application.* John Wiley & Sons, Ltd, Chichester, West Sussex, England.

Law, M., Cooper, B., Strong, S., Stewart, D., Rigby, P. & Letts, L. (1996) The person-environment-occupation model: a transactive approach to occupational performance. *Canadian Journal of Occupational Therapy*, **63**(1), 9–23. https://doi.org/10.1177/000841749606300103

Lee, J.H., Gamarel, K.E., Bryant, K.J., Zaller, N.D. & Operario, D. (2016) Discrimination, mental health, and substance use disorders among sexual minority populations. *LGBT Health*, **3**(4), 258–265. https://doi.org/10.1089/lgbt.2015.0135

Life, C. (2023) *Workplace strategies for mental health.* https://www.workplacestrategiesformentalhealth.com/about-us (accessed 08 March 2024)

Lukersmith, S., Hartley, S., Kuipers, P., Madden, R., Llewellyn, G. & Dune, T. (2013) Community-based rehabilitation (CBR) monitoring and evaluation methods and tools: a literature review. *Disability and Rehabilitation*, **35**(23), 1941–1953. https://doi.org/10.3109/09638288.2013.770078

Memish, K., Martin, A., Bartlett, L., Dawkins, S. & Sanderson, K. (2017) Workplace mental health: an international review of guidelines. *Preventive Medicine*, **101**, 213–222. https://doi.org/10.1016/j.ypmed.2017.03.017

NIDA (2021) *National Institute of Drug Abuse. Why is there comorbidity between substance use disorders and mental illnesses?* https://nida.nih.gov/publications/research-reports/common-comorbidities-substance-use-disorders/why-there-comorbidity-between-substance-use-disorders-mental-illnesses (accessed 08 March 2024)

Nirmala, B.P., Roy, T., Naik, V. & Srikanth, P. (2020) Employability of people with mental illness and substance use problems: field realities. *Journal of Family Medicine and Primary Care*, **9**(7), 3405–3410. https://doi.org/10.4103/jfmpc.jfmpc_212_20

Robertson, E. (2021) A pilot study to develop a VR case review instrument for WIOA performance measure data collection. *Rehabilitation Counselors and Educators Journal*, **10**(2). https://doi.org/10.52017/001c.29555

Robinson, H. & Botha, A. (2013) Quality management in occupational therapy. *South African Journal of Occupational Therapy*, **43**(3), 8–18.

Ross, J. (2007) *Occupational Therapy and Vocational Rehabilitation.* John Wiley & Sons, Chichester, West Sussex, England.

Rössler, W., Ujeyl, M., Kawohl, W. *et al* (2019) Predictors of employment for people with mental illness: results of a multicenter randomized trial on the effectiveness of placement budgets for supported employment. *Frontiers in Psychiatry*, **10**, 518. https://doi.org/10.3389/fpsyt.2019.00518

Sevak, P. & Khan, S. (2017) Psychiatric versus physical disabilities: a comparison of barriers and facilitators to employment. *Psychiatric Rehabilitation Journal*, **40**(2), 163–171. https://doi.org/10.1037/prj0000236

Strong, S., Rigby, P., Stewart, D., Law, M., Letts, L. & Cooper, B. (1999) Application of the person-environment-occupation model: a practical tool. *Canadian Journal of Occupational Therapy*, **66**(3), 122–133. https://doi.org/doi.org/10.1177/000841749906600304

Sun, J., Sarfraz, M., Ivascu, L., Iqbal, K. & Mansoor, A. (2022) How did work-related depression, anxiety, and stress hamper healthcare employee performance during COVID-19? The mediating role of job burnout and mental health. *International Journal of Environmental Research and Public Health*, **19**(16) https://doi.org/10.3390/ijerph191610359

Thompson, A., Fugard, M.I. & Kirsh, B. (2021) Organizational workplace mental health: an emerging role for occupational therapy. *Occupational Therapy in Mental Health*, **37**, 240–263. https://doi.org/10.1080/0164212X.2021.1908925

Torous, J., Jän Myrick, K., Rauseo-Ricupero, N. & Firth, J. (2020) Digital mental health and COVID-19: using technology today to accelerate the curve on access and quality tomorrow. *JMIR Mental Health*, **7**(3), e18848. https://doi.org/10.2196/18848

UDHR (1948) *Article 23 of the universal declaration of human rights.* https://www.humanrights.com/course/lesson/articles-19-25/read-article-23.html (accessed 08 March 2024)

van Niekerk, L. (2009) Participation in work: a source of wellness for people with psychiatric disability. *Work*, **32**(4), 455–465. https://doi.org/10.3233/WOR-2009-0856

van Niekerk, L. (2016) Identity construction and participation in work: learning from the experiences of persons with psychiatric disability. *Scandinavian Journal of Occupational Therapy*, **23**(2), 107–114. https://doi.org/10.3109/11038128.2015.1091895

van Niekerk, L., Casteleijn, D., Govindjee, A., Holness, W., Oberholster, J. & Grobler, C. (2020) Conceptualising disability: health and legal perspectives related to psychosocial disability and work. *South African Journal of Bioethics and Law*, **13**(1), 43–51. https://doi.org/10.7196/SAJBL.2020.v13i1.689

van Niekerk, L., Coetzee, Z., Engelbrecht, M., Hajwani, Z. & Terreblanche, S. (2015) Time utilisation trends of supported employment services by persons with mental disability in South Africa. *Work*, **52**(4), 825–833. https://doi.org/10.3233/wor-152149

Waghorn, G. & Lloyd, C. (2005) The employment of people with mental illness. *Australian e-Journal for the Advancement of Mental Health*, **4**(2), 129–171. https://doi.org/10.5172/jamh.4.2.129

Wallace, S., Nazroo, J. & Bécares, L. (2016) Cumulative effect of racial discrimination on the mental health of ethnic minorities in the United Kingdom. *American Journal of Public Health*, **106**(7), 1294–12300. https://doi.org/10.2105/ajph.2016.303121

WFOT (2021) *Position statement occupational therapy and telehealth.* https://wfot.org/resources/occupational-therapy-and-telehealth

WHO (2001) *International Classification of Functioning, Disability and Health: ICF.* World Health Organization, Geneva, Switzerland.

WHO (2021) *Mental Health Atlas 2020: Country Profiles.* WHO Press, Geneva, Switzerland. https://www.who.int/publications/i/item/9789240036703 (accessed 08 March 2024)

WHO (2022a) *Guidelines on mental health at work.* World Health Organization. https://www.who.int/news-room/fact-sheets/detail/mental-health-at-work (accessed 08 March 2024)

WHO (2022b) *World mental health report: transforming mental health for all*. World Health Organization. https://www.who.int/publications/i/item/9789240049338 (accessed 08 March 2024)

WHO (2023) *ATC classification index with DDDs*. World Health Organization Collaborating Centre for Drug Statistics Methodology. https://www.who.int/tools/atc-ddd-toolkit/atc-classification (accessed 08 March 2024)

Wilhelm, K., Kovess, V., Rios-Seidel, C. & Finch, A. (2004) Work and mental health. *Social Psychiatry and Psychiatric Epidemiology*, **39(11)**, 866–873. https://doi.org/10.1007/s00127-004-0869-7

Zafar, N., Rotenberg, M. & Rudnick, A. (2019) A systematic review of work accommodations for people with mental disorders. *Work*, **64(3)**, 461–475. https://doi.org/10.3233/wor-193008

Zhang, G.F., Tsui, C.M., Lu, A.J.B., Yu, L.B., Tsang, H.W.H. & Li, D. (2017) Integrated supported employment for people with schizophrenia in Mainland, China: a randomized controlled trial. *American Journal of Occupational Therapy*, **71(6)**, 21–28. https://doi.org/10.5014/ajot.2017.024802

Psychiatric Occupational Therapy in the Corporate, Insurance and Medicolegal Sectors

CHAPTER 14

Lee Randall

SAMRC/Wits Centre for Health Economics & Decision Science-Priceless SA, School of Public Health, University of the Witwatersrand, Gauteng, South Africa

KEY LEARNING POINTS

- Psychiatric illness and disability affect people's day-to-day functioning and work capacity.

- Loss of functional capacity and work capacity forms the basis for many insurance and compensation claims and presents challenges to employees and employers.

- Occupational therapists are well placed to evaluate residual functional capacity and work capacity in people with psychiatric conditions and offer professional opinions and recommendations to employers,

- insurers, attorneys and the court system in different countries around the world.

- Offering corporate, insurance and medicolegal services demands additional skills and sensitivities, including moving from a client-centred to a justice-centred frame of reference.

- Clear communication of occupational therapists' domain of expertise is critical, to avoid misconceptions and inappropriate expectations.

INTRODUCTION

Psychiatric illness and disability can have devastating consequences for people's day-to-day functioning, of concern for them, their families, their employers and also their disability insurers. Stigma and discrimination are rife in the labour market (Papakonstantinou 2018) along with lack of appropriate employee supports (Dong et al. 2021), and the Covid-19 pandemic has worsened existing psychiatric conditions and increased the incidence of new conditions (Byrne et al. 2021). Occupational therapists' expertise in functional capacity evaluation and activity analysis makes them a valuable source of independent, objective expertise, able to match individuals' abilities and limitations to jobs, self-care tasks, home management activities and leisure pursuits to determine their level of impairment or disability. Occupational therapy opinions help corporates to make decisions regarding affected employees' work situations, insurers to process disability claims and lawyers to quantify compensation claims and civil cases. This chapter sets out key principles for working in the corporate, insurance and medicolegal sectors and is complemented by other chapters especially those on human rights and ethics (Chapter 4), forensic occupational therapy (Chapter 9) and work and vocational rehabilitation (Chapter 13). Chapter 6 is also relevant, dealing with clinical reasoning as well as epistemic fluency (the ability to articulate expertise using language everyone can understand and excluding occupational therapy-specific jargon).

Crouch and Alers Occupational Therapy in Psychiatry and Mental Health, Sixth Edition.
Edited by Rosemary Crouch, Tania Buys, Enos Morankoana Ramano, Matty van Niekerk and Lisa Wegner.
© 2025 John Wiley & Sons Ltd. Published 2025 by John Wiley & Sons Ltd.

PREREQUISITES FOR EFFECTIVE WORK IN THE CORPORATE, INSURANCE AND MEDICOLEGAL SECTORS

Occupational therapists stepping into these sectors should be confident in their roles and adept at explaining what they do and how they do it. They also need to equip themselves with additional skills and knowledge (Byrne 2003), given that basic occupational therapy training does not fully prepare one for the responsibilities of being a gatekeeper in relation to benefits, equipment or compensation awards (Barclay *et al.* 2020). Occupational therapists with advanced knowledge and skill in psychiatry face particular challenges given common public misconceptions that the profession focuses only on physical rehabilitation, paediatrics or geriatrics – resulting in employers, insurers, lawyers, judges and juries underestimating their depth of mental health training. In addition, at times, their expertise is confused with that of occupational health practitioners and that of industrial psychologists and occupational social workers, so a clear understanding is needed in relation to the intersections with those disciplines. Having been trained in multidisciplinary health care settings which typically employ client-centred approaches, occupational therapists must make a conceptual leap when entering corporate, insurance and medicolegal work which is more justice-centred, requiring knowledge of the law and labour market realities and a sense of the greater good. Whilst there remains a duty of care to the client, there is no therapist–client relationship in the traditional sense – instead, services are rendered primarily to the referring employer, insurer or lawyer, and in the case of medicolegal work, the occupational therapist's highest duty is towards the court system. A successful transition into these spheres of work requires maturity, flexibility, further training (Byrne 2003) and, ideally, mentoring by a more experienced practitioner (Van Biljon 2013). It is thus highly unwise for a newly qualified occupational therapist to try and step straight into this practice niche.

Van Niekerk *et al.* (2004, p. 3) point out that individuals with psychiatric disabilities face 'numerous barriers at the human, family, organisational and societal levels' which 'prevent [them] from performing their work roles in accordance with their own needs'. Determining loss of work capacity and broader functional capacity, or the degree to which people's functional abilities are mismatched with task demands (Gold & Shuman 2009), is the most common reason for occupational therapists being called on by corporates, insurers and lawyers. They have over the years acquired good international standing as functional experts – for instance, in South Africa, they have been called on as expert witnesses in Road Accident Fund compensation claims, medical malpractice matters and civil cases since the 1990s (Randall & Crosbie 2004). South African occupational therapists have also been involved in the insurance sector for the better part of three decades, including as claims assessors, independent evaluators, case managers and vocational rehabilitation providers (Byrne 2003).

A strength of occupational therapists is that they are viewed as able to provide well-substantiated and unbiased opinions with no vested interest in the outcome of the matter. The tools of trade consist of evaluation processes, methods and tests which are utilised to measure human functioning against relevant norms and standards, together with interviews, documentary review, sourcing of occupational data and collateral information and (where appropriate) conducting home and/or work visits. The data derived through these means allow the therapist to formulate rigorous and robust opinions, with the finished product taking the form of a written report which may also be accompanied by oral testimony. The report is typically forwarded directly to the referral agent (from whom the client may request a copy) (Van Niekerk 2019) and may become a matter of public record through court processes in disputes and medicolegal claims. At times, there is a need to include cost estimations; as noted by Duncan *et al.* (2011, p. 62), 'mental illness, in particular psychotic disorders that are untreated or poorly managed, introduces a range of costs that may fall under the radar of health economists and mental health service providers'. By demonstrating thoroughness, objectivity and independence, along with sensitivity to corporate, insurance and medicolegal needs and nuances, an occupational therapist serves as an ambassador for the profession.

When entering these sectors, the occupational therapist should understand and appreciate the following:

- Possible outcomes of **common psychiatric conditions** – i.e. their symptom constellations, treatment prognoses and so-called 'natural course'.

- Methods used to evaluate **functional capacity** (and particularly **work capacity**) against relevant yardsticks including job descriptions and task analyses.

- The wide-ranging nature of **real-life work and home settings**, within which people with psychiatric conditions function, including the differing roles, cultures, norms, practicalities and access to resources associated with different settings.

- The spectrum of **interventions, equipment, assistive devices, human assistance and task modifications** which can help maximise day-to-day and workplace functioning for people with psychiatric conditions, and the likely costs thereof.

- Relevant **legislation, policies, labour market practices and court procedures**.

More specific requirements are detailed below.

IN THE CORPORATE SECTOR

Occupational therapists must appreciate the difficulties faced by both employer and employee and grasp the realities of the particular business and type of job which is under scrutiny, being sensitive to the concept that 'time is money'. They need a good understanding of the labour market legislation which applies in the country in which they practise – in particular, legislation related to employment conditions, employees' rights, privacy of personal information and disability in the workplace. They must be able to differentiate clearly between illness and disability and between the different norms and requirements of work settings versus rehabilitation settings. The chapter on work and vocational rehabilitation provides a great deal of further information which the reader will find helpful.

IN THE INSURANCE SECTOR

Insurance work requires a broad understanding of the purpose and limitations of a range of disability and income replacement policies as well as of concepts like *temporary* and *permanent* disability, *partial* and *total* disability, *lump sum payments, monthly benefits* and *top-up benefits*. Occupational therapists should be aware of the vested interests of different parties, especially those of insurers and claimants and their families, but also those of employers. An accurate grasp is needed of the roles of stakeholders, including brokers, claimants/policyholders, claims assessors, chief medical officers employed by insurance companies, company doctors and nurses, human resource practitioners, line managers and claimants' treating practitioners. Various legal and ethical requirements must be followed when releasing information derived from claimant evaluations, with awareness of the broader protective mechanisms available to insurance consumers, such as an ombuds for long-term insurance. Due to reportedly high levels of fraudulent or spurious disability insurance claims and the possibility that large financial incentives may lead claimants to distort their symptoms, occupational therapists must be vigilant in relation to symptom exaggeration and inconsistencies in the information presented, gathering sufficient data including collateral evidence to satisfy themselves that they have reached a full and fair understanding of the functional status of the claimant. Where guidelines have been provided by the disability insurer, these need to be followed scrupulously, with deviations only for sound reasons which are clearly explained.

IN THE MEDICOLEGAL SECTOR

In a medicolegal setting, occupational therapists need to present themselves in a way which shows appreciation of their role in serving the ends of justice – i.e. as an expert witness or advisor within the court system or alternative dispute resolution forum. It is crucial that they avoid being 'hired guns', overly influenced by one party in a dispute which seeks to exploit their expertise to achieve its own ends. It must be clear that they have formulated objective opinions free of bias, regardless of the instructing party (Luke 2009). This rests on a grasp of the roles and vested interests of a large number of role players including lawyers, claimants and their families, claims handlers, compensation systems (e.g. motor vehicle accident funds) and other expert witnesses including occupational therapists and those from other disciplines. It is important to understand what is sometimes termed *compensationitis* – i.e. the tendency for claimants, consciously or unconsciously, to exaggerate their symptoms or complaints in the hope of

maximising their monetary awards. A grasp of basic legal language is imperative, including terms such as *plaintiff* and *defendant, special and general damages, loss of earnings, loss of amenities of life, undertakings, possibility* versus *probability, pleadings, summons, apportionment* and *contingency*. The terms used for lawyers in the country in which the occupational therapist practises must be known and understood – for instance, what are known as attorneys and advocates in some countries may be referred to as solicitors and barristers in others. Finally, it is important to understand the features of the applicable legal system: while some countries have jury systems, others do not and judges are the sole decision-makers. Each country also has its own system of lower and higher courts and courts of last resort, with specific names and duties prescribed for their presiding officers.

COMMON TO ALL THREE SECTORS

While occupational therapists in these spheres of work must step aside from a client-centred therapist or 'advocate' role into an objective, independent evaluator role which recognises the 'greater good', this does not mean they should abandon their client handling skills, such as establishing rapport and validating the individual's worth during the evaluation. If one feels ambivalent about this, it helps to focus on the role played in ensuring that society has productive and law-abiding corporates, fair disability insurance products and compensation systems which pay out on legitimate claims only. Occupational therapists should guard against confusing or conflicting 'multiple relationships' – for instance, they should *not* evaluate individuals they already know personally or have treated, and they should limit social interactions with referring parties like employers, insurance company staff and lawyers lest these influence their professional opinions. Finally, as noted by Watson and Buchanan (2005), like all other occupational therapists those working in the corporate, insurance and medicolegal sectors should embrace evidence-based practice and draw on the best available evidence when formulating professional opinions which have a real-life impact on clients. This requires lifelong learning in relation to new developments and keeping abreast of legal and labour market changes.

REASONS FOR REFERRAL

It is vitally important that occupational therapists understand the underlying reasons for referral and the specific questions which they are expected to answer through their evaluations and reports. Some examples are shown below:

IN THE CORPORATE SECTOR

- When employees have been off work due to a psychiatric condition, their managers and human resource practitioners need to know if they have sufficient work capacity to resume their usual duties and, if so, whether they need a graded return-to-work (e.g. working half-days initially and later reverting to full-time).

- As employees with invisible disabilities face a 'predicament of disclosure' (Prince 2017, p. 80) and people with psychiatric conditions who need accommodations may be hesitant to ask for these (Dong *et al.* 2021), it can be difficult for people like line managers, human resource practitioners and company doctors to identify potential options which would be reasonable rather than causing unjustifiable hardship to the company, and to determine whether accommodations will be needed on a temporary or permanent basis as well as at what intervals their effectiveness should be reviewed.

- When employees have insufficient residual work capacity to return to their usual duties, it is important to establish whether there are other roles available into which they can be realigned, matching their qualifications, experience and potential for vocational retraining or reskilling.

IN THE INSURANCE SECTOR

- When employees with psychiatric illnesses are off work for some time, their managers, human resource practitioners, company doctors or wellness practitioners may wish to explore whether a disability insurance claim would be appropriate.

- Risk managers rendering disability and absenteeism management services to insurers may request work capacity evaluations for employees with a history of taking excessive sick leave on psychiatric grounds. This could be as part of a *pre-claims screening* or *early intervention* process, designed to avert inappropriate disability claims.

- Once an insurance claim is lodged, claims assessors need expert opinions on the impact of the psychiatric condition on claimants' functional capacity and work capacity and their long-term functional prognoses. This assists with processing claims and determining whether it is appropriate to pay out disability benefits and on what basis – for instance, full or partial ('salary top-up') and temporary or longer term.

- When claimants are placed on disability benefits, claims assessors require periodic reviews to determine their functional trajectories and whether they can return to work and be taken off benefits.

IN THE MEDICOLEGAL SECTOR

- Lawyers representing clients who are claiming compensation (for instance, for injuries and psychiatric sequelae from road crashes, or for psychiatric illness allegedly caused by another person or event) need to know how those clients have been affected functionally. This includes how functional limitations affect their performance of day-to-day tasks, work roles and leisure pursuits, as well as their general amenities like quality of life and ability to engage in and enjoy previously valued activities.

- In matters like divorces and child custody disputes, the legal parties and judge (as well as the jury, where relevant) may need to understand the impact of psychiatric conditions on individuals' day-to-day functioning (self-care, home management and parenting tasks) as well as their work capacity. This helps with decision-making with regards to, for instance, spousal support and awarding of custodial parenting rights.

- Judges require detailed information on claimants' functional abilities in relation to both paid and unpaid tasks, and Kennedy (1997a p. 2) notes that 'changes in the law regarding compensation for loss of capacity to perform household services have led to increased demand for occupational therapists' assessment skills to determine the impact of impairment upon individuals' abilities to perform unpaid labour such as housekeeping, child care or yard work and the cost of replacing this labour. In addition, individuals such as entrepreneurs or farm wives, whose work is multidimensional, can benefit from the occupational therapist's ability to analyse and describe their jobs and relate this to their past, present and potential function'.

STAGES IN CORPORATE, INSURANCE AND MEDICOLEGAL WORK

PRELIMINARY WORK – RECEIVING REFERRALS AND PREPARING FOR THE EVALUATION

Before plunging into a piece of corporate, insurance or medicolegal work, occupational therapists should screen referrals to check the appropriateness thereof and that they are the best placed experts to answer the referrer's questions. This usually involves obtaining a clear letter of instruction as well as a set of background documentation, well in advance of any appointment scheduled for an evaluation. When reviewing the documentation, they should note whether any unusual arrangements need to be made. For instance, if the individuals to be evaluated may not be able to provide a full or coherent history, there may be a need to request that a family member accompanies them to the appointment, and if an interpreter is required this should be discussed with the referring party with agreement reached on how one will be secured and at whose cost. The therapist should explain to referrer and client that the evaluation will be in-depth and provide practical details such as the likely duration and what items (e.g. spectacles, list of medication) should be brought by the client. It is helpful to confirm in writing the time, date and address of the evaluation, and to reconfirm telephonically a day or two before the appointment.

Report deadlines should be negotiated, bearing in mind the likely depth and length of the finished product and allowing contingency time for unexpected delays – for instance, due to difficulties in obtaining collateral information, waiting periods for additional documentation, or slow turnaround times in obtaining quotes for particular interventions or pieces of equipment. It is especially important to clarify court-mandated deadlines when it comes to medicolegal work, due to the time-sensitive nature of case preparation and, in some countries, the need for lawyers to gather all their evidence together before a trial date can even be allocated. Finally, billing arrangements should be clarified and agreed with the referrer, including details such as whether the therapist charges an hourly rate or a flat amount, what disbursements may be charged for (e.g. printing, mileage and telecommunications costs), whether a surcharge will apply for urgent or after-hours work, and whether or not the occupational therapist is registered for tax purposes depending on the registration requirements of the country in which he or she practises.

INFORMED CONSENT AND THE EVALUATION PROCESS

Clients arriving for an evaluation need to be advised of its purpose and what the process will consist of, as well as who will be covering the costs. They should be requested to give their written informed consent both for the evaluation and for the preparation of a report which will be released to a designated person or organisation. For those under the age of legal majority (18 in many countries), consent must be obtained from someone with decisional capacity, such as a parent (Gillespie 2011). Consent is especially important in the medicolegal sector, as anything divulged or found during the evaluation process may effectively become a matter of public record through proceedings in open court. Occupational therapists must be scrupulously ethical with regard to releasing personal information derived from client evaluations and must reassure clients that they will comply with relevant legislation relating to data and personal information protection. If a client is unwilling to proceed with the evaluation, this should be fully documented and communicated to the referring party. It is inappropriate to coerce a client into participating, and in any event, this would yield invalid functional results.

Clients need a clear understanding of the relationship between referrers and occupational therapists, with the latter often being independent service providers who are paid for services rendered. Misunderstandings about the relationship can, at best, lead to inappropriate requests – for instance, the therapist may be asked to pass on a change of address to the insurance company or lawyer – and at worst could lead to clients doubting his or her objectivity or venting emotions towards the therapist which should instead be directed elsewhere. It is worth spending time on a good preamble at the start of appointments to help clients fully understand that the occupational therapist is effectively an information gatherer who will provide an objective professional opinion to the referring party – that is, that he or she is not a *decision-maker* in relation to the client's employment situation, disability insurance claim or medicolegal matter.

The evaluation process typically consists of:

- An interview
- Completion of self-report questionnaires by the client (if appropriate)
- Practical assessment tasks (including basic functional screening, standardised tests, non-standardised tests and job samples)

Notes made during the evaluation should be detailed and well organised to provide a contemporaneous account of what happened during the session. Tests should be scored and all raw data (e.g. interview notes, completed questionnaires, score sheets and writing samples) should be placed in the client file. Photographs (taken with the client's permission) can provide a valuable record, especially when the evaluation includes a home or work visit. During or after the evaluation, it may be appropriate to gather collateral information (e.g. from family members, treating practitioners or the employer) and the reason for this should be explained to the client, with permission obtained along with the names and contact numbers of relevant people. The occupational therapist should take care, whilst obtaining collateral information, not to inappropriately reveal sensitive issues and must carefully record the information obtained, from whom and on what date. With regards to functional testing, the most thorough testing that is possible and appropriate under the circumstances must be conducted, with a written record made in relation to any limitations, such as a need to omit certain assessment tasks and the grounds for this. Leaving out relevant assessments weakens the base of information from which occupational therapists draw their professional conclusions, and this can reflect adversely on their credibility if not properly explained in their reports.

At times, it is appropriate to conduct a home or work visit or both, either separately from the evaluation session or incorporating the evaluation. This must be cleared with the referrer upfront due to the extra costs involved and the following considerations should be borne in mind:

Home visits yield valuable information and clarify the client's circumstances but they can create challenges when it comes to structuring evaluations, potentially affecting the validity of test results. They may require one to venture into unknown and potentially dangerous areas or to be alone with unpredictable clients who may or may not welcome being evaluated. Occupational therapists may bear the brunt of clients' displeasure with their employer, insurer or lawyer, and may be subjected to attempts to influence their opinions, such as being offered gifts or meals. Home visits can also be difficult to schedule due to uncertainty about travel time and visit duration, and being unsure of how to behave in the homes of people from different cultures may result in an inadvertent social *faux pas* – like sitting down in the presence of elderly people when cultural norms require a younger person to stay standing (Lubbe 2009). Tools like navigation apps and mobile phones are vital in case the therapist experiences vehicle breakdowns, delays or difficulties locating the address. It is wise to try and get an advance description of the home and plan for the best evaluation location, ideally a quiet and private room which may need to be the client's bedroom. Finally, if a family member or interpreter needs to be present, this should be arranged in advance.

Work visits involve greater formality than home visits and there may be more severe professional consequences if things go wrong. When arranging a work visit, the occupational therapist should establish who will host it (e.g. line manager, human resource practitioner or occupational health nurse) and request permission to take items like test equipment, laptop or camera into the workplace. The purpose of the visit needs to be clearly communicated in advance, along with requests for facilities like a private interview room or quiet testing area. Requirements unique to the job site should be established, such as dress codes and personal protection equipment – including whether items like safety boots, hard hats or overalls will be supplied on arrival. Work hours must be considered as it may be inappropriate to schedule a work visit for knocking-off time, shift change-overs, lunch breaks etc. It is important that occupational therapists should not overstay their welcome or be over-demanding of people's time, and they should be polite, friendly and respectful to everyone encountered. If asked for their professional opinion, they should tactfully note that they will provide a formal report (and specify to whom) only after processing the evaluation results.

REPORT WRITING AND SUBMISSION

After the evaluation, occupational therapists process all data, triangulated from various sources, formulate a professional opinion and present this (including recommendations and costs when necessary) in a written report. It is important to use non-confusing terminology which can be understood by someone from outside of the profession to report on *all* aspects of the evaluations. If a particular assessment tool did not yield a valid and usable score (for instance, if clients were unable to grasp the instructions, could not complete the test or provided information which was clearly not in keeping with reality), this must be explained. Therapists may need to substantiate their professional opinions to a variety of readers, including non-health professionals such as employers, managers, human resources officers, claims assessors, lawyers and judges. Thus, their professional reasoning must be sound, meeting the 'reasonable person' standard – that is, they should not expound weird or wonderful ideas, venture into what has been termed 'the twilight zone of expertise' (Meintjies-van der Walt 2003), paint an unrealistic picture or make outrageously extravagant or conservative recommendations. As already noted, they must also not allow themselves to be influenced and should reach as objective an opinion as possible, regardless

of the consequences. They should take special care never to step outside their scope of expertise or encroach on another profession's domain; where appropriate, they should be willing to defer to other experts' opinions. Whereas reports by treating occupational therapists often focus on clients' assets and downplay their impairments, in keeping with a rehabilitation philosophy, reports written for the corporate, insurance or medicolegal sectors must consider 'the possibility of a less than optimal scenario' (Kennedy 1997b), as failure to do so could result in inappropriate decision-making or undercompensation. Practitioners must clearly understand for whom they are preparing the report, to ensure that the content does not contravene any ethical or legal principles. For instance, a report containing in-depth information on an employee's psychiatric difficulties would not be released to a line manager but could be released to an occupational health practitioner bound by the Hippocratic Oath – when needed, a shorter report can be written for the manager which simply contains job-related recommendations.

It is useful to have a standard template for reports which can be tailor-made as needed. In general, occupational therapists should follow these style guidelines:

- Reports should be succinct, reader-friendly and clearly structured, broken up with headings and numbering for easy reference and to avoid confusion (e.g. when testifying in court).

- Proofreading, spell-checking and grammar-checking should be carried out to ensure that the final product is as error-free as possible. Common grammatical and syntax errors arise from (over-) use of passive voice and overly long sentences.

- Particular care should be taken over critical information. This includes, for instance, the client's full name, age and address; dates of injuries or illness onset, hospitalisations and medical/surgical/psychiatric interventions; period of time off work (when relevant) and pertinent details like policy numbers, claim numbers or case reference numbers. Where clients use more than one name (for instance, a maiden name and married name, or an official name and nickname or short version) this should be reflected.

- Key information like the author's name and professional designation, client's name and date of the report can be contained in headers and footers.

- Longer reports can benefit from the addition of a list of contents and an executive summary. To keep the main body of the report concise, supplementary information like photographs, job descriptions and reference lists can be provided in the form of footnotes, appendices and attachments. A full report including attachments may run from a few pages in the case of a straightforward corporate or insurance case, to 50–60 pages or more in relation to a large or complex medicolegal claim. It is helpful to obtain a clear brief from the referring party as to the depth of information required.

- Bear in mind that it is often a waste to replicate lengthy passages from the documentation received – these can simply be referred to, and the main points summarised as needed.

- The conclusion should not contain new information, instead drawing together the threads from earlier sections in the report and making sense of them collectively. Recommendations can be provided (along with costs, where appropriate) either within the main body of the report or in an appendix or attachment.

The specific content of a report will vary from one situation to another but typical items are reflected in Table 14.1, showing the differences between reports produced for the corporate, insurance and medicolegal sectors. When possible, reports for corporates and insurers should be produced within two to four weeks. Medicolegal reports can sometimes only be finalised once additional documentation has been received – for instance, documentary evidence of the client's past work history, treating therapists' reports or expert medical opinions without which we cannot accurately predict the client's future functional status and needs. Delayed reports can cause problems for corporates which need to make decisions about employees, lead to suspension of disability insurance benefits and infringe court requirements; thus, the report-writing process must be efficiently managed. Particularly in the medicolegal sector, there may be a need for update reports and addenda – for instance, if two years or more elapse

Table 14.1   Typical contents of reports.

Corporate sector	Insurance sector	Medicolegal sector
Author details:	Author details:	Author details:
Name	Name	Name
Qualifications	Qualifications	Qualifications
Contact details	Contact details	Contact details
Client details:	Client details:	Client details:
Name	Name	Name
Age/date of birth	Age/date of birth	Age/date of birth
Home address	Home address	Home address
Job title	Job title	Job title
Name of employer	Name of employer	Name of employer
Date of injury/illness	Date of injury/illness	Date of injury/incident
Diagnosis/diagnoses	Diagnosis/diagnoses	Diagnosis/diagnoses
Employee no.	Policy and claim no.	Case or claim no.
Evaluation details:	Evaluation details:	Evaluation details:
Date of referral	Date of referral	Date of referral
Name of referrer	Name of referrer	Name of referrer
Referrer's ref. no.	Referrer's ref. no.	Referrer's ref. no.
Date of evaluation	Date of evaluation	Date of evaluation
Place of evaluation	Place of evaluation	Place of evaluation
Accompanying persons	Accompanying persons	Accompanying persons
Language(s) utilised	Language(s) utilised	Language(s) utilised
File ref. number	File ref. number	File ref. number
Purpose of evaluation	Purpose of evaluation	Purpose of evaluation
Methods used	Methods used	Methods used
List of background documentation received	List of background documentation received	List of background documentation received
Background information (brief):	Background information (brief):	Background information (in depth):
Social circumstances	Social circumstances	Social circumstances
Education and work history (as needed) Medical/psychiatric condition(s)	Educational history	Educational history
	Work history	Work history
	Medical/psychiatric history	Leisure pursuits
		Medical/psychiatric history including incident for which claim has been lodged

(continued)

Table 14.1 (*Continued*)

Corporate sector	Insurance sector	Medicolegal sector
Assessment findings:	Assessment findings:	Assessment findings:
Physical function	Physical function	Physical function
Psychosocial function	Psychosocial function	Psychosocial function
Brief information on occupational performance in the:	Brief information on occupational performance in the:	Detailed information on occupational performance in the:
– Self-care sphere	– Self-care sphere	– Self-care sphere
– Home management sphere	– Home management sphere	– Home management sphere
– Survival activities sphere	– Survival activities sphere	– Survival activities sphere
– Leisure sphere	– Leisure sphere	– Leisure sphere
Detailed information on residual work capacity	Detailed information on residual work capacity	Detailed information on residual work capacity with particular reference to pre-incident occupation(s)
Comment on job accommodations and/or alternative occupations (if requested)	Comment on job accommodations and/or alternative occupations (if requested)	Review of possible alternative or future occupation(s) (as relevant)
		Loss of amenities of life
Conclusion and recommendations (with costing as required)	Conclusion and recommendations (with costing as required)	Conclusion and recommendations (with costing as required)

from the time a client was evaluated, and functional test results have become 'stale', or if further information comes to light which causes a need for the occupational therapist to refine his or her opinions or recommendations. In the corporate sector, there may be a need to provide two reports – a more medically-oriented one for a company doctor or human resources practitioner, and a strictly job-oriented report for the line manager. Reports are customarily sent to the appropriate person via electronic means, using secure measures which prevent interception by unauthorised people or alteration of their contents. They should never be provided to the client directly – instead, the client should request a copy from the referrer.

In addition to adhering to their country's laws relating to the protection of personal information, occupational therapists may need to follow specific professional guidelines, such as the medicolegal guidelines available in the United Kingdom (College of Occupational Therapists 2009), or to undergo special training and certification (for instance, all expert witnesses in the United Kingdom must be trained in relation to Civil Procedure Rules).

FOLLOW-ON TASKS

Referrals from the corporate, insurance and medicolegal sector may require occupational therapists to perform follow-on tasks after evaluating a client and providing a report. This is commonly true in the medicolegal sector, where the report forms part of a set of evidence which goes forward to the court system or alternative dispute resolution process. Taking on a medicolegal case binds the therapist to see it through until settlement, according to the legal requirements of compensation claims and civil court procedures in the relevant country.

Follow-on tasks for occupational therapists offering medicolegal services can include taking part in multidisciplinary expert meetings or clarifying aspects of their reports through addenda or discussions with senior lawyers who will be taking the case to court. Very often, they also receive written instructions to hold a joint discussion with the occupational therapist appointed by the opposing side, producing a document known as a joint minute or joint statement which outlines their areas of agreement and disagreement. This helps narrow the issues in dispute and potentially shortens legal proceedings, facilitates settlements and contains costs. With or without a joint minute having been produced, occupational therapists may be called on to give oral testimony in court or an alternative dispute resolution forum, following key principles to testify effectively and maintain professional credibility (Allen *et al.* 2010).

It must be reiterated that medicolegal work should not be undertaken by new graduates, and this chapter provides only an overview of this sector of work. Expert witnesses are privileged to be allowed to express professional opinions (which are a form of hearsay evidence which is ordinarily disallowed in trials), as ordinary witnesses are only allowed to testify about facts. Occupational therapists acquire authority as expert witnesses not only from their specialised training but also from a depth of experience coupled with an ability to convey their knowledge to the 'fact finders' (judges and, in some countries, juries) to help them make fair decisions (Meintjies-van der Walt 2003; Robbins 2010). It may be necessary to provide a curriculum vitae (resumé) to substantiate one's professional experience and postgraduate qualifications. If the occupational therapist is seen to overstep his or her expertise, there is a risk of being publicly chastised and damage to one's professional reputation, leading to fewer referrals for medicolegal work. To help avoid this, there is a need to prepare thoroughly prior to testifying, including ensuring a sound grasp of other experts' opinions which have a bearing on the occupational therapy viewpoint. Whilst on the stand, therapists should avoid volunteering information or elaborating when not asked to do so, confining themselves to answering the questions put to them. They may need to prepare themselves to quote or provide their sources, where their opinions are based on literature or statistics (Luke 2009).

Finally, familiarity with the trial tactics used by lawyers and an ability to remain emotionally neutral is helpful, and the occupational therapist should remain calm and reasoned and guard against anger or defensiveness.

ADMINISTRATIVE INFRASTRUCTURE

An occupational therapist offering corporate, insurance and medicolegal services requires a sound administrative infrastructure, consulting rooms with a professional appearance and features such as wheelchair-friendliness, accurate contact details and information and communication technology including email, voicemail, telephony and internet connectivity. In countries where occupational therapists are regulated by a professional board or other statutory body, their practices' business formats must conform to requirements and they should hold appropriate indemnity (malpractice) insurance (Pepper & Slabbert 2011). Written documents need to be produced to a high standard, preferably using up-to-date software (word processing, spreadsheets and graphics) and with hard copies printed out in strong black ink on good quality white paper. Records storage is an important consideration, whether hard copy-based or electronic, with all client data needing to be stored in a secure and confidential way, in adherence to data protection legislation such as the General Data Protection Regulations of the European Union and the Protection of Personal Information Act of South Africa; password-protected cloud-based systems are less vulnerable to hardware malfunctions and data breaches but other options can be used such as external hard drives stored off-site. Client files should be kept in lockable rooms away from public access and in fireproof housing (e.g. metal filing cabinets). The period for which records should be retained depends on the country in which the occupational therapist is practicing as well as other considerations such as the age of the client or nature of the case. Reference systems should make it easy to retrieve files and track them to archives, if relevant. Each client file or electronic folder must include letters of instruction, correspondence and background documentation as well as raw data from the evaluation (interview notes, test scores, questionnaires, assessment forms, photographs and the like). Disposing of such items can be seen as 'sanitising' the file and may call into question the credibility and substantiveness of the therapist's reports and opinions. It should be borne in mind that what may appear to be a once-off involvement (e.g. a single request to perform an insurance evaluation) can always lead to further work down the line. In the case of multi-therapist facilities, the practice owner or chief therapist must also be able to handle queries when the original evaluating therapist is no longer available.

Some degree of administrative support may be needed in relation to filing, printing, correspondence, bookings, billing, report generation and other clerical tasks. Support staff also provide continuity while the occupational therapist is away at home or work visits, attending meetings or testifying in court.

CONCLUSION

Corporate, insurance and medicolegal sector roles are amongst the most challenging which can be taken on by an occupational therapist. Employers, insurance claims assessors, lawyers, judges and (where relevant) juries become frustrated when therapists do not appreciate business realities, have naïve or utopian expectations, lack an appreciation of contemporary labour market conditions or show ignorance of occupational health and safety principles, labour legislation and the purpose and limitations of a range of disability and income replacement policies. Thus, high standards of professionalism and advanced skills and knowledge are required to succeed in these sectors. However, together with the challenge can go a high level of job satisfaction, particularly for those who enjoy intellectual stimulation. It can be immensely pleasing for occupational therapists to explain and substantiate their professional opinions in a court of law, before a layperson such as an employer or for the benefit of a public figure like an insurance ombuds, with confidence and in a way which leads to a fair outcome. This type of work is arguably the 'gold standard' of professional competence and judgement, placing the practitioner in a position of prominence in spheres beyond the health care sector where most occupational therapists are found.

CASE STUDY

This case study, loosely based around a real-life case in South Africa, illustrates the role of psychiatric occupational therapists within the corporate, insurance and medicolegal sectors. It also shows how their roles dovetail with those of treating occupational therapists in a multidisciplinary psychiatric inpatient and outpatient unit.

Mr M (58 years), a senior financial manager for a major corporate in a large city, experienced a number of traumatic events over a six-month period in 2018. He had several periods of compassionate and family responsibility leave from work and was eventually diagnosed with post-traumatic stress disorder with concomitant depression and anxiety. Despite a period of inpatient treatment in a multidisciplinary psychiatric unit, followed by extensive outpatient psychotherapy, occupational therapy, psychiatric follow-up and use of prescribed medication, his functional status remained poor. He made two attempts to return to work but was unable to cope with his previous duties, and his employer requested that his treating occupational therapist provide vocational rehabilitation services. She reviewed the possibilities of his being aligned into an alternative occupation with fewer interpersonal and cognitive demands and recommended a graded return-to-work. The human resources department identified a lower-level, part-time and behind-the-scenes role in a different branch of the company, and he proceeded with a transitional work programme overseen by the occupational therapist. Since the alternative position was at a lower salary level, a temporary partial disability claim was submitted to the company's group disability insurer, which paid him top-up benefits. Unfortunately, after a further traumatic incident Mr M experienced a marked psychiatric relapse and was unable to continue working to any extent. The human resources department and insurer concluded that he met the definition of permanent disability, his employment was terminated on the grounds of incapacity and the insurer began paying him a full monthly disability benefit.

Being aware that he also held a policy with a private disability insurer, Mr M's family helped him lodge a claim against it. The claims assessor reviewed the documentation they supplied, noting the nature of his condition and confirming that he held appropriate cover for his designated occupation. He referred Mr M to an independent occupational therapist with psychiatric experience for a functional capacity evaluation. The ensuing report indicated that Mr M lacked the functional capacity to meet the demands of his usual occupation and, in response to a specific question from the claims assessor, the occupational therapist also indicated that his functional limitations would preclude him from working in any related occupation for which he possessed the necessary education, qualifications and work experience. Despite having been furnished with this opinion, as well as the opinions of Mr M's psychiatrist and an independent psychiatrist to the effect that his prognosis was very poor and he was permanently incapacitated, the insurer opted to repudiate the claim. This was explained on grounds that an inadequate passage of

time had elapsed to definitively establish the permanency of his condition.

Mr M and his family unsuccessfully used internal channels to dispute the insurer's decision, then decided to turn to the courts for resolution. Their lawyer appointed several relevant experts who conducted thorough medicolegal evaluations and provided in-depth written reports expressing professional opinions substantiated by their findings on standardised and non-standardised measures. These experts included an independent occupational therapist with many years of experience both in the field of psychiatric occupational therapy and in the medicolegal sphere. In her report, she expressed the view that over the 18-month period which had elapsed since Mr M's diagnosis, he had shown a downwards functional trajectory. She based this on the available documentation from his inpatient and outpatient treatment as well as records from his workplace attesting to his failed attempts to resume his usual occupation or a less demanding realigned occupation, coupled with her contemporaneous assessment findings. She noted that the chronicity and severity of his symptoms, coupled with factors like marked loss of self-esteem and -confidence, suggested a very poor functional prognosis. Thus, in her view, even with further multidisciplinary treatment, he had a negligible chance of regaining sufficient work capacity to return to any form of open labour market work, let alone his previous highly demanding occupation.

The lawyers appointed to defend the insurance company also briefed a medicolegal occupational therapist who had significantly less experience than the plaintiff occupational therapist in relation to psychiatric conditions. He duly evaluated Mr M and produced a medicolegal report in which he expressed a tentative view with regards to Mr M's long-term prognosis, but firmly indicated that his current functional status was incompatible with his usual occupation or any alternate occupation in the financial sector. Once a trial date had been allocated, both occupational therapists were instructed by their lawyers to meet and produce a joint minute. During their ensuing discussion, they found no discrepancies between their respective evaluation findings and conclusions as to Mr M's residual functional capacity, but the defendant occupational therapist reiterated that, with his limited experience in the psychiatric field, he felt unable to comment on whether Mr M had a permanent loss of work capacity. He indicated that he was willing to concede to the views of the more experienced plaintiff occupational therapist in this respect. In court, the judge noted this and also noted that the psychiatrist appointed by the defence appeared to display bias in expressing the opinion (after a very short examination of Mr M) that he was not permanently disabled, without adequately substantiating this.

Ultimately, the judge found in favour of Mr M, pointing out that the defendant experts were less credible and reliable sources of evidence than the plaintiff experts and concluding that the insurance company had acted unreasonably in repudiating the claim. He ordered the insurer to pay Mr M a large sum of money, with interest payable from the date on which it would have been reasonable to deem his disability as permanent in nature. The judge set this date as the date on which his company, having made multiple reasonable attempts to accommodate his residual limitations after affording him the necessary leave to seek treatment, concluded that his employment should be terminated on grounds of ill-health incapacity. The judge noted that Mr M had striven to mitigate his losses by being fully compliant with various phases of multidisciplinary treatment and making several attempts to resume work in either his own occupation or in a less demanding realigned role.

Although Mr M was distressed by the unexpectedly early termination of his career, he was satisfied with how he had been treated from a corporate perspective and medicolegal perspective. He and his family were also pleased and relieved that ultimately his private insurer was compelled to act in concert with how he had been treated by the group disability insurer which provided cover for the company where he had been employed at the onset of his psychiatric problems. With the resolution of his medicolegal case his anxiety symptoms improved substantially, which enhanced his quality of life despite his unremitting psychiatric difficulties on a day-to-day level.

QUESTIONS

1. Give six instances when an occupational therapist may be called on to act as an expert advisor/consultant/evaluator in the corporate, insurance or medicolegal sectors.

2. Discuss the general prerequisites for working in these sectors.

3. Outline the type of preliminary work which may be required when accepting a corporate, insurance or medicolegal referral.

4. Discuss the features of written communications which are produced whilst rendering corporate, insurance and medicolegal occupational therapy services.

5. Describe the possible pitfalls associated with conducting home visits and work visits, and how best to address these.

6. Highlight the most important features of the administrative infrastructure required in an occupational therapy practice which offers corporate, insurance and medicolegal services.

REFERENCES

Allen, S., Ownsworth, T., Carlson, G. & Strong, J. (2010) Occupational therapists as expert witnesses on work capacity. *Australian Journal of Occupational Therapy,* **57** (2), 88–94.

Barclay, L., Callaway, L. & Pope, K. (2020) Perspectives of individuals receiving occupational therapy services through the national disability insurance scheme: implications for occupational therapy educators. *Australian Occupational Therapy Journal,* **67**, 39–48. https://doi.org/10.1111/1440-1630.12620

Byrne, L.J. (2003) The current and future role of occupational therapists in the South African group life insurance industry. *South African Journal of Occupational Therapy,* **33** (2), 2–10.

Byrne, A., Barber, R. & Lim, C.H. (2021) Impact of the Covid-19 pandemic – a mental health service perspective. *Progress in Neurology and Psychiatric,* **25** (2), 27–33b.

College of Occupational Therapists Specialist Section: Independent Practice (2009) *Medico-Legal Forum Standards for Practice for Expert Witnesses.* College of Occupational Therapists, London.

Dong, S., Eto, O. & Spitz, C. (2021) Barriers and facilitators to requesting accommodation among individuals with psychiatric disabilities: a qualitative approach. *Journal of Vocational Rehabilitation,* **55**, 207–218 https://doi.org/10.3233/JVR-211157

Duncan, M., Swartz, L. & Kathard, H. (2011) The burden of psychiatric disability on chronically poor households: part 1 (costs). *South African Journal of Occupational Therapy,* **41** (3), 55–63.

Gillespie, G. (2011) Considering the issue of consent. *Newsletter of the Institute for Occupational Therapists in Private Practice,* **2**, 12–13.

Gold, L.H. & Shuman, D.W. (2009) *Evaluating Mental Health Disability in the Workplace: Model, Process, and Analysis.* Springer, New York.

Kennedy, L. (1997a) *The role of the occupational therapist in personal injury litigation – Part I. The Expert Witness Newsletter,* **2** (3). http://www.economica.ca/ew02_3p3.htm (accessed on 27 January 2014)

Kennedy, L. (1997b) *The role of the occupational therapist in personal injury litigation – Part II. The Expert Witness Newsletter,* **2** (4). http://www.economica.ca/ew02_4p2.htm (accessed on 27 January 2014)

Lubbe, G. (2009) *Simply Ask! A Guide to Religious Sensitivity for Healthcare Professionals.* Desmond Tutu Diversity Trust, Johannesburg.

Luke, G.B. (2009) *The Expert Witness: An Occupational Therapist's Perspective.* Arima Publishing, Suffolk.

Meintjies-van der Walt, L. (2003) The proof of the pudding: the presentation and proof of expert evidence in South Africa. *Journal of African Law,* **47** (1), 88–106.

Papakonstantinou, D. (2018) Why should employers be interested in hiring people with mental illness? A review for occupational therapists. *Journal of Vocational Rehabilitation,* **49**, 217–226. https://doi.org/10.3233/JVR-180967

Pepper, M.S. & Slabbert, M.N. (2011) Is South Africa on the verge of a medical malpractice litigation storm? *South African Journal of Bioethics and Law,* **4** (1), 29–35.

Prince, M.J. (2017) Persons with invisible disabilities and workplace accommodation: findings from a scoping literature review. *Journal of Vocational Rehabilitation,* **46**, 75–86. https://doi.org/10.3233/JVR-160844

Randall, L. & Crosbie, A. (2004) *Medicolegal evaluations and expert testimony: critical skills and ethical principles for occupational therapists entering this field. Workshop Presented at OTASA National Congress May.* Cape Town.

Robbins, J. (2010) *Expert Witness Training: Profit from your Expertise.* Presentation Dynamics, Ashland.

Van Biljon, H. (2013) Occupational therapists in medico-legal work – South African experiences and opinions. *South African Journal of Occupational Therapy,* **43** (**2**), 27–33.

Van Niekerk, M. (2019) Providing claimants with access to information: a comparative analysis of the POPIA, PAIA and HPCSA guidelines. *South African Journal of Bioethics and Law,* **12** (**1**), 32–37. https://doi .org/10.7196/SAJBL.2019.v12i1.656

Van Niekerk, L., Furnaux, M., Percy, S., Roberts, C. & Seider, L. (2004) Influences on the experience of work of employees with psychiatric disabilities: a collective case study. *South African Journal of Occupational Therapy,* **34** (**3**), 3–9.

Watson, R. & Buchanan, H. (2005) Making our practice evidence-based. *South African Journal of Occupational Therapy,* **35** (**3**), 14–19.

Spirituality and Mental Health
An Occupational Therapy Perspective

CHAPTER 15

Thuli Godfrey Mthembu[1] and Louise Fouché[2]

[1]Department of Occupational Therapy, Faculty of Community and Health Sciences, University of the Western Cape, Bellville, South Africa

[2]Occuptional Therapist in Private Practice, Founder and director of OTGrow, Tulbagh, South Africa

KEY LEARNING POINTS

- Spirituality in occupational therapy.
- Holistic approach in mental health.
- Spirituality in mental health.
- Therapeutic relationship in mental health.
- Spiritual history assessment.
- Occupational therapy models related to spirituality and mental health.
- Spiritual development.

INTRODUCTION

Spirituality is a phenomenon that provides meaning to life. Spirituality can help a person cope with mental illness. Spiritual beliefs can make everyday occupations more meaningful and health enhancing. Some people find it valuable to engage in shared occupations that focus on spirituality

(Wilding 2007, p. 67).

The chapter sets out to provide occupational therapists with frameworks, models and guidelines to incorporate spirituality as part of intervention in a confident manner. Although occupational therapists have long advocated for a holistic approach, spirituality has been the last frontier to be crossed, with therapists shying away from this sensitive topic, unsure how to broach the topic without consciously or unconsciously showing bias to a specific religion or spirituality.

SPIRITUALITY IN OCCUPATIONAL THERAPY

It necessary to clarify the differences between spirituality and religion to address the confusions, misunderstanding and personal meaning of these terms, which may influence occupational therapists in practice (Arrey *et al.* 2016). Religion involves the organised beliefs and practices related to a higher power or God that are shared by people who belong in a community or group (Arrey *et al.* 2016). In religion, spirituality is viewed as an essential part of faith and hope and often includes beliefs. It is important to understand that religion helps people to connect spiritually because of the rules and regulations that are practiced in the organisations where everyone worships the same God. For instance, clients and families in times of difficulties tend rely on their religion for solutions and support. Hence, it is valued as part of the people's approach in occupational therapy services because of its foundation in the belief systems.

In contrast, spirituality is a personal factor that focuses on self, which is an I-consciousness that enables an individual to search for a meaning and purpose in life. This is important in occupational therapy because a person's identity is grounded in self. Therefore, occupational therapy students and occupational therapists need to assist individuals to meet their needs of meaning, purpose, transcendence and relatedness. These needs assist clients to ascertain their direction in life when they are facing challenges related to tension,

Crouch and Alers Occupational Therapy in Psychiatry and Mental Health, Sixth Edition.
Edited by Rosemary Crouch, Tania Buys, Enos Morankoana Ramano, Matty van Niekerk and Lisa Wegner.
© 2025 John Wiley & Sons Ltd. Published 2025 by John Wiley & Sons Ltd.

disharmony, disequilibrium and stress. Consequently, clients who believe in the importance of spirituality tend to have opportunities to enhance their health, well-being and quality of life. Therefore, occupational therapists are in good position to use themselves as therapeutic tools for intervention (Solman & Clouston 2016). In existential perspective, spirituality is the element that helps people revive their capacities of self-awareness that guides them to identify who they are as individuals, which provides direction to the actions needed for promoting the quality of life through engagement in diverse occupations in life. Spirituality is an intangible thing that is entrenched in the human existential to guide therapeutic relationships and connections, which are valued in occupational therapy (Mthembu *et al.* 2017a).

Therefore, both religion and spirituality are valued and considered within occupational therapy. Although clients tend to place more emphasis on one or the other, and they will indicate their preference through the words and concepts they convey, when they are asked to elaborate on their spirituality.

THERAPEUTIC RELATIONSHIP IN MENTAL HEALTH AND OCCUPATIONAL THERAPY

In occupational therapy, spirituality promotes Batho Pele (People's First) and *Ubuntu* philosophy that deals with humanity, interdependence, inclusion, dignity and respect, which guides occupational therapists to build therapeutic relationships with self, family, community, society and nature (Mthembu *et al.* 2017b). Occupational therapists who have an encounter with mental health users provide interventions that are designed to preserve human dignity. Therapists might ask themselves why they need to have an insight into spirituality; however, it is an element of person-centred care that illuminates people's motivation and actions needed to flourish in life during difficulties. The relationship considers mental health users, therapists and students to navigate the influences of the mental health conditions, adversity and hardships on their well-being, engagement in occupations and health. Social interactions and participation are conduits for the therapists to provide a conducive environment that enables the mental health users to express their beliefs, values, traditions and practices, as part of conserving dignity.

Occupational therapists are professionally responsible to have contact with one another and others (i.e. mental health users and their families) to promote living in mutual relation through therapeutic relationship (Hess & Ramugondo 2014; Mthembu *et al.* 2017a; Horton *et al.* 2021). In explaining the significance of therapeutic relationship, Tolosa-Merlos *et al.* (2023) highlight that attitudinal, practices and contextual factors should be considered in mental health. In relation to *attitudinal factors*, it has been suggested that occupational therapists should be open and willing to adapt to the client factors that involve values, beliefs and spirituality (AOTA 2020). These client factors form the core of the mental health users'

lives and influence their performance in a variety of occupations. Regarding *practice factors*, occupational therapists need to form a collaborative partnership with the mental health users and their families to promote health management, which facilitates care and recovery. Concerning *contextual factors*, occupational therapists identify the facilitating factors of spirituality and clients' beliefs (AOTA 2020). Overall, occupational therapists and students have the responsibility to modify their attitudes and behaviours so that they can be compassionate to the needs of the clients by engaging in dialogue that promotes personhood and totality.

HOLISTIC APPROACH IN MENTAL HEALTH CARE

Occupational therapists have a mandate through the scope of practice to espouse mental health as the 'state of mental well-being that enables people to cope with the stresses of life, realize their abilities, learn well and work well, and contribute to their community' (World Health Organisation [WHO] 2022a). The need for action on mental health is indisputable, which indicates that occupational therapy interventions should be designed with an intention to promote holistic mental health care (Moreira-Almeida *et al.* 2014; Mthembu *et al.* 2017a). Therefore, occupational therapists and students need to address mental health users' needs, which are grounded in a positive vision that integrates physical, emotional, mental, spiritual and social well-being (WHO 2022b). This is part of the positive vision supported by Beng's (2004) biopsychosocial-spiritual model of care that acknowledges the 'totality of the patient's relational existence-physical, psychological, social and spiritual' (p. 1). Results from earlier studies demonstrate that the biopsychosocial-spiritual model should guide a good mental health clinical practice (Sallam *et al.* 2022; Van Denend *et al.* 2022). This is important for the occupational therapists because they need to have a better understanding of the religious/spiritual beliefs, values and practices of the mental health users and their families and communities (American Occupational Therapy Association [AOTA] 2020). These factors have influence on the occupational patterns and engagement of the mental health users.

Occupational therapists like other health professionals have an obligation to ensure that they perform a spiritual assessment for each mental health user and to recognise the value of appropriate referral to relevant members of the interprofessional team (Soomar *et al.* 2018; AOTA 2020). This is supported by Janse van Rensburg (2014) and Van der Watt *et al.* (2018), who indicated that referral arrangements could be facilitated with the involvement of other members of the interprofessional team such as traditional and faith healers. Hence, the Gyimah *et al.* (2023) study explored the experiences of persons with mental illness receiving care in a faith-based setting in Ghana, which found that mental health users engaged in religious activities such as meditation, Bible study and deliverance services. However, Hamer and colleagues

(2017) and Gyimah *et al.* (2023) raised concern about the importance of human rights of the mental health users in the faith-based institutions and their inclusion, which needs to be attended to address their abuse and restore human dignity.

In the occupational therapy profession, the patterns and engagement play an important role in the spiritual occupations that mental health users may engage in daily in their lives. This is in resonance with Forrester-Jones *et al.* (2018) who discover whether and in what ways a spirituality support group mediated mental well-being from the viewpoint of the attendees. The results of Forrester-Jones *et al.*'s (2018) study revealed that attending spiritual support groups enabled mental health users to structure their week so that they could engage in valued spiritual/religious activities and enhance social networks. The spiritual occupations are perceived as 'a variety of activities specifically imbued with spiritual meanings and effects that have been performed by human beings over many generations and across all cultures . . . [which] can be enacted at both individual and community levels' (Kang 2003, pp. 95–96). Consequently, it is crucial that occupational therapists should consider the spiritual occupations because they add value in the promotion of well-being and quality of life of mental health users (Forrester-Jones *et al.* 2018; Garssen *et al.* 2021).

The WHO (2023) refers to well-being as the ability of people and societies to contribute to the world with a sense of meaning and purpose. This is in line with goal three (i.e. Ensure healthy lives and promote well-being for all at all ages) of the Agenda 2030 Sustainable Development Goal (United Nations 2023). Therefore, occupational therapists should strengthen and enable the mental health users to be resilient, builds capacity for action and be prepared to transcend challenges emanating from the mental health conditions (Wilding *et al.* 2005). It is essential that occupational therapists acknowledge spirituality of the mental health users and their family and community so that they can use it as part of the coping strategies to manage stress (Wilding *et al.* 2005; Najafi *et al.* 2022). It has been reported that health professionals should identify mental health users' spiritual needs and provide appropriate interventions to address challenges related to mental health conditions.

Occupational therapists promote the well-being of the mental health users and their families as highlighted in the three of five action areas of the Geneva Charter (WHO 2022b). The action areas include designing an equitable economy that serves human development within planetary boundaries, creating public policy for the common good and achieving universal health coverage (WHO 2022b). These action areas add value to the integration of spirituality as part of the mental health services. In considering spirituality as part of self-care activities, occupational therapists will enable the mental health users to enhance their self-esteem and motivation. Spirituality contributes to self-care activities that enhance people's volition and motivation that governs actions to do, be, belong and become (Martin *et al.* 2023). For instance, spirituality connects the mind and body so that people can still use their potential to engage in activities that regenerate their humanity.

SPIRITUALITY IN MENTAL HEALTH

The role of spirituality in psychiatry has received increased attention across a number of disciplines in recent years including occupational therapy (Wilding *et al.* 2005; Wilding 2007; Hess & Ramugondo 2014; Janse van Rensburg *et al.* 2015; Janse van Rensburg 2014). Therefore, the growing body of literature further recognises that occupational therapists consider the importance of spirituality in improving the quality of life and functional outcomes of people with mental health conditions (Wilding *et al.* 2005; Wilding 2007; Hess & Ramugondo 2014). While a variety of definitions of the term spirituality have been suggested, this chapter will use the South African definition suggested by Janse van Rensburg *et al.* (2015) who perceive it as:

'progressive individual or collective inner capacity, consciousness or awareness of transcendence. It also consists of relational aspects or connectedness and essentially exists as a process, representing growth, or a journey. This capacity, consciousness and connectedness provide the motivating drive for living and constitute the source from which meaning and purpose is derived'.

Janse van Rensburg *et al.*'s (2015) definition highlights the importance of individual and collective inner capacities. However, it has been highlighted that the inner capacities of the mental health users who have been diagnosed with conditions such as depression, anxiety, drug and alcohol misuse; bipolar disorders and psychosis tend to be affected, which result in occupational disruption (Wilding 2007). Occupational disruption refers to the temporary disturbances that influence a person's usual pattern of occupational performance and occupational engagement (AOTA 2020). This indicates that occupational therapists should ensure that mental health users' occupational potential is enhanced so that their 'capacity to do what they are required and have opportunity to do, to become who they have the potential to be' (Wicks 2005).

Spirituality is identified as a catalyst that assists mental health users to cope with their mental health conditions so that they can be able to engage in different activities and participate in a variety of occupations in community (Wilding *et al.* 2005). An observational longitudinal six-month study conducted to assess the role of spirituality on outcomes of patients with major depressive disorder in Egypt has shown that there was a relationship between spirituality and functional outcomes (Sallam *et al.* 2022). The evidence in Sallam *et al.*'s study supported Wilding (2007) that health professionals such as occupational therapists should consider spirituality as a part of therapeutic route to enhance interventions, quality of life and occupational engagement of mental health users. This is important in occupational therapy and mental health because spirituality forms part of the client factors and performance patterns related to beliefs, values, rituals, traditions and practices (Puchalski *et al.* 2014; AOTA 2020). The consideration of spirituality in occupational therapy profession and mental health contributes to a biopsychosocial-spiritual model that underpins holistic approach and people-centred (Beng 2004; Moreira-Almeida *et al.* 2014).

The advantage of the integration of spirituality in mental health is that it 'serves as a key factor of resilience' (Manning *et al.* 2019, p. 168). Mental health users can benefit from spirituality because it supports their actions and efforts to deal with the adversity and hardship of having mental health conditions. Therefore, occupational therapists may enhance interventions by using spirituality as a client factor that facilitates relationships, coping and commitment to spiritual values and practices (Hess & Ramugondo 2014; Manning *et al.* 2019; AOTA 2020). Integration of spirituality in mental health strengthens spiritual resilience, which is considered as 'the ability to sustain one's sense of self and purpose through a set of beliefs, principles, or values while encountering adversity, stress, and trauma by using internal and external spiritual resources' (Manning *et al.* 2019, p. 172). In enabling spiritual resilience, occupational therapists need to invest in therapeutic relationships when providing mental health services. This indicates that occupational therapists should put a premium on serving the community, lifting others and finding joy in empowering others to address mental health problems that influence their health, well-being and quality of life.

SPIRITUAL HISTORY ASSESSMENT

In occupation therapy, occupational therapists and students need to adopt compassion while engaging in dialogue that promotes mental health users' personhood and identity grounded in their beliefs, spiritual and cultural values as well as practices. Integration of spirituality in occupational therapy has grown importance in light of the loss of meaning and purpose in life that appeared to emanate from various mental health conditions (Mthembu *et al.* 2017a). It has been reported that there are therapeutic implications of conducting spiritual history assessment with people living with mental health conditions (Moreira-Almeida *et al.* 2014). This indicates that occupational therapists should also endeavour to conduct spiritual history assessment so that they may engage in open-ended spiritual history discussion with the mental health users, families and communities to conserve their dignity (Kelso-Wright 2012; Hemphill 2015). The spiritual history discussions are significant in occupational therapy and mental health because they contribute to the client factors related to values, beliefs and spirituality as well as rituals with symbolic actions with spiritual, cultural and social meaning (AOTA 2020). Understanding the perceptions and practices of spirituality from the mental health users and their families might be useful for occupational therapists who provide services in the different levels of care.

It is very important that occupational therapist should have insight into the differences between spirituality and religion as explained in the beginning of this chapter. A number of studies have begun to examine how spiritual history assessment is conducted in occupational therapy (Kelso-Wright 2012; Hemphill 2015). The studies indicate that there are diverse spiritual history assessments that can be conducted with mental health users such as Faith (Belief and Meaning), Importance and Influence, Community, and Address/Action in Care (FICA) (Puchalski & Romer 2000); HOPE (Anandarajah and Hight 2001) and SPIRIT (Maugans 1996) to name a few. Although we have highlighted the spiritual history assessments, for the purpose of this chapter, we opted to focus more on FICA©. It is a spiritual history assessment developed to be used by health professionals such as occupational therapists who aim to promote holistic and client-centred approach. The FICA© is an acronym used for Faith (Belief and Meaning), Importance and Influence, Community, and Address/Action in Care, which is more applicable for occupational therapists (Puchalski & Romer 2000). Kelso-Wright (2012) highlights that the FICA© is relevant for occupational therapy because it enables 'clients and clinicians to discuss spiritual occupations or beliefs' (p. 11) and guides occupational therapy intervention. Moreover, FICA© is indispensable because occupational therapists can evaluate mental health users' commitment to spiritual values and practices. Occupational therapists may conduct the spiritual history assessment using the specific questions developed by Puchalski and Romer (2000) and evaluated by Borneman *et al.* (2010) to facilitate the spiritual discussions in occupational therapy. The specific questions are structured based on the FICA© acronym as presented in Table 15.1.

These questions are significant in occupational therapy practice because they provide information that can be incorporated in the occupational profile and analysis of the mental health users. Furthermore, the mental health users' response to the spiritual assessment questions can be used with the model of spirituality in occupational therapy.

OCCUPATIONAL THERAPY MODELS RELATED TO SPIRITUALITY AND MENTAL HEALTH

There are two models from the occupational therapy stock of models, which undergird the understanding of spirituality, namely Canadian Model of Occupational Performance and Engagement (CMOP-E) and Vona du Toit Model of Creative Ability (VdTMoCA).

RELEVANCE OF CMOP-E IN OCCUPATIONAL THERAPY AND SPIRITUALITY

In the occupational therapy literature, CMOP-E is used to have a better understanding of the occupational performance and engagement as an interdependent relationship between the person, the environment and their occupations (Polatajko *et al.* 2007). In the CMOP-E, spirituality is recognised as a core of the person, which is shaped by the environment and provides meaning through engagement in occupation (Duncan 2011; Hall *et al.* 2015). The CMOP-E acknowledges that the person is made up of cognitive, affective and physical elements, which necessitates occupational therapists to assess

Table 15.1 FICA© questions for spiritual history assessment.

F – Faith, Belief, Meaning	• Do you consider yourself to be spiritual? or 'Is spirituality something important to you?'
	• Do you have spiritual beliefs, practices or values that help you to cope with stress, difficult times or what you are going through right now? (contextualise to visit)
	• What gives your life meaning?
I – Importance and Influence	What importance does spirituality have in your life?
	Has your spirituality influenced how you take care of yourself particularly regarding your health?
	Does your spirituality affect your healthcare decision-making?
C – Community	• Are you part of a spiritual community?
	• Is your community of support to you and how?
	• For people who don't identify with a community consider asking 'Is there a group of people you really love or who are important to you?'
	• (Communities such as churches, temples, mosques, family, groups of like-minded friends, or yoga or similar groups can serve as strong support systems for some patients.)
A – Address/ Action in Care	• How would you like me, as your healthcare provider, to address spiritual issues in your healthcare? (With newer models, including the diagnosis of spiritual distress, 'A' also refers to the 'Assessment and Plan' for patient spiritual distress, needs and or resources within a treatment or care plan.)

these elements. In relation to the environment, Polatajko *et al.* (2007) share that physical, institutional, cultural and social are part of the environment. Occupational therapists can also assess the environmental factors so they could make sense of its influence in occupational performance and engagement. However, the occupation component not only includes generic self-care, productivity and leisure but also other areas of occupation such as social participation, rest and sleep, health management, play, education and instrumental activities of daily living (Polatajko *et al.* 2007; AOTA 2020). Therefore, occupational therapists need to assess mental health users' occupational performance. In summary, CMOP-E highlights that occupational performance and engagement is the result of the interactions of the person, the environment and their occupation. However, occupational therapists need to be aware of the function-dysfunction continuum of the CMOP-E.

FUNCTION-DYSFUNCTION CONTINUUM

CMOP-E is essential in occupational therapy because of its connection with the occupation-based and client-centred practice,

which is needed as part of integrating spirituality in mental health care. Despite its long clinical success, it is imperative that CMOP-E should be used to gain insight into the function-dysfunction continuum. In relation to *function* in mental health, mental health users may experience occupational harmony because there is an interdependent relationship between their occupation and environment (Liu *et al.* 2023). This indicates that occupational therapists should facilitate equilibrium between the mental health users and social engagement to enable harmony with others and with self, which is supported by their spirituality. Hence, Liu *et al.* (2023) assert that through engagement with others tends to provide social and spiritual support, which is necessary for mental health users so that they cope with the challenges related to their conditions, activity limitations and participation restrictions. Furthermore, occupational therapists may assist mental health users to meet their wellbeing needs of maintenance, self-care and safety through engagement in valued occupations and target the drivers of dysfunction as Patel (2015) highlights.

Dysfunction among mental health users is one of the concerning issues in the public mental health that needs occupational therapists to 'equip people and communities to better cope with the stressors' (Patel 2015, p. 44). People living with mental health conditions tend to experience dysfunction and inability to produce adaptive response due to influences of personal factors or environmental factors (Partti-Enkenberg 2022). It is evident that mental health users experience occupational injustices, disparities and disruptions (Hamer *et al.* 2017; Kearns Murphy & Shiel 2019; Partti-Enkenberg 2022). Recent examples of research into occupational injustices include environmental barriers, lack of opportunities for engaging in meaningful activities, positive identity, self-esteem and stigma that influence mental health users (Hamer *et al.* 2017; Kearns Murphy & Shiel 2019; Partti-Enkenberg 2022). In relation to institutional injustices, Kearns Murphy and Shiel (2019) report that mental health users were restricted to engagement in activities, got less opportunities for occupations and lacked productive roles, which affected their occupational choice and autonomy. Regarding practices of exclusions, it was evident that the mental health users tend to experience occupational marginalisation, which makes them to be disempowered to make choices and decisions (WHO 2021, 2022a; Partti-Enkenberg 2022). Therefore, it is propound that social and occupational justice should be considered to support mental health users' right quality of life and 'wellbeing, and the right to live good lives, as citizens and productive members of their communities' (Hamer et al. 2017, p. 85). This is important because mental health users also have responsibilities to contribute and connect with others, which promotes a sense of belongingness and spirituality (Hamer *et al.* 2017; WHO 2021).

In using the FICA© with occupational therapy assessments, occupational therapists can be able to identify which areas of occupation are affected by the mental health conditions. Furthermore, occupational therapists will need to assess how the environment may result in activity limitation and occupational opportunities for the mental health users. This is important so that occupational therapists will be able to figure out what strategies to use for environmental modifications and adaptations. In occupational therapy practice, there is a need for occupational therapists to accompany their clients through the spiritual growth and journey by availing the opportunities for the mental health users to engage in spiritual assessment guided by the questions from the FICA© and conceptualisation with the CMOP-E. Thus, it is important that spiritual development should be considered as part of occupational therapy practice.

RELEVANCE OF SPIRITUALITY IN Vona du Toit MODEL OF CREATIVE ABILITY

Spirituality is promoted in occupational therapy as an intrinsic motivational factor in life that can be adopted as part of the person-centred approach for individuals with mental health conditions who need to overcome challenging situations (Rogers & Wattis 2020). In relation to VdTMoCA, spirituality is congruent with the volition that governs actions of creative ability among mental health users and other people (Joubert 2019). Motivation refers to a driving force that gives purpose or direction to behaviour and it operates at both conscious and unconscious levels among humans (Nandika & Nagalakshmi 2022). This equates with the spiritual elements of meaning, purpose and direction to life journey. Similar to motivation, spirituality can be perceived as part of VdTMoCA levels of motivation with different actions, which influences people's creative ability. Therefore, VdTMoCA not only focuses on the importance of physical and mental health of individuals but also the contribution of spirituality in the creative response, adaptive and act. Four occupational performance areas may facilitate the integration of spirituality, namely personal management, work ability, use of free time and social ability. These occupations are bridges to the levels of creative ability, which include tone, self-differentiation, self-presentation, passive participation, imitative participation and active participation (Joubert 2019).

SPIRITUAL DEVELOPMENT MODEL

An emphasis has been highlighted that occupational therapists should not bring their own religious beliefs and spirituality into the therapy context. However, it is recommended that any therapist who is drawn to working psycho-spiritually with clients have their own spiritual practices within their own beliefs. This enables the therapist to be grounded in spirituality. It is also recommended that the therapist be one level higher on the spiritual development model than the clients she/he is facilitating. It is crucial that the therapist ensures that the client determines the goals for treatment and that a process is facilitated. Working psycho-spiritually does not entail providing information or giving advice but guides a process of experiences that the client makes sense of within their own spiritual beliefs and experience. It is imperative that at no time does the client feel judged, as they will close down. Occupational therapists can determine the client's level of spiritual development, by asking them to give a brief description of their spiritual journey throughout their life. The two psycho-spiritual models that can be considered when working with the mental health users' spirituality include psychoanalytic theories such Jung and Rohr's work on spiritual development. These models are important in occupational therapy because they provide guidelines for the therapeutic intervention along the spiritual journey.

JUNG'S PROCESS OF INDIVIDUATION

Carl Jung is a psychoanalytic theorist who has an interesting background and his father was a staunch Lutheran pastor (Jung 1990). Due to Jung's poor relationship with his father and traumatic incidents with religion, he wanted nothing to do with religion and was drawn to psychology, working under Freud (Jung 1990). Although Jung was anti-religious, most of his life, work and writings have a deep fascination with spirituality. In the later part of his life, he travelled to the east to find out more about alchemy and eastern spiritual practices to help inform his thoughts on individuation (Jung 1990). Jung coined terms like the false self and the True Self, shadow work, synchronicity and the collective unconscious, which form foundational concepts in psycho-spiritual intervention. However, due to the scope of this chapter, the focus is on Jung's theory of individuation, which highlights that each person has a state of selfhood through the process of individuation. The Individuation process consists of letting go of the persona, which is seen as the mask a person wears to fit into society and the conscious self represents the person behind the mask (Fouché 2021). These first two levels of a person's psyche are within the conscious realm and can be accessed by the rational mind.

However, Jung believed that there were three additional levels of a person's psyche, which are seated in the unconscious, namely shadows, which are the parts of the self that have been suppressed in order to be accepted by society. The anima and animus represent a balance of both masculine and feminine energies to reach the True Self (also referred to as the divine self or soul). A person would need to embrace and integrate their shadows and anima/animus to become fully human, to live a life true to their soul. Jung was of the opinion that these last three levels of the psyche, which were mostly in the unconscious, could only be accessed or given a voice through stories, dreams, myths and symbols (Fouché 2021). He believed in archetypal folklores and parables that held wisdom not easily understood by the conscious mind. After Jung moved to the lake, he lived for a large portion of his life in solitude and would draw a mandala on a daily basis to observe his psyche's transformation.

Within an occupational therapy context, working psycho-spiritually, Jung's individuation process can be viewed as a spiritual progressive process, facilitating the client through the different psyche levels to ultimately reach a state of selfhood or to live from their True Self. Progression through these levels can take years to complete and cannot be rushed, else it runs the risk of becoming a conscious, intellectual experience, remaining on a conscious level, never allowing the person to drop down into the unconscious. The second valuable guide for occupational therapists is the need to NOT work in the intellectual, cognitive realm when working psycho-spiritually, but rather to make use of art, storytelling and projective techniques like the right-left hand dialogue, where the unconscious is constantly engaged in the activities. Only afterwards does the client try to find the words, because at times our unconscious has already processed something that our conscious has not even properly conceived or has the words for yet.

ROHR'S MODEL OF SPIRITUAL DEVELOPMENT

Richard Rohr developed a model for Spiritual Development (Rohr 2009) and he is a Franciscan father who studied psychology and was a spiritual director to people for many years (Fouché 2021). He later developed a model from all the years of accompanying people on their spiritual journey and realised there was a developmental nature to everyone's journey. He described nine levels in his spiritual development model. In this chapter, the first six levels are described as the clients seen by occupational therapists will most probably fall within the first six levels of spiritual development. This model is in line with other psycho-spiritual developmental models but has the added advantage of incorporating both Jung's theory and provides more detail to enable therapists to facilitate or provide opportunities for psycho-spiritual development.

Level 1: Physical development: The client is focused on physical development and does not yet possess a concept of spirituality, neither have they experienced their spirit or God/the Universe/the Creator/the Divine.

Level 2: Group identity: The client identifies with a group's beliefs, which prescribes their spirituality. People on this spiritual development level tend to have a more religious identity than spiritual. The laws, dogmas and rituals of the group are seen as the ultimate truth to spirituality. A lot of emphasis is placed on participating in the rituals and religious practices as explained by the religious leaders. People feel it is unacceptable to question religious beliefs or practices prescribed.

Level 3: Individual awareness: The client starts to question the rituals, laws and dogmas of their religion and starts to choose their own beliefs. There is a process where the person defines their own beliefs and dares to move away from the group's prescriptions. The client on this level becomes aware of the

influence of their emotions, thoughts and behaviours and realises their spirituality is something more than their thoughts, behaviours and emotions or religion.

SHOCK POINT

Rohr explains that the majority of people will spend most of their life on level 3, unless something traumatic happens that makes them deeply question their beliefs, life and/or the meaning of life. He described these trigger events as a shock point. In this no-man's land, between levels 3 and 4, people struggle to voice deeply held beliefs which are directly opposed to their own life experience that leads them to question the meaning of life. A common belief is that 'good things happen to good people' . . . then their child dies. An internal struggle is set in motion: Am I not a good person? If I were a good person, why would God/life allow this to happen? What is the point of being a good person, if bad things still happen to me? Is God not powerful enough to stop bad things? What did I do to cause this? What is life really about, if there is pain? Can I still trust God/the Divine? Where does this tragic incident leave me in life? These questions are difficult to answer with a level 3 spiritual development and facilitate clients to mature to a level 4, which enables them to explore these deeper questions.

Level 4: Aware of their spirit: The client becomes aware of spiritual experiences and moves to a personal relationship with their God/the Universe/the Creator/the Divine. The spiritual experiences are outside the confines of prayer time/church/spiritual practices. The client experiences their spirit as something other than their thoughts, behaviours and emotions and allows themselves to be guided by their spirit. Often this guidance is not rational but allows greater awareness. Clients become aware of synchronicity, (i.e. unexplainable 'co-incidences') which enables them to find answers (Roxburgh *et al.* 2016). It becomes a space to explore the meaning of life questions with more ease as the spirit can hold mystery easier than the rational mind. This level of spiritual development allows a person to hold contradictory paradoxes and move away from dualistic thinking, which is required to make meaning. People become more comfortable with holding questions, rather than frantically looking for answers.

Level 5: Integrating shadows: The client is ready now to work on their shadows, recognising, embracing and integrating all parts of the self they have disowned due to socialisation as a young child. Normally, anxiety levels increase on this level, as clients take more risks in trusting their spirit to guide them in their decision-making but are still unsure if their spirit or God/the Universe/the Creator can be fully trusted. Psychodrama, projective techniques, creative arts and storytelling are the mediums of choice on this level, as the rational mind does not have the capacity to work on deeper levels. The aim of integrating the shadows is to strive for the psyche to be whole and to love rather than strive to be 'right' or 'perfect' or 'beautiful' or 'good' or 'holy' – which are all relative concepts, defined by context. They are at peace with their flaws and understand their need for others, seeking deeper connections, allowing others to have flaws and being less judgemental.

Level 6: Finding life purpose: After clients have integrated their shadow, they are closer to living from their True Self. New parameters are found to make sense of life. A person on this level tends to become more detached to earthly things, more responsive (instead of reactive) and more focused on living in the now. They start to let go of control, trusting their spirit and God/the Universe/ the Creator/the Divine. They are more in tune with who they truly are, including their talents, characteristics, gifts etc. as well as their flaws and their spirit guides them to finding a calling or purpose, which is usually larger than themselves, in which they are called to love and serve others. This does not mean it has to be a religious calling. For example, it may be being an empathetic hairdresser, where people leave the salon feeling inspired and hopeful, and good about themselves. They have settled the question of the meaning of life for themselves and allow others to follow their own journey.

At this point in the spiritual development, Rohr describes the person *surrendering* to life, to spirit, to God/the Universe/ the Creator/the Divine. Levels 7–9 in spiritual development describe the person letting go more and more of their humanness and becoming more spiritual within society. Here the mystics and spiritual leaders are found. They focus on uplifting society and are willing to make sacrifices for a greater good. Unlike level 3, there is no resentment and they do not suffer burn-out despite hardships. It is like they are plugged into God/the Universe/the Creator/the Divine. They inspire others just by their way of being, and others are naturally drawn to them. Again, it is important to realise it is unlikely that therapists will encounter people on this spiritual developmental level in their consulting rooms.

OCCUPATIONAL THERAPIST WITH MRS H IN PRACTICE

During the first consultation, Mrs H struggled to explain her history systematically and coherently and it seemed her thoughts were confused and contradictory as she tried to make sense of her past. She felt it was impacting her relationship with both daughters and did not have the capacity to take care of her mother, who was suffering from a cognitive disorder. She emphasised that God was important to her, but that God had become distant and she wanted to understand why God would allow the accident to happen.

As Mrs H specifically asked to work spiritually, she selected her own treatment goals, which were to forgive the people responsible for the accident and to draw closer to God as her relationship with God was important to her. As Mrs H was on a spiritual development levels 3–4, the therapist decided to facilitate an adapted 3-step process of forgiveness, as described by Tipping (2009). The therapist used the 3-step process of letter writing combined with hot pen technique. The first step focuses on giving pain a voice. The second step on balancing the two perspectives of being a victim and attempting to put yourself into the 'perpetrator's shoes'. The third step is where God writes a letter to you, from God's perspective. The therapist had included a step 2b – where the client is asked to consider what the client will need to let go of, in order to forgive. For example, give up being self-righteous; give up the victim role and give up external locus of control.

Mrs H attended four therapy sessions, where each forgiveness step was facilitated at each session. The sessions were spread across two months. Mrs H was encouraged to keep a

---

CASE STUDY 1

Mrs H was referred to the therapist because the client wanted a therapist that incorporated spirituality within the treatment context. Her family was concerned that Mrs H was showing the signs of depression and they felt she had not 'dealt with' her daughter's accident. The first consultation focused on obtaining a full history, understanding her beliefs and assessing her level of spiritual development. The assessment revealed:

Her daughter had a tragic accident at age 13 that required multiple operations for internal, abdominal damage, broken pelvis etc. Her daughter had rehabilitation for a long period afterwards learning to walk again. This occurred over 25 years ago. While talking about the accident, it was observed that there were still raw emotions that had not been given a voice.

- Mrs H found out her daughter was pregnant, which she considered a miracle, but was fearful that due to her daughter's previous internal damage she would not carry the baby to term.

- Mrs H felt guilty and blamed herself for the accident.

- Mrs H felt it was time to forgive the people that she held responsible for the accident and whom she had resented and been angry with for almost 25 years.

- Mrs H's background history revealed a lot of changes and loss since the accident.

Taking a closer look at Mrs H's spiritual development, it was found she had experienced a shock point (the first of a string of losses, beginning with her daughter's accident) and she seemed to be stuck between spiritual development levels 3 and 4.

journal to write her thoughts and feelings during the week. Interestingly, as the therapy progressed, Mrs H's focus shifted to forgiving herself. Her last letter from God to her was deeply cathartic, and she shared that she thought all her losses throughout her life were a punishment because of 'her role' (her perception) in her daughter's accident. She believed deep down, which she could never verbalise before, that her life would have been perfect, if she just did not make that terrible mistake of sending her daughter to play with a friend. Her letter from God described how he had been present at each stage, but she did not recognise him through her pain. After the last session, Mrs H felt closer to God and her thoughts, emotions and beliefs settled and found their 'right place'. Therapy was terminated.

PS: It is important to note this adapted 3-step process of forgiveness may not be suitable for all clients. Some clients are so angry that they cannot progress to the second step. Forgiveness cannot be forced and clients are then encouraged to find a way of expressing their anger through multi-medium art. Another caution is that the hot pen technique dedicates that the clients write the letters from their heart and not from their mind. The last letter is difficult to write from a mind space, because 'we don't know what God thinks'.

OCCUPATIONAL THERAPIST WITH MRS A IN PRACTICE

Mrs A's religion was part of her identity; moving further along her spiritual development would be problematic. On level 2, all the group's norms and dictates, in this case her religion, are slavishly followed, and the belief held is *to be a good or holy person, I need to comply*. However, the paradox is that deeply spiritual people and mystics are people who have navigated their way through doubt and have come full circle with a burning heart for God and people.

Mrs A would self-righteously bring religion in her conflict situations, which exacerbated the conflict with her family and community members. She would not allow herself to experience emotions, believing they were 'bad' and her actions were often followed by resentment, doing the 'right thing' for others continuously left her unfulfilled. This in turn made her feel guilty and left to try harder to be 'good' or 'holy'.

Mrs A's therapy was focused on allowing her to become aware of her emotions, of expressing her emotions through creativity and later to verbalise them. These aims were reached through multi-medium collages as an expressive technique. Conflict resolution strategies and tools were imparted, taking time to practice the 'I-language' in conflict situations, focusing on her own feelings and explaining the impact of the other person's behaviour on her. Therapy also facilitated Mrs A to discover her identity in a range of different areas, using collage making with an emphasis on selecting pictures that 'jump out at her', rather than a conscious selection. This taps into the unconscious, as suggested by Jung. Other activities included the 'inside-outside box', uncompleted sentences and using the junk box as projective technique. The activities were used to explore and discover who she was, so that her identity was not exclusively defined by her religion. Other fields of interests and passions were also highlighted. One session focused on different types of prayer, meditation, contemplation, mindful awareness etc. and experiencing samples of these. This was to encourage Mrs A to participate in spiritual practices that did not focus on the 'rules' and did not work for rewards but rather focused on 'just sitting' in God's presence.

As Mrs A's moved to a spiritual development level 3, her anxiety decreased. She implemented the conflict resolution

CASE STUDY 2

A client, Mrs A contacted me requesting to work psycho-spiritually. She said she was in need of healing, and through her explanation, it was observed that her religion was part of her identity. She had attended numerous therapies, but despite all the tools and techniques she had been taught, her anxiety levels remained high. She was often in conflict with her husband, her children and her community members and wanted assistance to know what life choices she needed to make. Her psycho-spiritual development indicated she was on level 2, moving towards level 3 and although there had been a lot of drama in her life, there was no specific shock point.

CASE STUDY 3

Mr P, who is a pastor and was experiencing a crisis of faith, came to seek assistance. He was at the point of leaving his job. He heard that the therapist facilitated healing retreats and wanted to attend. The healing retreat program is designed to facilitate people that have experienced a shock point to move from spiritual development level 3 to level 4. The program focuses on exploring each person's uniqueness, taking a closer look at the image of the divine held by each participant and the impact it has on their spirituality. The retreat exposes retreatants to different types of spiritual practices, creative arts as a dialogue with the divine, forgiveness and drawing closer to the divine and making sense of each person's life story from a spiritual perspective. People from all spiritual beliefs are welcome.

strategies and her relationships improved significantly. She became involved in a support group for women she ran from her home on Friday mornings. Her communication with her husband improved immeasurably as she could verbalise her feelings and use 'I-language' in conflict situations. She was able to stop smothering her children, allowing them more autonomy.

Her treatment lasted about eight months. She attended sessions once every second week for two months, then graded down to once a month and the last two sessions were once every six weeks.

OCCUPATIONAL THERAPIST WITH MR P IN PRACTICE

In one of the first sessions, Mr P became aware that his image of the divine is one of a punitive figure. This was established through the making of a collage with 'My sense of God' as the instruction. The consequence being that Mr P was constantly trying to earn the divine's favour, which he felt could not be achieved. Mr P was asked to write a 'soul letter' and to engage in a left-right hand dialogue with his expressive art, to explore more unconscious material around this experience of the divine and his spirituality. The creative arts dialogue with the divine had the greatest impact on Mr P, as he had a profound spiritual experience of the divine's love for him. Using the life graph exercise, Mr P took a closer look at his life story from a spiritual perspective, which allowed him to view his deeply unhappy childhood with fresh eyes, finding meaning and a renewed purpose for his job. As he put it, '*I found a new calling, within my old job*'. Subsequently, he has flourished moving into a different field within his job, coming out of his shell by not trying to be who others expect him to be, and has a sense of peace surrounding him that others have observed and commented on.

CONCLUSION

This chapter was undertaken to highlight the importance of spirituality and mental health. The relevance of holistic approach in connecting the body, mind and spirit is clearly supported by this chapter. This approach will prove useful in expanding our understanding of how the components are related to each other. The evidence from this chapter suggests that spirituality plays an important role in enhancing mental health, well-being and quality of life. It has been highlighted that therapeutic relationships in mental health enable occupational therapists to collaborate with the mental health users and their families during interventions. This work contributes to existing knowledge of occupational therapy practice by providing possible spiritual history assessment that occupational therapists could use to integrate spirituality in mental health such as FICA©. The chapter adds to the rapidly expanding field of spirituality and mental health by highlighting how occupational therapy models such as CMOP-E could be used to conceptualise the mental health user by considering the person, the environment and the occupations. The insights gained from this chapter may be of assistance to occupational therapists when providing intervention by considering the spiritual journey through the spiritual development theories.

QUESTIONS

1. Explain why holistic approach is important in mental health.

2. What are the benefits of considering spirituality in mental health?

3. Why do therapeutic relationships play an important role in mental health and occupational therapy?

4. What is the spiritual history assessment recommended for occupational therapy and why?

5. Describe why spirituality is a core of the CMOP-E.

6. How can the model be used in mental health?

7. Explain the relevance of the spiritual development model in occupational therapy and mental health.

REFERENCES

American Occupational Therapy Association (AOTA) (2020) Occupational therapy practice framework: domain and process. 4th edn. *American Journal of Occupational Therapy*, **74** (Suppl. 2), 7412410010. https://doi.org/10.5014/ajot.2020.74S2001

Anandarajah, G. & Hight, E. (2001). Spirituality and medical practice: using the HOPE questions as a practical tool for spiritual assessment. *American Family Physician*, **63**(1), 81–89.

Arrey, A.E., Bilsen, J., Lacor, P. & Deschepper, R. (2016) Spirituality/religiosity: a cultural and psychological resource among Sub-Saharan African migrant women with HIV/AIDS in Belgium. *PloS One*, **11**(7), e0159488. https://doi.org/10.1371/journal.pone.0159488

Beng, K.S. (2004) The last hours and days of life: a biopsychosocial-spiritual model of care. *Asia Pacific Family Medicine*, **4**, 1–3.

Borneman, T., Ferrell, B. & Puchalski, C.M. (2010) Evaluation of the FICA tool for spiritual assessment. *Journal of Pain and Symptom Management*, **40**(2), 163–173. https://doi.org/10.1016/j.jpainsymman.2009.12.019

Duncan, E.A.S. (2011) *Foundations for Practice in Occupational Therapy*, 5th edn. Elsevier, Churchill Livingstone.

Forrester-Jones, R., Dietzfelbinger, L., Stedman, D. & Richmond, P. (2018) Including the 'spiritual' within mental health care in the UK, from the experiences of people with mental health problems. *Journal of Religion and Health*, **57**, 384–407. https://doi.org/10.1007/s10943-017-0502-1

Fouché, L. (2021) Transformation through creativity. In: S. Sherwood (ed), *Perspectives on the Vona du Toit Model of Creative Ability*, pp. 196–218. International Creative Ability Network, Great Britain.

Garssen, B., Visser, A. & Pool, G. (2021) Does spirituality or religion positively affect mental health? Meta-analysis of longitudinal studies. *The International Journal for the Psychology of Religion*, **31**(1), 4–20. https://doi.org/10.1080/10508619.2020.1729570

Gyimah, L., Ofori-Atta, A., Asafo, S. & Curry, L. (2023) Seeking healing for a mental illness: understanding the care experiences of service users at a prayer camp in Ghana. *Journal of Religion and Health*, **62**, 1853–1871. https://doi.org/10.1007/s10943-022-01643-0

Hall, S., McKinstry, C. & Hyett, N. (2015) An occupational perspective of youth positive mental health: a critical review. *British Journal of Occupational Therapy*, **78**(5), 276–285. https://doi.org/10.1177/0308022615573540

Hamer, H.P., Kidd, J., Clarke, S., Butler, R. & Lampshire, D. (2017) Citizens uninterrupted: practices of inclusion by mental health service users. *Journal of Occupational Science*, **24**(1), 76–87. https://doi.org/10.1080/14427591.2016.1253497

Hess, K.Y. & Ramugondo, E. (2014) Clinical reasoning used by occupational therapists to determine the nature of spiritual occupations in relation to psychiatric pathology. *British Journal of Occupational Therapy*, **77**(5), 234–242. https://doi.org/10.4276/030802214X13990455043449

Horton, A., Hebson, G. & Holman, D. (2021) A longitudinal study of the turning points and trajectories of therapeutic relationship development in occupational and physical therapy. *BMC Health Services Research*, **21**, 97. https://doi.org/10.1186/s12913-021-06095-y

Hemphill, B. (2015) Spiritual assessments in occupational therapy. *The Open Journal of Occupational Therapy*, **3**(3). https://doi.org/10.15453/2168-6408.1159

Janse van Rensburg, A.B., Poggenpoel, M., Myburgh, C.P. & Szabo, C.P. (2015) Defining and measuring spirituality in South African specialist psychiatry. *Journal of Religion and Health*, **54**(5), 1839–1855. https://doi.org/10.1007/s10943-014-9943-y

Janse van Rensburg, A.B.R. (2014) Integrating spirituality in the approach to psychiatric practice. *South African Journal of Psychiatry*, **20**(4), 131. https://doi.org/10.4102/sajpsychiatry.v20i4.594

Joubert, R. (2019) Theoretical paradigms and influences underpinning the development of the Vona du Toit model of creative ability. In D. van der Reyden, W. Sherwood, & P. de Witt (eds), *VdTMoCA: The Vona du Toit Model of Creative Ability: Origins, Constructs, Principles and Application in Occupational Therapy*, pp. 44–57. The Vona du Toit and Marié du Toit Foundation, Pretoria.

Jung, C.G. (1990) *Memories, Dreams, Reflections*, 7th edn. Flamingo, Glasgow.

Kang, C. (2003) A psychospiritual integration frame of reference for occupational therapy. Part 1: conceptual foundation. *Australian Occupational Therapy Journal*, **50**(2), 92–103.

Kearns Murphy, C. & Shiel, A. (2019) Institutional injustices? Exploring engagement in occupations in a residential mental health facility. *Journal of Occupational Science*, **26**(1), 115–127. https://doi.org/10.1080/14427591.2018.1531780

Kelso-Wright, P. (2012). *Spiritual History Assessment and Occupational Therapy: Students Using FICA*. Masters Thesis. University of Puget Sound, Tacoma, Washington.

Liu, Y., Zemke, R., Liang, L. & Gray, J.M. (2023) Occupational harmony: embracing the complexity of occupational balance. *Journal of Occupational Science*, **30**(2), 145–159, https://doi.org/10.1080/14427591.2021.1881592

Manning, L., Ferris, M., Rosario, C.N., Prues, M. & Bouchard, L. (2019) Spiritual resilience: understanding the protection and promotion of well-being in the later life. *Journal of Religion, Spirituality & Aging*, **31**(2), 168–186. https://doi.org/10.1080/15528030.2018.1532859

Martin, E., Hocking, C. & Sandham, M. (2023) Doing, being, becoming, and belonging: experiences transitioning from bowel cancer patient to survivor. *Journal of Occupational Science*, **30**(2), 277–290. https://doi.org/10.1080/14427591.2020.1827017

Maugans, T. A. (1996) The SPIRITual history. *Archives of Family Medicine*, **5**(1), 11–16. https://doi.org/10.1001/archfami.5.1.11

Moreira-Almeida, A., Koenig, H.G. & Lucchetti, G. (2014) Clinical implications of spirituality to mental health: review of evidence and practical guidelines. *Revista Brasileira de Psiquiatria*, **36**, 176–182.

Mthembu, T.G., Wegner, L. & Roman, N.V. (2017a) Exploring occupational therapy students' perceptions of spirituality in occupational therapy groups. A qualitative study. *Journal of Occupational Therapy in Mental Health*, **33**(2), 141–167. https://doi.org/10.1080/0164212X.2016.1245595

Mthembu, T.G., Wegner, L. & Roman, N.V. (2017b) Spirituality in the occupational therapy community fieldwork process: a qualitative study in the South African context. *South African Journal of Occupational Therapy*, **47**(1), 16–23. https://dx.doi.org/10.17159/2310-3833/2016/v46n3a4

Najafi, K., Khoshab, H., Rahimi, N. & Jahanara, A. (2022) Relationship between spiritual health with stress, anxiety and depression in patients with chronic diseases. *International Journal of Africa Nursing Sciences*, **17**, 100463. https://doi.org/10.1016/j.ijans.2022.100463

Nandika, S.R. & Nagalakshmi, K. (2022) Spirituality as intrinsic motivational factor and health related quality of life among hospitalized male patients practicing Hinduism in India. *Industrial Psychiatry Journal*, **31**(1), 120–125. https://doi.org/10.4103/ipj.ipj_222_20

Patel V. (2015) Addressing social injustice: a key public mental health strategy. *World Psychiatry: Official Journal of the World Psychiatric Association (WPA)*, **14**(1), 43–44. https://doi.org/10.1002/wps.20179

Partti-Enkenberg, S. (2022) *Occupational Justice and Injustice in Persons with Mental Disorder – a Scoping Review*. Thesis Jönköping University School of Health and Welfare, Sweden.

Polatajko, H.J., Townsend, E.A. & Craik, J. (2007) Canadian model of occupational performance and engagement (CMOP-E). In: E.A. Townsend, H.J. Polatajko (eds), *Enabling Occupation II: Advancing an Occupational Therapy Vision of Health, Well-being, & Justice through Occupation*, pp. 22–36. CAOT Publications ACE, Ottawa.

Puchalski, C.M., Vitillo, R., Hull, S.K. & Reller, N. (2014) Improving the spiritual dimension of whole person care: reaching national and international consensus. *Journal of Palliative Medicine*, **17**(6), 642–656. https://doi.org/10.1089/jpm.2014.9427

Puchalski, C. & Romer, A.L. (2000) Taking a spiritual history allows clinicians to understand patients more fully. *Journal of Palliative Medicine*, **3**(1), 129–137. https://doi.org/10.1089/jpm.2000.3.129

Rohr, R. (2009) *Where You are, is Where I'll Meet You: A Guide for Spiritual Directors*. Centre for Action and Contemplation, Albuquerque.

Rogers, M., & Wattis, J. (2020) Understanding the role of spirituality in providing person-centred care. *Nursing Standard (Royal College of Nursing (Great Britain): 1987)*, **35**(9), 25–30. https://doi.org/10.7748/ns.2020.e11342

Roxburgh, E., Ridgway, S. & Roe, C. (2016) Synchronicity in the therapeutic setting: a survey of practitioners. *Counselling and Psychotherapy Research*, **16**, 44–53. https://doi.org/10.1002/capr.12057

Sallam, E.E., El-Sheshtawy, E.A.M., Amr, M.A.M., El-Bahaey, W.A.H. & Okasha, A.M. (2022) The power of spirituality in symptomatic and functional outcomes of patients with major depressive disorder in an Egyptian sample. *Journal of Spirituality in Mental Health*, **25**(3), 232–242. https://doi.org/10.1080/19349637.2022.2130851

Solman, B. & Clouston, T. (2016) Occupational therapy and the therapeutic use of self. *British Journal of Occupational Therapy*, **79**(8), 514–516. https://doi.org/10.1177/0308022616638675

Soomar, N., Mthembu, T.G. & Ramugondo, E. (2018) Occupational therapy association South Africa (OTASA) position statement: spirituality in occupational therapy. *South African Journal of Occupational Therapy*, **48**(3), 64–65.

Tipping, C. (2009) *Radical Forgiveness*. Sounds True, Canada.

Tolosa-Merlos, D., Moreno-Poyato, A.R., González-Palau, F. *et al* (2023) Exploring the therapeutic relationship through the reflective practice of nurses in acute mental health units: a qualitative study. *Journal of Clinical Nursing*, **32**, 253–263. https://doi.org/10.1111/jocn.16223

United Nations (2023) *Sustainable development goals*. Goal 3: Ensure health lives and promote well-being for all at all ages. https://www.un.org/sustainabledevelopment/health/ (accessed 31 May 2023)

Van Denend, J., Ford, K., Berg, P., Edens, E.L. & Cooke, J. (2022) The body, the mind, and the spirit: including the spiritual domain in mental health care. *Journal of Religion and Health*, **61**(5), 3571–3588. https://doi.org/10.1007/s10943-022-01609-2

Van der Watt, A.S.J., van de Water, T., Nortje, G. *et al* (2018) The perceived effectiveness of traditional and faith healing in the treatment of mental illness: a systematic review of qualitative studies. *Social Psychiatry and Psychiatric Epidemiology*, **53**(6), 555–566. https://doi.org/10.1007/s00127-018-1519-9

Wicks, A. (2005) Understanding occupational potential. *Journal of Occupational Science*, **12**(3), 130-139. https://doi.org/10.1080/14427591.2005.9686556

Wilding C. (2007) Spirituality as sustenance for mental health and meaningful doing: a case illustration. *The Medical Journal of Australia*, **186**(S10), S67–S69. https://doi.org/10.5694/j.1326-5377.2007.tb01046.x

Wilding, C., May, E. & Muir-Cochrane, E. (2005) Experience of spirituality, mental illness and occupation: a life-sustaining phenomenon. *Australian Occupational Therapy Journal*, **52**, 2–9. https://doi.org/10.1111/j.1440-1630.2005.00462.x

World Health Organisation (2023) *Promoting wellbeing*. https://www.who.int/activities/promoting-well-being (accessed 19 June 2024)

World Health Organisation (2022a) *The geneva charter for wellbeing*. https://cdn.who.int/media/docs/default-source/health-promotion/geneva-charter-4-march-2022.pdf?sfvrsn=f55dec7_21&download=true (accessed 31 May 2023)

World Health Organisation (2022b) *Mental health*. https://www.who.int/news-room/fact-sheets/detail/mental-health-strengthening-our-response (accessed 31 May 2023)

World Health Organisation (2021) *Comprehensive Mental Health Action Plan 2013–2030*. World Health Organisation, Geneva. file:///C:/Users/Admin/Downloads/9789240031029-eng.pdf (accessed 31 May 2023)

Children, Adolescents and Adults

Early Intervention for Young Children at Risk for Developmental Mental Health Disorders

CHAPTER 16

Kerry Wallace

Therapy SPOT, Early Intervention Centre, Perth, Australia
SPOTlight Trust SA, Cape Town, South Africa
DIR→:FCD™ Trainer's certificate

KEY LEARNING POINTS

- Evidence-based practice in the treatment of developmental disorders.

- An axis-based diagnosis to provide a roadmap for intervention through the life span.

- The role of occupational therapists in early intervention.

- Occupational therapy assessment of children with developmental disorders.

- Framework for occupational therapy intervention.

INTRODUCTION

Providing a framework for identifying and early intervention for infants and young children at risk for developmental and mental health disorders (0–4 years) requires a broad knowledge base. Many factors could influence the child's ability to participate in age-appropriate occupations, including activities of daily living, rest, sleep, play and social participation across home, preschool, and community environments. Underlying sensory, motor, social and process skills, considering their biological differences in body structures and functions, need to be investigated (AOTA 2020).

RATIONALE FOR EARLY INTERVENTION

During infancy and early childhood, the brain grows fast, forming the relationships between its components to form synaptic connections (Siegel 1999; Tierney & Nelson 2009). A wealth of behavioural markers is now identifiable during the first two years of life, indicating a significant likelihood that an infant might be diagnosed with a neurodevelopmental condition (Zwaigenbaum et al. 2005). Early intervention induces accelerated learning, capitalising on neuroplasticity (changes in neural pathways and synapses) (Ratey 2002).

EVIDENCE-BASED PRACTICE

In the 21st century, there has been a plethora of new information in this field supporting the need for evidence-based practice. Treatment models are abundant for children at risk for mental health and neurodevelopmental conditions. Still, every child is unique, and no one approach is suitable for all children as they grow. Too often, parents making important choices for their children are overwhelmed by various options. Other parents may need access to more resources in their area where practitioners are trained in only one approach, for example, an outdated behavioural model (American Medical Association House of Delegates [AMA] 2023), rather than

Crouch and Alers Occupational Therapy in Psychiatry and Mental Health, Sixth Edition.
Edited by Rosemary Crouch, Tania Buys, Enos Morankoana Ramano, Matty van Niekerk and Lisa Wegner.
© 2025 John Wiley & Sons Ltd. Published 2025 by John Wiley & Sons Ltd.

across several disciplines and models. Developmental models individualised to the child's specific differences in sensory processing, motor and emotional development that are relationship-based effectively address functional developmental delays (Sandbank *et al.* 2020). The intervention must be age-appropriate and symptom-specific to minimise maladaptive plasticity (Novak *et al.* 2017). The Autism Cooperative Research Centre's umbrella review provides a list of interventions that stand up to peer review (Whitehouse *et al.* 2020).

ETIOLOGICAL EVIDENCE

The origin of mental health conditions is largely polygenetic and frequently present in conjunction with an emotional regulatory disorder, persistent attention deficits and a sensory processing disorder (Bayrami *et al.* 2007). Epigenetic factors are also highly significant in understanding the cause of challenging behaviours. These include prenatal exposure to toxins or stress, prematurity and infants subjected to trauma or deprivation very early in life when the brain is developing most rapidly (Fagiolini *et al.* 2009).

THE NEUROSCIENCE EVIDENCE

Methodological advances have provided new insights and much-needed evidence for long-held occupational therapy treatment assumptions since most brain connections develop postnatally. Intensive early intervention programs that focus on treating underlying issues such as sensory processing (Lane & Schaaf 2010), motor development (Damiano & Longo 2021), emotional development (Cullinane 2020) and the development of caregiver–child attachment can forge neurological changes that can affect long-term functionality. Treatment of the infant/child and parent dyad in their natural environments as they participate in the everyday routines makes occupational therapy intervention one of the first lines of treatment.

THE NEUROPSYCHOLOGICAL EVIDENCE

Research shows that a consistent relationship with an attuned caregiver can repair social–emotional deficits caused by genetic or environmental factors (Tronick & Beeghly 2011). This primary relationship is the model for future relationships, and everyday experiences build the foundation for thought and language development in young children. These emotionally rich experiences build the brain architecture (Ratey 2002). Understanding the functional, emotional developmental stages seen in typically developing children enables occupational therapists to identify how to intervene and support families when there are social–emotional challenges (Harvard University 2011). Understanding the reasons behind their child's behaviour enables the occupational therapist to provide parental support and strategies to address early signs of mental health issues.

A DEVELOPMENTAL HYPOTHESIS FOR THE MANIFESTATION OF PSYCHIATRIC DISORDERS

The Interdisciplinary Council for Developmental and Learning Disorders hypothesises that symptoms among children with special needs come from the same core but with different variations (ICDL-DMIC 2005). The concept of co-morbidity, which creates the illusion that these are separate and distinct biomedical diseases, is unnecessary, as in most instances, there is no known specific genetic cause for each pattern. The theory of epigenetic phenomena, 'nurture', which turns genes on and off, for example environmental factors, which operate when 'nature' has prepared the way, is supported. Motor, sensory and affective processing difficulties are often the manifestation of genetic-biological differences. The emphasis is placed on the role of parents with genetically vulnerable children to change the children's developmental trajectory and optimise their developmental potential (Greenspan & Wieder 2006).

DEVELOPMENTAL PATHWAY TO ANXIETY

Anxiety is a common yet misunderstood symptom whose origin we need to understand so that it does not become a lifelong mental health problem. Firstly, is anxiety primarily related to child–caregiver interactions? When a known stressor or trauma has occurred, a traumatic stress disorder diagnosis takes precedence. Secondly, is the anxiety primarily related to anticipated developmental transitions or tasks the child has difficulty mastering? Or thirdly, is the anxiety associated with a regulatory sensory processing disorder? Hypersensitivity towards the environment leads to anxiety (Lane *et al.* 2012). Often, children with difficulties in multiple sensory processing areas (Dunn & Brown 1997) show increased anxiety. In addressing the issue, when a toddler experiences anxiety, the adult caregiver, who also becomes alarmed and anxious, makes the child feel more anxious. Alternatively, the caregiver can counterbalance the anxiety by calming the child down (ICDL-DMIC 2005).

DEVELOPMENTAL PATHWAY TO DEPRESSION

The biological tendency of over-reactivity, related to sensory sensitivity, is often seen in children predisposed to depression. When a child overreacts, the caregiver may freeze and be expressionless. Poor pattern recognition results and the child feels isolated and alone. Alternatively, the caregiver shows empathy towards the child using a soothing affect so the child can tolerate their discomfort. The latter outcome is very different because there is pattern recognition, as the child feels nurtured and understood. The child can begin to rely on these feelings, the warm internal security blanket, when feeling empty or lonely and feels disappointment and sadness instead of depression. Suppose the problem is not dealt with appropriately at this early stage. In that case, it can escalate through the functional developmental stages and manifest in a full depressive episode in later life (ICDL-DMIC 2005).

DEVELOPMENTAL PATHWAY TO BIPOLAR PATTERNS

The biological tendency of a fluctuating pattern that swings from under-reactivity to over-reactivity to sensation leads to anxiety. Instead of sensory avoidance, there tends to be a switch to sensory craving patterns, particularly in the vestibular system. These children tend to have stronger auditory and language processing capacities than visual-spatial capacities (Dunn & Brown 1997). They also show difficulties mastering co-regulated affective signalling with their caregivers in the first and second years of life. These tendencies, coupled with caregivers that struggle to contain their emotional lability sufficiently, lead to hyper-reactivity and mood swings or bipolar patterns (Greenspan & Glovinski 2002; ICDL-DMIC 2005).

DEVELOPMENTAL PATHWAY TO ATTENTION DEFICIT HYPERACTIVITY DISORDER (ADHD)

The biological tendency of craving sensation in a child with associated motor planning and sequencing challenges (Dunn & Brown 1997; Lane *et al.* 2012) is common in children later diagnosed with ADHD. When the child becomes very active and has sensory cravings, the caregiver can become frazzled and ignore the child, resulting in the child being over-reactive. Alternatively, suppose the caregiver plays regulating games at the child's activity level. In that case, the child learns self-regulation by slowing down the child's activity and teaching them how to regulate and control their activity level. In addition, through occupational therapy, the child's motor planning and sequencing abilities can be increased by engaging in long chains of interactions. Unpredictable caregiving patterns can also result in high activity and distractibility. In contrast, under-reactive children are more likely to live in a fantasy world and struggle to develop authentic relationships, becoming inattentive. These children need to be energised and engaged in long chains of communication (ICDL-DMIC 2005).

DEVELOPMENTAL PATHWAY TO OBSESSIVE-COMPULSIVE DISORDER

The biological tendency of hypersensitivity, with strengths in visual-spatial capacities, manifests in children who want to control the world. Power struggles with a caregiver can develop when a child desires control and manifest in rigidity, stubborn behaviour, negativism, inflexibility and obsessive or compulsive patterns. Alternatively, the caregiver can counterbalance the controlling response by negotiating, resulting in more flexibility and the child feeling more in charge of their own body and environment (ICDL-DMIC 2005).

DEVELOPMENTAL PATHWAY TO OPPOSITIONAL-DEFIANT DISORDER

The biological tendency of a sensory craving pattern, but occasionally over-reactivity to sensation, can manifest in aggression due to fear. The child with sensory craving patterns who experiences punitive caregiving, or perhaps isolation, as in foster homes, where there is no intimacy, may turn to aggressive behaviours without consciousness of the effect of their behaviour and lack compassion for others. This child needs long chains of interactions, counterbalancing games and setting limits early in life so that it does not lead to aggression later. Limit setting or boundaries give barriers for containment and, thus, safety, but must be done appropriately (ICDL-DMIC 2005).

DEVELOPMENTAL PATHWAY TO AUTISM SPECTRUM DISORDER

The biological tendency is of an extreme sensory craving pattern (Dunn & Brown 1997) or extreme sensory hyper-responsivity (Lane *et al.* 2012), coupled with severe motor planning problems and visual-spatial processing difficulties or auditory–language difficulties. The pathway between affect and motor planning is poorly developed (Lane *et al.* 2012; Boshoff *et al.* 2020).

A COMPREHENSIVE FUNCTIONAL INTERVENTION PLAN

EARLY IDENTIFICATION

The following red flags help occupational therapists assess at-risk children in the 0- to 4-year age group who need early intervention (Table 16.1). The Bayley Scales of Infant and Toddler Development Fourth Edition enables an OT to assess cognitive, language, motor, social-emotional development and adaptive behaviour. It includes the Greenspan Social-emotional Growth Chart (2004) to document the social–emotional developmental trajectory from 0 to 4 years. When signs of a plateau or regression occur, refer them to an appropriate therapist for evaluation and therapy (Greenspan 2004).

DIAGNOSIS

Parents whose children are later diagnosed with developmental disorders relate that before their child's first birthday, they suspected something was amiss. A 'wait and see' attitude is counter-productive because providing intervention to these children will likely deliver better outcomes in reducing long-term disability than waiting until diagnostic behavioural symptoms emerge in later years (Zwaigenbaum *et al.* 2015). Paediatricians, general family practitioners and nurses who run well-baby clinics could identify at-risk children. The first step is a medical investigation to rule out a treatable condition. Irrespective of a diagnosis, for these children to achieve cost-effective, long-term, positive functional outcomes, a referral to a paediatric occupational, physical or speech and language therapist who can provide family support and swift, symptom-specific early intervention is the following step (Chasson *et al.* 2007; Peters-Scheffer *et al.* 2012).

Table 16.1 Red flags indicating the need for early assessment and intervention.

Sensory hyper-responsiveness (defensive)

Mother cannot soothe her child

Colic beyond six months or reflux

Poor regulation of sleep/wake cycles

Picky eater, gags at sight, smell and taste of food

Cries to noise, shields eyes to lights

Labile in situations with lots of people, noise and movement

Demonstrates fight, flight or freeze behaviour

Refuses to walk on sand and grass, uncomfortable getting messy or dirty

Gets wild with loud music, high energy and high affect

Sensory under-responsiveness

It needs high affect and high energy interactions to respond.

High pain tolerance

Misses visual or auditory cues

Sensory avoidant

Withdrawn and self-absorbed, seems lost

Slow to wake and lethargic

Sensory seeking

Excessive self-rocking, jumping, pounding, making sounds

Overfills mouth, poor chewing and swallowing, craves extreme tastes

Seeks extreme sensations, even those that are painful

Crashes into objects and people

Self-stimulates on visual or motor actions

Postural control and motor difficulties

Low muscle tone, floppy and sluggish

Head lag, weak neck muscles

Poor eye contact, neck and eye control

Clumsy, uncoordinated

Awkward body positioning – does not self-correct

Cannot stand or sit still without leaning against objects or people.

Can run and may climb but struggles to learn ball skills.

Poor hand usage for manipulating objects.

Poorly coordinated use of two hands.

Poor planning and organisation

Cries in new situations, shy, fearful, cautious

Tolerates transitions poorly

Rigid, inflexible and repetitive behaviours

Poor imitation of gestures, finger or facial play

Immature play routines, limited play repertoire, repeats familiar scenarios.

Difficulty following instructions, can't track time sequences

Poor organisation of space, organisation of belongings and construction

Due to the overlap between the symptoms of the various neurodevelopmental conditions, the diagnosis is less important because the symptoms change as development unfolds. Over time, the changing support needs of the child and family require a long-term transdiagnostic approach and collaboration between various healthcare professionals (Evans *et al.* 2022). A holistic multidisciplinary assessment, followed by a clinical formulation and recommendations for a comprehensive intervention programme that is both individual and family-centred, with a lifespan perspective, takes time to formulate (Autism CRC 2021).

Parents described a five-stage journey before, during and after a diagnosis of a neurodevelopmental condition. They progressed through 'searching' for an explanation, 'waiting' for the diagnostic evaluation, 'investigating' the signs and symptoms, 'knowing' that their child has a neurodevelopmental condition and 'accessing' support (Evans *et al.* 2022). They experience frustration due to their lack of understanding of the process, so they need collaboration between professionals and targeted support through this process. Parents experience grief and loss at the time of diagnosis or 'high-risk' notification, and therefore, communication with a family should be a series of well-planned and compassionate conversations. Communication should be face-to-face, with both parents or caregivers present (where appropriate), private, honest, jargon-free, with empathic communication tailored to the family, followed by written information, identification of strengths, the invitation to ask questions, discussion of feelings, recommendations to use parent-to-parent support and arrangement of early intervention (Novak *et al.* 2017).

A TRANSDISCIPLINARY APPROACH

As healthcare practitioners have become more specialised, transferring information, knowledge and skills across disciplines can alleviate many issues. In a trans-disciplinary approach (King *et al.* 2009), assessments are carried out as 'an arena evaluation' so all members see the same sample of behaviour.

The designated case manager takes a detailed case history and transcribes or takes video footage of a play-based assessment in the child's natural environment in the company of familiar family members. In this way, a sample of the child's best functioning level is seen and indicates the child's prognosis. In contrast, exposing a young child to unfamiliar faces and an unfamiliar environment using standardised tests can create heightened anxiety and highlight the child's worst level of functioning with possibly an unrealistically unfavourable prognosis. Treatment of the young child needs to be within the context of their family because of the safety that this relationship affords. The OT forms a working alliance with the family regarding their expectations, hopes and dreams for their child. Therapists must be fully present in body and mind and emotionally available, with the child as the sole focus of attention, so a therapeutic relationship is possible.

The trans-disciplinary team uses the following principles:

- Through active listening and clarification, reflect helpful information to the family.

- Affirmation of the parents' observations.

- The OT contains emotions by being present through negative emotions without changing anything.

- Mindfulness, being attuned and responding contingently to the child's emotions.

- The OT needs to manage professional boundaries.

- The OT must stay present in the moment within the relationship (King et al. 2009).

COMPONENTS OF A MULTIDISCIPLINARY ASSESSMENT

A review of the child's current functioning with parents and caregivers, looking at both presenting problems and the child's adaptive capacities, should include:

- A detailed prenatal, perinatal, and postnatal developmental history.

- A developmental history with details of the child's functioning in all areas of their life.

- A family history of mental health issues.

- Discussion around functional developmental capacities is the child's capacity for shared attention, engagement, communication, play and thinking.

- Discuss the child's processing capacities, for example, sensory modulation, auditory processing capacities, motor planning, sequencing and visuospatial capacities.

- Discussion around variations in relevant contexts, for example at home with caregivers and siblings, with peers and in educational settings.

- Two or more observations of the child and caregiver interactions for 45 minutes.

The clinicians develop a hypothesis about the child's functional emotional developmental capacities, individual sensory processing, motor planning differences and interactive family patterns and prioritise the child and family's needs. A referral to the appropriate therapist is the next step in the process. The choice of a key therapist would be based on the parent's priorities and could be an OT, speech or physiotherapist or psychologist.

THE OCCUPATIONAL THERAPIST'S ROLE IN THE ASSESSMENT PROCESS

The occupational therapist's role encompasses a consultant, a model and a coach to the significant adults, including the child's parents and teachers, in natural environments. Therefore, the assessment may not only occur in a therapy centre but also in the child's home, on the playground, in the classroom, in the shopping centre or at the beach, wherever the child faces difficulties due to their specific challenges.

A parent meeting is necessary so the parents can voice their concerns and provide more detailed information about their child's medical, developmental, sensory processing and social history. These could include an infant's sleep behaviour, where when and how and sleep positions or parental expectations for acceptable levels of night waking. There is a variation between different cultural groups. Issues such as the child being carried by the parent and at what age toilet training is the norm vary. The culture of play, namely, who plays with the children, is also a variable. Some parents do not play with their children and expect peers, older or younger children, to play with the child.

Observing the young child in unstructured play with their parents/caregivers helps ascertain the child's best level of function and determine the intervention's starting point. The Functional Emotional Assessment Scales (FEAS) is a valuable assessment tool whereby video footage of the child in the clinic and their familiar home environment is analysed to gain a more comprehensive and realistic overall impression of the child's best level of function and challenges (Greenspan & Wieder 2006).

Cultural factors, including societal norms and expectations surrounding a family's habits and daily routines, must be considered. The OT may take the case manager role when working in isolation or in an under-resourced community. Consultation with a psychologist or a speech and language therapist may be necessary. However, as the primary therapist, the OT would share their recommendations with the family.

FRAMEWORK FOR ASSESSMENT

Occupational therapists working in this age group with children at risk for mental health challenges need to assess the child's specific sensory and motor differences that are biologically based and the child's social-emotional development.

SYNCHRONY OF SENSORY PROCESSING AND REGULATORY CAPACITIES

Behaviour reflects the child's neurobiological state in response to stimuli from their body and environment during social interaction. Therefore, a deep understanding of the child's differences in sensory processing and the effect on regulating behaviour is critical. The child's physiological and emotional responses to the sense of touch, sense of movement or muscle and joint action, awareness of position in space, as well as reactions to the sights and sounds of the world and sense of taste and smell will manifest emotionally in their behaviour, which is how infants and young children communicate. The parent's capacity for emotional co-regulation through emotional texture and affective tone will determine the child's ability to tolerate and eventually self-regulate their response to extreme sensations and emotions. The child's development of a feeling of control will foster a sense of self-confidence and the capacity for self-regulation across a range of emotions and circumstances (White 2010). Parent consultation, observations and the use of standardised instruments such as the Infant-Toddler Sensory Profile provide this information (Dunn 2014).

MOTOR CONTROL FOR FUNCTION

Understanding the child's differences in postural development and motor control, which enable the child to regulate and direct the mechanisms essential to movement, is vital. Motor control develops in the context of the rhythms of interaction with an available and responsive caregiver who responds to the intent of the infant and the developing child. Motor control encompasses the development of a body schema, an internal sense of the relationship of the body parts to each other and the response to their base of support. It enables the child to explore their environment and sets the stage for praxis, and intentional action (White 2010). Assessment is through parent consultation, observations and standardised assessment tools such as Bayley Scales of Infant and Toddler Development-4 (Bayley & Aylward 2020).

PRAXIS AND EXECUTIVE FUNCTIONS

Sensory perceptions and motor control lay the foundation for voluntary movement and praxis, encompassing motor planning, sequencing, execution and adaptability. Ideation requires thinking and conceiving an idea with clear goals and purpose (executive functions) (Schaaf & Smith-Roley 2006). Motor planning is the ability to plan and organise the sequence of the steps necessary to successfully execute the idea (executive function) (Schaaf & Smith-Roley 2006). Both ideation and planning depend on accurate information from the body and environment, including vision, sound, touch and muscle and joint information. Motor execution requires initiating and coordinating the motor actions related to an idea or motor plan. Adaption constantly occurs as one compares feedback from the body with the initial plan and enables the child to adapt throughout the ongoing process (Schaaf & Smith-Roley 2006; White 2010). Assessment is through consultation with parents and observations.

FRAMEWORK FOR OCCUPATIONAL THERAPY INTERVENTION

Treatment options are abundant for the range of symptoms, applicable at different stages of the child's development with varying levels of evidence (Whitehouse *et al.* 2020). The therapist is responsible for providing this information to the child's caregivers so they can make an informed decision about what suits their child and family's needs.

Within family-centred practice, the occupational therapist's role has broadened. They are the child's therapist, the playmate who models interactions at their developmental level and supports parents, siblings, teachers and extended family members in fostering therapeutic interactions in natural environments so they can implement therapeutic principles across all settings. The OT is a counsellor to the caregivers, enabling them to understand and manage their child's behaviour. The OT is also an advocate for child and family services. Interventions must be embedded in the child's natural home and school environments to achieve functional outcomes, including the parents and caregivers in the therapeutic process, empowering them to apply treatment principles to all routines and aspects of the child's daily life to enable the generalisation of skills. Flexibility in the treatment environment can range from consultations in the therapy clinic to conducting sessions in natural settings, the child's home, classroom, playground or wherever challenges present and facilitation is required. The OT must constantly reflect on their approach as the child progresses and as the child's needs change, continually adjusting the goals to move in the direction of age-appropriate activities that would be part of the routines of a typically developing child.

GENERAL PRINCIPLES OF TREATMENT

For the process of emotional maturation to unfold and for the child to function optimally, the child needs to be able to self-regulate arousal, attention and affect, to execute the action (Williams & Anzalone 2001).

REGULATION OF AROUSAL STATE

To engage with others, have meaningful relationships and learn, the child needs to be in an optimal state between quiet and active alert. If the child is under-aroused (drowsy) or tired, he requires intensity, touch, facial expression, tone of voice and movement to increase alertness. When the child is over-aroused, anxious or overexcited, rhythmical movement, calming touch and a soothing tone of voice will help lower their arousal state.

MASTERY OF ACTIVITIES OF DAILY LIVING

Interoception is the sensory system that gives human beings information regarding body-emotion connections. It enables people to feel many significant sensations, including pain, body temperature, itch, hunger, thirst, heart rate, breathing rates, muscle tension, sleepiness, sensory overload, the need to use the toilet and sexual arousal are crucial in functional adaptation to the demands of daily life (Mahler 2017). Interoceptive awareness helps humans notice body signals and connect them to emotions, excitement, joy, fear, safety, love and anxiety. An infant who feels hungry or thirsty communicates his discomfort by crying. The responsive caregiver meets his needs and is rewarded by the infant smiling.

Thus, interoceptive awareness is the foundation that drives the attachment process.

Conversely, adult caregivers may not understand the child's reduced awareness or oversensitivity to interoceptive signals. Emotional dysregulation or social challenges can be mistakenly attributed to behaviour instead of understanding the child's physiology and can disrupt the attachment process (Flipetti 2021). Building interoceptive awareness can enhance self-regulation strategies (Kuypers 2021) by developing a clear and timely urge for action. It is about developing that intuitive understanding of what an internal signal means and what is causing it. It is about creating the ability to comfort and balance, which is when true independence can occur. Therefore, in many cases, it is imperative to consider an individual's level of interoceptive awareness during the OT evaluation and treatment process (Mahler 2017).

SHARED ATTENTION

To be able to pay attention, the child needs to be alert and orientated to the person and task and have the capacity for shared attention with another person, as was first experienced in the intimacy of relationships with primary caregivers. The next step is to experience joint attention on a desirable object with another person. Typically, this occurs between 15 and 24 months of age and is a stepping-stone to shift attention (Reddy 2007).

AFFECT-BASED INTERACTIONS

Central to the approach is the principle of affect-based interactions throughout all aspects of the child's life, ensuring that all interventions facilitate the child's development and support family functioning. Regulation of affect is one of the most critical aspects of high-risk infants and young children. Affect involves the emotional response to sensory input and social-based emotions in relationships (Duncan & Barrett 2007). There can be atypical heightened or depressed responses to sensory input. These responses can influence the formation of primary attachment relationships or disrupt the child's ability to be influenced by their social environment, not only because of the atypical responses but also because of how the parents may interpret the child's responses (Holloway 1998). As the child develops intentions and ideas in co-regulated interactions with others, he will become more adaptable across a broader range of experiences and environments. Regulation of behaviour is, therefore, a balance between self and co-regulation with an attuned caregiver (Holloway 1998).

PLAY

Play is the vehicle for intervention as children learn to think and develop language (Vygotsky 1978). Occupational therapy should be child-directed and the OT should follow the child's lead and interests. The goal is to increase interaction in emotionally meaningful learning experiences, characterised by high interest and motivation. The OT needs to be flexible to get optimal participation and to stop the game when it is no longer fun. Building real-life experiences based on what is meaningful for the child fulfils the aim of building functional developmental capacities. Therapy, therefore, needs to be embedded into the child's daily routines and all interactions. Development is complex, cumulative, and reliant on experiences and spirals in an upward and outward direction, so a constant review is necessary.

The formation of attachment relationships, purposeful communication, understanding causal relationships and the development of self-initiated organised behaviours depend on the modulation of sensory reactivity, emotional responsiveness, attention and praxis (Williams & Anzalone 2001).

FACILITATE FUNCTIONAL, EMOTIONAL AND DEVELOPMENT

Children with special needs grow through the same levels as any other children, except children with developmental delays will go through each stage at a later chronological age. The first six stages of the functional emotional development of the child typically unfold during the first four years of life. They are:

Stage 1: Regulation and Shared Attention (0–3 months),
Stage 2: Engagement and Relating (4–5 months),
Stage 3: Purposeful Emotional Interactions (6–9 months),
Stage 4: Social Problem Solving (10–18 months),
Stage 5: Symbols, Words and Ideas (19–30 months),
Stage 6: Building Bridges between Ideas (31–42 months)
  (Greenspan *et al.* 2003; DelaHooke 2019).

Affect-based learning is critical to enable the child to simultaneously mobilise all the first four goals and strengthen underlying functional capacities that are only partially mastered (Greenspan 2004). Recognising these levels gives vital clues on engaging effectively with each child. The occupational therapist's role is to support the parents to join their child at their developmental level. Their job is to read the child's cues and gestures, which can often be very subtle, like reading body language, expression in the eyes, language, or sounds. Often, these factors give clues as to which activities the therapist could offer the child.

Reading the child's mood or expressed feelings and responding in an attuned manner are essential. Following the child's lead, parents learn how to be with their child, 'to wait and watch' so that the child can express interests and anticipate engagement with others. Some parents have their agenda for how their child will spend their time and shifting to child-led play will take practice.

When a child is at a lower level of functioning, the focus is on 'engagement and regulation of feelings', so the child might play physical games that stimulate the sensory-motor system. Parents must concentrate their efforts on the child's mutual attention and engagement. By calmly joining the child's activity by gently connecting with them, they will not only enjoy the experience but may invite others to join in. Parents can work on securing and maintaining attention and strengthening bonds of engagement and intimacy.

In a child-centred developmental approach, the child customises their play based on their interests and abilities. In responding to individual attention, the child initiates interaction to meet their needs through simple non-verbal communication. In the higher levels of functioning, the child is learning to think symbolically, and adults might present problems for the child to solve. In the ability to sustain a long continuous flow of interaction with another person, the emerging 'sense of self' and the capacity to be a 'problem solver' are supported. The emergence of language symbols underlies the ability to represent. It is the foundation for developing symbolic play, supporting logical connections and abstract thinking.

Increasing or decreasing the intensity enables the child to be calm and regulated. The OT needs to be empathetic and mirror the child's feelings, whether they are positive or negative. By working up the functional and emotional development levels, the child will reach a point where thinking and multiple problem-solving can occur. Creating a solid emotional–social foundation aims to facilitate thought and affect-based learning rather than rote learning (Greenspan & Wieder 1997, 2006).

ADDRESSING INDIVIDUAL DIFFERENCES IN SENSORY PROCESSING AND MOTOR PLANNING

The OT is primarily responsible for managing the child's underlying individual differences in sensory processing and motor planning that affect development on all levels.

The therapist needs to constantly adjust the intensity of sensory challenges to suit the child's differences, considering slow processing and motor planning challenges, so pacing is crucial. The OT uses her body to create physical gestural problems for the child to solve. By building logical sequences and scaffolding, communication and thinking will follow. The objectives are to increase the child's range of experiences, including gestures and behaviours, mediate the process through communication, and aim for a long, continuous flow in the interaction. The therapist's role is to elaborate on the child's play and deepen the plot, encouraging the child to respond. By reflecting on what the child is doing or thinking rather than asking questions, an expansion of the child's problem-solving skills will be supported (White 2010).

OCCUPATIONAL THERAPY IN THE CONTEXT OF RELATIONSHIPS

The infant's primary survival drive is to develop a relationship with a highly attuned caregiver who can co-regulate interactions with their world through physiological maturation, caregiver responsiveness and the infant's adaption to environmental demands. The occupational therapist's role is to model sensory–affective modulation, starting with shared attention, engagement, reciprocity, development of a sense of self and representational and symbolic play. Coaching parents to enable them to support their children in moving up the developmental ladder is important (Kasari *et al.* 2006). Solid foundations pave the way for interactions with peers and emotionally robust relationships.

BEHAVIOURAL STRATEGIES

Behaviour can be a response to a disturbance in the external or internal environment of the child and is an opportunity for parents to help their child problem-solve what is stimulating this response. Assume a child's behaviour expresses emotional needs, pleasure, or discomfort. Negative behaviour is often due to dysregulation or an assault on their system. Essentially, it is a cry for help! Punishing or ignoring often makes things worse as the underlying reason for the behaviour remains unresolved. This results in the negative behaviour escalating. Understanding the behaviour as a way of communicating an emotional need is critical.

Porges (2011) developed the 'Polyvagal Theory' to describe the process in which the child's neural circuits (autonomic nervous system) read cues of safety, danger, or life threat in the environment, a term he called 'neuroception'. 'Neuroception is the nervous system's way of sensing what is happening in the body, environment and between two people in a relationship' (Porges 2011, pp. 193–194). Trauma interrupts the process of building the autonomic circuitry of safe connection and side-tracks the development of regulation and resilience. Polyvagal theory gives therapists a neurophysiological framework to consider how children act in the ways they do (Dana 2018).

When ventral vagal activation occurs, the child will exhibit 'Social engagement' cues that their adult caregivers can understand. These include bright, shiny eyes, direct eye contact, smiling, laughing, a relaxed posture, good muscle tone and coordinated movements. The child is at ease and has the attitude that they can manage whatever comes their way. They feel safe, empowered and connected. They can see the 'big picture' and connect to the world and its people (Dana 2018).

When there is sympathetic activation of the ventral vagal system, an alarm is triggered, and the child will be frantic, agitated and mobilised. 'Fight or flight' cues include high-pitched crying, out-of-control laughing, body tension, biting, hitting, kicking, and clenched jaw and teeth, indicating the sympathetic nervous system takes over. The child feels overwhelmed and is having a hard time keeping up. They feel anxious and irritated, and their world seems dangerous, chaotic and unfriendly (Dana 2018).

When dorsal vagal activation occurs, the child feels numb, collapsed and may shut down. 'Shutdown' cues include gaze aversion, a flat facial expression, a slumped posture, and a frozen or slow-moving rate of movement when the parasympathetic system is activated. The child feels buried under a considerable load and cannot escape. They feel alone in their despair. The world is empty, dead and dark (Dana 2018).

Behaviours are just the tip of the iceberg and are signals of what children are experiencing inside of their bodies and brains (Delahooke 2019). Negative behaviour is usually not wilful. When children act out, aggressive behaviour that may result in harm causes remorse later. Children with developmental disorders tend to respond in an extreme way, such as engaging in aggressive or self-injurious behaviour out of frustration. They may use repetitive behaviour to soothe themselves or self-absorption in the case of flicking wheels. Performance anxiety may instigate oppositional behaviour triggered by demands. Learning as much as possible about the environment, the child's internal and external world and what might be stimulating the behaviour should provide the necessary clues for intervention. Exploring the issue requires thoughtful investigation by the therapist and adult caregiver (Robinson 2011).

If stress-related behaviour increases, ask the parents to keep a log record of this on a calendar and note when it occurs. Identify the time of day, week, weekends or school holidays. Note whether these episodes are related to challenges the child faces in the school environment that may need extra support. Identify whether it is a new or old pattern of behaviour. If it is a new behaviour, rule out any medical problem and review anxiety caused by environmental changes. A family event, teacher, classroom or seating change, a new child acting out, or bullying that makes the child uncomfortable could be the trigger. The increased academic challenge also has a significant influence. Changes in the sensory environment, primarily visual and auditory stimuli, are most disruptive, especially where sensory defensiveness is apparent. A collaborative, proactive problem-solving approach that includes the child and parent or teacher is required to understand and resolve the underlying reason for the problem (Greene 2021).

Encourage the caregivers to prepare a 'rescue kit'. These include brushes, weighted items, videos, books, music and favourite toys that can be left in the car or taken to school in the child's schoolbag for emergency self-regulation (Robinson 2011).

CONCLUSION

Current evidence based on research, as well as a functional, developmental model for understanding and dealing with young children with developmental and mental health disorders, has been explored. Based on this framework, the OT develops a hypothesis using the information available and uses clinical reasoning abilities to formulate a broad intervention plan. In this age group, the child's caregivers need to be at the epicentre of the multidisciplinary team, and their cultural values, hopes, dreams and expectations need to be heard and considered in tailor-making a roadmap to address their child's support needs. Typically, different professionals support the child and the family's ever-changing needs, enabling each child to reach their potential.

CASE STUDY

Background information: John was a timid child and slow to warm up. He is the elder in a family of two children. His mother was very concerned about his social difficulties, as she was outgoing and proactive, but his father tended to be anxious, shy, inflexible and moody. John exhibited severe separation anxiety when he and his mother attended mother and toddler groups, with crying, moodiness and extreme social anxiety from infancy. He hated social occasions, especially birthday parties, spending the whole time clinging to his mother. At preschool, John isolated himself, as he could not adapt to the games his peers played in the preschool, which resulted in him wandering alone at break time. John watched children's videos at home and collected characters to play out stories repetitively.

Reasons for referral: John was referred for occupational therapy at the age of four years due to crying, clinging to his mother when he was at preschool or social events and being unable to play with his peers. He could not go on play invitations and showed selective mutism at preschool.

AXIS-BASED DIAGNOSIS (ICDL-DMIC 2005)

Axis I: Interactive disorder

Axis II, type 1: Difficulties with self-regulation, dependent on mother as a co-regulator. Poor engagement, non-verbal communication and difficulties sustaining continuous interaction, especially in peer groups.

Axis III: Sensory regulatory disorder, significant sensory regulation difficulties with gravitational insecurity, tactile sensitivity and proprioceptive seeking behaviour during testing and in the background history.

Axis IV: Subtle speech and language difficulties apparent, and a history of early expressive language development delays, including a lisp associated with developmental articulation difficulties.

Axis V: Gravitational insecurity limited his exploration of his environment and led to visual-spatial challenges.

Axis VI: He has a supportive family, but his father experienced similar difficulties with social anxiety.

Axis VII: Stress associated with unfamiliar environments and expectations manifests in anxiety and selective mutism.

Axis VIII: No known medical, immunological or allergic co-morbidities.

Behaviour during initial therapy sessions: John and his mother attended the occupational therapy sessions together. The opportunities afforded by the multi-sensory and emotionally safe

(continued)

CASE STUDY *(Continued)*

therapeutic environment and the absence of expectation to communicate verbally, with facilitated self-regulation, enabled him to engage with the therapist non-verbally from the first session.

SHORT-TERM GOALS

1. Improve emotional and sensory regulation to become functional in his roles as a playmate and learner in the classroom by reducing his anxiety level. Greenspan and Wieder developed principles in the DIR®: Floortime™ model, such as following the child's lead, engaging his imagination, joining him in his interests and using affect to engage him and reduce his anxiety are employed. Start sessions with his feet firmly on the ground with his head upright. Then, practise falling to the sides and slightly raised surfaces, increasing the height and instability of the equipment.

2. Stay engaged in a long continuous interaction flow and expand his thinking through play. Start where the child is currently with his interests and encourage him to bring his toys. Initially, let him play out scripts of movies and books and expand the themes, deepening the emotional range and tone.

3. Facilitate language in a natural setting, initially communicate non-verbally and then expand on his ideas to engage him in a meaningful social interaction using gesture, facial expression, tone of voice and vocalisations. Follow the child's lead and interests, affirming his ideas and sustaining a long continuous flow of interaction.

4. Facilitate purposeful interaction with an adult therapist as a play partner and the environment through movement and motor planning, supporting the development of a sense of self. Initially, work on visual-spatial and vestibular processing challenges in getting him to solve problems about space and time in the context of the activity. Expand the play by utilising various therapeutic equipment to build the scene, enabling the child to explore and move through three-dimensional space using scooter boards, hammocks or swings.

5. Build bridges between his ideas in playing with peers and grade from adult interaction to facilitated interaction with a peer in a therapy session. The OT encourages the children to develop their ideas and games and promotes engagement between them in problem-solving, making joint decisions and taking turns. They need to work towards understanding another person's point of view and compromise for the benefit of the relationship. During free play, his OT can provide self-regulating activities that meet his need for proprioceptive input, for example swinging in a hammock.

LONG-TERM OCCUPATIONAL PERFORMANCE GOALS

1. Facilitate socialisation within his peer group by providing emotional scaffolding to enhance function on the playground through facilitated peer interactions and during group activities/discussions in the classroom. Support should be faded as it is no longer required.

2. Encourage participation in his occupational role as a scholar. The OT must address this child's praxis and sensory processing challenges affecting function, including gross motor, eye–hand and oral-motor coordination, and visual-motor difficulties. Predictable routines, individualised schedules and physical organisation of materials using visual strategies are helpful.

3. Encourage adaptability in a variety of environments. Home and school visits are critical to identify the child's specific challenges. Based on observations, the OT provides a 24-hour sensory diet to enable the child to regulate his arousal levels. Parent/teacher education helps create an awareness of children's individual differences in arousal levels and teaches self-regulation strategies, such as using stress balls and movement breaks, social stories and social skills groups.

4. Modify daily routines for optimal functioning. The occupational therapist's role includes making suggestions regarding adaptations to routines at home, encouraging diversity in play with siblings, facilitating interactions on play invitations and recommending limits on activities that discourage interaction, especially screens. As the child can maintain self-regulation and engagement in his safe home environment, he is ready for new experiences by using predictable transitions, like the OT accompanying the child and his friend to the park.

RESULTS

After six months of individual therapy, John was encouraged to invite his family, teacher and school friends into his safe therapy environment to demonstrate his emerging social engagement capacities and non-verbal and verbal communication. Following on, John was encouraged to invite some friends home for play invitations, initially one at a time and to their surprise, they discovered that he could talk. The next step would be going to a friend's house to play invitations himself.

In the classroom, John slowly started moving into the group, whispering answers to his teacher and was less dependent on his toys as anchors in the conversation. By the end of the year, he was starting to volunteer when questions were asked by raising his hand. He moved into the group with the rest of his peers, coping well with the transition. Occupational therapy sessions were terminated after nine months. Feedback from the family a year later was positive. John had made a smooth transition into grade one as a gentle boy but confident enough to participate fully in the classroom and extracurricular activities. By the following year, John was taking on a leadership role in his peer group and appointed cricket team captain.

QUESTIONS

1. Discuss the factors that have influenced occupational therapy practice in the 21st century.

2. Describe how an anxious child's individual differences in sensory and affective dysregulation influence their behaviour and could manifest in depression, obsessive–compulsive disorder or conduct disorder.

3. A toddler of 18 months is referred to you by the paediatrician due to delayed language development and poor sleeping. His parents cannot leave him with caregivers, including his grandparents. Describe the assessment process. Where, how, and what tools would you use, and which other multidisciplinary team members would you confer with to formulate a comprehensive intervention plan for this family?

4. You are a rural hospital's only allied health care professional. A mother presents her three-year-old, breastfed, eating only porridge and carried on his mother's back. Recently, the mother unsuccessfully tried to place him in a crèche so she could find a job as a domestic worker. The teacher reported that she could not get him to participate in the daily programme, and he spent the morning lying on the floor, rolling, screaming, bashing his head and biting anybody who tried to approach him. Describe the approach you would take in assessing this child's needs and the recommendations you would make regarding handling principles, changes to the environment and routine to shift his developmental trajectory.

REFERENCES

American Medical Association House of Delegates (AMA) (2023) *Removal of A.M.A support for applied behavior analysis*. Resolution:706 (A-23).

AOTA (2020) Occupational therapy practice framework: domain and process-fourth edition. *American Journal Occupational Therapy*, **74** (**Supplement_2**), 7412410010p1-7412410010p87. https://doi.org/10.5014/ajot.2020.74S2001

Autism CRC (2021) *Supporting young children and their families early to reach their full potential*. Submission to the Australian Government in response to National Disability Insurance Agency Consultation Paper. https:\\www.autismcrc.com.au (accessed 24 October 2023).

Bayley, M.N. & Aylward, G.P. (2020) *Bayley Scales of Infant and Toddler Development*, 4th edn. Pearson Clinical, Bloomington.

Bayrami, L., Greenspan, S.I. & Casenheiser, D. (2007) *Early identification study*. 11th ICDL International Conference, Minneapolis.

Boshoff, K., Bowen, H., Paton, H. et al (2020) Child development outcomes of DIR/Floortime™-based programs: a systematic review. *Canadian Journal of Occupational Therapy*, **87**, 153–164.

Chasson, G., Harris, G. & Neely, W. (2007) Cost comparison of early intensive behavioral intervention and special education for children with autism. *Journal of Child and Family Studies*, **16**, 401–413.

Cullinane, D. (2020) *Evidence base for the DIR→: Floortime™ approach*. accessed from https://cdikids.org>2020/11>DIR-research-2020 (accessed 16 June 2024)

Damiano, D.L. & Longo, E. (2021) Early intervention evidence for infants with or at risk for cerebral palsy: an overview of systematic reviews. *Developmental Medicine and Child Neurology*, **63**(7), 771–784.

Dana, D. (2018) *The Polyvagal Theory in Therapy: Engaging the Rhythm of Regulation*. W.W. Norton, New York.

Delahooke, M. (2019) *Beyond Behaviors: Using Brain Science and Compassion to Understand and Solve Children's Behavioral Challenges*. PESI Publishing and Media, Eau Claire, WI.

Duncan, S. & Barrett L.F. (2007) Affect is a form of cognition: a neurobiological analysis. *Cognition and Emotion*, **21**(6), 1184–1211. https://doi.org/10.1080/02699930701437931

Dunn, W. (2014) *Sensory Profile-2*. Pearson Assessments, Bloomington.

Dunn, W. & Brown, C. (1997) Factor analysis on the sensory profile from a national sample of children without disabilities. *American Journal of Occupational Therapy*, **51**, 490–495.

Evans, K., Afsharnejad, B., Finlay-Jones, A. et al (2022) Improving the journey, before, during and after diagnosis of a neurodevelopmental condition: suggestions from a sample of Australian consumers and professionals. *Advances in Neurodevelopmental Disorders*, **6**, 397–406. https://doi.org/10.1007/s41252-022-00289-z

Fagiolini, M., Jensen, C.L. & Champagne, F.A. (2009) Epigenetic influences on brain development and plasticity. *Current Opinion in Neurobiology*, **19**(2), 207–212.

Flipetti, M.L. (2021) Being in tune with your body: the emergence of interoceptive caregiver-infant feeding interactions. *Child Development Perspectives*, **15**(3), 182–188.

Greene, R. (2021) *The Explosive Child (Sixth Edition): A New Approach for Understanding and Parenting Easily Frustrated, Chronically Inflexible Children*. Harper Collins Publishers Inc., New York.

Greenspan, S.I. (2004) *The Greenspan Social Emotional Growth Chart: A Screening Questionnaire for Infants and Young Children*. Psych Corp (Harcourt Assessment), San Antonio, Texas.

Greenspan, S.I., DeGangi, G. & Wieder, S. (2003) *The Functional Emotional Assessment Scale for Infancy and Early Childhood: Clinical and Research Applications*, 2nd edn. ICDL, Bethesda, Maryland.

Greenspan, S.I. & Glovinski, I. (2002) *Bipolar Patterns in Children, New Perspectives on Developmental Pathways and a Comprehensive Approach to Prevention and Treatment*. ICDL, Bethesda, Maryland.

Greenspan, S.I. & Wieder, S. (1997) Developmental patterns and outcomes for infants and children with disorders in relating and communicating: a chart review of 200 cases of children with autistic spectrum diagnoses receiving a DIR: Floortime approach. *Journal of Developmental and Learning Disorders*, **1**, 87–141.

Greenspan, S.I. & Wieder, S. (2006) *Engaging Autism*. DaCapo Press, Cambridge, Massachusetts.

Harvard University, Centre for the Developing Child (2011) *Building the brain's "air traffic control" system: how early experiences shape the development of executive function.* Cambridge, MA. https://developingchild.harvard.edu/resources/building-the-brains-air-traffic-control-system-how-early-experiences-shape-the-development-of-executive-function/ (accessed on 16 October 2022)

Holloway, E. (1998) Early emotional development and sensory processing. In: J. Case-Smith (ed), *Pediatric Occupational Therapy and Early Intervention*, pp. 167–187. Butterworth-Heinemann, Boston.

ICDL-DMIC (2005) *ICDL Diagnostic Manual from Infancy and Early Childhood.* Interdisciplinary Council for Developmental and Learning Disorders, Bethesda, Maryland.

Kasari, C., Freeman, S. & Paparella, T. (2006) Joint attention and symbolic play in young children with autism: a randomised controlled intervention study. *Journal of Child Psychology and Psychiatry*, **47**(**6**), 611–620.

King, G., Strachan, D., Tucker, M., Duwyn, B., Deserud, S. & Shillington, M. (2009) The application of a transdisciplinary model for early intervention services. *Infants and Young Children,* **22**(**3**), 211–223.

Kuypers, L.M. (2021) *The Zones of Regulation.* Social Thinking, Minneapolis.

Lane, S.A., Reynolds, S. & Dumenci, L. (2012) Sensory over-responsivity and anxiety in typically developing children and children with autism and attention deficit hyperactivity disorder: cause or coexistence? *American Journal of Occupational Therapy*, **66**, 595–603.

Lane S.J. & Schaaf R.C. (2010) Examining the neuroscience evidence for sensory-driven neuroplasticity: implications for sensory-based occupational therapy for children and adolescents. *American Journal Occupational Therapy*, **64**(**3**), 375–390. https://doi.org/10.5014/ajot.2010.09069.

Mahler, K. (2017) *Interoception – The Eighth Sensory System.* APC Publishing, Lenexa, KS.

Novak, I., Morgan, C., Adde, L. *et al* (2017) Early, accurate diagnosis and early intervention in cerebral palsy: advances in diagnosis and treatment. *Journal American Medical Association Pediatrics*, **171**, 897–907.

Peters-Scheffer, N., Didden, R., Korzilius, H. & Matson, J. (2012) Cost comparison of early intensive behavioural intervention and treatment as usual for children with autism spectrum disorder in the Netherlands. *Research in Developmental Disabilities*, **33**, 1763–1772.

Porges, S. (2011) *The Polyvagal Theory*, pp. 193–194. W.W. Norton & Co, New York.

Ratey, J. (2002) *The User's Guide to the Brain.* First Vintage Books Edition, London.

Reddy, V. (2007) Mind knowledge in the first year: understanding attention and intention. In: G. Bremner & A. Fogel (eds), *Blackwell Handbook of Infant Development*, pp. 241–264. Blackwell Publishing Ltd., Oxford.

Robinson, R. (2011) *Autism Solutions: How to Create a Healthy and Meaningful Life for your Child: Innovative Strategies for Developing the Right Treatment Plan.* Harlequin, Don Mills.

Sandbank, M., Bottema-Beutel, K., Crowley, S. *et al* (2020) Project AIM: autism intervention meta-analysis for studies of young children. *Psychological Bulletin*, **16**(**1**), 1–29. https://doi.org/10.1037/bul0000215

Schaaf, R.C. & Smith-Roley, S. (2006) *Sensory Integration: Applying Clinical Reasoning to Practice with Diverse Populations.* Pro-Ed, Austin.

Siegel, D. (1999) *The Developing Mind: How Relationships and the Brain Interact to Shape Who We Are.* Guildford Press, New York.

Tierney, A.L. & Nelson, C.A. 3rd. (2009). Brain development and the role of experience in the early years. *Zero to Three*, **30**(**2**), 9–13.

Tronick, E. & Beeghly, M. (2011) Infants meaning-making and the development of mental health problems. *American Psychologist,* **66**(**2**), 107–119. https://doi.org/10.1037/a0021631

Vygotsky, L.S. (1978) *Mind in Society: The Development of Higher Psychological Processes.* Harvard University Press, Massachusetts.

White, R. 2010 *NDRC – Neurodevelopmental disorders of relating and communicating functional emotional developmental capacities.* DIR→: Floortime™ Conference, Cape Town, South Africa.

Whitehouse, A., Varcin, K., Waddington, H. *et al* (2020) *Interventions for Children on the Autism Spectrum: A Synthesis of Research Evidence.* Autism CRC, Brisbane.

Williams, G.G. & Anzalone, M.E. (2001) *Helping Infants and Young Children Interact with Their Environment: Improving Sensory Integration and Self-Regulation.* Zero to Three, Washington, DC.

Zwaigenbaum, L., Bauman, M.L., Choueiri, R. *et al* (2015) Early intervention for children with autism spectrum disorder under three years of age: recommendations for practice and research. *Pediatrics*, **136**, 60–81.

Zwaigenbaum, L., Bryson, S., Rogers, T. *et al* (2005) Behavioral manifestations of autism in the first year of life. *International Journal of Developmental Neuroscience*, **23**(**2–3**), 143–152.

Occupational Therapy with Children with Psycho-social Disorders and Autism

CHAPTER 17

Marie Clare (Mush) Perrins Gendron

Occupational Therapist, Cape Town, South Africa

KEY LEARNING POINTS

- Knowledge and skills required by occupational therapists working with children with psycho-social disorders and autism.

- Methodology regarding the assessment and interpretation of results of children with psycho-social disorders and autism.

NOTES ON TERMINOLOGY

The term child will be used to represent child and adolescent age ranges in this chapter, as many of the behaviours start in childhood and continue into adolescence, for example those relating to autism. Psycho-social conditions specific to adolescence will be covered in Chapter 18. Children grow up with a variety of caregivers, which may be one, or many parents, guardians, caregivers or the child-head of a child-headed household. For practicality, this chapter will use the term parents, but it should be read to include any other caregiver, unless otherwise specified. Intervention is the umbrella term for what to attend to when working together with the child. It could include treatment from different specialists, contacting a school teacher, educating parents etc. The reader is advised to refer to the DSM-5 (American Psychiatric Association 2013), or subsequent DSM, for the latest diagnostic criteria.

GENERAL GUIDING PRINCIPLES TO CONSIDER WHEN WORKING WITH CHILDREN

CONTEXTUAL

Working with children in any area of intervention cannot be carried out in isolation: the family, community and school environments are integral components, with careful, non-judgmental attention paid to the social, cultural and religious contexts within which the individual is raised.

To illustrate the latter contexts:

- Due to practitioners' lack of awareness of the contextual situation of children living on the street, who sniff glue to get high, unintentionally using contact glue in a psychodynamic collage activity in a day drug rehabilitation programme for these children is not therapeutic.

Crouch and Alers Occupational Therapy in Psychiatry and Mental Health, Sixth Edition.
Edited by Rosemary Crouch, Tania Buys, Enos Morankoana Ramano, Matty van Niekerk and Lisa Wegner.
© 2025 John Wiley & Sons Ltd. Published 2025 by John Wiley & Sons Ltd.

– An adolescent Xhosa male wanting to participate in the traditional initiation rite of passage to which his Christian parents were vehemently opposed, was admitted to hospital with sudden onset of paralysis. A diagnosis of pseudo-paralysis was made, and he was referred to a neuro-psychiatric centre for intervention. The rehabilitation team then needs to be sensitive to his cultural preference within the context of his parents' religious beliefs and values and help mediate tolerance of both beliefs with all parties.

It is essential to establish how the child's psycho-social behaviour impacts the lives of other family members, both from an emotional and financial aspect. The occupational therapist can raise awareness of areas of potential concern with the family members and suggest ways to manage these.

SIBLINGS

Siblings who are considered neuro-typical by their parents often feel guilty about this and may become resentful of their neuro-atypical sibling who is demanding all of the parents' time, energy and money. The siblings may also become depressed (Gold 1993).

Parents can take time to regularly check in with the siblings as to how they are doing, and to just listen. Parents could write a letter to the siblings stating what they see as wonderful about that specific sibling. If it is recognised that a sibling has stepped back to allow the index child to get the attention they need, this must be acknowledged. Parents can try giving daily compliments to each family member, validating that they have been seen carrying out tasks, even if it was expected of them, such as thanking them for putting their clothes in the wash basket or helping make supper.

PARENTS

Many marriages take strain, often ending in separation or divorce (Steinhagen 2013). A couple once reflected to an occupational therapist who had sincerely asked how they were doing that she was the first health professional of the many who had seen their child who had asked this important question.

Single parents might try to find a back-up support system for child-minding or have adult conversations with friends.

Asking for help is very difficult for many people, as one's sense of dignity is impacted by the imagined perception of not being strong enough to cope. Therefore, factor in a reciprocal action that one can manage, so it can be considered a transaction, rather than a favour. This also reduces the heavy burden of guilt or feeling one is a nuisance, which may inhibit one from making use of the help as often as is required.

Parents should plan and include at least one hour a week for re-charging their batteries with activities that are important to them, such as, sleeping, watching a series without interruptions, gardening, reading, taking a walk or going for a run. Holiday or respite care for the child may be required when the parents are exhausted. This could be the child staying with a family member or being cared for in the child's home by a family member or friend. Parents could ask within local community networks, as some hospitals, church and care organisations offer respite care.

CAREGIVERS AND SUPERVISORS

The occupational therapist should also be aware of potential burnout with child caregivers and their supervisors, for example, carers in children's homes, or hospital staff. They often have children of their own and give so much to their work that they are depleted when they go home. If support is not in place, support sessions, either one-on-one or in a group, should be built into the programme.

DEVELOPMENTAL CONSIDERATIONS

The occupational therapist working with children requires an understanding of all aspects of neuro-typical development, as for example, muscle tone concerns could affect speech production, self-esteem and feeding, which in turn could impact social integration with peers. As development is a step-by-step process of laying down foundation skills that subsequent stages are built upon, particularly in children one would address the underlying contributing or causative concern(s) where possible (i.e. foundation skill development), rather than only just focusing on the presenting concern(s) (which would result in splinter skill development). The underlying concern(s) could be biological as in the muscle tone example noted above, or skills-based such as under-developed sensory modulation causing a child to hit out in a busy school environment and/or contextual, such as a very disorganised mother resulting in the child presenting with heightened anxiety, as nothing is predictable. The various developmental skills are interwoven and inter-relate.

Another challenge when working with most children is that their development continues to change, and this is even more rapid in the younger child. So, what the occupational therapist assessed last week may be different this week. The occupational therapist also has to critically evaluate if the changes seen in the child after intervention are due to the intervention, or developmental maturation and/or both. Early intervention is recommended as brain plasticity is lifelong, but more flexible the younger one is. Habits can become entrenched and therefore are harder to change the longer the habit is reinforced (Doidge 2016).

Occupational therapists working with children need to understand what is neuro-typical developmentally appropriate behaviour (such as temper tantrums in the two-year-old), concerning behaviours that can be addressed in occupational therapy (for example becoming dysregulated or 'meltdowns', learnt helplessness, low self-esteem, rudeness), and those behaviours that require intervention from other specialists and/or a team of specialists that includes the occupational therapist (for example, eating disorders and autism).

An in-depth understanding of play and the inter-relatedness of play and learning is crucial in assessment and intervention when working with children.

SETTINGS WHERE OCCUPATIONAL THERAPISTS WORK WITH CHILDREN WITH PSYCHO-SOCIAL DISORDERS AND AUTISM

Occupational therapy settings when working with children range from the child's home, schools, clinics, hospitals, institutions (such as children's homes, orphanages, places of safety, juvenile detention centres), non-governmental organisations (NGOs), non-profit organisations (NPOs) and the private sector.

In the Global South, posts in governmental health departments for occupational therapists are scarce. As an example, in 2018, only 25% of occupational therapists working in South Africa were employed in governmental health departments (Ned et al. 2020). Due to this ongoing limited number of posts available in the governmental sector in many countries, the trend has been for younger occupational therapists to work in, or start up their own, private practice or work for NGOs or NPOs. This has led to a skewed distribution of service delivery. The high workload of occupational therapists working in governmental settings may lead to these occupational therapists feeling frustrated about not being able to administer a high-quality, comprehensive assessment due to time constraints. This then impacts on the accuracy of the intervention. Experienced occupational therapists would be better equipped in this context, but it is often the junior or novice occupational therapist who has this responsibility.

OCCUPATIONAL THERAPY INTERVENTION WITH CHILDREN WITH PSYCHO-SOCIAL DISORDERS AND AUTISM

Various models of occupational therapy can be applied in the intervention with children with psycho-social disorder and autism, to inform best practice that is most suited to the service user/s and the specific therapist (see Figure 17.1 below) (Crouch & Alers 2014; Taylor et al. 2023; Christiansen & Baum 2015; Schultz & Schkade 1992; Dunn et al. 1994; Doble & Magill-Evans 1992).

CASE STUDY 1	Application of Two Models

Kielhofner's Model of Human Occupation – Kielhofner 1995 (Taylor et al. 2023) and Model of Creative Ability – Vona du Toit 2005 (Crouch & Alers 2014). Please refer to Chapters 1 and 2 for further information on these models.

Adam is a five-year-old child presenting with delayed speech development, fluctuating moods (ranging from being aloof to having aggressive outbursts), being slow to warm-up in new situations, hyper-focusing on stereotypical play with toy trains and becoming very distressed when this is interfered with, only assisting in dressing, and still in nappies. Causative concerns established after assessment were sensory modulation, concentration, and spinal alignment. These concerns were interlinked, as concentration energy is necessary for the child's sensory filter to operate effectively, sensory modulation concerns can erode concentration energy and spinal alignment concerns can increase sensory irritability and erode concentration. Concentration concerns could impact not listening to internal signals, like needing to go to the toilet. Many of the presenting concerns could be associated with a diagnosis of autism.

Models of OT

Model of creative ability (Vona Du Toit 2005)

Model of human occupation (Kielhofner 1995)

Person environment occupational performance model (Christiansen & Baum 1991)

Occupational adaptation model (Schkade & Schultz 1992)

Ecology of human performance (Dunn, et al. 1994)

In addition

Model of social interaction (Doble & Magill-Evans 1992)

FIGURE 17.1   Models of occupational therapy applicable when working with children with psycho-social and autism.

APPLYING THE MODEL OF HUMAN OCCUPATION

Only implementing environmental adaptations to suit Adam will not enable him to function optimally in the long term. One would rather address his sensory modulation and spinal alignment concerns, so that he would become more habituated rather than alerted to incoming sensations (habituation). This would allow him to re-direct his energy to playing and learning (volition and occupational performance capacity), starting with his safe space of playing with his familiar trains to sustain his motivation and decrease his anxiety. Include in his daily routine calming, deep pressure activities, scaffolding them onto the daily tasks in his home and school, such as giving him the heaviest bag to bring into the home/classroom, sweeping the yard and watering the plants. Educate his parents and teachers regarding sensory modulation and Adam's sensory-based behaviours, and how they could address these (such as speaking quietly to him, guiding him to a quieter environment when he becomes overwhelmed in a busy and noisy one – environmental adaptations). Guide Adam to recognise what stresses him and strategise together as to what he can do to manage this in a socially appropriate way (self-organisation). Do regular monitoring of this and praise his efforts (volition). Adam's self-organisation would be facilitated by using specific, not vague questions. A vague question like: 'What do you need?' would increase his anxiety, whereas: 'What types of blocks from these choices do you need to build a railway station next to this railway track?' would allow him to know exactly to what to answer, and on what to act.

APPLYING THE MODEL OF CREATIVE ABILITY

Adam presents with a scattered profile of being between the Motivational levels of self-differentiation (ego-centric), self-presentation and imitative participation (in school and occupational therapy). His Action levels are unconstructive for toileting, incidentally constructive for dressing, social and school ability, and constructive for play. Intervention would start by addressing his spinal alignment and sensory modulation (see above), as these are the barriers that prevent him from engaging more effectively with the materials, objects and people in his world. His current sensory profile and its impact on his behaviour must be constantly factored into his occupational therapy in order to limit his anxiety and distress. The therapeutic activities should therefore be graded from his area of familiarity and comfort gradually, and incrementally linking and expanding on the activities. Then bring in similarly related activities, where relevant. Examples are a toileting programme where he has the familiarity of having a nappy on, then stably sitting on the toilet with the familiar comfort of his nappy on, graded to over time slowly loosening the nappy until it is off; encouraging independent dressing, starting with the occupational therapist dressing him, then incrementally adding in that he must start and finish the dressing of one item of clothing (implementing the circle of task completion), with the occupational therapist executing the in-between bit, grading off how much is done as his skill increases. This grading also develops his action level, by including more steps in the activity and developing an end product, namely toileting and dressing independently. Regarding developing product-centred play, start with the familiar trains, grade on to building the train station, to bringing in cars coming to and from the station, to including people in the cars and trains, then conversations of these people as to their purpose (going to school, to the shops or on holiday), to drawing the story of his play. Also facilitate his exploration of new play items, by including them in familiar play activities. In order to work on his egocentric volition, the occupational therapist would grade the interaction during play with Adam by slowly adding in other trains and then acting out a storyline in congruence, and then gradually diverting from his stereotypical way of playing. In addressing his aggressive outbursts, one would direct him to evacuate or channel this through activities such as hitting a suspended ball, bashing or jumping on an egg box, weeding, blowing a Vuvuzela trumpet, blowing destructive feelings into a balloon that one then releases, and/or drawing or writing destructive feelings down and then tearing the paper up. One would then progressively guide the child as to how they could apply safe, socially appropriate evacuation actions independently when not in therapy. Using social stories would be helpful in developing his awareness of socially appropriate behaviour.

For both models, referrals would be made to a speech and language therapist and a paediatrician for a diagnosis, school placement, and support recommendations.

SKILLS SET FOR ASSESSMENT AND INTERVENTION

Occupational therapists need to draw on a variety of practice skills in order to effectively assess and treat children with psycho-social concerns and those living with autism (See Figure 17.2.)

PLAY

Considering Nancy Takata's Taxonomy of Play that includes sensory-motor, construction, dramatic, symbolic, gameplay and recreation, play is a lifelong occupation, and is the primary occupation of children (Parham & Fazio 2008; Perrins Gendron et al. 2022). Using play as an assessment and treatment tool would thus be relevant and essential when working with children.

True free play is intrinsically motivated, internally controlled, and not based on objective reality (where an object can be anything one would want it to be, such as spoons representing family figures in a role-play activity) (Parham & Fazio 2008; Bruwer & Tzanos 2016; Weenink-Schoonover & O'Brien 2020). Play and playfulness could be a tool to achieve a specific

Skills set for assessment and treatment – understanding of and training in:

Observation skills

Task analysis

Proficient in administering standardized assessments

Neuro-typical development

Play and playfulness

Neuro-developmental therapy

Sensory integration, in particular sensory modulation

Communication skills

Educative techniques

Cognitive interventions

Psycho-social interventions

Medical conditions

Side effects of medication

Social, cultural, and religious rules and values

Working with a team with a clear understanding of each team member's role

FIGURE 17.2   Skills set for occupational therapy assessment and treatment.

outcome, such as a play dough activity to develop hand strength or playfully putting the shoe on one's ear asking if that is where it goes, to engage the child in the dressing activity (Parham & Fazio 2008; Whitebread 2012; Weenink-Schoonover & O'Brien 2020). Being able to play or to be playful could be the intended outcome, such as facilitating the engagement and communication of a parent and child in a shared shopping game (Parham & Fazio 2008; Whitebread 2012; Weenink-Schoonover & O'Brien 2020; Perrins Gendron *et al.* 2022).

ASSESSMENT

An in-depth assessment provides the occupational therapist with the necessary information to conduct a well-reasoned clinical analysis, clarifying the individual's strengths and teasing out the causative concerns that contribute to the presenting concerns. In paediatrics, the causative concerns are the prime focus of the intervention where possible, with the inclusion of the presenting concerns for holistic therapy.

The assessment comprises of:

• In-depth interview with the parents that includes the history of firstly, the child's strengths, then the areas of concern, behaviour and handling techniques used, birth, any miscarriages, any post-partum depression in the mother, child's health, medications, schooling, play, outline of the child's daily occupational activities that would include electronic media engagement (devices/apps, amount of daily time spent, when in daily schedule, child's behaviour when the electronic media play is stopped), sensory seeking behaviours and reactions to sensory input (if not using a specific sensory assessment).

The child is in the room during the interview, with age-appropriate activities present for the child to engage with. This inclusion facilitates the development of the interpersonal relationships, allowing the adults, and subsequently the child, to relax. The child could also listen in to how others perceive their behaviour. The occupational therapist can also observe the child's interaction with the available activities and the interaction between the child and parents during the interview. If the child does not engage with the available toys, encourage the parents to offer the child a food item.

- Developmental assessment with clinical observations of the child, to ascertain the developmental strengths and areas of concern. Include play/recreation, a range of movement assessment (particularly of the spinal alignment, as this may increase sensory irritability and impact on effective motor function), visual skills screening, and emotional check-in (is the child happy, sad, mad, anxious and/or scared?). Also include the three wishes from the genie's magic lamp (they can change anything about themselves or the world, or ask for anything), three things the child knows they are good at and three things they wish could be better at. If the child is not that engaged and/or becomes overstimulated, it is best to split the assessment over two or more sessions. Allow movement, a healthy snack, water drinking, and toilet breaks.

- School visits are useful if the child's behaviour at school and/ or the teacher's management thereof are a concern. The school visit should comprise of observing the child in the classroom and playground, looking through work files and books if relevant, and privately chatting to those working with the child in the school about the child's strengths and concerns, and difficulties they have in managing the child in that setting. Always follow this up with a summary of your observations and suggestions of what might help, sent to parents and school (with parental permission).

ANALYSIS AND SYNTHESIS OF ASSESSMENT RESULTS

The analysis and synthesis of assessment results is core for a successful intervention plan, which includes the structuring of an individualised, appropriate treatment plan. Always ask: Why is this concern presenting? What could be contributing to it? With recent changes in behaviour, was there a trigger, such as a new baby sibling in the home and the 3½-year-old child now presenting with hitting and screaming? Thinking out-of-the-box is highly recommended at this stage, as it stimulates trains of clinical reasoning that when linked together with the assessment evidence, can produce an accurate and effective intervention plan. Structuring the analysis varies from using headings regarding components of function (underlying concern/s), occupational performance, or both, usually referencing the reasons for referral (presenting concern). It may be helpful to refer to Bunty McDougall's The Wall, Part 1 (McDougall 2012), the Interpretation sheet of Jean Ayres (Ayres 2005), and Mush Perrins Gendron's Interpretation Sheet (Perrins Gendron 2016–2023: see Figure 17.3). Clinical reasoning is deepened through mapping and rethinking causative to presenting concerns, facilitated through report writing.

Report copies are given to the parents at the feedback session. In the feedback session, emphasise that the parents

fundamentally know the child better than the occupational therapist in many ways, having spent more time with the child than the occupational therapist. What professionals offer is other insights into the child, allowing the parents to understand the child better, which can help them in the management of the child's behaviour. Guidance from the professionals should expand on the parents' skills further. Extracting out recommendations included in the report onto a Suggested Strategies to Apply at Home and School hand-out is helpful for the parents and teachers.

It is a good idea to allow parents about one week to get back to the occupational therapist with corrections on the report and inclusions of their comments if the child performed differently in the assessment than what they know the child does at home or school. This is important, as any occupational therapy report must accurately reflect what the child is able to do and what they struggle with. The report is a legal document that would be considered valid in a court of law. Furthermore, occupational therapists should consider their country's protection of personal information laws regarding the collection and storage of personal information on clients and how and for how long this information must be kept, as children and adolescents are considered minors.

Home-based assessments are invaluable, as 'one picture says a thousand words', and enable the occupational therapist to meet other people involved in the child's life and get an understanding of the context in order to provide more appropriate recommendations and suggestions for the report and home programme. One example was observing a pristine white lounge area, where one would not recommend finger painting as a home programme activity idea.

INTERVENTION

Treatment aims are extracted from the findings, focusing on the underlying causative concerns where possible, and scaffolding the presenting concerns onto the causative concerns through the grading of the treatment programme. For example, first start work on improving the sensory modulation of a child who presents with fussy eating, before introducing a new food to eat, but including both as the sessions progress.

Choose relevant treatment techniques, principles and grading, appropriate for the child's developmental age and situation in their lived environments. Be aware of the social, cultural, or religious rules and values. For example, avoid using dry food materials like pasta or barley as a sensory treatment medium in a community where food is scarce and rather find a non-food alternative as the treatment medium; using playing cards to develop mathematical concepts in a family ascribing to the Muslim faith where cards could represent gambling – rather choose an alternative game.

Should there be clashes of expectations, treatment methods or materials used, discuss and respectfully negotiate these with the parents. The foundational premise should always be what is in the best interest of the child. For example,

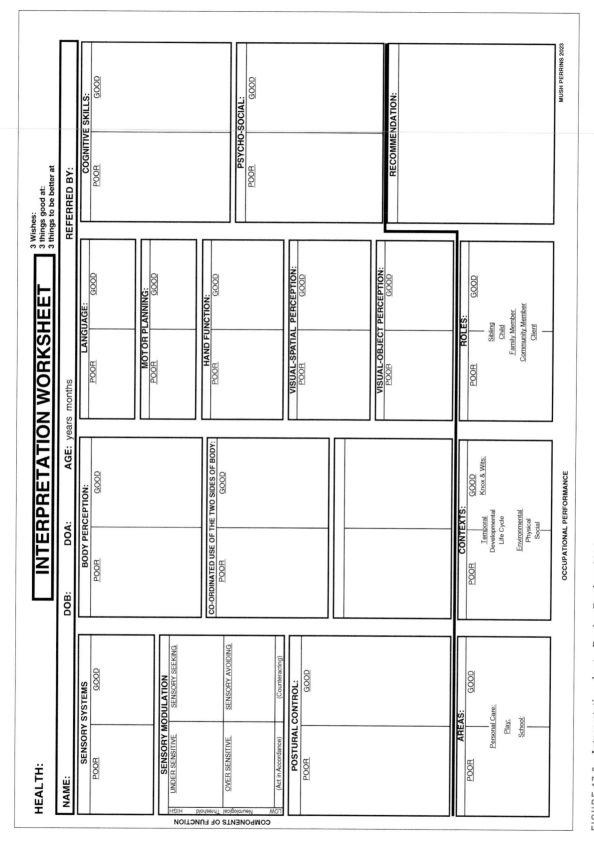

FIGURE 17.3   Interpretation sheet – Perrins Gendron 2016.

255

parents emphasising that the child must be silent and obey, where the child is feeling threatened by decisions made for them – explain how the child is feeling to the parents, exploring how the parents were treated and felt as children, negotiating respect boundaries from both sides and discussing the possible long-term effects of the child not having a voice.

When working with a team that includes the parents, teacher and other health professionals, ascertain:

• Who takes responsibility for what, as there can be an overlap (e.g. feeding).

• Ensure input by various team members is not contradictory, as this can confuse the child.

• Phasing of interventions. This is important to not overwhelm the child or the parents and their finances (cost of interventions, transport and time off from work).

Book in a follow-up session. This could be in person, where one has to consider the time required by parents to be taken off from work and transport costs. Using lower-tech telerehabilitation (e.g. telephonically) to follow-up is cost- and time-effective, as it connects parents and the occupational therapist wherever they are, permitting real-time communication (Kubheka *et al.* 2020). Bear in mind that this may not be that effective if hands-on input, guidance and/or more nonverbal observations are required.

ASSESSMENT AND TREATMENT OF SPECIFIC PRESENTING AND CAUSATIVE CONCERNS

This section will be discussed on two levels: Level 1 is where pharmacological intervention is not the first intervention required; Level 2 is where pharmacological intervention is the first intervention required, with various other interventions following on.

Level 1:

A. *Interpersonal concerns (rudeness, swearing, poor reciprocation, disregard of others and/or gaze avoidance).*

Explore if the behaviour is learnt at home, school, from peers and/or electronic media, in reaction to how others have treated the child or part of a condition. Regarding being part of a condition, difficulty in inhibiting an impulse (related to a concentration concern, tiredness resulting from a health condition) can result in the child saying or doing things they would not like to, or intentionally mean to. Individuals living with Tourette's Syndrome may swear as one of their anxiety tics, so allow them opportunities to evacuate this anxiety by, for example, swearing all the worst words they could think of in a safe space. Some children will deliberately test one or want to provoke a reaction by being rude or using 'toilet talk'. In this case, quietly reflect back to them that you noticed what they are doing and you wondered why this is so. Explore if others have behaved like that with them and how this made them feel.

Intervention:

• Allow evacuation of pent-up feelings through therapeutic activities.

• Reflect back to the child as noted earlier and/or use social stories to explore how they would feel if you or others behaved rudely to them. If it is learnt behaviour from the home, discuss this with the parents.

• Set rules that apply to everyone regarding expected behaviour in the occupational therapy space. Explain that clear, fair rules make everyone feel safe. Limit the rules to three, such as no deliberate hurting with words or actions (apologising if one hurts by accident); the child is welcome to say how they feel using the 'I messages' ('I feel so angry when you talk over me' not 'You make me so mad!'), and regarding what equipment is not allowed to be used without the occupational therapist's permission and presence in the space. Have fair consequences for deliberately thwarting the rules, such as losing five minutes of free play in the session.

• Board games: There are various commercially available board games that help in developing emotionally expressive children. One South African product is the Smart Heart, a board game, developed by psychologists, for children to: Identify and communicate feelings – Foster assertiveness – Talk about serious issues playfully – Think independently (Kritzas & Bytheway 2015).

B. *Learnt Helplessness/Indulged Child:*

Explore the background history for any contributing circumstances, such as a premature or difficult birth, medical conditions (in particular those that were potentially life-threatening for the child or where the parents felt sorry for the child), parents wanting to prolong the dependency stage longer than is developmentally appropriate, different cultural rearing norms, reduced endurance (mental, muscular or physiological) and/or laziness.

CASE HISTORY

An eight-year-old boy who had his leg amputated when a runaway lorry/truck drove into his backyard and over his leg. With occupational- and physio-therapy, he was fully functional using his crutches. When his family visited, he sat in a wheelchair and acted sad and helpless, manipulating the situation to make his family feel sorry for him, which was working for him. On him wanting to go the toilet, the family was discussing how to lift him when the occupational therapist intervened, informing the family of his capabilities, whilst the child angrily stared at the therapist. A frank discussion ensued, regarding the best way for him to feel 'normal' was for them to apply those expectations of him, which included appropriately disciplining him as they disciplined his siblings.

Intervention always depends on the causative factors. Counsel regarding the developmental stages of competency with the child and the parents and co-develop strategies on how to achieve these levels of competency, being sensitive regarding cultural norms. If the reason is the parents are prolonging the dependency stage, this may require referring the parents to counselling or psychotherapy.

C. *Bossy or Controlling Child*

Explore if this is learnt and/or facilitated behaviour, part of a condition like autism, sensory modulation concerns (need to control to feel sensory safe), motor planning or poor skills-based concerns (need to control so they appear competent) and/or a personality or inherited trait.

Address the underlying concern(s) where feasible. Increase the child's self-awareness through reflection of their behaviour and/or social stories on how it feels to be on the receiving end of being bossed around. Discuss strategies with the child and parents, such as giving two choices to give the child an element of control or teaching them how to share leadership/toys.

D. *Skill-specific Decreased Self-confidence*

Explore, identify and address the underlying skill causing the decreased self-confidence. Apply techniques such as task analysis, occupational scaffolding and the 'just right challenge', appropriate praise for effort, and reflecting back on progress achieved in the skill (keep dated examples of these where possible). Chat about the beauty of everyone being unique regarding their strengths and areas of concern. The book 'Accidental Genius' by Richard Gaughan (2010) describes how mistakes resulted in amazing inventions like penicillin and glass. Chat to the child about this, and it being okay to make mistakes, as one could come up with a better way of doing things and/or learn a valuable lesson from the mistake.

E. *Low Self-esteem*

Explore the underlying causes and address these causes. As above, apply the 'just right challenge' technique, chat about being unique, and give appropriate praise for effort.

F. *Bullying*

Bullying behaviour is perpetrated on a person considered being weaker or less powerful than the perpetrator (Imuta *et al.* 2022). Bullying may be verbal, social, physical, or cyberbullying (Thiart 2020). Low self-esteem, being different or over-reactive to input, especially if there are sensory modulation concerns, can be triggers for one to be bullied and can also result in low self-esteem. A meta-analytic review regarding bullying found the incidence of bullying in adolescents worldwide as being between 30.5% and 35% across socio-economic communities, with regional and country variations (Imuta *et al.* 2022). A report in the South African # Stop Bullying anti-bullying programme noted that about 57% of South African high-school learners have been bullied (Thiart 2020).

For the person being bullied and the person doing the bullying, initially explore the underlying causes and address these where possible. If the bullying occurs in the school environment, initiate a team meeting to discuss the incident/s and together put strategies in place to address the bullying. These include creating a culture of tolerance, mindfulness and empathy, appropriate communication and assertiveness, assisting in conflict resolution, devising and spreading a bullying prevention plan and education around bullying for learners, parents and local communities. Where possible, use available local anti-bullying resources (Thiart 2020; Imuta *et al.* 2022).

G. *Aggressive Child*

Provide appropriate evacuation therapeutic activities for the aggression and explore and address the underlying causes, for example impulse control.

In therapy, discuss rules of behaviour. Understand and address the child's triggers for aggressive behaviour. If the aggression is potentially dangerous to persons in the occupational therapy space, call for back-up help to enter when called into the space, if necessary, evacuate others, use a low-toned, slow voice and actions to try and calm the child, staying out of their reach until they have calmed down.

H. *Self-regulation Difficulties*

Ascertain the underlying causes, and address where possible. For example, sensory modulation concerns can result in fluctuating moods of varied intensity. Other underlying causes that might increase irritability and trigger difficulties in

CASE STUDY 2

Ethan was a five-year-old child referred for aggressive behaviour at school. Exploration through play therapy only indicated some gouging out of a figurine's eyes, but there was no history of visual trauma or operations. The occupational therapist administered the Ayre's Clinical Observations, the first test item being the screening of visual skills. This assessment, coupled with asking Ethan whether he could see clearly or not (he said things were blurry), pointed to visual difficulties, which were confirmed by the behavioural optometrist. On addressing the visual difficulties, the aggression stopped.

impulse control are health issues, allergies, medications, spinal alignment concerns, concentration concerns, brain injuries and conditions, lack of sleep, tiredness, hormones and/or poor nutrition.

Consider the child's daily structure and routines. Predictability of events helps the child to self-regulate. Too many events one after the other can negatively impact self-regulation as there is no time to quieten down and self-regulate. Babies use what has been termed protective apathy (Als *et al.* 1996), where they turn their heads away from noise and activity and start to yawn, presenting these signals for one to stop interacting with them, thus allowing time to quieten down and self-regulate. However, if a child shuts down, adults normally up their input to get the child's attention, pushing the child further into shutdown. Strategise together with the child and the parents where feasible, regarding what could help the child to self-regulate in the home, at school and social events.

I. *Fussy Feeder*

The prevalence of fussy eaters varied across studies, with reports of between 5.6 and 59% (Wolstenholme *et al.* 2020). A meta-analysis study noted that an estimated 22% of children over 30 months were fussy eaters (Wolstenholme *et al.* 2020), with approximately a 30–80% prevalence rate in children with developmental disorders (Freeman *et al.* 2015).

In exploring the underlying causes, consider the following:

- The family history of any feeding concerns (choking, bulimia and anorexia), gastro-oesophageal reflux, food intolerances and food allergies.

- If the child saw a medical practitioner to rule out health concerns, like a mineral deficiency (for example iron), constipation or tonsillitis.

- Ascertain documented possible side-effects of medication the child is on.

- Is there an established diagnosis, such as autism?

- Sensory profile. Look in particular at the smells, textures, tastes and temperature of food the individual tolerates, dislikes and cannot tolerate (colder foods have less smell). Can the child tolerate teeth brushing (taste, texture and action of brush)? Do they suck to feed (could indicate a mechanical obstruction to swallowing a bolus of food), and do they hate the dressing and undressing the top half of their body (which could indicate an upper spinal alignment concern)?

- Spinal alignment: Check if the child had a fall that could cause spinal alignment concerns. Spinal alignment concerns of C1–C2 could impact the vagal nerve that innervates the gut, which could result in gastro-oesophageal reflux. Spinal alignment concerns could increase sensory irritability. It is also difficult to swallow a bolus of food if one's neck is retracted, with the hyoid bone and associated muscles then also not being correctly positioned to assist in the swallowing action.

- Tolerance of wearing a seat belt and the position of the child in the car seat, and whether the car seat straps are exerting pressure on the neck and shoulder muscles. A more flexed, banana-shaped positioning can squash up the contents of the gut, which could exacerbate gastro-oesophageal reflux incidences.

- Does the child cry suddenly outside of a cry-inducing stimulus, especially when being placed in the lying position?

- Acid-smelling breath.

- Husky, gravelly voice.

- As a baby, the child had to be held upright for most of the day.

  (The last six presentations could be indicative of gastro-oesophageal reflux, which makes the sufferer feel bilious, mostly wanting to eat dry foods or those with a crust on it, having foods separated on the plate so they are easily identifiable and drinking a lot of fluid to ease the pain caused by acid having been in the throat and oesophagus.)

- Manipulation of adults by the child to get what they want.

- Family expectations around food and eating.

- Past and current handling of fussy eating, especially any incidents of forced feeding.

- Levels of stress around mealtimes.

- The parents' sense of competency in feeding the child.

- Whether the child eats better with certain people or in specific spaces.

- Parental awareness of child's hunger and satiety cues.

Intervention:

The occupational therapists can address the underlying cause(s), such as sensory modulation, more upright positioning in the car seat, expectations around food and mealtimes, managing manipulative behaviour from the child. The child can be referred to the following team members: (i) a chiropractor if there are spinal alignment concerns. Suggest muscle-strengthening activities to prevent repeat spinal malalignment concerns. (ii) A medical practitioner if gastro-oesophageal reflux is suspected. (iii) A dietician if the child is losing weight, has stopped eating a food, and shows shrinking food choices. (iv) A swallowing expert speech therapist if there are swallowing co-ordination difficulties. (v) A specialist unit dealing with eating disorders if anorexia or bulimia is suspected in the school-going child.

Stress to parents that no forced feeding should occur, as this can have negative psychological repercussions. If bottle feeds or breastfeeding is still in place beyond when reasonable, wean off bottle or breastfeeding as the solid meals are simultaneously increased. Place new food on a tray to play with before the meal, so the child becomes accustomed to the sight, smell, and feel of the new food item. Placing food into one's mouth can be quite intrusive if it is not acceptable to the individual. Food in bowls and on a plate is for eating. Continue to present the rejected food over time. Model eating food and enjoying it. Have healthy snacks or a meal to share when the child's friends come around, placing the food in central bowls for all to share. Change where and how meals are presented. Eat together as a family if possible, reducing other sensory input. Switch off electronic media, unless one is playing calming music and use candles or dim lighting to reduce visual sensory input. Place the various foods in separate bowls on the table. The child dishes out for themselves to allow them some element of control, but they have to take some food from each bowl. Have short matter-of-fact discussions about the health benefits of each food. The child may take more food if they are still hungry once the plate is empty. No snacks are allowed until the scheduled snack time. Use a matter-of-fact approach to eating, with no bribing or begging around eating the food, thus reducing the potential to be manipulated through food. Encourage the child to help cook the meal, so you can spend time together during the food preparation. This increases the amount of time the child is exposed to the food. Watch cooking shows together on electronic media. This reduces the smell and taste components of food, but highlights the visual, bonding and enjoyment aspects of food. The last two suggestions can help the child acclimatise to a variety of foods.

J. *Sleep Concerns*

Various issues can impact the ability of the child to go to sleep, stay asleep and wake up rested, having had sufficient REM sleep. These include health concerns such as mineral deficiencies and worm infestation, sensory modulation, spinal alignment, lack of daily physical activity, safety concerns, emotional concerns, exposure to electronic media such as big flat screens, rapidly changing images, blue light that suppresses melatonin (West *et al.* 2011) and hyper-arouses the brain (LeBourgeois *et al.* 2017).

Intervention:

Address the underlying concerns. According to Giampapa (2023), intervention for sleep concerns includes considering the daily and weekly activity profile of the child to evaluate if there is too much, too little or an imbalance of healthy activities in the day and if it is an unpredictable routine from day to day. Discuss suitable strategies to address any concerns here, such as no visual electronic media one to three hours before bedtime, some physical exercise such as a walk around the block during the day, and a predictable supper time.

Structure a regular going-to-bed routine that includes less excitatory activities, the evening meal, toileting, washing, teeth brushing, bonding activities such as cuddling and storytelling, or reading from a printed book for the older child and lights out. Ten minutes of time to chat with the trusted parent after story time and reading can be the safe space for the child to share what they need to. Some children will try to manipulate the parent to stay up later with all sorts of requests, the most common being that they are thirsty. Use a firm, matter-of-fact approach, laced with the importance for children to have enough sleep at night to allow their brain and body to recuperate and be ready for the challenges of the next day. Casually mention if there was a link between the child having a better day after a good night's sleep.

For those children who really struggle to fall asleep, the following strategies may be helpful. Drinking a cup of Chamomile tea, or warm milk as part of the bedtime routine. Using a health-based stress-reducing product or one prescribed by the medical practitioner. Do not tell or read exciting stories at bedtime. Try finger milking (pulling a finger as deep pressure is applied to the skin, from the metacarpal joint to the fingertip) or giving a hand, foot or body massage or administering the Wilbarger Protocol (Lynch *et al.* 2011) (as recommended and shown how to administer by a Sensory Integration trained occupational therapist), if tolerated by the child. Do deep breathing together, trying to slow the breathing down and imagining the body sinking into the bed as one breathes out, deeper with each breath. Try using a weighted blanket or tuck the child's bedding around the abdominal and solar plexus area, or where and how the child prefers. For those who do not tolerate the added warmth the weighted blanket may provide, place it only over the abdominal and solar plexus area, leaving the arms, head, and feet free to cool. Ensure the room and bedding are not too hot or too cold, if possible. Melatonin is produced if the body temperature drops, which is why on long airplane flights, the air temperature is cooled when it is time for the passengers to sleep. Try placing your clothing of the day with your personal odour on it into the child's pillowcase, if the child likes how you smell. Smell is very comforting, as it is the endorphin oxytocin one secretes that facilitates attachment (Scatliffe *et al.* 2019). Together with the child, tidy the room to be slept in, check under the bed and in the cupboards, making sure the cupboard doors are closed properly with no gaps showing, so there are no new or hiding objects, or shadows that can frighten the child if they wake up in the night. There should be no light on in the room, but leave the passage light on, with the door partially open. Have a touch light or torch next to the bed, for the child to switch on if they wake up scared in the night. One could cut out all electronic media for a week to see the effect of this on the sleep of the child. Some children like protection in the form of their religious or spiritual icons placed next to their bed at night.

K. *Repressed Child*

If after this has been highlighted as a concern and discussed with the parents (see the example under 'Assessment'), with discussed strategies then not being implemented, referral to a psychologist is recommended.

L. *Concentration*

A detailed evidence-based description of Attention-Deficit Hyperactivity Disorder (ADHD) can be found in 'Changes in the Definition of ADHD in DSM-5: Subtle but important' (Epstein & Loren 2013). If difficulty in concentration is the only concern, an assessment by an educational psychologist is the first line of assessment, as occupational therapists are not professionally allowed to administer concentration-specific assessments. Health, tiredness, visual, hearing, sensory modulation, postural control, stress and emotional concerns can erode concentration energy.

Intervention:

Address the underlying causes. Include activities within the theme the child has chosen and grade them to the 'just right challenge' to increase the motivational drive of the child. Also include a motor component as it is better to focus and stay focused when one is engaged in a physical activity as both motor and multiple sensory areas of the brain are activated during a physical activity, compared to a purely mental activity. Give feedback on any improvement, stasis, or regression of the child's concentration to the child and other involved parties.

To ensure that the child takes in what one is saying, first softly call the child's name, wait for them to respond, and gently touch the arm to get their attention if they have not yet responded. Only then give the request. Shouting can result in the child choosing to shut one out, or they could go into shutdown. Advising the child that one can generally see if someone is lying when you look into their eyes is a good way to encourage eye contact (apart from those that find eye contact too sensory threatening).

A true concentration difficulty is due to the insufficiency of the neuro-transmitters in the brain. Research has shown that the most effective method to address properly diagnosed concentration difficulties is a combination of behavioural modification and medication, the second best is medication and the final and not so effective method is behavioural modification (Brown *et al.* 2005). If the child is on medication to address their concentration, give feedback to the parents regarding how the medication has impacted the child's ability to focus and work during the session. Getting the correct dosage of the correct medication for that specific child is crucial. Chat with the child about how their brains are functioning, what the medication does and ask how the medication is currently impacting their occupational performance across all areas. Handwriting, social skills (Brown *et al.* 2005) (particularly regarding reading other's non-verbal cues), awareness of one's own internal cues like needing to go to the toilet, and sports skills (Moran 2008) appear to improve if the concentration difficulty is correctly addressed.

M. *Autism*

The prevalence of autism since the year 2000 has increased by 178% (Schiller 2022). In the United States in 2018, one in 44 children aged eight years and older presented with a diagnosis of autism (Maenner *et al.* 2021). In 2022, Qatar had the highest incidence at 151 per 10 000 children, with the lowest being in France at 69 per 10 000 children. The prevalence in South Africa was 83 per 10 000 children (World Population Review 2023). Four times more boys than girls have autism (Schiller 2022).

A diagnosis for autism is usually only made after the child is three years of age by a medical practitioner, psychologist, or psychiatrist. If the child's occupational therapist sees symptoms of autism behaviour in a child, it is always best to refer the family for a diagnosis. This is to start the provision of guidance in sourcing the most suitable childcare, play group and schooling, relevant support systems (financial and support groups), and to commence any relevant therapies. This diagnosis can be very threatening and scary for many families. It is helpful to gently ask what the parents feel about the child's presenting behaviour. This can guide the occupational therapist in establishing the parents' thoughts and feelings about referral to obtain a diagnosis, support and guidance.

The awareness and acceptance of autism is assisted by the dissemination of information about autism through interested parties and various reality television shows looking at people living with autism, such as 'Love on the Spectrum' (Netflix©).

Assessment:

Be sensitive and adaptable to the child's tolerance of the assessment process, as it can be very threatening for them. One may need to split the assessment into shorter sessions. Home-based assessments can be extremely helpful as the environment is familiar, and the occupational therapist and assessment materials are the only new sensory input. As many formal assessments have numerous language-based test items, it is wise to initially ask what receptive and verbal production language skills the child has, so the most appropriate assessment tool can be selected. Also ascertain beforehand the child's favourite activity so this activity can be used in the assessment to get their attention and engagement, and/or as a reward for their participation. Initially use a calm, low-toned approach to reduce the amount of sensory input. Some parents see the value of the child becoming dysregulated in the assessment, as the occupational therapist then has a clear picture of what they have to manage on a regular basis, and various calming strategies can then be tried out.

It is important to remember that autism has varied presentations and individualised behaviours. Many individuals who present as being higher-functioning have commented that they felt off-kilter with their peers and society as a whole, which can result in anxiety and depression (Lake *et al.* 2014), particularly in the pre-teen and teenage years. Receiving a diagnosis helped them understand why they behave and feel the way they do, and that this is inherently who they are (Aylott 2000; Lake *et al.* 2014).

It is important to be aware that an attachment disorder can present as autism (see below for attachment disorder).

Intervention:

This depends on what areas of concern are established in the assessment. Early intervention is best, to reduce the inculcation of habit patterns that are harder to break, as individuals with autism often have an incredible, exact memory of what was a positive or negative experience, and that can stretch back many years. This excellent memory can impede engagement with activities, affecting all areas of occupational performance.

Intervention is usually multi-faceted. Often the child gets referred first to occupational therapy to address the sensory-based behaviour, which then allows the child to engage more effectively with the other intervention therapies and professionals. Quarterly or biannual team meetings are extremely useful for the parents and the other team members to gain insight into how the child manages in the various settings and regarding the different intervention techniques. Progress, stasis or regression can then be discussed, and techniques can then be streamlined to effect more relevant and cohesive intervention. Medical doctors also address present and emerging concerns like concentration, sleep, eating, anxiety and depression.

N. *Attachment Disorder*

Three attachment styles have been described, namely: Secure, Ambivalent (or contact-resistant, anxious-ambivalent, or resistant) and Defensive (or proximity-avoidant, anxious-avoidant or avoidant) (Tyminski 2021). There are two categories of attachment disorders, reactive attachment disorder and disinhibited social engagement disorder. Both disorders present with a difficulty in relating to other people appropriately. Underlying the attachment disorders is a deprivation of parental care-giving behaviours (Forshee 2015; Tyminski 2021).

The occupational therapist should ascertain the underlying causes. Possible contributing factors to a difficulty in attachment could be a depressed mother (such a post-partum depression and low iron levels) (Murray-Kolb & Beard 2009), parents with attachment disorder themselves, and/or a mismatch of the sensory profiles of the child and the parent. Examples of Attachment Disorders follow:

- A baby was referred for feeding and sensory defensive behaviours, as reported by his mother. During the home-based assessment, it was observed by the mother, occupational therapist, and childminder present, that the baby calmed and took the bottle easily with the childminder, but not with the mother. At the end of the session, the mother slowly turned to the occupational therapist and softly said: 'I was adopted . . . I now realise I have not dealt with this. I need to see a psychotherapist'.

- A mother pregnant with her fourth child, together with the other children, witnessed the sudden, unexpected passing of her husband/the children's father, of a stroke. Dealing with this loss and highly active, grieving children, having low iron levels and feeling exhausted all the time, she was unable to react appropriately to her children's, or her own, needs.

- A mother who was very sensory defensive regarding touch, had a baby who needed lots of deep pressure and touch, which she could not tolerate, so she pushed the baby away.

- A baby who was very over-reactive to touch and deep pressure, calmed only if left to lie on the mat to self-regulate. His mother was desperate to hold and cuddle her baby to help her bond with him.

- Many babies suffering from gastro-oesophageal reflux arch out of being cuddled, which the parents can perceive as rejection.

Intervention depends on the underlying causes. With children, recommendations include psychotherapy, such as play therapy and emotion-focused therapy where the emotions are named and validated (Laurence 2023), counselling and parenting guidance (Kinniburgh *et al.* 2005). The very anxious child may require medication.

Level 2:

These disorders require pharmacological intervention prescribed and monitored by a paediatric psychiatrist. Intervention may also include psychotherapy, speech and language and occupational therapy. Occupational therapy would focus on increasing contact with reality, task analysis, addressing occupational performance and applying the Creative Ability Model (Sherwood 2011).

A. *Anxiety Disorders*

B. *Conduct and Defiant Oppositional Disorders*

C. *Bipolar Mood and Unipolar Depression Disorders*

D. *Elective Mutism*

This is best addressed by behavioural treatment plus medication to reduce underlying anxiety (Black & Uhde 1994). One example was a three-year-old girl from a very rural community who was admitted to a burns unit with 65% burns to her body, where she remained for seven months. Her parents were unfortunately unable to stay for the full length of her treatment and rehabilitation. She stopped talking and all efforts by the varied staff to encourage and entice her to talk were met with silence. The psychologist established that the only control she had, where everything else was taken away from her (from her self-care, nutrition, freedom to do what she wanted when she wanted to, no family who understood her), was to stop talking. Intervention included arranging for regular family stays, medication and providing choices within her daily activities.

E. *Psychotic Disorders*

In a child presenting with signs of psychosis and considering today's current pre-occupation with electronic media, it is important to investigate if the child is suffering from true psychosis or is it the influence of the child's electronic gaming. Electronic gaming can impact on the child's inner world, filling it with images from the engaged-with fantasy world. Enmeshment of the fantasy world with perceived reality can occur. Thus, a disorder of thought perception and delusion disorder of gaming could be established, which would impact on which intervention strategies would be relevant.

QUESTIONS

1. When working with children, what other components and contexts does one have to take cognisance of?

2. Why is it important to understand all aspects of neuro-typical development when working in this field?

3. What is the difference between foundation and splinter skill development, and what should receive priority in therapy in children?

4. What skills set would help you as an occupational therapist when working in this field?

REFERENCES

Als, H., Duffy, F.H. & McAnulty, G.B. (1996) Effectiveness of individualized neurodevelopmental care in the newborn intensive care unit (NICU). *Acta Paediatrica, International Journal of Paediatrics, Supplement*, **85**(**s416**), 21–30. https://doi.org/10.1111/j.1651-2227.1996.tb14273.x

American Psychiatric Association (2013). *Diagnostic and Statistical Manual of Mental Disorders*, 5th edn. American Psychiatric Association, Arlington, VA.

Aylott, J. (2000) Autism in adulthood: the concepts of identity and difference. *British Journal of Nursing*, **9**(**13**), 851–858. https://doi.org/10.12968/bjon.2000.9.13.5513

Ayres, J.A. (2005) *Sensory integration and the child*. p. 213. https://books.google.co.uk/books?hl=en&lr=&id=-7NeFNFswo0C&oi=fnd&pg=PR9&dq=proprioception+causes+difficulty+learning+to+read&ots=iKkuwiQ5Mi&sig=da1L2-YEScUa7LL1cravwgwZ0Ts#v=onepage&q=proprioceptioncausesdifficultylearningtoread&f=false (accessed 22 March 2023)

Black, B. & Uhde, T. (1994) Treatment of elective mutism with fluoxetine: a double-blind, placebo-controlled study. *Journal of the American Academy of Child and Adolescent Psychiatry*, **33**(**7**), 1000–1006. https://doi.org/10.1097/00004583-199409000-00010

Brown, R.T., Amler, R.W., Freeman, W.S. *et al* (2005) American Academy of Pediatrics Technical Report treatment of attention-deficit/hyperactivity disorder: overview of the evidence. *Pediatrics*, **115**(**6**), e749–e757. https://doi.org/10.1542/peds.2004-2560

Bruwer, L. & Tzanos, C. (2016) *Play - a child's primary occupation*. INSTOPP Newsletter, pp. 10–13.

Christiansen, C.H., Baum, C.M. & Bass, J.D. (2015) *Occupational Therapy: Performance, Participation, and Well-Being*, 4th edn. Slack Incorporated, Thorofare, New Jersey.

Crouch, R. & Alers, V. (2014) *Occupational Therapy in Psychiatry and Mental Health*, 5th edn. John Wiley & Sons, Ltd. https://doi.org/10.1002/9781118913536

Doble, S. & Magill-Evans, J. (1992) A model of social interaction to guide occupational therapy practice. *Canadian Journal of Occupational Therapy*, **59**(**3**).

Doidge, N. (2016) *The Brain's Way of Healing: Stories of Remarkable Recoveries and Discoveries*, 1st edn. Penguin Random House UK.

Dunn, W., Brown, C. & McGuigan, A. (1994) The ecology of human performance: a framework for considering the effect of context. *The American Journal of Occupational Therapy _ American Occupational Therapy Association*, **48**(**7**), 595–607. https://doi.org/10.5014/ajot.48.7.595

Epstein, J.N. & Loren, R.E.A. (2013) Changes in the definition of ADHD in DSM-5: subtle but important. *Neuropsychiatry*, **3**(**5**), 455–458. https://doi.org/10.2217/npy.13.59

Forshee, D.L. (2015) *Vagus nerve stimulation for reactive attachment disorder*. Dissertation Abstracts International: Section B: The Sciences and Engineering, 76(2-B(E)), p. Not-Specified. http://ovidsp.ovid.com/ovidweb.cgi?T=JS&PAGE=reference&D=psyc12&NEWS=N&AN=2015-99160-274 (accessed 23 March 2023).

Freeman, H., Reedy, A. & Schalow, A. (2015) *There is limited evidence supporting the use of the SOS approach to feeding with mixed results on the effectiveness to improve eating*. pp. 1–23. www.UWLAX.EDU/OT (accessed 08 March 2023).

Gaughan, R. (2010) *Accidental Genius*. Zebra Press, Cape-Town.

Giampapa, V. (2023) *How to Sleep Better_ 12 Pro Tips for Better Sleep Tonight – Healthycell*. Healthycell. https://www.healthycell.com/blogs/articles/12-pro-tips-for-better-sleep-tonight (accessed 29 March 2023)

Gold, N. (1993) Depression and social adjustment in siblings of boys with autism. *Journal of Autism and Developmental Disorders*, **23**(**1**), 147–163. https://doi.org/10.1007/BF01066424

Imuta, K., Song, S., Henry, J.D. *et al* (2022) A meta-analytic review on the social–emotional intelligence correlates of the six bullying roles: bullies, followers, victims, bully-victims, defenders, and outsiders. *Psychological Bulletin*, **148**(**3–4**), 199–226. https://doi.org/10.1037/bul0000364

Kinniburgh, K.J., Blaustein, M., Spinazzola, J. & van der Kolk, B.A. (2005) Attachment, self-regulation, and competency. *Psychiatric Annals*, **35**(**5**), 424–430. https://doi.org/10.3928/00485713-20050501-08

Kritzas, C. & Bytheway, J. (2015) *Smart heart - the big box board games*. https://www.thebigbox.co.za/game/smart-heart/ (accessed 22 March 2023)

Kubheka, B.Z., Carter, V. & Mwaura, J. (2020) Social media health promotion in South Africa: opportunities and challenges. *African Journal of Primary Health Care and Family Medicine*, **12**(**1**), e1–e7. https://doi.org/10.4102/PHCFM.V12I1.2389

Lake, J.K., Perry, A. & Lunsky, Y. (2014) Mental health services for individuals with high functioning autism spectrum disorder. *Autism Research and Treatment*, **2014**, 1–9. https://doi.org/10.1155/2014/502420

Laurence, E.R.S. (2023) *Attachment disorder: signs, symptoms and treatments – Forbes Health*. https://www.forbes.com/health/mind/what-is-attachment-disorder/ (accessed 25 March 2023)

LeBourgeois, M.K., Hale L., Chang, A.-M., Akacem, L.D., Montgomery-Downs, H.E. & Buxton, O.M. (2017) Digital media and sleep in childhood and adolescence. *Pediatrics*. American Academy of Pediatrics, **140** (Supplement_2 November 2017), S92–S96. https://doi.org/10.1542/peds.2016-1758J

Lynch, K.M., Kimball, J.G., Williams, N.E., Thomas, M.A., Atwood, K.D. & Stewart, K.C. (2011) Using salivary cortisol to measure the effects of a Wilbarger protocol-based procedure on sympathetic arousal: a pilot study. *American Journal of Occupational Therapy*. https://doi.org/10.5014/ajot.61.406

Maenner, M.J., Shaw, K.A., Bakian, A.V. *et al* (2021) Prevalence and characteristics of autism spectrum disorder among children aged 8 years — autism and developmental disabilities monitoring network, 11 sites, United States, 2018. *MMWR Surveillance Summaries*, **70(11)**, 1–16. https://doi.org/10.15585/MMWR.SS7011A1

McDougall, B. (2012) *The wall model of occupational performance | Bunty's Wall*. https://thehappyhandwriter.co.za/wall-model-occupational-performance/ (accessed 22 March 2023)

Moran, A. (2008) *Attention in Sport–A Review*, 1st edn. Routledge.

Murray-Kolb, L.E. & Beard, J.L. (2009) Iron deficiency and child and maternal health 1–4. The *American Journal of Clinical Nutrition*, **89(3)**, 946–950. https://doi.org/10.3945/ajcn.2008.26692D.946S

Ned, L., Tiwari, R., Buchanan, H., Van Niekerk, L., Sherry, K. & Chikte, U. (2020) Changing demographic trends among South African occupational therapists: 2002 to 2018. *Human Resources for Health*, **18(1)**, 1–12. https://doi.org/10.1186/s12960-020-0464-3

Parham, L.D. & Fazio, L.S. (2008) *Play in Occupational Therapy for Children*. Mosby Elsevier, St. Louis. https://doi.org/10.1016/B978-0-323-02954-4.X0001-3

Perrins Gendron, M. (2016–2023). Interpretation sheet. Presented at Paediatric Courses held SA, Namibia, Kenya.

Perrins Gendron, M.M.C., Van Niekerk, L. & Cloete, L. (2022) The use and value of play: perspectives from the continent of Africa–a scoping review. *Scandinavian Journal of Occupational Therapy*, **29(3)**. https://doi.org/10.1080/11038128.2022.2043433

Scatliffe, N. Casavant, S., Vittner, D., Cong, X. (2019) Oxytocin and early parent-infant interactions: a systematic review. *International Journal of Nursing Sciences*, **6(4)**, 445–453. https://doi.org/10.1016/j.ijnss.2019.09.009

Schiller, J. (2022) *Autism statistics & facts: how many people have autism*. The Treetop Therapy © 2023.

Schultz, J.K. & Schkade, S. (1992) Occupational adaptation: toward a holistic approach for contemporary practice, part 1. *The American Journal of Occupational Therapy, American Occupational Therapy Association.*, **46(9)**, 829–837. https://doi.org/10.5014/ajot.46.9.829

Sherwood, W. (2011) An introduction to the Vona Du Toit Model of creative ability. *Revista Electrónica de Terapia Ocupacional Galicia, TOG*, **8(14)**, 1–26.

Taylor, R., Bower, P. & Fisher, G. (2023) *Kielhofner's Model of Human Occupation*, 6th edn. Lippincott Williams & Wilkins.

Thiart, T. (2020) *About us - anti bullying programme*. www.1000women.co.za (accessed 25 March 2023)

Tyminski, Q. (2021) Psychosocial occupational therapy. *Occupational Therapy in Health Care*, **36(2)**, 1–2. https://doi.org/10.1080/07380577.2021.1983239

Weenink-Schoonover, J. & O'Brien, J. (2020) *Case-Smith's Occupational Therapy for Children and Adolescents*. Mosby.

West, K.E. Jablonski, M.R., Warfield, B. *et al* (2011) Blue light from light-emitting diodes elicits a dose-dependent suppression of melatonin in humans. *Journal of Applied Physiology*, **110(3)**, 619–626. https://doi.org/10.1152/japplphysiol.01413.2009

Whitebread, D.D. (2012) *The importance of play*, Toy Industries of Europe, (April), pp. 1–55. https://doi.org/10.5455/msm.2015.27.438-441

Wolstenholme, H. Kelly, C., Hennessy, M. & Heary, C. (2020) Childhood fussy/picky eating behaviours: a systematic review and synthesis of qualitative studies. *International Journal of Behavioural Nutrition and Physical Activity*, **17(1)**, pp. 1–22. https://doi.org/10.1186/s12966-019-0899-x

World Population Review (2023) *World population review: autism rates by Country 2023*. https://worldpopulationreview.com.about (accessed 15 May 2023)

CHAPTER 18

Occupational Therapy Intervention with Adolescents Experiencing Mental Health Distress

Lisa Wegner[1], Elvin Williams[2] and Marlene van den Berg[3]

[1]Department of Occupational Therapy, Faculty of Community and Health Sciences, University of the Western Cape, Bellville, South Africa

[2]Division of Occupational Therapy and Arts Therapies, School of Health Sciences, Queen Margaret University, Edinburgh, Scotland

[3]Akeso Montrose Manor, Specialist Eating Disorder Clinic & Healing Spaces Wellness, Mental Health Community, Constantia, South Africa

KEY LEARNING POINTS

- A theoretical understanding of adolescent mental health and distress.

- Application of the Occupational Therapy Practice Framework: Domain and Process (OTPF-4).

- Legislation for adolescent mental health.

- Value of the therapeutic relationship in adolescent care.

- Contextual and evidence-based assessment in adolescent mental health.

- Occupational therapy intervention in adolescent mental health and distress.

- Intervention planning and principles in adolescent mental health.

- Aftercare.

INTRODUCTION

Adolescence can be described as the time between childhood and adulthood, and comes from the Latin word 'adolescere', which means 'to grow up' or 'to grow to adulthood'. Generally, the adolescent phase is from 12 to 18 years for girls and 13 to 20 years for boys (Cherry 2013). Adolescence can be divided up further into three stages: early phase (11–14 years), middle phase (14–17 years) and late phase (17–19 years); however, these divisions are arbitrary, as growth and development occur along a continuum that varies from person to person (Boland *et al.* 2021). The rapid physical and developmental changes that take place during the adolescents' life phase play a major role in their specific needs, behaviours and problems.

Therefore, it is essential that mental health services for adolescents are separated from services for children and adults. The transition to adulthood and ease with which the adolescent makes the transition are dependent on a multitude of different factors, which are outlined in this chapter.

A THEORETICAL UNDERSTANDING OF ADOLESCENT MENTAL HEALTH AND DISTRESS

The multifaceted, interactive effects of personal and environmental factors on adolescent mental health can be understood through the application of theory, for example Life Course theory (Elder *et al.* 2003), Ecological Systems theory (Bronfenbrenner 1995) and the Socio-Ecological Model (SEM) (Centers for Disease Control and Prevention 2019). Adopting a life course approach to adolescent mental health means that to understand adolescent behaviour, it is essential to consider events prior to, during and post, adolescence. The life course approach aligns with Bronfenbrenner's Ecological Systems theory (1995), which proposes that development takes place in four nested systems:

- the microsystem which is the layer closest to the adolescent containing the structures with which the adolescent has contact and interacts (e.g. family, school and community);

- the mesosystem which includes connections between structures of the microsystem;

- the exosystem, which is the larger social system or external environment which indirectly influences development;

- the macrosystem which is the broad socio-cultural context such as culture, politics, values, customs and laws.

Each level has a cascading effect and interacts with the other systems. Examples of factors that influence adolescent health and well-being include personality and parental involvement (microsystem); school curricula, extracurricular programmes and community resources (mesosystem); safety issues in communities that influence access to certain leisure pursuits (exosystem) and cultural beliefs (macrosystem).

Similarly, the SEM examines the individual, relationship, societal and community factors that place individuals at risk. Majee *et al.* (2021) used the SEM to describe factors influencing substance use and other risk behaviour in youth aged 18–34 years living in rural communities in South Africa. Majee *et al.* (2021) found that rural youth experienced challenges at an individual level, for example, hopelessness and lack of motivation; in relationships with others, for example, a lack of adult role models including fathers; at a community level, for example, lack of built environmental resources and educational opportunities; and at a societal level, for example, unemployment.

Occupational therapists work with adolescents in a variety of different settings and it is essential to consider their mental health and potential distress. Globally, research highlights the multitude of challenges faced by adolescents. Challenges negatively affect adolescent mental health and result in mental distress and disorders. Exacerbating the situation are global human ecosystem disasters such as the COVID-19 pandemic, earthquakes, floods and wars, in conjunction with widespread poverty and youth unemployment. Youth in low-to middle-income countries such as South Africa, tend to bear the brunt of such challenges, amidst the burgeoning growth of the youth population.

Occupational therapists gain a holistic perspective of their adolescent clients using theories such as those mentioned above. In addition, there is the Occupational Therapy Practice Framework: Domain and Process (OTPF-4) that was developed by the American Occupational Therapy Association (AOTA) (2020). The OTPF-4 is based on systems theory and is a useful way to view occupational therapy intervention with adolescents experiencing mental health distress.

APPLICATION OF THE OCCUPATIONAL THERAPY PRACTICE FRAMEWORK: DOMAIN AND PROCESS

The OTPF-4 (AOTA 2020) provides a structure to describe concepts that guide occupational therapy practice and can be applied in any setting. The OTPF-4 is divided into two sections: (i) the domain, which is the scope of the occupational therapy profession's knowledge and expertise, and (ii) the process, which are the steps implemented to carry out the practice of occupational therapy. The aspect of 'domain' includes occupations, contexts, performance patterns, performance skills and client factors (AOTA 2020).

OCCUPATIONS

When working with adolescents, occupational therapists consider areas of occupation including activities of daily living (ADL), instrumental ADL (IADL), health management, rest and sleep, education, work, play, leisure, civic and social participation (AOTA 2020). Engagement in these areas provides opportunities for adolescents to develop knowledge and skills, and shapes attitudes. For example, education is central to adolescent development as it enables the adolescent to practise performance skills such as process skills and social interaction, and develop performance patterns such as daily routine. Occupational performance priorities amongst adolescents with learning difficulties included productivity (studying, attending classes and doing a part-time job), pleasure (playing games, listening to music, attending a party, playing sport, going on holiday, spending time with family) and restoration (eating, taking a shower, other hygiene occupations and exercising) (Marx *et al.* 2023). Truancy and premature school leaving or 'drop-out' are indicators of problems in the occupation of education and are associated with substance use (Wegner *et al.* 2006) and leisure boredom (Wegner *et al.* 2008).

As adolescents explore the occupation of leisure, they identify interests, experiment with different activities and search for resources in their community, whilst leisure participation promotes autonomy, motivation, decision-making and social skills, and enhances self-confidence. However, leisure also provides a context for adolescents to engage in negative, unhealthy leisure activities such as substance use (Wegner 2011). This places adolescents at-risk of mental health distress and disorders. Occupations such as substance use that are not prosocial, healthy or productive and do not promote health and well-being are known as 'dark occupations'; these include violence and other anti-social behaviours (Twinley & Addidle 2012; Twinley 2013).

During adolescence, peer groups are important, enabling adolescents to practise social skills as they learn to build relationships with others, and forming the foundation of intimate relationships in adult life. Peer groups are a mini-society in which adolescents can experiment with social behaviour and relationships because they usually provide a safe environment. On the other hand, bullying and cyberbullying in adolescent peer groups is a phenomenon that may cause mental distress. Typically, in the early phase, adolescents may form friendships and intimate relationships within a spectrum of gender identities that are not limited to a binary understanding. Because adolescence can also be a time of experimentation with sexuality, these experiences of friendships and intimate relationships vary widely and may be influenced by individual, cultural and societal factors. Due to the emotional and cognitive development that occurs as they search for identity and develop independence, adolescents may conflict with parents, educators and those in authority. Finally, it is essential to consider the development of prevocational skills in preparation for further education and work.

CONTEXTS

Environmental and Personal Factors

Occupational therapists believe that participation in life through active engagement in occupation promotes health and well-being. Participation involves engagement in, and performance of, occupations, that occurs as a transaction between the person, the context and the occupation (Law et al. 1996; Christiansen & Baum 1997). Occupational therapists facilitate optimal performance in meaningful occupations. To do this, they consider context in terms of the environmental and personal factors that act either as facilitators or barriers to performance. Environmental factors are aspects of the physical, social and attitudinal context, for example, natural environment, technology, support, attitudes, services and policies (AOTA 2020). Personal factors are the unique features of a person that are not part of health, for example, demographic information, but also include customs, beliefs, spirituality and expectations accepted by the society or culture of a person (AOTA 2020).

Adolescents face many challenges from environmental factors that can be regarded as occupational injustices (Wilcock 1998) and increase the risk of experiencing mental distress. Examples of these challenges include poverty, unemployment, violence, gangsterism, substance use, HIV infection and teenage pregnancy. Many adolescents grow up in unsupportive families, where parents lack parenting skills or are absent. Some adolescents have their own children to care for, or are forced to take on a parenting role for younger siblings; this comes with additional responsibilities. Risk factors such as substance use, learning problems, antisocial behaviour and difficulty negotiating peer pressure may increase the likelihood of gang involvement and violent or delinquent behaviour (Cooper & Ward 2012). Schools should be safe contexts for adolescents, but unfortunately, this is not always the case as can be seen by the high prevalence of bullying, gang activity, educator-on-learner abuse and sexual violence (Gevers & Flisher 2012). Cyberbullying is a form of aggression using electronic means such as mobile phones, social networking sites, personal webpages and photos to inflict harm, and is associated with psychological, behavioural and health problems including suicide risk (Brochado et al. 2017).

It is essential for occupational therapists to consider the influence of personal factors on adolescent health and mental distress. During adolescence, individuals engage in an active process of exploring their sense of self, which includes exploring various roles and values related to their sexual self and gender identity. While there is growing recognition that gender identity is a non-binary, complex and diverse concept, it is also acknowledged that gender diversity in adolescents likely causes tension because of being outside of society's binary expectations and that this can therefore be closely related to their experience of mental health, well-being and distress (Potter et al. 2020). In their large-scale study investigating the prevalence of gender diversity and its connection with mental health problems amongst youth, Potter et al. (2020) found that compared to their peers, transgender youth aged between 9 and 11 years old had notably higher rates of recurrent thoughts of death and self-injurious behaviour. These findings are in line with previous research conducted by Turban and Ehrensaft (2017), which demonstrated that transgender and gender-diverse (TGD) youth have higher rates of depression, anxiety, and suicidality when compared to their cisgender peers. These studies have important implications for occupational therapy in terms of providing, and advocating for, an inclusive, person-centred practice and profession that embraces occupational justice.

PERFORMANCE PATTERNS

Habits, Routines, Roles and Rituals

Performance patterns (habits, routines, roles and rituals) are acquired through consistent engagement in occupations over time (AOTA 2020). These patterns develop throughout life and structure the use of time. They can either facilitate or hinder performance, therefore influencing mental health. For example, poor time management can be stressful and anxiety-provoking for adolescents. In addition to the basic roles of childhood such as son/daughter, sibling, learner and friend, adolescents develop more diverse and far-reaching roles, for example member of a sports team, boyfriend/girlfriend, volunteer and casual worker. These new roles contribute to the adolescent's identity and provide a framework for establishing new performance patterns and skills.

PERFORMANCE SKILLS

Motor Skills, Process Skills and Social Interaction Skills

Performance skills are observable, goal-directed actions comprising motor, process and social interaction skills (AOTA 2020). The occupational therapist evaluates the client's ability to perform an activity through the performance of the relevant skills and actions. Motor skills include movement of self and objects, and positioning of the body. Process skills include applying knowledge and organising self, time, space and objects. Social interaction includes verbal and non-verbal skills to communicate.

Emotional regulation skills are an important part of adolescent development that influence social interaction. Due to the influence of hormonal changes on emotions, the adolescent phase is fraught with frequent emotional instability and lability. Adolescents find it difficult to regulate their emotions. They may be aggressive one moment and in tears the next, to the astonishment of the people around them. Due to their egocentrism, they are more focused on their own emotional experiences. The changes in their bodies and expectations and responsibilities around them may leave them feeling out of control and confused. However, occupational therapists should remember that this is part of normal development and does not necessarily indicate the presence of pathology.

CLIENT FACTORS

According to the OTPF-4 (AOTA 2020), client factors are specific capacities and characteristics present in a person that influence occupational performance and include values, beliefs, spirituality, body functions and body structures. These elements cannot be directly seen through the performance of actions as they reside within the individual. Client factors are affected by illness, disability, life stages, life experiences, occupations, contexts, performance patterns and performance skills (AOTA 2020).

Values, Beliefs and Spirituality

During this developmental phase, adolescents start to internalise their values and beliefs. They often question the values, beliefs and spirituality prescribed by those around them, for example parents and educators, which may lead to conflict. Adolescents whose behaviour is incongruent with their internalised values are at risk of developing mental distress such as depression and anxiety.

Body Functions and Structures

Occupational therapists working with adolescents should consider the body structure and functional changes that occur during puberty. Due to hormonal changes, adolescents' bodies change, their growth rate increases and they develop secondary sexual characteristics. These physiological changes require energy, and adolescents therefore often present with an apathy or lethargic nature, which could easily be labelled as laziness. Their bodies may not change or grow proportionally, and they often appear gangly or feel clumsy. These body changes affect their body image, which needs to be adjusted continually. Adolescents may become self-conscious about their bodies, and physical appearance becomes very important.

According to Piaget's (McLeod 2009) theory, adolescents' cognitive development is described as formal operational thought. As adolescents develop abstract thought processes, they develop the ability to formulate a logical argument and speculate. Their ability to plan improves as well as their metacognitive ability, which enables them to evaluate their own thinking. The development of the ability to think creatively improves their problem-solving abilities. Adolescents enjoy formulating, testing and evaluating hypotheses. For example, they may debate the political situation with their parents or choose to change their religion. This may result in conflict arising as the adolescent practises their newfound skills and abilities. Adolescents' cognitive development includes self-centred thought, and their egocentrism often causes conflict with others around them.

POLICIES FOR ADOLESCENT MENTAL HEALTH

It is imperative for occupational therapists to have a comprehensive understanding of the policies that influence the provision of person-centred care to young people experiencing mental health distress or who are at risk of developing mental health concerns (Brooks & Bannigan 2018). By understanding the relevant mental health policies, occupational therapists can provide evidence-based interventions that are effective and aligned with the health system realities impacting care provision. By staying informed about mental health policies, occupational therapists can advocate for, and enable, self-advocacy for the adolescent and family to facilitate access to services that support health, well-being and participation. Occupational therapists utilise their knowledge and understanding of mental health policies to collaborate effectively with team members across the health, social, education and work sectors to ensure that service provision extends beyond medical, curative care to include issues of access to school, leisure and social participation in communities and vocational exploration, as well as health promotion and health prevention initiatives that enable their overall health and well-being.

VALUE OF THE THERAPEUTIC RELATIONSHIP IN ADOLESCENT CARE

Forming a dynamic and inclusive relationship is a prerequisite for effectively engaging with, and understanding, adolescents (Labouliere et al. 2017; Ryan et al. 2021). Establishing trust and rapport is a foundation for effective treatment (Fraser et al. 2019). Occupational therapists should recognise that they may be one of the most stable and consistent adults in the life of their adolescent clients. Although adolescents may initially display defensive behaviour, occupational therapists are trained to overcome resistance and establish and maintain a transparent, effective therapeutic rapport.

To support the development of a therapeutic relationship with adolescents, the following strategies are recommended. Firstly, occupational therapists should remain authentic while adhering to professional, therapeutic boundaries. Adolescents value clinicians who are honest and do not adjust themselves to conform to the adolescent's expectations (Fraser *et al.* 2019; Ryan *et al.* 2021). Clinicians should aim to create a non-judgmental environment where adolescents feel safe and cared for as they 'open up'. Secondly, occupation and engagement are crucial for effective occupational therapy. Bueno *et al.* (2021) describe the concept of 'occupation as a path' and suggest that occupational therapists consider this when selecting activities. Adolescents should be brought into the therapeutic alliance through collaborative work with the therapist to strengthen the therapeutic bond (Bueno *et al.* 2021). Clinicians should avoid using a didactic approach and instead view themselves as partners in the therapeutic process. Thirdly, the therapeutic relationship with an adolescent requires a high level of intuitive responsiveness. Occupational therapists should not rely solely on frameworks, strategies and activities, but instead remain alert to the unique characteristics, life circumstances and interpersonal dynamics of each client (Bueno *et al.* 2021). Lastly, occupational therapists should not underestimate the abilities of adolescents during therapy sessions. They should support them in completing the tasks of therapy themselves, which reinforces the development of life skills and a sense of autonomy and empowerment (Witty 2007; Schlapobersky 2016). An adolescent who feels trusted, respected and validated for their ability within the therapeutic relationship will be able to transfer this experience to their interactions for the rest of their lives.

CONTEXTUAL AND EVIDENCE-BASED ASSESSMENT IN ADOLESCENT MENTAL HEALTH

ASSESSMENT METHODS

Assessments are essential for effective treatment. Furthermore, without a good assessment, occupational therapists cannot provide evidence of quality treatment. Time should be taken to conduct a comprehensive assessment, with a focus on occupation-based assessments in order to create an occupational profile. In short, all aspects of the OTPF-4 (AOTA 2020) need to be assessed although other practice models may be selected to form an integrated client assessment. The different assessment methods include interviews, collateral information, participation in occupation-based activities, observations in structured and unstructured situations and formal/standardised and informal tests. The occupational therapist should investigate the

advantages of each assessment and decide which would work best within the specific practice context. Importantly, any assessment needs to be used and interpreted using clinical reasoning. Occupational therapists liaise with the multidisciplinary team to present their assessment findings and determine the impact of the mental health distress on the occupational functioning of the adolescent, and plan relevant intervention.

Interviewing

The interview is an essential part of the assessment process. It supports the gathering of information, and assists with establishing therapeutic relationships. Since interviewing is a generic skill, it can be performed by different members of the multidisciplinary team depending on the role division within the team. The occupational therapist is well suited to interview the client, with a focus on all aspects of the OTPF-4 providing a holistic perspective of the obstacles to recovery.

Part of the interview should be conducted with the parents (even if divorced) present. The occupational therapist can gain valuable insight by observing the client's relationship with both parents and their relationship with each other. Whilst the parents are present the occupational therapist can ask open-ended questions regarding milestones and general background history, as well as school functioning or decline.

After the parents have been asked to leave, the interview will continue with the client. It is important to reassure the client of confidentiality, explaining that the information will be shared with all the team members to ensure optimal treatment but that the parents will not be informed unless the adolescent gives permission. Only then is it more likely that the personal information concerning sexual development, relationship with peers, suicidal ideation and attempts, self-harm behaviour and use of substances will yield truthful answers. The way the questions are posed and the occupational therapist's non-verbal communication are important when sensitive questions are asked. The therapist should ask engaging and open-ended questions, for example, 'What do you do after school?' and 'What would your best friends say if I asked them about you?', and avoid leading questions like 'You haven't used drugs before, have you?'

Collateral Information

The occupational therapist should select appropriate people to verify information by making use of collateral information. The nursing staff who observe the client continuously in the ward can offer valuable information. If possible, collateral information can also be obtained from family members and/or educators, but always with the permission of the client and the parents.

Participation in Occupation-based Activities

Using activities is an essential part of occupational therapy assessment. Poor insight and poor self-concept on the part of the client may cause inaccurate accounts of abilities during interviewing, therefore, participation in activities yields a wealth of information. The manner in which adolescents approach and carry out an activity may be indicative of the way they lead their lives. For example, adolescents who find it difficult to make decisions within a craft activity may exhibit problems concerning decision-making in their schoolwork or in relationships. The same may hold true for other performance skills which can be observed during the activity.

An example of an assessment activity is making a collage about oneself and then explaining it. This assessment is useful because it covers many performance patterns and skills within the occupational areas, and provides insight into pre-vocational skills, especially work competency, which includes planning, neatness, accuracy, ability to evaluate one's work, ability to recognise mistakes and perseverance. It is also an easy and affordable assessment. The themes of the collage provide an indication of issues that are uppermost in the client's mind. Another advantage of a collage is that it is non-threatening to adolescents and they can express themselves freely and creatively.

Occupational group therapy is highly recommended as a method of assessing adolescents as peer relationships are essential to their development. Adolescents should be introduced to unstructured and structured groups as part of their assessment providing the occupational therapist with opportunities to observe social interaction and other skills.

Observation in Structured and Unstructured Situations

During assessments, the occupational therapist should observe both content (what is the client saying) and process (e.g. what do they avoid? What body language is portrayed?). Additional observations can be made when the client is in an unstructured situation, for example eating lunch and playing outside in free time or during sports. These observations may bring new insights. It is especially useful when assessing clients with anxiety disorders as their anxiety can influence test results.

Standardised Tests and Informal Tests

Occupational therapists must ensure that the standardised tests used during assessments are suitable for the client's culture as well as their developmental level. Assessment results of tests standardised for adults or younger children cannot simply be generalised to adolescents. For example, the Developmental Test of Visual-Motor Integration (Beery 1997) is reliable for adolescents only up to the ceiling age of 15 years (Boyt Schell *et al.* 2013). Tests like the Canadian Occupational Performance Measure (COPM) (Law *et al.* 1999), Hospital Anxiety and Depression Scale (HADS) (Milne 1992), Inventory of Interpersonal Problems (Milne 1992), Coping Responses Inventory (Milne 1992) and Cognitive Assessment of Minnesota (CAM) (Rustad *et al.* 1993) are tests that occupational therapists may administer with adolescents. Repeated mood assessments over time are more accurate (Morrison & Anders 1999). Numerous informal questionnaires are available on the Internet but should be used with caution. The clients may also be referred to a counselling psychologist for additional tests, for example, personality, aptitude and study skills assessments.

ASSESSMENT OF OCCUPATIONAL PERFORMANCE AREAS

LEISURE

Adolescents may engage in both active and passive leisure activities. The clinician should assess the type of leisure activities engaged in, as well as the subjective meaning and experience of the engagement. Negative leisure, dysfunctional leisure, or non-constructive leisure activities, including risky sexual behaviour or substance use, should be explored, although the clinician should note that a client may not volunteer this information without feeling safe within the therapeutic relationship. Occupational therapists should avoid judging or criticising the adolescent's leisure activities and rather ascertain what underlying motivation (or potential indication of pathology) underpins the leisure pursuits of the client.

EDUCATION

Assessing the performance area of education, specifically school functioning, is essential. If a school teacher or educational psychologist is part of the multidisciplinary team, they could assess this area. The adolescent experiencing mental distress or illness may struggle to complete their academic work, due to overwhelming anxiety, drive, behaviour, mood or other emotional and psychological difficulties. Traumatic experiences and the adolescent's relationships with peers and teachers should also be assessed and discussed.

WORK

For most adolescent clients, school or educational pursuits may constitute their primary performance area. However, adolescence is also the stage of life where individuals develop their capacity for entering the open labour market, even if on a part-time or voluntary basis. Occupational therapists should consider both pre-vocational and vocational skills, especially work endurance, work habits (which include personal and social presentation and work competency) and work motivation. Refer to Chapter 13 of this book.

ACTIVITIES OF DAILY LIVING (ADL)

Typically developing adolescents should be able to manage their ADL independently. This includes bathing, showering, toileting, dressing, eating, feeding, mobility, personal device care, personal hygiene and grooming. If problem areas surface from the interview or collateral information, the occupational therapist should assess the execution of the ADL to determine the exact problem. Occupational therapists should not shy away from enquiring about the sexual activities of an adolescent, but should approach this with sensitivity considering the adolescent's level of development. For some, this may be mastering the activity of grooming, cosmetics, shaving and managing menstruation; whilst others may be curious about sexual intimacy, or possibly engaging in risky behaviour. It should also be noted that the adolescent's physical abilities to perform ADL's may be intact, but underlying causes of an emotional nature, i.e. lack of motivation, poor sense of self-worth or rebellion may lie beneath the negation of ADL performance.

INSTRUMENTAL ACTIVITIES OF DAILY LIVING (IADL)

The more complex ADL, otherwise known as IADL (AOTA 2020), are those orientated towards interacting with the environment and include caring for others, child-rearing, care of pets, communication device use, community mobility, financial management, health management and maintenance, home establishment and management, meal preparation and clean-up, safety procedures, emergency responses and shopping. The assumption of caregiving and home management roles by adolescents, when necessitated by conditions of extreme poverty, unemployment, or child-headed households, can significantly impact their developmental trajectory, limiting opportunities for education and personal growth, and can potentially lead to a variety of occupational risk factors, such an occupational imbalance and occupational deprivation. Occupational therapists should understand their role as advocates in this regard and should work towards facilitating occupational balance and enabling occupational choice for educational and economic support. In addition, occupational therapist may work with parents or guardians to identify potential IADLS that may bring physical or emotional harm to the adolescent. Assessment could further include determining where the client needs assistance and support and what resources are available in their contexts that support their occupational engagement.

HEALTH MANAGEMENT

The occupational therapist should asses the adolescent's understanding and insight of, and ability to manage, their social and emotional health, specific conditions and symptoms, medication management, physical activity, nutrition management and personal care device management.

SOCIAL PARTICIPATION

Social participation and acceptance, and the experience of belonging are a major part of adolescent development. Social skills and experiences gained in this phase may either positively or negatively transfer to all the remaining life phases. Problems experienced in developing social participation will have a detrimental impact on all aspects of the client's life in the next phase. Social participation assessment includes all

aspects of social skills with peers, siblings, parents, educators and within the community. It should also review the adolescent's social participation history to determine whether unhelpful patterns in the past or previous traumatic experiences are currently hindering social inclusion. Verbal and non-verbal communication as well as the more subtle aspects of social skills, like reciprocity and nuances, should be assessed. The ability to reciprocate in a relationship can be observed within a group setting. Observation of the adolescent's non-verbal communication should assess whether it is congruent with verbal skills. The occupational therapist should assess if the adolescent is able to look beyond themselves and focus on others by giving support, listening, taking turns and being able to give and receive in a relationship. When observed within a group setting, the adolescent's ability to be assertive will be reflected more realistically. With the ever-expanding use of technology and socialising via electronic social media, adolescents may be at-risk of not developing effective social participation skills required in relationships. The use of social media should therefore form part of the occupational therapy assessment.

SLEEP/REST

Adolescents often report feelings of exhaustion, which may be mistakenly perceived as 'laziness', 'unwillingness to help' or being 'unmotivated'. However, research has shown that adolescents have a biological delay in their circadian rhythms, which causes them to feel tired later and go to bed much later. Due to still needing to rise early for school, adolescents experience significant sleep deprivation during their teenage years, which can affect their neurological development (Bruce et al. 2017). The occupational therapist should expect some sleep difficulties, and anticipate parents/guardians complaining about the ongoing tiredness and lethargy with which the adolescent presents. The assessment needs to take into account context, normative development, and hidden pathology. Assessment should explore whether stressors, mood and cognitive factors, trauma or substance use play a role in sleep/rest disruption (Bruce et al. 2017). Collateral information and sleep tracking can also be helpful in assessing sleep and rest performance. When assessing sleep, it is important to consider all activities and habits that the adolescent engages in during the day, including practical factors, for example, using energy drinks or lack of exercise, and emotional factors, for example, anxiety or trauma, that may affect sleep (Bruce et al. 2017).

OCCUPATIONAL THERAPY INTERVENTION IN ADOLESCENT MENTAL HEALTH AND DISTRESS

INTERVENTION PROGRAMMES

When planning treatment, the occupational therapist should consider the most relevant focus of intervention. The level of insight and stage of recovery plays a role in the format of

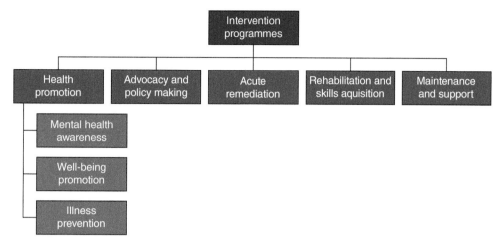

DIAGRAM 18.1 Types of intervention programmes.

treatment. Diagram 18.1 shows the type of programmes that can be considered when working with adolescents. Intervention can be directed towards one programme type or include a combination of programmes, for instance, acute remediation will be the appropriate programme when working with the psychotic adolescent admitted in hospital, whilst a health promotion programme on mental health awareness and skills acquisition can be used when presenting leadership groups in a school setting.

INTERVENTION SETTINGS

Equipped with a multifaceted skill set and a broad understanding of functioning across various areas of life, occupational therapists can expertly step into different roles and work seamlessly in diverse settings including schools, hospitals, community centres, places of safety and private practice and out-of-school contexts (Wegner & Caldwell 2012). Diagrams 18.2–18.4 show the health, education and social welfare settings where occupational therapists can work with adolescents.

CONSIDERATIONS FOR INTERVENTION

A comprehensive assessment by the team should ascertain the treatment focus and order of treatment priorities. Treating adolescent clients involves holding many parts of their lives and their inner worlds, whilst rooted in an understanding of therapy. Occupational therapists can often fixate on the aspect that

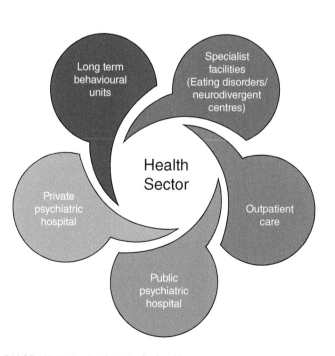

DIAGRAM 18.2 Settings in the health sector.

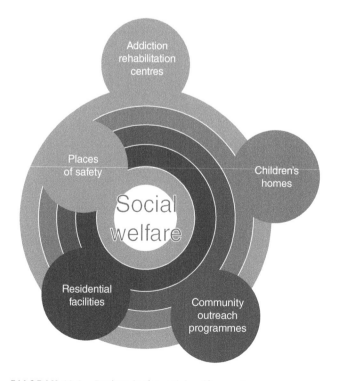

DIAGRAM 18.3 Settings in the social welfare sector.

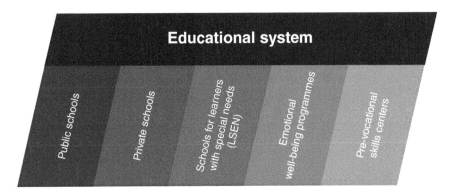

DIAGRAM 18.4   Settings in the education system.

brought the client into therapy, but a comprehensive treatment plan is required to support the adolescent's progress from distress to mental well-being. The next section integrates the well-proven foundations of occupational therapy and occupational performance areas with a contemporary perspective on what is observed and experienced in the practice of working with adolescents. The following areas of intervention can be used as a guideline for clinicians in their planning process.

Symptom Alleviation

Adolescents often arrive in the therapy room with high levels of distress. Occupational therapy should offer immediate symptom alleviation and post-session containment strategies. Due to the normative adolescent experience of feeling misunderstood and separated from others (Hazen et al. 2008), a client who feels validated and guided to implement containment strategies in action is more likely to commit to ongoing therapy. Occupational therapists should consider appropriate and evidence-based symptom alleviation techniques, approaches and frameworks, for example, Dialectical Behavioural Therapy (DBT), Sensory Integration, Neurophysiology and the Behaviouristic approach (discussed below). Sessions should start, and end, with activities that facilitate emotional regulation and instil hope to enhance the positive outcomes of intervention.

Developing a Sense of Self

Adolescence can be a time of insecurity, with issues such as fear of judgement, validation seeking, poor self-worth and identity confusion prevalent in both pathological and non-pathological cases (Caskey & Anfara 2007). It is crucial for therapists to understand this developmental challenge and focus on strengthening an adolescent's sense of self before addressing other therapeutic goals. If an occupational therapist prematurely focuses on problem-solving and skill development with a depressed adolescent, they may face resistance and sessions that spiral into negative self-talk (Waszczuk et al. 2016). Therefore, intervention aimed at promoting self-worth and identity formation should be facilitated in addition to symptom alleviation (Hazen et al. 2008). Rather than striving towards a fixed identity for the client, the therapist should

empower them to invest in a lifelong process of self-discovery (Fernández-Berrocal et al. 2006). By equipping adolescents with emotional intelligence and interpersonal skills, they will be better equipped to manage mental illness and future obstacles (Fernández-Berrocal et al. 2006).

Developing Skills

Occupational therapists often receive requests from parents and adults to equip their adolescent clients with mental health management 'tools'. However, therapists should not pursue this hastily and superficially, but rather ground skill development in careful clinical reasoning and client commitment to implementation. In order to achieve this, therapists help clients understand the purpose and benefits of the skill and co-create practical, individualised ways of implementing it in the adolescent's everyday life. Learning skills is most effective for adolescents through experiential and interactive methods, not a teacher-student relationship (Paul-Ward et al. 2014). Thus, occupational therapists should enable meaningful engagement, using 'learning through doing' at the centre of adolescent intervention (Bueno et al. 2021). Playful activities that allow for experimentation, self-recognition, and creative expression are highly recommended to promote behaviour change and skill acquisition (Bueno et al. 2021).

Identifying Therapeutic Spaces

Occupational therapists must recognise that intervening with adolescents can occur in non-formal therapeutic settings (Caskey & Anfara 2007). Adolescents require spaces where they can connect with others, receive validation and engage in health-promoting activities (Bueno et al. 2021). To facilitate helpful occupation, therapists and clients can creatively identify activities that meet the individualised therapeutic aims. Therapeutic spaces can include, for example, drama or art clubs that allow for self-expression, while sports activities or video game groups foster social inclusion and a sense of community (Yalom & Leszcz 2020). These groups offer potential for meeting secondary therapeutic objectives and complement individual sessions. Occupational therapists should conduct a thorough activity analysis of therapeutic spaces for adolescents to grow and thrive with others, and are instrumental in setting up, and facilitating, such spaces (Bueno *et al.* 2021).

TREATMENT APPROACHES WITH ADOLESCENTS

Selecting the appropriate treatment approach is essential to building an effective therapeutic plan. Occupational therapists should caution against using the same approach with each client as context, level of function and therapeutic aims will influence the most optimal treatment approach. A sound theoretical knowledge base of various approaches combined with thorough client assessment and an accurate sense of what the client needs to function will assist the selection of a relevant treatment approach. Occupational therapists may also choose to work in an eclectic way by choosing multiple approaches within the treatment process.

Developmental Approach

Adopting a developmental approach implies possessing a good understanding of the developmental changes and challenges faced by an adolescent, and is part of a life course approach. The developmental approach provides the theoretical lens through which the client is viewed, whilst secondary approaches are selected for framing the treatment approach.

Humanistic Approach

The humanistic/client-centred approach developed by Rogers (1951) is a helpful framework to use in developing a therapeutic relationship with adolescents. The framework encourages a horizontal engagement between client and therapist, allowing the client to use their own experience, knowledge and internal understanding with the occupational therapist in a collaborative attempt to make meaning of life (Gunnarsson 2008). In this approach, the occupational therapist allows for transparency, genuine warmth, authenticity and autonomy to validate the client's innate ability to think, reason, and be. Through this, the client can take ownership of their therapeutic process and life responsibilities. Allowing choice, reflection and full engagement through mutual dialogue empowers the adolescent client. The occupational therapist can make use of different creative activities to encourage spontaneous expressions, thereby enabling clients to reach their potential and improve their self-esteem. Sufficient cognitive abilities, especially the potential for intellectual insight, are a prerequisite for selecting the humanistic approach for adolescent clients.

Psychosocial Interactive Approach

The adolescent developmental stage largely revolves around social evolution, with maturing in relationships and belonging to a group being key tasks to master (Caskey & Anfara 2007; Hazen *et al.* 2008). The psychosocial interactive group is therefore a vital approach in adolescent occupational therapy. During occupational group therapy, adolescents are exposed to simulated 'peer groups' and can learn to experiment and

practise their social skills within the safe, therapeutic group context. The group offers a platform for acquiring skills and expressing emotions, but in itself is a valuable rehabilitation tool. Specific feedback concerning the client's maladaptive behaviour can be facilitated by the group members. Skills learned during group therapy are transferred over to society once the adolescent is discharged (Yalom 1985).

Cognitive Approach

To use the cognitive approach the adolescent's cognitive development should have reached a stage where they are able to reason abstractly. As different complex thoughts develop during the adolescent phase, this approach may be implemented with success. However, care should be taken that the adolescent does not intellectualise. This may happen as cognitive abilities develop faster than emotional abilities. The cognitive approach should be used as a tool for psycho-education and engagement. Interactive discussions based on theoretical understandings, whilst using interactive learning principles, should be implemented in the process of challenging negative thoughts and replacing them with more rational thoughts or insightful realisations.

Cognitive Behavioural Approach

Cognitive-behavioural therapy (CBT) is an effective social learning model in adolescent treatment, attributed to its concrete therapeutic techniques (Cornelius *et al.* 2011). The three-step CBT process involves identifying feelings, clarifying irrational thoughts, and adjusting behaviour through the acquisition of new coping skills (James *et al.* 2015). The functional problem-solving nature of CBT aligns with the skill set of occupational therapists, making it an ideal approach for intervention (Henderson 1998). CBT can be applied successfully for life skills, prevocational and vocational skills training, and with the use of experiential strategies such as role-play.

Dialectical Behavioural Therapy

Although DBT was designed to treat individuals with Borderline Personality Disorder, it has shown efficacy in reducing levels of distress and emotional dysregulation (Lynch *et al.* 2013). DBT offers a framework of thinking and practical tools to assist the client in managing themselves internally, as well as managing themselves within the world. DBT has shown positive results in harm reduction with regards to suicidality and self-harm behaviour (McCauley *et al.* 2018). DBT is well suited to the occupational therapist's skill set due to the practical nature of its intervention, although additional training is advised to use this approach effectively.

Neurophysiological Approach

Adolescents are frequently passive and have low energy, therefore, by stimulating the vestibular system, their activity levels increase. This provides feedback about their new body image and helps to develop their self-concept (which is part of identity).

Adolescent clients often have internalised aggression, and the aggression can be channelled by means of physical activities to help them dissipate emotional energy. Physical activity has a significant effect in reducing depression, anxiety, psychological distress and emotional disturbance, and improving self-esteem in children and adolescents (Ahn & Fedewa 2011), indicating the effectiveness of a neurophysiological approach for adolescents with mood disorders. Neurophysiological principles are helpful in teaching distress tolerance and emotional regulation skills.

Behavioural Approach

A behavioural approach can be used to change a specific maladaptive behaviour, for example, self-mutilating behaviour, or to increase weight in clients with eating disorders. However, the behavioural approach can cause the therapeutic relationship to suffer as the clinician may be required to confront the client about their maladaptive behaviour. When selecting this approach, it is suggested that the client is equally engaged in, and understands, the rationale of the approach. An alternative clinician can monitor and enforce the behavioural programme to safeguard the original therapeutic relationship.

Sensory Integration

The popular occupational therapy framework of Sensory Integration (Ayres 1972) is increasingly supported by evidence as having validity in the treatment process of clients with mental health disorders (Moore 2016). Occupational therapists can utilise their specialised understanding of the body as a sensory system to offer psycho-education and regulation tools to clients experiencing anxiety or trauma. Sensory Integration provides a framework not only for emotional regulation but also for re-establishing the individual's relationship with their body and self, thereby destigmatising symptoms and illness in adolescents. Moreover, sensory integration strategies can be implemented indirectly through sensory habits or sensory rooms, which are valuable in mental health maintenance strategies (Moore 2016).

Trauma-based Intervention

Research in the field of childhood trauma has expanded the understanding of mental health disorders and indicates the significant impact of trauma on the adolescent population (Evarist 2018; Distel *et al.* 2019). Mental health clinicians cannot ignore the need to be trauma-centred and culturally sensitive in their intervention (Elswick *et al.* 2022). Trauma-focused Cognitive Behavioural Therapy (TF-CBT), Sensory Motor Arousal Regulation Therapy (SMART), Attachment Regulation and Competence (ARC), and other somatic interventions are newly researched modalities developed for trauma-specific treatment (Finn *et al.* 2018; Palfrey *et al.* 2022). The occupational therapist trained in these techniques can effectively implement these modalities, along with helpful activity choices, whilst untrained therapists should mindfully maintain a trauma-informed lens when working with traumatised clients.

INTERVENTION IN OCCUPATIONAL PERFORMANCE AREAS

LEISURE

Discussing the adolescent's leisure time assessment results with them is essential to start addressing dysfunction or imbalance. However, adding more leisure activities may not resolve pathological limitations. Sometimes, working on occupational performance skills must come before participating in a leisure activity, for example improving self-esteem and social skills before joining the school choir. Grading therapeutic input and engagement in leisure activities can help adolescents feel confident in their progress. As adolescents fear failure, motivating them to attend extracurricular activities or social clubs requires careful consideration. Occupational therapists can prepare and model behaviour for the client within therapeutic sessions, such as introducing music for an adolescent who wants to join the choir. Occupational therapists should select meaningful and fulfilling leisure activities that are appropriate for the client's culture and finances, and investigate participation in inexpensive and accessible extracurricular activities at school, prioritising activities that encourage movement, social inclusion and creative expression for the benefit of mental well-being.

EDUCATION

Occupational therapists can support the development of pre-vocational, vocational and academic management skills. They can assist with time management by setting up a weekly timetable and teaching distress tolerance skills to manage anxiety. Additionally, occupational therapists can help clients with psychosocial issues that contribute to scholastic difficulties, including managing conflict, being assertive and regulating mood and energy for optimal focus. They can also teach study techniques and compensation methods for learning challenges. Occupational therapists can collaborate with the multidisciplinary team by advising educators on ways to adapt to the client's scholastic difficulties, writing reports recommending reasonable accommodations such as additional examination time, or referring clients to educational psychologists for guidance on career and subject choices.

WORK

Intervention for pre-vocational and vocational development with the adolescent focuses on developing life skills and abilities to manage the intra- and interpersonal pressures of engaging in a work environment. These may include improving time management, planning and scheduling skills, stress management skills, conflict management skills, emotional regulation, and the development of values and an ethical code. Additionally, promoting the development of an internal locus of control prepares the adolescent for the real world of work and supports them in the management of their mental illness. Activities can include games, therapeutic tasks, simulated school or work environments, or experiential exposure through volunteering, casual jobs or part-time positions.

ACTIVITIES OF DAILY LIVING

ADL limitations can be addressed in various ways. An occupational therapist may educate on health-promoting ADL behaviour or facilitate experiential ADL skill acquisition, either individually or in a group. For example, a client group may exchange make-up tips, or clients with eating disorders may receive coaching on regular meal times. ADL activities offer therapeutic potential, for example, depressed adolescents engaging in self-care skills experience positive emotions and boosted self-esteem. ADLs can serve as a means to an end and teach life skills such as value clarification, motivating independence and healthy sexual relationships. Clients with mental health issues often struggle with basic tasks and benefit from successfully performing them with support; thus, ADLs are essential tools for therapists.

INSTRUMENTAL ACTIVITIES OF DAILY LIVING

Intervention for IADLs depends on each adolescent's mastery and their unique context. The occupational therapist may need to advocate for the client by addressing inappropriate IADL performance with caregivers. However, should the client be required to complete these tasks, the occupational therapist can guide the adolescent to helpful exposure and learning of IADL skills, for example, cooking or meal preparation. As the adolescent becomes more comfortable they can be encouraged to experiment for themselves. Various age-appropriate IADLs can be included in the treatment plan, for example learning to budget, obtaining learner's driving licences, using public transport, responsible social media use and complying with treatment appointments and medication. IADLs are often successfully incorporated into schedules and can be addressed within the structure and boundaries of a treatment programme or clinic setting.

SOCIAL PARTICIPATION

Addressing social skills, social participation mobilisation and initiating and maintaining reciprocal relationships takes up a significant portion of any intervention with adolescents. Adolescents often find themselves on one end of the social spectrum, struggling with social ineptitude and exclusion or managing the pressures of popularity. In order to address these issues, occupational therapists should focus on enabling their clients to practise social skills within real-life situations and in group therapy settings, such as processing groups or social activity groups.

Group therapy can be a powerful tool for addressing social participation and promoting positive social development in adolescents. The value of group therapy lies in the feedback adolescents receive from their peers, which can have a greater impact than education alone. With the guidance of a therapist, constructive and respectful feedback on unhelpful behavioural patterns can help adolescents learn mature conflict resolution and communication skills, co-create solutions and engage in supportive therapeutic experiments. Activities that require the group to work together, such as treasure hunts, poster-making, community building, theatrical play-writing and group debates, can further promote a sense of belonging and unity within the group, ultimately boosting resilience and motivation for social functioning in other areas of their lives. In order to facilitate this unity within the group, occupational therapists must remain mindful of the importance of facilitating mutual connection and a sense of worth and companionship. By providing opportunities for adolescents to experience this within the group, therapists can help them develop a sense of cohesion and transfer social skills to functioning outside of treatment. The book *Occupational Group Therapy* provides a useful, practical guide to occupational therapists to develop their group skills and apply different models of group therapy in various settings (Crouch 2021).

SLEEP/REST

Interventions for sleep with adolescents start with providing psycho-education around the sleep-wake cycle and how brain waves reflect this phenomenon. This provides the client with a clear understanding of why healthy routines during the day and a structured sleep habit with good sleep hygiene would support better sleep. Adolescents (and their parents/guardians) should be informed that some sleep deprivation is normal. The occupational therapist and adolescent can use the newly established knowledge of sleep as a platform to co-create solutions and routines for improved sleep. Sleep/rest interventions cannot be a once-off treatment goal and should be revisited in therapy often to ensure the adolescent remains responsible for implementing strategies or modifying routines when necessary. It is also important to note that around the time of exams and additional studying or during times of emotional distress, such as a break-up or issues with friends, sleep will be more disrupted and additional support to maintain sleep routines should be provided.

HEALTH MANAGEMENT

It is important that adolescents learn to take responsibility for their health by carrying out activities and routines related to developing, managing and maintaining health and wellness (AOTA 2020). This self-management of health becomes even more important when an adolescent is living with a health-related challenge such as diabetes or anxiety, which may be lifelong and for which they need to take over responsibility from their parents. Intervention focuses on supporting the adolescent to take responsibility for the self-management of social and emotional health, specific conditions and symptoms, medication management, physical activity, nutrition management and personal care device management.

INTERVENTION PLANNING AND PRINCIPLES

ACTIVITY ANALYSIS AND SELECTION

The occupational therapist faces a daunting task in selecting activities for adolescent clients or groups. The adolescent's natural tendency to rebel and defy (Zhang & Li 2022) needs to be skilfully mediated and circumvented by the clinician. In order to do this, it is helpful to have a robust commitment to the therapeutic use of self, a limitless catalogue of activities and an extensive aptitude for activity analysis. A starting point for selecting activities for working with adolescents can be found in the United Nations International Children's Emergency Fund (UNICEF) Foundational Guide: The Adolescent Kit for Expression and Innovation. UNICEF draws attention to ten key approaches in working with adolescents that appear in Table 18.1.

These approaches are closely aligned with the principles of occupational therapy intervention when working with adolescents and can be summarised in the following helpful questions when activities are selected:

1. Will the activity elicit energy, movement and engagement?

    Adolescents participate best in the therapeutic process or activity when they are fully engaged in the process. Occupational therapists can achieve this by adapting activities to be interactive, fun, and involve movement. By incorporating physical elements, therapists can stimulate adolescents' limbic systems, activate their psychomotor levels and reduce anxiety, thereby addressing their passive nature. Through activity selection, therapists can encourage adolescents to move beyond cognitive engagement and into their bodies, emotions and experiences, breaking down defence mechanisms like denial and intellectualisation. Activities should encourage creativity, imagination, exploration and experimentation, so adolescents are fully present and generating energy for emotional processing later in the session.

    Activities that can be considered are active warm-ups, interactive icebreakers, team-building activities, movement games, dancing, socio-drama activities, group tasks, projects and obstacle courses.

2. Does the activity provide a safe container and boundaries?

Adolescents need firm, yet subtle boundaries from occupational therapists. Rigid norms and clear consequences may increase the adolescent's need for rebellion and defiance, as they navigate the developmental experience of identity formation versus separation (Hazen *et al.* 2008). The occupational therapist should view the adolescent's defensive behaviour as rooted in fear and respond with honest reflection, clear communication and supportive guidance towards corrective behaviour. Setting group norms can help establish behavioural expectations, and building boundaries in the activity is key. Explicit norms around harm and disrespect are essential, but therapists should also create a safe space for exploration and expression. This may involve processing unruly behaviour with the client during the session.

Activities that can be helpful here are establishing group or individual values, facilitating regular conversations about integrity towards these values, exploring the internal and external dynamics of rule-breaking behaviour and supporting debate about fair consequences. The occupational therapist should carefully consider the structuring of groups to create safety and boundaries. Setting up activities prior to clients entering the room, using music, furnishings, candles to create a required atmosphere, managing dangerous items and creating containment through instructions and support can be beneficial therapeutic tools.

3. Will the activity support cohesion, validation and self- and other-recognition?

Activities, in group and individual sessions, should instil a sense of belonging and strengthen the adolescent's self-concept. Therapists should be mindful to facilitate universality and self-statements whilst empowering the clients to collectively explore personal attributes. In group therapy, adolescents hold an incredible, healing power, when they are able to connect to each other and work together to resolve inter- and intrapersonal issues. This enables them to gain hope, motivation and responsibility, and this can be applied to other areas of their lives.

Activities must encourage teamwork, meaningful dialogue and free, respectful feedback between adolescents. The occupational therapist should facilitate this process by promoting the identification of unhelpful behaviour patterns, acknowledging growth and encouraging experiments to enhance skills. In individual sessions, clients may reflect on their progress and development after each session. Projective techniques, life stories, life puzzles, self-portraits or art therapy work well within the group or with the individual client to elicit these experiences. Adolescents also respond well to projective work with music, poetry, images, reflective questions or wisdom cards.

Table 18.1 Ten key approaches in working with adolescents (UNICEF).

Reach out to all adolescents	Provide structure and support	Listen to adolescents	Let adolescents take the lead	Include all adolescents
Make space for expression and creativity	Challenge and encourage adolescents	Improvise and adapt	Build connections	Build on the positive

4. Will the adolescent grasp the concept and rationale of the activity?

The adolescent is not fooled by meaningless activities and the occupational therapist should not underestimate their ability to reason. The occupational therapist should be creative about the use of themes and the adaptation of activities to bring across the theme in the session. The adolescent who grasps and connects to the concept of the session is more likely to retain and implement the intervention in future. Activities should be designed to offer some form of challenge, whilst taking care not to overwhelm the adolescent or the group. Adolescents require challenges to learn and grow, and by selecting activities that present an appropriate level of challenge, the occupational therapist can support the adolescent in building a sense of mastery and competence. The goal is to provide an opportunity for the adolescent to experience success in a safe and structured environment, which will translate to feelings of confidence and self-efficacy in other areas of their life. In addition, activities that keep adolescents intrigued and engaged, whilst encouraging self-expression and creativity can be particularly effective in helping adolescents to explore their emotions and experiences, and to communicate these in a safe and supportive environment.

Activities that are helpful to facilitate concepts and themes include board games (for example, Jenga, Pick-Up Sticks, Go Fish, The Ultimate Werewolf), art games (such as painting with the non-dominant hand and drawing on head), adapted icebreakers and team building games, obstacle courses and physical activities (group juggle, human knot, balloon volleyball, sock hockey). The effective use of these activities depends on the appropriate selection and activity adaptation by the occupational therapist and how well the concept is facilitated in the post-activity discussion. It is further helpful to consider a variety of activities for the post-activity discussion. Adolescents enjoy debates; discussing in buzz-groups or pairs; designing questions for each other based on the activity; writing letters, poems or sentences about it; creating their own tool cards or intention reminders; and role playing or unpacking the concepts with the use of words and diagrams. Adolescents find metaphors, stories and analogies valuable in the sense-making process.

5. Will the activity allow for expression of identity or emotions?

Adolescents tend to internalise their emotional, psychological and social struggles, leading to a higher prevalence of mental health and psychosomatic issues (Duberg et al. 2016). Expression of self and emotions in occupational therapy interventions is crucial. The occupational therapist must create a safe space where adolescents can co-create their treatment and express their authentic selves. The therapist should curate activities that promote expression, such as dance and physical activities (MacLennan & Dies 1992; Duberg et al. 2016; Healey et al. 2016). Throughout activity engagement, the therapist should guide the adolescent towards reflection, insight and the making of self-statements, to relieve them of unexpressed emotions.

Activities for emotional expression should allow for elements of movement, creativity and co-creation of the therapist and the adolescent or the group (Duberg et al. 2016). Reflective journaling (Wegner et al. 2017), storytelling, music, movement and dancing, acting and putting on plays, projective techniques, art as therapy and community rituals like a daily gratitude practice or reflective space can be effectively used to encourage emotional expression. Exposing the adolescent to positive role models and other adolescents who engage in personal reflection and self-expression will assist the client in building courage towards expression as it will lead to a sense of belonging (Healey et al. 2016). It is therefore recommended to consider group therapy or facilitated interactions for adolescents with nurturing adults or peers.

6. Will the activity guide the adolescent to concrete insights or steps?

It is crucial that all activities and intervention strategies have a specific aim in mind and that this aim is named and focused on during the activity. Very often occupational therapists and clients get involved in the activity, but negate the crucial aspect of framing the activity for the client in terms of therapeutic growth. This will lead to clients being confused about the purpose of therapy and to the idea that occupational therapy is just 'fun activities'. The occupational therapist should create space within the activity for feedback on the purpose and process of the activity, and dialogue the theme, concept or aim of the activity. The client should leave a session having either a concrete step to implement at home or an insight with which to further explore or experiment.

It is helpful for clients to end all sessions with a cue card of their goal for the week or a set of practical steps that they can implement. This in itself can be a creative extension of the therapeutic process depending on the client's level of functioning and aims. Clients may, during the course of therapy, develop a therapy book with notes and ideas, they may work on building towards a balanced schedule and each week adding an element, they may create affirmation cards, with a new affirmation or quote each week or they may work on trying various social, emotional and life experiments every week to provide feedback at the next session. The occupational therapist may also use sensory-based activities such as art, music or sensory exploration to help clients process emotions and experiences. Outdoor activities, such as hiking or camping, can also be a valuable tool in helping clients develop self-awareness, self-esteem and social skills. If the occupational therapist guides the clients towards concrete steps and insights, therapy will be transferred more easily beyond the bounds of the session itself. By helping clients set and achieve goals, the occupational therapist can help them develop a sense of agency and autonomy, which can lead to increased motivation and confidence in their ability to navigate life's challenges.

TREATMENT PRINCIPLES

In addition to the above-mentioned questions, occupational therapists can refer to the following intervention principles when selecting, adapting and implementing activities with adolescents:

HANDLING PRINCIPLES

- Balance authority and friendliness through a good therapeutic relationship that allows honesty and firmness, yet encourages spontaneity and fun interactions.

- Set boundaries for unacceptable behaviour through discussion with the client. Explore the reason for breaking the boundary, whilst consistently, fairly and immediately implementing the consequence.

- Be encouraging and motivational, especially when the client lacks confidence.

- Encourage and validate positive interaction and therapeutic growth, whilst providing truthful feedback on areas of struggle with the aim to support ongoing effort.

- Use appropriate self-disclosure, to support a horizontal relationship with the client. Be prepared to express your beliefs without influencing the client's beliefs.

- Be mindful of where the client elicits a power struggle or unhelpful dynamic, reflect on this without getting hooked into unhealthy relational patterns.

- Be approachable and warm at all times. Remain calm and avoid overreacting. Clearly express emotions and feelings in an appropriate manner.

- Be a constant, secure point of reference. Allow the client to access the clinician as a healthy, nurturing and supportive adult in their life.

- Although adolescents engage well in social banter, be mindful of being sensitive to their feelings, appearance, issues and socio-economic circumstances. Keep interaction casual, but professional at all times.

- Always seek opportunities to assist the adolescent in defining their opinions, values and sense of self.

- Be a role model in all aspects of functioning. Dress appropriately and neatly, act with respect and manage one's own mental health, boundaries and time effectively.

ACTIVITY SELECTION PRINCIPLES

- Refer to the previously mentioned questions as an outline for activity selection.

- Activities should allow for autonomy and choice.

- Activities should be contextually relevant and be appropriate to the clients' interest, level of functioning, cultural background and socio-economic status.

- Activities should ensure self-efficacy and the experience of success or the experience of grasping the concept presented.

- Activities should allow for feedback and ongoing therapeutic discussion.

- Allow for activities to be changed or adapted in action. Make sure to have alternative plans that can accommodate low mood and energy or resistance from the adolescent.

STRUCTURING PRINCIPLES

- Ensure the room is set out prior to the client's arrival and is warm, neat, interesting, calming and welcoming.

- Rooms should be well ventilated, light and have space to move and engage in expressive, creative activities.

- Conduct intervention in appropriate spaces; for instance do yoga in the garden or cook in the kitchen, not in the therapy room.

- Allow the adolescent to sit in a manner that is comfortable yet appropriate; for example art activities may be done on the floor, or discussion can occur whilst sitting on bean bags.

- Ensure all the correct and appropriate material is at hand. Always have stationery and paper available when activities are adapted or explained in a more concrete way.

- Allow for freedom of movement and expression, but ensure the client remains emotionally and physically safe at all times.

- Keep a close eye on sharp and/or dangerous equipment and materials, for example, scissors, glue, mosaic tiles, glass shards and thinners.

GROUP THERAPY AS INTERVENTION

Irrespective of the activities used, groups are a good medium of choice for adolescents as it can help clients develop their social and life skills in action. Group therapy allows adolescents to interact with peers in a safe and healthy environment. The therapist should always lead from behind and facilitate curative factors (Yalom 1985) throughout the group.

Cohesion and universality are essential in adolescent groups, as these allow them to try out social and interpersonal risks in a supported and safe environment. The therapist should also facilitate the imparting of information, as adolescents value advice and solutions offered by their peers more than those offered by therapists or parents. Facilitating existential factors can also be curative for adolescents, as it helps them realise that they are responsible for their own choices.

CASE STUDY

Kay, a 15-year-old female, has been brought to the community wellness centre by her mother. Kay is reluctant to be there, but her mother is desperate as Kay has been missing school, is becoming more argumentative and aggressive and is often found isolated in her room gaming violent video games. Kay's mother reports that she struggles to get her out of bed in the mornings, that she rarely eats proper meals and that she has stopped engaging in all her previous leisure activities.

About a year ago, Kay still had an active social circle, played soccer and was part of the drama club at school. Her marks have dropped over the last six months, with her teacher reporting her behaviour to have drastically changed, with outbursts of insolence and rudeness. Kay's style and clothes have also changed. She used to wear dresses, but now mostly wears baggy clothes bought at the second-hand market. Kay's mother is very upset as Kay is claiming she does not want to be a female anymore and wants her name to be changed from Kaylene to Kay. Before coming to the community centre, Kay was seen by her house doctor who referred Kay to a psychiatrist as she feels that Kay may be depressed and undergoing a gender identity crisis.

Kay's mother, as a single parent, is struggling to find the money for this appointment.

Kay's father passed away in a traumatic motor vehicle accident when she was 12 years old. The police reported that he was highly intoxicated at the time of the accident and was most probably the cause of the accident in which a family of three were severely injured. Kay reports never liking her dad and being glad that he is gone as he was always drinking and verbally abusing her mother. Recently Kay's mother started dating again. The man she is now seeing occasionally drinks, but Kay explains that she does not know him as she makes sure she locks her room and plays a video game when he is around.

The community wellness centre where you work offers affordable services to a low-income community. The centre staff includes two occupational therapists, a psychiatric nurse, a social worker, a psychologist, and psychiatrist part-time. The centre offers individual support and a wellness programme with various activities, run by the staff or volunteers. The centre director asked you as the occupational therapist to see Kay for assessment and intervention for ten sessions.

If the adolescent's peer group is destructive, the therapist should work with them to gain insight into the unhealthy behaviour pattern and guide the group to find a healthier way of engaging. All incidents within the group should be seen as a learning opportunity. It is also helpful if adolescents state their social skill goals within the group, so that they can assist each other in achieving these goals therapeutically. The occupational therapist should continuously be aware of defences that may arise in an individual member or the group as a whole, for example low group energy may be a sign of resistance or a client may respond with a positive outlook providing the answers that they think are correct. These incidents are rich in therapeutic content and should be explored and resolved within the group.

FAMILY INVOLVEMENT IN THERAPY

There is a recognised gap in the mental health profession's ability to include families in the care of individuals with severe mental illness (Kim & Salyers 2008). The parent-teen relationship is particularly complex, and parental involvement can be difficult, especially when working with adolescents (Tian *et al.* 2019). When providing occupational therapy services, it is essential to maintain a therapeutic relationship with the client while liaising with parents. Providing psycho-education to the family on the diagnosis and methods to support the client can positively impact intervention outcomes (McFarlane *et al.* 2003). If the relationship between the parent and adolescent is irreparable, the occupational therapist can

support the adolescent in forming healthy relationships with other role models in the community. However, occupational therapists must remain mindful of their scope of practice and refer intensive family therapy to a suitable professional.

QUESTIONS

1. When Kay arrives in the therapy room for the first time, she is clearly reluctant to be there and very uncomfortable. Explain how you will approach the first session in terms of your approach, principles, assessment activities and therapeutic relationship.

2. The centre director requires a thorough report and treatment plan after the second session. Discuss how you will approach the assessment of Kay and what assessments you will use.

3. You refer Kay to the psychiatrist, who confirms a diagnosis of Depression and Complex Post-Traumatic Stress Disorder. Frame Kay's case through the use of the Occupational Therapy Practice Framework (OTPF-4).

4. With regard to your specific context, discuss which legislative policies should be considered when working with Kay.

5. Discuss your treatment aims for intervention indicating which treatment approaches will be best suited to achieve those aims.

6. Develop a treatment plan using a diagram or table, indicating your session aims, activity choices and activity analysis rationale for each of the remaining eight sessions.

7. Kay is a highly traumatised individual, who currently struggles with grief and trust and is reluctant to open up in therapy. Discuss what handling principles you will implement in your work with Kay.

8. Present an outline of an occupational therapy group session in which one of Kay's main problems is addressed.

9. Kay's absenteeism at school has become highly problematic. The school has requested a meeting with you and Kay's mother. Plan your comprehensive input for this meeting to support Kay's return to school.

10. Kay has, due to her trauma and depression, struggled with her personal and gender identity. Explain how you will address this in the treatment process.

11. The community wellness centre hosts a number of wellness activities and projects. Explain why and how you will include these activities in Kay's treatment process.

12. One year after treatment Kay has achieved good recovery. She has worked through her trauma, returned to school and resumed her hobbies. She has remained an active member of the wellness centre. She still experiences anxiety and bouts of depression but uses her tools and a monthly session with you to maintain her recovery. She is still working on her relationship with her mother and her mother's fiancé. Kay indicates a need to give back and support other children in her school and wants to start a mental health awareness campaign. Explain how you will guide and support Kay with this project.

REFERENCES

Ahn, S. & Fedewa, A. (2011) A meta-analysis of the relationship between children's physical activity and mental health. *Journal of Pediatric Psychology*, **36**(4), 385–397. https://doi.org/10.1093/jpepsy/jsq107.jsq107

American Occupational Therapy Association (AOTA) (2020) Occupational therapy practice framework: domain and process (4th ed.). *American Journal of Occupational Therapy*, 74 (**Suppl. 2**), 7412410010. https://doi.org/10.5014/ajot.2020.74S2001

Ayres, A.J. (1972) Treatment of sensory integrative dysfunction. *Australian Occupational Therapy Journal*, **19**, 88–88. https://doi.org/10.1111/j.1440-1630.1972.tb00547.x

Beery, K.E. (1997) *The Beery-Buktenica Developmental Test of Visual-Motor Integration: VMI, with Supplemental Developmental Tests of Visual Perception and Motor Coordination: Administration, Scoring and Testing Manual*, 4th edn, rev edn. Modern Curriculum Press, Parsippany.

Boland, R., Verduin, M. & Ruiz, P. (2021) *Kaplan and Sadock's Synopsis of Psychiatry*, 12th edn. Wolters Kluwer Health, USA.

Boyt Schell, B.A., Gillen, G., Scaffa, M. & Cohn, E. (2013) *Willard and Spackman's Occupational Therapy*. Lippincott Williams & Wilkins, Baltimore.

Brochado, S., Soares, S. & Fraga, S. (2017) A scoping review on studies of cyberbullying prevalence among adolescents. *Trauma, Violence, & Abuse*, **18**(5), 523–531.

Bronfenbrenner, U. (1995) Developmental ecology through space and time: a future perspective. In: P. Moen, G.H. Elder, Jr. & K. Lüscher (eds), *Examining Lives in Context: Perspectives on the Ecology of Human Development*, pp. 619–647. American Psychological Association, Washington, DC. https://doi.org/10.1037/10176-018

Brooks, R. & Bannigan, K. (2018) Occupational therapy interventions in child and adolescent mental health. *JBI Database of Systematic Reviews and Implementation Reports*, **16**(9), 1764–1771. https://doi.org/10.11124/jbisrir-2017-003612

Bruce, E.S., Lunt, L. & McDonagh, J.E. (2017) Sleep in adolescents and young adults. *Clinical Medicine*, **17**(5), 424–428. https://doi.org/10.7861/clinmedicine.17-5-424

Bueno, K.M.P., Almeida, S.C., Sales, M.M. & Salgado, M.F. (2021) Occupational therapy practices in the child and adolescent mental health network. *Cadernos Brasileiros de Terapia Ocupacional*, **29**, e2877. https://doi.org/10.1590/2526-8910.ctoAO2173

Caskey, M.M. & Anfara, V.A., Jr. (2007) *Research summary: young adolescents' developmental characteristics*. http://www.nmsa.org/Research/ResearchSummaries/DevelopmentalCharacteristics/tabid/1414/Default.aspx (accessed on 14 June 2013)

Centers for Disease Control and Prevention (2019) *The social-ecological model: a framework for violence prevention*. https://www.cdc.gov/violenceprevention/pdf/sem_framewrk-a.pdf (accessed 9 March 2023)

Cherry, K. (2013) *Introduction to theories of development*. http://psychology.about.com/od/developmentecourse/a/dev_intro.htm (accessed on 30 January 2014)

Christiansen, C. & Baum, C. (1997) *Occupational Therapy: Enabling Function and Well-Being*. SLACK Inc., Thorofare, New Jersey.

Cooper, A. & Ward, C. (2012) Intervening with youth in gangs. In: C.L. Ward, A. van der Merwe & A. Dawes (eds), *Youth Violence: Sources and Solutions in South Africa*, pp. 23–51. UCT Press, Cape Town.

Cornelius, J.R., Douaihy, A., Bukstein, O.G. et al (2011) Evaluation of cognitive-behavioral therapy/motivational enhancement therapy (CBT/MET) in a treatment trial of comorbid MDD/AUD adolescents. *Addictive Behaviors*, **36**(8), 843–848. https://doi.org/10.1016/j.addbeh.2011.03.016

Crouch, R. (2021) *Occupational Group Therapy*. Wiley Blackwell, Oxford.

Distel, L.M.L., Torres, S.A., Ros, A.M. et al (2019) Evaluating the implementation of bounce back: clinicians' perspectives on a school-based trauma intervention. *Evidence-Based Practice in Child and Adolescent Mental Health*, **4**, 72–88. https://doi.org/10.1080/23794925.2019.1565501

Duberg, A., Möller, M. & Sunvisson, H. (2016) "I feel free": experiences of a dance intervention for adolescent girls with internalizing problems. *International Journal of Qualitative Studies on Health and Well-being*, **11**(1), 31946. https://doi.org/10.3402/qhw.v11.31946

Elder, G.H., Jr., Johnson, M.K. & Crosnoe, R. (2003) The emergence and development of life course theory. In: J.T. Mortimer & M.J. Shanahan (eds), *Handbook of the Life Course*, pp. 3–22. Kluwer Academic/Plenum, New York.

Elswick, S., Washington, G., Mangrum-Apple, H. *et al* (2022) Trauma healing club: utilizing culturally responsive processes in the implementation of an after-school group intervention to address trauma among African refugees. *Journal of Child and Adolescent Trauma,* **15**, 155–166. https://doi.org/10.1007/s40653-021-00387-5

Evarist, A. (2018) Adolescent trauma and psychosocial wellbeing in Entebbe-Uganda. *Universal Journal of Psychology, 6*(**3**), 67–79. https://doi.org/10.13189/ujp.2018.060301

Fernández-Berrocal, P., Alcaide, R., Extremera, N. & Pizarro, D.A. (2006) The role of emotional intelligence in anxiety and depression among adolescents. *Individual Differences Research,* **4**, 16–27.

Finn, H., Warner, E., Price, M. & Spinazzola, J. (2018) The boy who was hit in the face: somatic regulation and processing of preverbal complex trauma. *Journal of Child and Adolescent Trauma,* **11**(3), 277–288. https://doi.org/10.1007/s40653-017-0165-9

Fraser, K., MacKenzie, D. & Versnel, J. (2019) What is the current state of occupational therapy practice with children and adolescents with complex trauma? *Occupational Therapy in Mental Health,* **35**(4), 317–338. https://doi.org/10.1080/0164212X.2019.1652132

Gevers, A. & Flisher, A.J. (2012) School-based youth violence prevention interventions. In: C.L. Ward, A. van der Merwe & A. Dawes (eds), *Youth Violence: Sources and Solutions in South Africa,* pp. 175–209. UCT Press, Cape Town.

Gunnarsson, B. (2008) *The tree theme method - an occupational therapy intervention applied in outpatient psychiatric care.* Doctoral Thesis (compilation), Sustainable Occupations and Health in a Life Course Perspective. Lund University, Division of Occupational Therapy and Gerontology, Lund, Sweden. www.arb.lu.se

Hazen, E., Schlozman, S. & Beresin, E. (2008) Adolescent psychological development: a review. *Pediatrics in Review,* **29**(5), 161. https://doi.org/10.1542/pir.29-5-161

Healey, G., Noah, J. & Mearns, C. (2016) The Eight Ujarait (Rocks) Model: supporting Inuit adolescent mental health with an intervention model based on Inuit knowledge and ways of knowing. *International Journal of Indigenous Health,* **11**(1), 14–43. https://doi.org/10.18357/ijih111201614394

Henderson, A. (1998) An occupational therapist's guide to cognitive-behavioral therapy. *American Journal of Occupational Therapy,* **52**(9), 737–744.

James, A.C., James, G., Cowdrey, F.A., Soler, A. & Choke, A. (2015) Cognitive behavioural therapy for anxiety disorders in children and adolescents. *Cochrane Database of Systematic Reviews,* **2**, CD004690. https://doi.org/10.1002/14651858.CD004690.pub4

Kim, H.W. & Salyers, M.P. (2008) Attitudes and perceived barriers to working with families of persons with severe mental illness: mental health professionals' perspectives. *Community Mental Health Journal,* **44**(5), 337–345. https://doi.org/10.1007/s10597-008-9135-x

Labouliere, C.D., Reyes, J.P., Shirk, S. & Karver, M. (2017) Therapeutic alliance with depressed adolescents: predictor or outcome? Disentangling temporal confounds to understand early improvement. *Journal of Clinical Child & Adolescent Psychology, 46*(4), 600–610. https://doi.org/10.1080/15374416.2015.1041594

Law, M., Baptiste, S., Carswell, A., Polatajko, H. & Pollock, N. (1999) *Canadian Occupational Performance Measure (COPM)*. CAOT Publications ACE, Ottawa.

Law, M., Cooper, B., Strong, S., Stewart, D., Rigby, P. & Letts, L. (1996) The person–environment–occupation model: a transactive approach to occupational performance. *Canadian Journal of Occupational Therapy, 63*, 9–23.

Lynch, T.R., Gray, K.L.H., Hempel, R.J., Titley, M., Chen, E.Y. & O'Mahen, H.A. (2013) Radically open-dialectical behavior therapy for adult anorexia nervosa: feasibility and outcomes from an inpatient program. *BMC Psychiatry,* **13**(1), 293. https://doi.org/10.1186/1471-244x-13-293

MacLennan, B.W. & Dies, K.R. (1992) *Group Counselling and Psychotherapy with Adolescents,* 2nd edn. Columbia University Press, New York.

Majee, W., Conteh, M., Jacobs, J.J., Jooste, K. & Wegner, L. (2021) Rural voices: a social-ecological perspective on youth substance use in rural South Africa. *Health & Social Care in the Community,* **29**, 1824–1832. https://doi.org/10.1111/hsc.13292

Marx, L., Franzsen, D. & Van Niekerk, M. (2023) Current and future occupational performance priorities of adolescents with learning difficulties and their parents. *Journal of Occupational Science,* **30**(2), 262–276. https://doi.org/10.1080/14427591.2021.1976667

McCauley, E., Berk, M.S., Asarnow, J.R. *et al* (2018) Efficacy of dialectical behavior therapy for adolescents at high risk for suicide: a randomized clinical trial. *JAMA Psychiatry,* **75**(8), 777–785. https://doi.org/10.1001/jamapsychiatry.2018.1109

McFarlane, W.R., Dixon, L., Lukens, E. & Lucksted, A. (2003) Family psychoeducation and schizophrenia: a review of the literature. *Journal of Marital and Family Therapy,* **29**(2), 223.

McLeod, S.A. (2009) *Jean Piaget: cognitive theory – simply psychology.* http://www.simplypsychology.org/piaget.html (accessed on 24 May 2023)

Milne, D. (1992) *Assessment: A Mental Health Portfolio.* NFER-Nelson Publishing Co Ltd, Glasgow.

Morrison, J. & Anders, T.F. (1999) *Interviewing Children and Adolescents.* The Guilford Press, New York.

Moore, K. (2016) *Following the evidence: sensory approaches in mental health* [online]. http://www.sensoryconnectionprogram.com/sensory_treatment.php (accessed on 11 March 2023)

Palfrey, N., Ryan, R. & Reay, R.E. (2022) Implementation of trauma-specific interventions in a child and adolescent mental health service. *Journal of Child and Family Studies,* **32**, 1722–1735. https://doi.org/10.1007/s10826-022-02467-y

Paul-Ward, A., Lambdin-Pattavina, C.A. & Haskell, A. (2014) Occupational therapy's emerging role with transitioning adolescents in foster care. *Occupational Therapy in Mental Health, 30*, 162–177.

Potter, A., Dube, S., Allgaier, N. *et al* (2020) Early adolescent gender diversity and mental health in the Adolescent Brain Cognitive Development study. *Journal of Child Psychology and Psychiatry,* **62**(2), 171–179. https://doi.org/10.1111/jcpp.13248

Rogers, C.R. (1951) *Client-centered Therapy: Its Current Practice, Implications and Theory.* Houghton Mifflin, Boston.

Rustad, R.A., DeGroot, T.L., Jungkunz, M.L. *et al* (1993) *Cognitive Assessment of Minnesota (CAM).* Therapy Skill Builders, San Antonio.

Ryan, R., Berry, K., Law, H. & Hartley, S. (2021) Therapeutic relationships in child and adolescent mental health services: a Delphi study with young people, carers and clinicians. *International Journal of Mental Health Nursing*, **30**(**4**), 982–992. https://doi.org/10.1111/inm.12857

Schlapobersky, J.R. (2016) *From the Couch to the Circle: Group-Analytic Psychotherapy in Practice*. Routledge, Washington, DC.

Tian, Y., Yu, C., Lin, S., Lu, J., Liu, Y. & Zhang, W. (2019) Parental psychological control and adolescent aggressive behavior: deviant peer affiliation as a mediator and school connectedness as a moderator. *Frontiers in Psychology, 10*, 358. https://doi.org/10.3389/fpsyg.2019.00358

Turban, J.L. & Ehrensaft, D. (2017) Research review: gender identity in youth: treatment paradigms and controversies. *Journal of Child Psychology and Psychiatry*, **59**(**12**), 1228–1243. https://doi.org/10.1111/jcpp.12833

Twinley, R. (2013) The dark side of occupation: a concept for consideration. *Australian Occupational Therapy Journal*. **60**(**4**):301–303. https://doi.org/10.1111/1440-1630.12026

Twinley, R. & Addidle, G. (2012) Considering violence: the dark side of occupation. *British Journal of Occupational Therapy*, **75**(**4**):202–204. https://doi.org/10.4276/030802212X13336366278257

Waszczuk, M.A., Zavos, H.M., Gregory, A.M. & Eley, T.C. (2016) The stability and change of etiological influences on depression, anxiety symptoms and their co-occurrence across adolescence and young adulthood. *Psychological Medicine*, **46**(**1**), 161–175. https://doi.org/10.1017/S0033291715001634

Wegner, L. (2011) Through the lens of a peer: understanding leisure boredom and risk behaviour in adolescence. *South African Journal of Occupational Therapy*, **41**(**1**), 18–24.

Wegner, L. & Caldwell, L.L. (2012) Interventions for out-of-school contexts. In: C.L. Ward, A. van der Merwe & A. Dawes (eds), *Youth Violence: Sources and Solutions in South Africa*, pp. 213–239. UCT Press, Cape Town.

Wegner, L., Flisher, A.J., Chikobvu, P., Lombard, C. & King, G. (2008) Leisure boredom and high school dropout in Cape Town, South Africa. *Journal of Adolescence, 31*(**3**), 421–431.

Wegner, L., Flisher, A.J., Muller, M. & Lombard, C. (2006) Leisure boredom and substance use amongst high school students in Cape Town. *Journal of Leisure Research,* **38**(**2**), 249–266.

Wegner, L., Struthers, P. & Mohamed, S. (2017) "The pen is a powerful weapon; it can make you change": exploring empowerment through reflective writing in adolescents. *South African Journal of Occupational Therapy,* **47**(**3**), 11–16. http://dx.doi.org/10.17159/2310-3833/2017/v47n3a3

Wilcock, A.A. (1998) *An Occupational Perspective of Health*. SLACK Inc., Thorofare, New Jersey.

Witty, M.C. (2007) Client-centered therapy. In: N. Kazantzis & L. L'Abate (eds), *Handbook of Homework Assignments in Psychotherapy*, pp. 35–50. Springer, Boston. https://doi.org/10.1007/978-0-387-29681-4_3

Yalom, I.D. (1985) *The Theory and Practice of Group Psychotherapy,* 4th edn. Basic Books, New York, NY.

Yalom, I.D. & Leszcz. M. (2020) *The Theory and Practice of Group Psychotherapy*, 6th edn. Basic Books, New York.

Zhang, Z. & Li, C. (2022) Adolescent rebellion; influencing factors; guiding strategies. *Science Insights,* **40**(**4**), 485–487. https://doi.org/10.15354/si.22.re050

Ayres Sensory Integration in Child Mental Health

CHAPTER 19

Annamarie van Jaarsveld[1] and Elize Janse van Rensburg[2]
[1]Department of Occupational Therapy, University of the Free State, Bloemfontein, South Africa
[2]Sensory Roots Occupational Therapy, Bloemfontein, South Africa

KEY LEARNING POINTS

- Sensory integration plays a critical role in function and in child mental health.

- There is ample evidence of sensory integration difficulties across various child mental health diagnoses and convincing evidence for ASI as an evidence-based intervention in child mental health conditions

- like autism. Clinical reasoning forms an integral part of sensory integration and intervention in child mental health.

- Intervention strategies/techniques rooted in Ayres Sensory Integration® can be used for specific behaviours seen in child mental health.

INTRODUCTION

The field of sensory integration (SI) remains to be evolving due to expanding, rigorous and on-going research within the field. The work Dr A.J. Ayres did between the late 1960s and the 1990s has confirmed the theoretical basis of SI and the developing child. This was achieved through the development of the theory of SI based on neuroscience, the development of assessment instruments, empirical research and the clinical application of SI theory in practice. With her work, Ayres endeavoured to explain the connection between sensory processing in the brain and behaviour that is observed (Bundy & Lane 2020a, p. xi) and the influence thereof on daily function. In 2007, the work of Ayres was trademarked as Ayres Sensory Integration® (ASI) in order 'to preserve the integrity of this work within occupational therapy' (Smith Roley et al. 2007, pp. CE-1). Since the late 1980s, scholars of Ayres as well as many other researchers have further contributed to ASI and now this 'body of work . . . includes theory, postulates about the mechanisms of sensory integration's effects, assessment strategies to identify challenges in sensory integration, intervention principles, a manualised intervention to guide treatment, and a

measure of fidelity that is used to support research and practice' (Lane et al. 2019, p. 2).

Ayres defined SI as 'the neurological process that organises sensations from one's body and the environment and makes it possible to use the body effectively in the environment' (Ayres 1989, p. 9). A model of the sensory integrative process developed by Ayres already in 1972 displays the importance of the interactions between the different sensory systems and the role that the processing of sensory information and the integration thereof plays in learning and behaviour (Ayres 1972). End products of SI represent abilities and skills such as concentration, organizing skills, academic learning abilities, self-esteem, self-control and self-confidence. The model demonstrates not only how sensory systems work together but also how sensory systems contribute to increasingly complex behaviours.

The relationship between SI and play is well recognised (Mailloux & Burke 2008). Play provides opportunities for the intake of sensory input, but SI forms an important foundation for the development of occupational performance components, motor skills and thus the abilities involved in play. Typically developing children have an innate drive to take part in

Crouch and Alers Occupational Therapy in Psychiatry and Mental Health, Sixth Edition.
Edited by Rosemary Crouch, Tania Buys, Enos Morankoana Ramano, Matty van Niekerk and Lisa Wegner.
© 2025 John Wiley & Sons Ltd. Published 2025 by John Wiley & Sons Ltd.

activities that provide in their sensory needs and that contribute to development (Schaaf & Smith-Roley 2006; Mailloux & Burke 2008). However, this innate drive may be restricted in children with sensory integration, developmental and mental health difficulties. The environment may also impact the development of a child's sensory integrative functions and adaptive behaviours. Studies have indicated that children growing up in under-resourced environments have a higher prevalence of SI difficulties/disorders (Van Jaarsveld *et al.* 2001b; Geyser 2022). We also know that children growing up in under-resourced environments who are exposed to programs using an SI approach do benefit in terms of improved sensory-motor components underlying learning (Van Jaarsveld *et al.* 2021).

In children with developmental and mental health conditions, there is no definitive answer yet as to whether SI deficits co-exist with the pathology or whether it is an integral part thereof. In conditions such as intellectual disability, attention disorders and developmental coordination disorders (DCD) sensory processing difficulties are described as part of the challenges these children experience as it does not form part of the diagnostic criteria. However, atypical sensory-based behaviours are included in the DSM-5 TR diagnostic criteria for autism (American Psychiatric Association 2022).

SENSORY INTEGRATION THEORY, FUNCTION AND DISORDERS

SENSORY SYSTEMS

In the theory of SI it is postulated that 'adequate processing of sensory information is an important foundation for adaptive behaviour' (Schaaf & Mailloux 2015, p. 5). Although all the sensory systems are crucial in typical development and function, the three sensory systems that are central in SI theory and practice are the tactile-, vestibular- and proprioceptive systems, also referred to as 'body-related' senses (Schaaf *et al.* 2010). These three systems play an important role in sensory reactivity, ocular control, postural stability, bilateral integration and praxis, which can influence development and thus how a child will engage in daily activities (Lane 2020). Ayres originally proposed the following on brain function, learning and behaviour based on her observations, interpretations and the neuroscientific literature:

- 'Perceptual awareness supports and facilitates occupational engagement.
- Motor learning is influenced by, if not dependent on, incoming sensations.
- Body awareness creates a postural model to understand visual-motor development.
- Postural control is essential for skilled academic and motor performance.

- Tactile, vestibular, proprioceptive and visual systems provide key data in the development of reading and writing.
- The ability to focus and maintain attention and to keep a steady level of activity and the way in which the nervous system responds to tactile sensation are related.
- The sensory systems develop in an integrated and dependent manner.
- Visual and auditory processing depends on foundational body-centred senses' (Smith Roley *et al.* 2007, p. 3).

What is important to note and in the words of Lane *et al.* (2019, p. 9) 'advances in neuroscience over the last several decades have allowed contemporary scientists to confirm and clarify some of the sensory integration and praxis patterns of sensory–motor functioning that emerged from Ayres' research on children with learning and behavioural difficulties'.

Although ASI theory and practice are complex and integrated, the authors of this chapter display SI in different levels (Figure 19.1) in an attempt to construct it in a more comprehensible manner, providing foundational knowledge for students and clinicians who are not trained in ASI. The different levels explain the processes involved in SI that support function. Although it is staggered hierarchically, these processes are interdependent and cannot always be separated as it is done theoretically.

The subconscious interaction and integration of the different sensory systems not only play an important role in how we make sense of daily sensory experiences (Schoen *et al.* 2020) but also provide an important foundation for learning and behaviour and is well described in SI literature based on the work of Ayres.

Mailloux *et al.* (2018) describe the key constructs of SI as was identified through many years of research by Ayers, her first-generation scholars and subsequently other occupational therapists. The four overarching constructs are those of Sensory Reactivity, Sensory Perception, Ocular, Postural and Bilateral Motor Integration and Praxis.

SENSORY REGISTRATION (DEPICTED IN LEVEL 1 OF FIGURE 19.1)

The construct of Sensory Reactivity has relevance for both this section as well as the section on sensory modulation. The processing of sensory information includes the perceiving, organising and interpretation thereof to make an adaptive response (Kilroy *et al.* 2019). Perceiving sensory information is also referred to as sensory registration, which refers to the point where the brain registers or becomes aware of incoming sensory information. Dunn (1999) proposed that the point where the brain registers sensory information is referred to as a neurological threshold. Neurological thresholds are viewed to be on a continuum, where on the one side of the continuum, a low neurological threshold would implicate that very little sensory information is needed before the brain registers

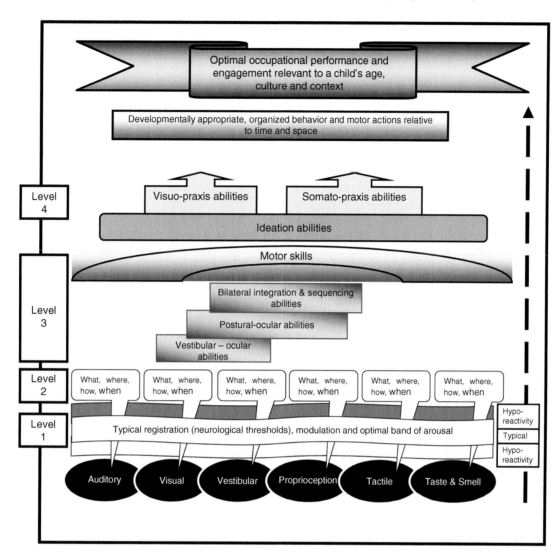

FIGURE 19.1   Basic model for understanding sensory integration and function. Level 1: Registration and modulation of sensory information and the effects of these processes on the maintenance of an optimal arousal state are functionally observed in the child's reactivity to sensory input. Level 2: Discrimination and perceptual functions are outcomes observed at this level. Level 3: Discrimination of spatial and temporal qualities becomes more accurate and advanced and is seen on ocular, postural and bilateral integration functions and the outcomes observed at this level and motor actions become more and more skilled. Level 4: Motor skills and praxis abilities for executing novel motor actions are the refined use outcomes observed at this level.

it, whereas, on the other side, a high neurological threshold would implicate that a lot of sensory information is needed before the brain registers it.

SENSORY MODULATION (DEPICTED IN LEVEL 1 OF FIGURE 19.1)

Ayres consistently associated modulation of sensory input with arousal, attention and activity levels, and contemporary research has evidenced associations between sensory reactivity and autonomic nervous system activity, sensory gating and differences in brain structures involved in multi-sensory integration (Lane *et al.* 2019). In this model, sensory reactivity is viewed as the observable responses associated with the individual's registration and modulation of sensory input.

Sensory modulation refers to the brain's ability to adapt or adjust sensory information (from inside the body or from the environment) in such a way that it supports optimal engagement in meaningful daily activities (Lane 2020). It includes the brain's ability to habituate to non-threatening/unimportant sensory information or sensitization to threatening/harmful and important sensory information. Modulation is also a brain function that needs to happen in relation to all the different sensory systems. Sensory modulation plays an important role in daily functioning, especially influencing the ability to focus, concentrate and be ready for engagement in tasks.

Adequate modulation of sensory information supports the capability of the individual to sustain engagement in activities despite variability within the body and/or the environment (Schaaf *et al.* 2010, p. 112) and it is thus of great importance in the learning process of a child. Sensory modulation also supports optimal levels of arousal to engage in activities. It further contributes to not only stability in emotions but also impacts on behaviour. Ayres originally postulated that sensory modulation is associated with the regulation of attention, arousal, activity level and affect (Lane et al. 2019) and specifically mentioned the limbic system as an important brain structure involved in the process of sensory modulation. Neuro-imaging and functional studies on functional connectivity have succeeded in proving Ayres's hypotheses in this regard (Kilroy et al. 2019) and these studies continue to increase our understanding of the neurophysiological processes that underpin the SI process.

Disorders in sensory modulation are reflected in behaviour. Disorders can be present in one or more of the sensory systems and can involve responses from internal or external sensations. Three distinct disorders were described by Ayres researched by several other authors. These are tactile defensiveness, gravitational insecurity and intolerance to movement. These three disorders are as follows:

Tactile defensiveness is linked to poor limbic or reticular processing within the brain and sympathetic nervous system reactions that are elicited by tactile sensations that others would consider non-noxious. This type of dysfunction is attributed to the antero-lateral system of the central nervous system. This system is responsible for the mediation of pain, crude touch, light touch and temperature. Most of the fibres of the antero-lateral system terminate in the reticular formation (Bundy et al. 2002). The reticular formation is responsible for arousal, emotional tone and autonomic regulation. Projections are sent from the reticular formation to the thalamus. The thalamus is also an integrating centre that assists with the coordination of information. From there, information is relayed to the cortex and the limbic system. The limbic system is responsible for emotional tone and motivational aspects of behaviour, arousal, attention and regulation.

Defensiveness can occur in any of the sensory systems and sensory defensiveness is an over-responsiveness to sensory stimulation causing the child to experience resultant anxiety, fear and aggression. Sensory defensive children often avoid activities that would expose them to the sensation to which they are defensive.

Ayres (1972) described a second sensory modulation disorder, namely gravitational insecurity. The child becomes fearful when their feet leave the ground or are on an unstable surface, or raised surface or when their head is tilted into 'unfamiliar' positions, especially into backward space. May Benson and Koomar (2007) have done further work on this type of SI dysfunction and have indicated that inadequate vestibulo-cerebellar interaction and possible decreased vestibular-ocular integration results in increased arousal levels and a fear response to sudden and/or unexpected movements.

Finally, intolerance or aversive response to movement occurs when the child is disorganised by any movements that are unfamiliar, which can lead to sympathetic nervous system reactions (Lane 2020). Although both gravitational insecurity and aversive response to movement dysfunctions are related to low neurological thresholds (over-responsivity/hyper-reactivity) within the vestibular system, the difference is that the child that experiences problems with gravitational insecurity likes movement, but their body needs to be secure in terms of gravitational pull. The child with aversion/intolerance to movement problems dislikes movement and is in general overwhelmed by movement.

Children experiencing sensory modulation difficulties can demonstrate hyper-responsivity (hyper-reactivity), hypo-responsivity (hypo-reactivity), or fluctuations in response to sensory stimuli. Children with sensory modulation difficulties are not only restricted in terms of processing sensory information but also in terms of their ability to attend and concentrate, their emotional control and activities of daily living such as toileting, dressing, feeding, bathing and socialising. Their levels of arousal not only impact their ability to engage in occupations, but also influence their emotions. Emotions that are seen include anxiety, lability, fear, aggression, depression and hostility.

SENSORY DISCRIMINATION AND PERCEPTION (DEPICTED IN LEVEL 2 OF FIGURE 19.1)

The construct of sensory perception has relevance in this section. The second and next level of SI is that of discrimination and perception which allow for a 'higher' and more involved level of participation in activities as cognitive involvement is also required. An example would be 'what am I touching?', 'what are the qualities of the object that I am touching?' and also 'when did I touch it?' and then 'how do I need to react?' Cognitive recognition, meaning and decision-making now form an important part of the process.

Sensory discriminatory abilities are supported by and dependent on all the different sensory systems. Discriminatory abilities allow for the individual to 'interpret and differentiate between the spatial and temporal qualities of sensory information' (Schaaf et al. 2010, p. 113). According to Lane and Reynolds (2020, p. 182) 'accuracy and efficiency in discrimination across all sensory systems contribute to an individual's ability to move through space, effectively interact with objects in the environment and perform daily occupations such as reading, eating and dressing, as well as fulfilling roles such as student, sibling and friend'. An example of discriminatory abilities within the tactile system would be when a child will be able to identify: where he/she has been touched?, what is it that touched him/her? and when did it touch him/her? In the process of discrimination, past experiences and memories need to be utilised to form associations about the spatial and or temporal qualities of what he/she is experiencing and then act on that information. Sensory discriminatory abilities add meaning to sensations and support the forming of perceptions.

Within the vestibular system, there are two discriminatory processes:

1. Otolithic processing is concerned with the pull of gravity and provides types of discrimination that have to do with postural accommodations together with where the body is in space when vision is excluded, for example whether up or down when in a swimming pool.

2. Semicircular canals processing is concerned with the detection of head movements through space. This type of processing contributes to three-dimensional spatial experiences and spatial orientation.

Proprioceptive discrimination is concerned with aspects where muscles, tendons and joints are working and where the brain needs to decide on actions such as adjusting posture when sitting in a chair, how hard to press when writing with a pencil or how far to stretch the elbow to pick up an object.

Discriminatory functions within the different sensory systems can vary from simple to very refined and these functions also evolve with development. Discriminatory functions can depend on only one sensory system but can also be dependent on combinations of sensory systems such as the visual and vestibular systems together to provide a stable visual field during head movements. Postural-ocular control involves the activations and coordinating of muscles 'in response to the position of the body relative to gravity and sustaining functional positions during transitions and while moving' (Schaaf *et al.* 2010, p. 114). Here the combination of the visual-, vestibular- and proprioceptive systems support function.

OCULAR, POSTURAL AND BILATERAL MOTOR INTEGRATION (DEPICTED IN LEVEL 3 OF FIGURE 19.1)

As the heading of this section indicates, the construct of Ocular, Postural and Bilateral integration has relevance. The third level in Figure 19.1 represents refined use, which is possible when integration of sensory information contributes to and supports motor skills as well as praxis. On this level, more advanced motor and cognitive functioning are required for successful interaction and engagement in activities. The requirements for successful participation also become more complex. An example of skilled action could be the ability to ride a bicycle and that of praxis the ability to perform new motor actions with a fair amount of success, for example, attempting to jump with a skipping rope for the first time. As soon as the action becomes learnt because of practice and repetition, it becomes a skill and no longer requires praxis abilities.

In terms of postural control poor processing of vestibular-proprioceptive input is believed to impede the development thereof (Lane & Reynolds 2020). A postural-ocular disorder is described as the behavioural manifestation of a vestibular-proprioceptive processing disorder and is hypothesised to be

the basis for the bilateral integration and sequencing (BIS) disorder. Difficulties with postural-related demands like righting and equilibrium reactions, flexion and extension postures, postural stability, and lateral flexion and rotation are experienced by these children. Poor ocular control impacts activities where a stable visual field is needed. When following an object with the eyes, visual fixation is needed with dissociation of the eyes from the head movements. Poor ocular control will also delay the development of form and space perception and eye-hand coordination.

In the literature, it is assumed that posture is the observable manifestation of vestibular and proprioceptive processing. There are also schools of thought that postural dysfunctions reflect the basis for deficits in BIS and sometimes for somatodyspraxia (Bundy & Lane 2020). Observable postural indicators include extensor muscle tone (observed in a standing position), prone extension, proximal stability, ability to move the neck into flexion against gravity (part of supine flexion), equilibrium and post-rotary nystagmus. This cluster of indicators is referred to in some cases as 'postural ocular' components. Postural control and stability are usually problematic for these children and they experience problems such as maintaining their posture and relying on their environment to support them with the postural demands. These children will lean against a wall when in the upright position, curl their legs and feet around chair legs, or assume a 'lying' position in a chair.

Postural-ocular abilities play important role in *motor skills* (depicted in level 3 of Figure 19.1) and especially so, in advanced postural-ocular abilities such as those used when riding a bicycle.

There is currently a debate on whether or not BIS are motor skill functions or functions supported by praxis abilities. The latest research indicates that a BIS dysfunction is a separate type of dysfunction from the visuo- and somato praxis factors that are identified in current research (Mailloux *et al.* 2011; Van Jaarsveld 2014). There is however consensus on what these functions entail and that it allows for:

- The effective use of the two sides of the body whether on a level of navigating the body through space or on a more skilled level.

- Similar use of the two hands, skilled in each, for example, skilled hand function and good hand function relative to hand skill.

- Cooperative use of hands together.

- Symmetrical rhythmic movements of arms, hands and feet.

- Coordinated bilateral asymmetric movements of limbs.

- Ability to coordinate rhythmic sequences of movements.

Children experiencing problems with BIS dysfunction will have difficulties in using the two sides of the body in a coordinated manner, crossing their midline and adequate establishment of dominance. Difficulties with the sequencing of motor actions, and specifically anticipatory projected movements, can be experienced. Anticipatory projected actions are very much feedforward dependent, meaning that they depend on past experiences and the ability to anticipate what is coming. Vestibular and proprioceptive system functions are the basis for adequate BIS actions and the visual system also plays an important role in directing motor actions (Cermak & May-Benson 2020). Children with BIS dysfunctions also suffer emotionally because of their inability to experience success in various everyday tasks and activities. They usually have low self-esteem and their motivation can be low.

In terms of other motor skills, many examples thereof are to be found in the literature. The important question is whether a child can perform skilled motor actions related to his/her age norm and to what extent it influences their function and engagement in occupations.

PRAXIS (DEPICTED IN LEVEL 4 OF FIGURE 19.1)

The construct of Praxis has relevance. Ayres defined developmental dyspraxia as a 'motor planning disorder' and as a 'disorder of SI interfering with the ability to plan and execute skilled or non-habitual motor tasks' (Ayres & Cermak 2011, p. 51). Praxis was also described by Ayres (1989) as the process that includes conceptualization or ideation, motor planning and execution of a novel or new motor action. Praxis abilities are crucial in successful interaction with the environment, to execute action plans and adapt/correct motor actions to achieve the desired outcomes (Schaaf & Smith-Roley 2006).

Ayres (1989) stated that the conceptualization or ideation part of the praxis process is a cognitive function, partially dependent on the integration of sensory information. She also described that children's knowledge of objects and their affordances (potential use) are dependent on the purposeful use of the body in activity and with objects in the environment. More work on the ideational component of the praxis process was done by May Benson and Cermak (2007), who developed the Test for Ideational Praxis (TIP). They state that 'ideation underlies planning, sequencing and organization of actions and ideational abilities may influence how a child engages in activities and occupations' (May Benson & Cermak, 2007, p. 152). Difficulties with ideation will present themselves in a child's inability to know or make use of the affordances of objects in three-dimensional (3D) space. Although Ayres' original assessment tools (the Southern California Sensory Integration Test [SCSIT] and later the Sensory Integration and Praxis Test [SIPT]) did not include specific tests of ideation, the new Evaluation in Ayres Sensory Integration (EASI) assessment instrument includes a test item Praxis: Ideation and aims to assess a child's ability to form and demonstrate ideas about possible actions using four everyday objects including the body (Mailloux et al. 2020, p. 20). The addition of ideational praxis to this test battery will in the future also generate new knowledge on the ideational component of praxis.

Visuo-praxis is mainly dependent on the visual system but also relies on the vestibular system in terms of providing a stable visual field. Somato-praxis is dependent on the support of the proprioceptive and tactile systems. Visuo- and somato-dyspraxia have been described in Ayres's original work on the SIPT. This is also one of the 'clusters' of dysfunctions that are described in the SIPT Manual (2004). These two types of dyspraxia are still seen as factors evolving from current research (Mailloux et al. 2011; Van Jaarsveld et al. 2014).

A child affected by poor SI abilities will experience difficulties with engaging in daily occupations during play, school, personal independence, recreation, sleep and interpersonal relations. The degree of difficulties can and will depend on the level/levels of the difficulties or dysfunctions as displayed in the Basic model for understanding sensory integration and function (Figure 19.1) and discussed above. A generalised SI dysfunction is also described in research as a combination of dysfunctions where a child obtains below-average scores within all the major areas tested by the SIPT (Ayres 1989).

Children with praxis dysfunctions can experience difficulties with body scheme, gross and fine motor skills and oral motor control (Lane 2012). They appear clumsy in performing motor actions, are accident-prone, may mouth objects or drool and depend on using their vision for the successful completion of tasks. Their behaviour varies from controlling and demanding to apathetic. Emotions that they frequently have to deal with include frustration, aggression or apathy. Academic problems such as perceptual and visual motor difficulties (inclusive of reading and writing) can also be a direct result of these disorders.

Visuo-dyspraxia is a deficit in visual perception abilities that affects constructional skills. The visual- as well as the proprioceptive systems are involved in this dysfunction. Children with visuo-dyspraxia experience difficulties with visually planning space on three-dimensional (3D) and two-dimensional (2D) levels, which impacts mapping space and organizing their own personal space (Lane 2012). Drawing and writing are usually problematic and can be observed in the management of their working space.

Somato-dyspraxia causes children to have difficulty with motor tasks in terms of creating ideas of the how or what is possible, the planning of the actions and the execution thereof. These children do not receive feedback from their body and the environment after the action was completed, namely, was it successful or unsuccessful and the quality of their feedforward mechanisms is also poor (before an action is carried out information is needed from the nervous system on the 'how' of the actions, for example in an action like catching a ball, the individual needs to get his/her limbs to a particular place in time to catch it). Any activity that depends on intact somato-sensory feedback (e.g. identifying shapes by touch, without seeing them) will pose problems for a child with dyspraxia. Fine motor abilities are often also affected (Schaaf et al. 2010).

FUNCTIONAL, ORGANISED BEHAVIOUR AND OCCUPATION (DEPICTED IN THE TOP LEVEL OF FIGURE 19.1)

Developmentally appropriate, organised behaviour and motor actions relative to time and space are what Ayres has termed 'end products' of sensory integration. This includes the ability to concentrate, ability to organise, good self-esteem, self-control and self-confidence, academic learning abilities, capacity for abstract thought and reasoning as well as specialisation of each side of the body and the brain (Schaaf *et al.* 2010, p. 100).This implies that when a child is able to participate meaningfully and developmentally appropriately in daily activities and occupations, sensory integration processes in the brain are supporting function.

SENSORY INTEGRATION DIFFICULTIES AND DYSFUNCTIONS IN CHILD MENTAL HEALTH CONDITIONS

Sensory integration difficulties and dysfunctions were originally described by Ayres within the population of children with developmental, learning and emotional difficulties (Ayres 1972), with a growing evidence base for SI difficulties and dysfunctions in various mental health conditions (Harrison *et al.* 2019). When the functional difficulties of children with developmental and mental health conditions are considered, through reasoning, it becomes clear that the processing and integration of sensory information contribute to the clinical picture. In Table 19.1 examples are given of common behavioural or functional difficulties that can relate to poor sensory integration.

For a child to perform optimally in daily occupations, they need to process sensory information throughout the day, and modulate the sensory information from all the different senses to attend and concentrate on all the activities they encounter. To participate in activities, they need the ability to discriminate sensory information, must have motor function and skills, and when challenged with new motor actions or sequences, need to be able to ideate, plan and execute actions. Therefore, it is evident that SI difficulties contribute to the functional problems experienced by children with child mental health conditions.

AUTISM SPECTRUM DISORDERS

Atypical sensory-based behaviours are included in one of the features for autism spectrum disorders (ASD) and is included under the 'restricted, repetitive patterns of behaviours, interests or activities' diagnostic criterion in the DSM-5-TR (American Psychiatric Association 2022). Prevalence rates for ASD vary in different geographical regions with a steady increase in autism rates reported universally over the past two

Table 19.1 Relating behaviour or functional problems to sensory integration problems.

Behaviour/functional difficulties	Possible difficulties contributing to sensory integration problem
Poor sleep-wake cycles that interfere with day routines and activities	May experience difficulties to self-regulate; cannot implement self-calming strategies and remains acutely aware of all the sensory information in his/her own body and in the environment
Poor attention abilities, always on the move	Difficulties with sensory reactivity (over- or under-reactivity); uses movement excessively in an attempt to regulate self or due to poor sensory perception or praxis
Difficulty in sustaining postures and poor physical endurance	Poor vestibular-proprioceptive processing that does not support muscle tone and postural mechanisms
Poor use of tools such as eating with a knife and fork	Poor development of the coordinated use of the upper extremities due to bilateral integration and sequencing dysfunction caused by insufficient integration of proprioceptive and vestibular functions
Engage with play materials in a restricted and repetitive way, do not engage in novel or new play situations	Praxis dysfunction; poor ability to recognise affordances of play materials (ideation difficulties), problems with planning and execution of motor actions during play

decades (Salari *et al.* 2022). Prevalence rates of 1 in 36 children are reported in eight-year-old children in the United States (Meanner *et al.* 2023). The prevalence of SI dysfunctions among autistic children is reported to be in the range of 88–96% (Pfeiffer *et al.* 2011; Marco *et al.* 2011; Schaaf *et al.* 2018). Functional difficulties of autistic children are often related to SI difficulties/dysfunctions. They experience difficulties with regulating responses in relation to sensations (often very specific stimuli) and they may use self-stimulation to compensate for limited input or to counter overstimulation.

Ayres wrote on the SI difficulties that children with autism experience in the 1980s (Ayres & Tickle 1980). She hypothesised that differences in sensory reactivity observed in autistic children related to limbic system functions, specifically the amygdala. Ayres also hypothesised about the effect of SI differences in autistic children on their motivation or their 'I want to do it part of the brain' (Kilroy *et al.* 2019, p. 8). Recent research has indicated that individuals with ASD show more than one type of SI difficulties as well as prominent sensory modulation symptoms across the ages and the spectrum of severity. These difficulties involve challenges in modulation, integration, organisation and discrimination of sensory input to such an extent that the person does not respond adaptively to the input and experiences disruptions in daily activities and emotional behaviour patterns (Ben-Sasson *et al.* 2009; Schaaf & Mailloux 2015).

Schaaf and Smith-Roley (2006, pp. 123–124) view the key considerations when using a sensory integration approach with children with ASD as follows:

- An inability to cope with unexpected or intense sensory input.

- Difficulty to register and attend to salient sensory information.

- Heightened sensory sensitivities.

- Variability in reactions to sensory input.

- Gravitational insecurity.

- Seeking and avoidant behaviours in relation to movement, auditory input, touch, smell and taste.

- Difficulties in processing multi-sensory information.

- Self-stimulatory behaviours.

- Difficulties with processing tactile input.

- Praxis difficulties.

- Strengths in visual memory and ability to visually manipulate objects.

The main intervention objectives when using an SI approach with children with ASD are to improve their ability to engage purposefully and successfully in daily activities, including the forming of meaningful social interactions and relationships. The objectives of therapy will include to help them in organising sensory information so that it has meaning for them; to help them to experience enhanced sensory feedback about their bodies and the environment; to support their sensory discrimination abilities so that the perceptions they form are more accurate; to broaden their motor skills that are supported by vestibular, proprioceptive and tactile functions; and to enhance their praxis abilities by providing enhanced opportunities for forming ideas, planning motor actions and executing them. Ensuring that their daily sensory needs are addressed will be crucial. This will also include human and environmental adaptations in those environments where they function on a daily basis.

Many studies have investigated the effectiveness of SI intervention in children with autism. A review study published in 2019 confirmed that Ayres Sensory Integration® intervention complies with the criteria of the Council for Exceptional Children (CEC) Standards for Evidence-based Practices in Special Education to be regarded as an evidence-based intervention for autistic children (Schoen *et al.* 2019).

ATTENTION DEFICIT HYPERACTIVE DISORDERS

The American Psychiatric Association (2022, p. 70) describes Attention Deficit Disorder (with Hyperactivity) (ADHD) as a disorder that 'is characterised by a persistent pattern of inattention and/or hyperactivity-impulsivity that interferes with functioning or development, diminished sustained attention

and higher levels of impulsivity in a child or adolescent than expected for someone of that age and developmental level'. Children with ADHD experience difficulties with perceptual-motor impairments, distractibility, completing tasks, organizational skills, motor and cognitive learning and controlling emotions. When using an SI approach, it will be important to assess which of the mentioned difficulties are caused or amplified by SI difficulties.

Schaaf and Miller (2005) reported different sympathetic markers of sensory reactivity and decreased responses of inhibition in the presence of typical sensory habituation, both indicative of sensory modulation difficulties, in children with ADHD. Budding (2012) discussed poor timing of behaviour that children with attention disorders experience. Lane (2012) reported that high comorbidity (50%) exists between children with attention deficit hyperactive disorder who also struggle with praxis dysfunctions. Work by Li *et al.* (2023) has shown that SI dysfunctions may play a mediating role in the executive function difficulties commonly experienced by children with ADHD.

Sensory integration difficulties and dysfunctions are highly prevalent among children with ADHD, although there is not yet consensus as to whether SI differences should be viewed as co-occurring conditions or as part of the core symptomatology of ADHD. Nonetheless, where children with ADHD present with functional difficulties related to sensory integrative functions, it is imperative that these should be addressed.

INTELLECTUAL DEVELOPMENTAL DISORDER (INTELLECTUAL DISABILITY)

Intellectual developmental disorder (intellectual disability) is defined by the DSM-5-TR as deficits in general mental (intellectual) abilities that affect adaptive functioning in conceptual, social and practical domains. The age of onset must be in the developmental period and the condition is considered lifelong. Intellectual disability can occur on its own or can co-occur with other mental health conditions like autism spectrum disorder or mood disorders (American Psychiatric Association 2022).

In developing adequate sensory integration, the child's ability to explore the environment plays an important role. Intellectual disability may influence the way in which children explore their environments on a sensory level. The importance of the contribution of sensory experiences to development cannot be emphasised enough. A sensory-rich environment, which can be freely used and explored, is a crucial element in the intervention plan for children with intellectual disabilities.

Children and adolescents with intellectual disability experience a wide variety of SI difficulties and dysfunctions, which include difficulties/dysfunction in sensory reactivity and modulation, difficulties with sensory perception, problems with motor skills as well as praxis dysfunctions. The degrees of the SI difficulties/dysfunctions vary from child to child. The functional outcomes of poor SI are prevalent in these children's performance in activities, and they are often dependent on environmental and social support for optimal functioning.

For some children with intellectual disabilities, repetitive or self-harming behaviours can have an adverse effect on their physical safety and occupational engagement (Smith *et al.* 2005). Differences in sensory processing have been shown to relate at least in part to these behaviours (Gal *et al.* 2010) and sensory integration-based interventions show promising results to influence repetitive or self-harming behaviours to increase occupational engagement (Smith *et al.* 2005; Mills *et al.* 2016) although more evidence is needed.

Targeting outcomes related to optimal motor function and skills is also an important focus of intervention for children with intellectual disabilities. Improved motor functions and skills could strengthen participation in occupations that can be fulfilling and potentially also provide a form of income. Differences in sensory reactivity, and motor difficulties/dysfunctions based in poor SI can thus be addressed through ASI therapy.

NEUROBEHAVIOURAL DISORDER ASSOCIATED WITH PRENATAL ALCOHOL EXPOSURE

Neurobehavioural disorder associated with prenatal alcohol exposure (ND-PAE), encompassing foetal alcohol spectrum disorders, refers to a wide range of neurobehavioural disabilities that are associated with more than minimal exposure to the teratogenic effects of alcohol in the gestational period (American Psychiatric Association 2022). It is characterised by deficits in neurocognitive functioning, self-regulation and adaptive functioning, and has a pervasive influence on a child's participation in daily life occupations. The mean prevalence of ND-PAE worldwide is estimated at 7.7% (American Psychiatric Association 2022), but much higher prevalence rates have been reported in certain communities. For example, in the Cape Winelands in South Africa, prevalence rates between 17 and 23% have been reported (May *et al.* 2016).

Several studies have demonstrated that children with ND-PAE present with a wide range of SI difficulties and dysfunctions (Jirokowic *et al.* 2008; Du Plooy 2017; Jirikowic *et al.* 2020). In a South African study conducted in the Cape Winelands, over- and under-reactivity across different sensory systems were reported, attesting to the diverse nature of SI difficulties that may occur among children with ND-PAE. When investigating patterns of SI dysfunction using results from the SIPT, the study demonstrated a high prevalence of visuo- and somatodyspraxia among children with ND-PAE (Du Plooy 2017).

With SI difficulties and dysfunctions being highly prevalent among children with ND-PAE and deficits in self-regulation being one of the defining features of the disorder, it stands to reason that intervention based on Ayres Sensory Integration® has an important role to play in the management of the disorder. Studies measuring the effectiveness of sensory integration-based interventions have shown promising results (Wilczynski & Zawada 2016; Wilczynski *et al.* 2018), and more robust research into the effectiveness of ASI intervention on children with ND-PAE will contribute to this field of practice.

DEVELOPMENTAL COORDINATION DISORDER

DCD is a serious impairment in the development of motor coordination that is not exclusively explainable in terms of general intellectual impairment or any specific congenital or acquired neurological disorder (American Psychiatric Association 2022). Neuro-developmental immaturity may be present, although no diagnosable neurological disorder is present, as well as definite signs of gross- and fine motor problems (Sadock & Sadock 2003). Motor coordination problems must interfere significantly with the child's academic performance. Poor performances in visuo-spatial cognitive tasks are also associated with DCD.

DCD prevalence rates are reported at around 5–6% of the general population (Blank *et al.* 2019). Children with DCD experience difficulties performing daily activities. They are clumsy, are at a higher risk of language and learning disorders and are often excluded by peers for poor performance in sports activities. This leads to difficulties with peer relationships.

There is a large overlap between dyspraxia and DCD from a SI perspective. Allen and Casey (2017) estimate that 88% of children with DCDs show differences in sensory processing and a study by Ringold *et al.* (2022) demonstrated sensory modulation difficulties in the form of sensory over-responsivity in at least 31% of children with DCD compared to autistic children (74%) and typically developing peers (4%). Delay of motor milestones, lack of motor abilities in sports, and problems with handwriting are commonly seen in both children with SI disorder with dyspraxia and DCD.

Unfortunately, evidence for the effectiveness of Ayres Sensory Integration® intervention for children with DCD is still sparse (Blank *et al.* 2019). Most guiding documents favour task-oriented approaches in the management of DCD (Blank *et al.* 2019; Caçola & Lage 2019). This emphasises the need for well-designed studies that adhere to fidelity criteria to ASI to evaluate effectiveness of ASI® in populations such as children with DCD (Schaaf *et al.* 2018).

ASSESSMENT

When using an SI frame of reference, the occupational therapist will collect information on the child's occupational profile. Depending on the child's age, abilities and context, decisions will be made regarding assessment instruments. The SIPT (Ayres 1989) remains one of the best assessment tools to identify SI and praxis dysfunctions. It is not always possible to use this instrument due to various reasons such as lack of training (formal training in the use of the SIPT is required), the age and/or intellectual abilities of the child, anxiety levels and also resources available. To address some of these challenges such as cost and accessibility, the EASI was developed in a large-scale international study. The EASI is an open-access, comprehensive assessment tool that aims to assess SI functions across all of the constructs that have emerged over the decades of research since Ayres first introduced SI theory. Normative data for the EASI were collected on more than 9000 children worldwide and included tests of functions not previously included in tests like the SIPT (such as objective measures of ideation and of reactivity). The constructs measured by the EASI include (Mailloux *et al.* 2018, p. 3):

- 'Sensory perception in the tactile, proprioceptive, vestibular and visual systems.

- Praxis based on somatosensory, language and visual-based functions.

- Postural, ocular and bilateral integration based on vestibular functions.

- Sensory over- and under-reactivity.'

For babies, the Test for Sensory Functions in Infants (DeGangi & Greenspan 1989) can be administered and for toddlers, the DeGangi-Berk test (DeGangi 1983) can be used. The Clinical observations are valuable assessments to assist in concluding the difficulties/dysfunctions of a child.

In addition to performance-based assessments like the SIPT and the EASI, parent-, teacher and self-report measures of SI are also available. The Sensory Profile (Dunn 1999, 2014) and the Sensory Processing Measures (Parham *et al.* 2006, 2021) are both now in their second editions, and are used to gather data regarding the child's sensory processing abilities as perceived by the child's caregivers and/or teachers and/or the (older) child themselves.

Clinical reasoning remains one of the critical components in the use of an SI framework, especially where standardised tests cannot be used and the therapist has to rely on history taking, checklists and clinical observations. The child's functional problems need to be related to the underlying sensory systems that are not supporting the child's functioning, in order to make conclusions on possible difficulties or dysfunctions and to plan intervention.

Comprehensive assessment forms a crucial part of the data-driven decision-making process when applying ASI theory as a frame of reference in clinical practice. The use of valid and reliable assessment tools is pivotal to this process and should always be done wherever possible (Schaaf & Mailloux 2015).

GENERAL SENSORY INTEGRATION TREATMENT PRINCIPLES

During intervention, the aim will always be to work towards the child making adaptive responses in areas that have been identified as problematic. An adaptive response is a purposeful action that responds to sensory information from the environment and the body in an appropriate and successful manner (Ayres 1972).

- The manner in which sensory information is processed needs to be experienced in a purposeful and meaningful way for learning to take place.

- When using activities that provide vestibular input: Angular movement stimulates the semicircular canals and facilitates phasic, fleeting postural reactions. Linear movements (up and down and forward and backwards) stimulate the utricle hair cells and facilitate tonic postural extension and increased muscle tone, which is needed in maintaining anti-gravity extensor postures. Whilst linear vestibular movements facilitate postural extension, only heavy work can promote postural flexion. First, work for total flexion through phasic fleeting movements and then grade to activities that promote tonic sustained flexion.

- Always work for an adaptive response, if only sensory stimulation is provided without active participation and adapted responses from the child, no integration and learning will take place.

- Where applicable, use short concrete language as the processing of verbal information places extra demands on the sensory systems. Both the mentally retarded child and the child with autistic spectrum disorders experience language difficulties.

- Routine and structure provide a lot of security to both the mentally retarded child and the child with autistic spectrum disorders, who especially experience challenges with change/transitions.

- Decrease anxiety as far as possible by allowing the treatment session to flow, keeping activities familiar (challenges within the activity could vary) and supporting children in anticipating change. This is especially applicable to children with autistic spectrum disorders.

- Notes must be kept on the child's responses to treatment and progress. Feedback on the child's progress should be given regularly to parents/caregivers and other members of the team.

AYRES SENSORY INTEGRATION THERAPY PRECAUTIONS

- A child can never be left unattended in a SI area. Apparatus used without supervision and guidance could cause serious injuries.

- Doctors, other staff members, parents/caregivers should always be informed that a child is exposed to SI treatment. Doctors should also be consulted about any condition that might be aggravated by especially vestibular stimulation (e.g. epilepsy and ventricular shunts). Feedback received from them plays a valuable part not only in the adaptation of the program but also in the success of the intervention.

- Sensory integration equipment must always be kept in a good condition and mattresses should always be placed under suspension apparatus to reduce the chance of injury. Polystyrene chips should be changed regularly as they disintegrate easily and the chances of ingesting pieces or getting them stuck in body cavities are a strong possibility.

- Sensory integration activities are never forced on a child. A golden rule of SI therapy is that if a child does not enjoy, his/her nervous system is not integrating and thus no learning will take place.

- As many children with more severe child psychiatric conditions are not able to communicate effectively, it is of the utmost importance to observe them very closely and according to Blackburn, who was a pioneer in SI in child mental health in South Africa, this observation should be continued by caregivers for at least two hours after treatment (Crouch & Alers, 1997). Any signs of distress, which indicate autonomic nervous system reactions, should be reported and treated accordingly. Signs of stress include the following: paleness, sweating, tachycardia, nausea or vomiting, extreme fear and/or agitation, constant yawning, over-excitement, constant crying, falling asleep or losing consciousness. Depending on the symptoms, the necessary intervention should be made. It must always be remembered that these children's nervous systems can be much more sensitive to sensory input and adverse reactions can easily occur.

SPECIFIC BEHAVIOURS AND TECHNIQUES DEVELOPED FROM SENSORY INTEGRATION THEORY

When working with children with child psychiatric conditions, one is often confronted with behaviour that is extremely challenging. Over the years various strategies, techniques or complementary programs have been developed from the work of Ayres that are not or do not necessarily adhere to ASI principles, but enhanced sensory input is inherent in the application thereof. That does not mean that it could not be applied, especially if it does improve behaviour and function (Van Jaarsveld 2014). It is strongly recommended that the strategies and techniques described in literature be used in combination with an ASI intervention program and closely monitored for effectiveness, as research into some of these strategies is sparse.

As authors we would like to acknowledge the treatment protocol that was developed by Joy Varney-Blackburn (1985) for the treatment of self-injurious behaviour in children with intellectual disabilities and ASD that is still used today. She also developed an oral stimulation program (Crouch & Alers, 1997). Both, as well as considerations regarding institutionalisation and the use of groups in SI therapy are described in detail in the chapter on Sensory Integration in Mental Health (Van Jaarsveld 2014). For purposes of updating, sensory seeking and self-stimulation behaviours are addressed in this edition.

SENSORY SEEKING AND SELF-STIMULATION BEHAVIOURS

Stereotypic, disruptive and self-stimulatory behaviours can occur among children with ASD and in children with intellectual disabilities and other mental health conditions. Examples of behaviours observed in children who are sensory seeking or who exhibit self-stimulatory behaviours include head banging, shaking of extremities, finger or ear flicking, scratching, biting (self or others), mouthing or chewing, grinding of teeth, rubbing of hands, rocking, spinning, scratching, humming (or any other form of vocalisation), smelling and sniffing of objects.

There are many reasons why a child may engage in these types of behaviours, but one of the reasons could be that the child has an SI disorder or difficulty. The cause of the behaviour could vary:

i. It could be that the sensation derived from the behaviour provides the child with enhanced sensory input, which provides in a need of the child.

ii. It may be a way for the child to communicate with his/her environment, in terms of attention received, obtained or avoided.

iii. It could provide the child with a manner to indicate his/her needs in terms of sensory input that is wanted (touch, vestibular, proprioceptive, auditory, visually, olfactory or smell).

Schaaf and Mailloux discuss a further four reasons why a child may have unusual sensory interests, which also needs to be considered and especially so if a child has an SI dysfunction (Schaaf & Mailloux 2015, p. 28):

i. A child may seek additional sensory input due to hypo-reactivity.

ii. A child with poor praxis will experience challenges to generate novel ideas and plans resulting in what may seem as seeking behaviours.

iii. A child with poor sensory perception may also seek additional sensory information in an effort to understand and interpret what is experienced.

iv. A child who is hyper-reactive to certain sensations may seek other sensory input in an effort to self-regulate.

The role of the occupational therapist will be to use clinical reasoning to analyse these behaviours by first identifying the reason for, and function of, the behaviour as mentioned above. The behaviour also needs to be analysed to identify which sensory systems are involved, e.g. where movement is involved like rocking, spinning and running – the child is providing him/her with vestibular input. The type of vestibular input should also be identified (linear, rotatory, angular, fast and slow). A child that hangs upside down or positions himself with his head in an inverted position seeks intense vestibular input. Where behaviours such as jumping, crashing, hitting, pinching, teeth grinding and chewing are involved, the child is providing him/herself with proprioceptive stimulation (some of the mentioned behaviours also have an element of vestibular stimulation). The type of proprioceptive input should also be identified, for example light proprioceptive or deep proprioceptive. Where behaviours such as scratching, biting, masturbating and headbanging are involved – the child is providing him/herself with tactile and proprioceptive input. The type of tactile stimulation should also be identified (light touch or deep touch). Where the child engages in activities such as finger or hand flicking, spinning him/herself with open eyes, there is an element of visual stimulation involved that needs attention. Behaviours which involve smelling and sniffing provide olfactory stimulation. Behaviours involving sounds provide auditory stimulation.

In autistic individuals, self-stimulatory (sometimes called 'stimming') behaviours often have a self-regulatory function and can be a way to express emotions or to release tension and provide distraction (Charlton *et al.* 2021). Suppressing stimming behaviours is reported to have negative emotional and cognitive consequences, and therefore sensory-seeking or self-stimulatory behaviours that do not cause harm to the person themselves or the people or environment around them seldom require attempts to diminish or redirect them. Still, an analysis of the sensory characteristics of the behaviour can assist in creating a varied 'sensory diet' that can make a meaningful contribution to the individual's quality of life if implemented in a person-centred manner. Analysis of these behaviours can also be valuable when considering environmental adaptations, assistive technologies and accommodations that may be of value to the child to enable them to participate meaningfully in their daily occupations.

In children with SI difficulties or dysfunctions that contribute to sensory seeking or self-stimulatory behaviours, applying principles of ASI therapy to assist the child to make adaptive responses through active engagement in functional and playful activities (as discussed earlier in the chapter) is beneficial to address the underlying difficulty or dysfunction.

CONCLUSION

The importance of SI in a developing child cannot be ignored. The impact of SI is not always recognised until a child experience problems. Although SI is but one of many aspects of human functioning, it needs to be considered when children experience developmental difficulties and when a mental health diagnosis is made. Sensory integration does not provide all the answers, but it can make a significant difference in not only the child's functioning but also in that of the family, caregivers, educators and other significant people in a child's life. Children are bombarded with visual and auditory stimuli, whilst tactile, vestibular and proprioceptive stimuli are often 'neglected' by our modern lifestyles. The impact of that alone can be detrimental in a developing child, so how much more would it be the case for a child with a diagnosis within the field of neurodevelopment and mental health? These children need to be understood and supported in terms of how they process and integrate sensory information from their own bodies and from the environment to be able to participate meaningfully in their occupations. As occupational therapists, we need to be 'sensory' advocates for these children.

QUESTIONS

1. Describe how SI influences play.

2. Describe the process of sensory registration and modulation and how it can impact a child's ability to engage in meaningful activities.

3. Describe in your own words what your understanding of sensory discrimination is and how that could impact perceptions.

4. Describe the symptoms that a child with praxis difficulties/dysfunction would display.

5. Describe how SI difficulties can affect:

   Sleeping patterns.

   Use of tools.

6. Explain why would children engage in sensory seeking and self-stimulatory behaviours.

7. Describe how would you address self-stimulatory behaviour in a child with intellectual disability.

8. Name examples of four assessment tools that were developed to measure sensory integration constructs.

9. Using your knowledge of children with autistic spectrum disorders, provide examples of behaviour that could be linked to poor sensory integration.

10. Explain why would children with child mental health conditions be more prone to SI difficulties than other children.

REFERENCES

Allen, S. & Casey, J. (2017) Developmental coordination disorders and sensory processing and integration: incidence, associations and co-morbidities. *British Journal of Occupational Therapy,* **80**(9), 549–557. https://doi.org/10.1177/0308022617709183

American Psychiatric Association (2022) *Diagnostic and Statistical Manual of Mental Disorders*, 5th edn. American Psychiatric Association, Washington, DC.

Ayres, A.J. (1972) *Sensory Integration and Learning Disorders.* Western Psychological Services, Los Angeles.

Ayres, A.J. (1989) *Sensory Integration and Praxis Tests.* Western Psychological Services, Los Angeles.

Ayres, A.J. & Cermak, S.A. (2011) *Ayres Dyspraxia Monograph.* Pediatric Therapy Network, Los Angeles.

Ayres, A.J. & Tickle, L.S. (1980) Hyper-responsivity to touch and vestibular stimuli as a predictor of positive response to sensory integration procedures by autistic children. *American Journal of Occupational Therapy, 34,* 375–381.

Ben-Sasson, A., Hen, L., Fluss, R., Cermak, S.A., Engel-Yeger, B. & Gal, E. (2009) A meta-analysis of sensory modulation symptoms in individuals with autism spectrum disorders. *Journal Autism & Developmental Disorders, 39,* 1–11.

Blank, R., Barnett, A.L., Cairney, J. *et al* (2019) International clinical practice recommendations on the definition, diagnosis, assessment, intervention, and psychosocial aspects of developmental coordination disorder. *Developmental Medicine & Child Neurology, 61,* 242–286. https://doi.org/10.1111/dmcn.14132

Budding, D. (2012) *Born to move: the inter-relation of cognitive and motor function.* Presentation at R2K Research Symposium. Unpublished, Los Angeles.

Bundy, A.C. & Lane, S. (2020a) Sensory integration: A. Jean Ayres' theory revisited. In: A.C. Bundy & S. Lane (eds), *Sensory Integration Theory and Practice,* 3rd edn, pp. 2–20. F.A. Davis, Philadelphia.

Bundy, A.C. & Lane, S.J. (2020b) Sensory Integration Theory and Practice, 3rd edn. F.A. Davis Company, Philadelphia.

Bundy, A.C., Lane, S.J., Murray, E.A. & Fisher, A.G. (2002) *Sensory Integration: Theory and Practice.* Mathewbooks, Philadelphia.

Caçola, P. & Lage, G. (2019) Developmental coordination disorder (DCD): an overview of the condition and research evidence. *Motriz: Revista de Educação Física, 25(2),* e101923. https://doi.org/10.1590/S1980-6574201900020001

Cermak, S. & May-Benson, T. (2020) Praxis and dyspraxia. In: A.C. Bundy & S. Lane (eds), *Sensory Integration Theory and Practice,* 3rd edn, pp. 115–150. F.A. Davis, Philadelphia.

Charlton, R., Entecott, T., Belova, E. & Nwaordu, G. (2021) "It feels like holding back something you need to say": autistic and non-autistic adults accounts of sensory experiences and stimming. *Research in Autism Spectrum Disorders, 89,* 101864. https://doi.org/10.1016/j.rasd.2021.101864

Crouch, R. & Alers, V. (1997) *Occupational Therapy in Psychiatry and Mental Health,* 3rd edn. Maskew Miller Longman (Pty.) Ltd., South Africa.

Crouch, R. & Alers, V. (2005) *Occupational Therapy in Mental Health,* 5th edn. Whurr Publishers, London.

DeGangi, G.A. (1983) *DeGangi-Berk Test of Sensory Integration (TSI).* Western Psychological Services, Los Angeles.

DeGangi, G. & Greenspan, S.I. (1989) *Test of Sensory Functions in Infants (TSFI) Manual.* Western Psychological Services, Los Angeles.

Du Plooy, M. (2017) *Sensory integration difficulties and dysfunctions in children with fetal alcohol spectrum disorders.* Master's Dissertation, University of the Free State, Bloemfontein.

Dunn, W. (1999) *The Sensory Profile: Examiner's Manual.* Physiological Corporation, San Antonio.

Dunn, W. (2014) *Sensory Profile 2.* Physiological Corporation, Bloomington, Minnesota

Gal, E., Dyck, M.J. & Passmore, A. (2010) Relationships between stereotyped movements and sensory processing disorders in children with and without developmental or sensory disorders. *American Journal of Occupational Therapy, 64,* 453–461. https://doi.org/10.5014/ajot.2010.09075

Geyser, E. (2022) *Guidelines for the Scoring and Interpretation of the evaluation of Ayres Sensory Integration® (EASI®) on a Typically Developing Paediatric Population in Gauteng.* University of the Free State, South Africa.

Harrison, L.A., Kats, A., Williams, M.E. & Aziz-Zadeh, L. (2019) The importance of sensory processing in mental health: a proposed addition to the research domain criteria (RDoC) and suggestions for RDoC 2.0. *Frontiers in Psychology, 10,* 1–15. https://doi.org/10.3389/fpsyg.2019.00103

Jirokowic, T.L., Olson, H.C. & Kartin, D. (2008) Sensory processing, school performance, and adaptive behaviour of young school-age children with fetal alcohol spectrum disorders. *Physical & Occupational Therapy in Pediatrics, 28(2),* 117–136. https://doi.org/10.1080/01942630802031800

Jirikowic, T.L., Thorne, J.C., McLaughlin, S.A., Waddington, T., Lee, A.K. & Astley Hemingway, S.J. (2020) Prevalence and patterns of sensory processing behaviors in a large clinical sample of children with prenatal alcohol exposure. *Research in Developmental Disabilities, 100,* 1–12. https://doi.org/10.1016/j.ridd.2020.103617

Kilroy, E., Aziz-Zadeh, L. & Cermak, C. (2019) Ayres theories of autism and sensory integration revisited: what contemporary neuroscience has to say. *Brain Sciences, 68(9),* 1–20. https://doi.org/10.3390/brainsci9030068

Lane, S.J. (2012) *Considerations in understanding praxis and dyspraxia* Unpublished, SAISI Workshop, Pretoria, Gauteng, South Africa.

Lane, S.J. (2020) Sensory modulation functions and disorders. In: A. Bundy & S. Lane (eds), *Sensory Integration Theory and Practice,* 3rd edn, pp. 151–180. F.A. Davis Company, Philadelphia.

Lane, S.J., Mailloux, Z., Schoen, S. *et al* (2019) Neural foundations of Ayres Sensory Integration®. *Brain Sciences, 9,* 153. https://doi.org/10.3390/brainsci9070153

Lane, S. & Reynolds, S. (2020) Sensory discrimination functions and disorders. In: A. Bundy & S. Lane (eds), *Sensory Integration Theory and Practice,* 3rd edn, pp. 181–205. F.A. Davis Company, Philadelphia.

Li, J., Wang, W., Cheng, J. *et al* (2023) Relationships between sensory integration and the core symptoms of attention-deficit/hyperactivity disorder: the mediating effect of executive function. *European Child & Adolescent Psychiatry, 32,* 2235–2246. https://doi.org/10.1007/s00787-022-02069-5

Mailloux, Z. & Burke, J.P. (2008) Play and the sensory integrative approach. In: L.D. Parham & L.S. Fasio (eds), *Play in Occupational Therapy for Children,* 2nd edn, pp. 263–299. Mosby; Elsevier, Missouri.

Mailloux, Z., Mulligan, S., Smith Roley, S. & Blanche, E. (2011) Verification and clarification of patterns of sensory integration dysfunctions. *American Journal of Occupational Therapy, 65(2),* 143–151.

Mailloux, Z., Parham, D.L. & Smith Roley, S. (2020) *EASI International Normative Data Collection Manual.* CLASI, Los Angeles.

Mailloux, Z., Parham, D.L., Smith Roley, S., Ruzzano, L. & Schaaf, R.C. (2018) Introduction to the evaluation in Ayres Sensory Integration®. *American Journal of Occupational Therapy, 72(1),* 1–7.

Marco, E.J., Hinkley, L.B., Hill, S.S. & Nagarajan, S. (2011) Sensory processing in autism: a review of neurophysiologic findings. *Pediatric Research*, **69**(5), 48R–54R.

May, P.A., Marais, A.S., De Vries, M.M. *et al* (2016) The continuum of fetal alcohol spectrum disorders in a community in South Africa: prevalence and characterization in a fifth sample. *Drug Alcohol Depend*, **168**, 274–286. https://doi.org/10.1016/j.drugalcdep.2016.09.025

May Benson, T.A. & Cermak, S.A. (2007) Development of an assessment for ideational praxis. *American Journal of Occupational Therapy*, **61**(2), 148–153.

May-Benson, T.A. & Koomar, J.A. (2007) Identifying gravitational insecurity in children: a pilot study. *American Journal of Occupational Therapy*, **61**(2), 142–147.

Meanner, M.J., Warren, Z., Williams, A.R. *et al* (2023) Prevalence and characteristics of autism spectrum disorder among children aged 8 years - autism and developmental disabilities monitoring network, 11 sites, United States, 2020. *MMWR Surveillance Summaries*, **72**(2), 1–14.

Mills, C., Chapparo, C. & Hinitt, J. (2016) The impact of an in-class sensory activity schedule on task performance of children with autism and intellectual disability: a pilot study. *British Journal of Occupational Therapy*, **79**(9), 530–539. https://doi.org/10.1177/0308022616639989

Parham, L.D., Ecker, C.L., Kuhaneck, H.M., Henry, D.A. & Glennon, T.J. (2006) *Sensory Processing Measure*. Western Psychological Services, Los Angeles.

Parham, L.D., Ecker, C.L., Kuhaneck, H.M., Henry, D.A. & Glennon, T.J. (2021) *Sensory Processing Measure, Second Edition (SPM-2)*. Western Psychological Services, Los Angeles.

Pfeiffer, B.A., Koenig, K., Kinnealey, M., Sheppard, M. & Henderson, L. (2011) Effectiveness of sensory integration interventions in children with autism spectrum disorders: a pilot study. *American Journal of Occupational Therapy*, **65**(1), 76–85.

Ringold, S.M., McGuire, R.W., Jayashankar, A. *et al* (2022) Sensory modulation in children with developmental coordination disorder compared to autism spectrum disorder and typically developing children. *Brain Sciences*, **12**, 1–24. https://doi.org/10.3390/brainsci12091171

Sadock, B.J. & Sadock, V.A. (2003) *Kaplan & Sadock's Synopsis of Psychiatry*, 9th edn. Lippincott Williams & Wilkens, Philadelphia.

Salari, N., Rasoulpoor, S., Rasoulpoor, S. *et al* (2022) The global prevalence of autism spectrum disorder: a comprehensive systematic review and meta-analysis. *Italian Journal of Pediatrics*, **48**(112), 1–16. https://doi.org/10.1186/s13052-022-01310-w

Schaaf, R.C., Dumont, R.L., Arbesman, M. & May-Benson, T.A. (2018) Efficacy of occupational therapy using Ayres Sensory Integration: a systematic review. *American Journal of Occupational Therapy*, **72**(1), 1–10. https://doi.org/10.5014/ajot.2018.028431

Schaaf, R. & Mailloux, Z. (2015) *Clinician's Guide for Implementing Ayres Sensory Integration*. American Occupational Therapy Association (AOTA Press).

Schaaf, R. & Miller, L.J. (2005) Novel therapies for developmental disabilities occupational therapy using a sensory integration approach. *Mental Retardation and Developmental Disabilities*, **11**(2), 1–5.

Schaaf, R.C., Schoen, A.S., Smith-Roley, S., Lane, S.J., Koomar, J. & Mey-Benson, A.T. (2010) A frame of reference for sensory integration.

In P. Kramer & J. Hinojosa, *Frames of Reference for Pediatric Occupational Therapy*, 3rd edn, pp. 99–186. Wolters Kluwer; Lippincott Williams & Wilkins, New York.

Schaaf, R.C. & Smith-Roley, S. (2006) *Sensory Integration: Applying Clinical Reasoning to Practice with Diverse Populations*. Pro-Ed, Texas.

Schoen, S.A., Lane, S.J., Mailloux, Z. *et al* (2019) A systematic review of Ayres Sensory Integration intervention for children with autism. *Autism Research*, **12**, 6–19. https://doi.org/10.1002/aur.2046

Schoen, S.A., Lane, S.J., Miller, L. & Reynolds, S. (2020) Advances in sensory integration research: basic science research. In: A. Bundy & S. Lane (eds), *Sensory Integration Theory and Practice*, 3rd edn, pp. 371–392. F.A. Davis Company, Philadelphia.

Smith, A.M., Roux, S., Naidoo, N.T. & Venter, D.J. (2005) Food choices of tactile defensive children. *Nutrition*, **21**, 14–19. https://doi.org/10.1016/j.nut.2004.09.004

Smith Roley, S., Mailloux, Z., Miller-Kuhaneck, H. & Glennon, T. (2007) *Understanding Ayres Sensory Integration*. American Occupational Therapy Association Continuing Education Article, OT Process, pp. 1–8.

Van Jaarsveld, A. (2014) Sensory integration in mental health. In: R. Crouch & V. Alers (eds), *Occupational Therapy in Psychiatry and Mental Health*, pp. 295–318. John Wiley & Sons.

Van Jaarsveld, A., Liebenberg, E., Van Rooyen, F.C. & Janse van Rensburg, E. (2021) Promoting the development of foundation phase learners in under-resourced environments using Ayres Sensory Integration® principles and custom-designed, low-cost playgrounds. *South African Journal of Occupational Therapy*, **51**(1), 9–17. https://doi.org/10.17159/2310-3833/2021/vol51n1a3

Van Jaarsveld, A., Mailloux, Z., Smith Roley, S. & Raubenheimer, J. (2014) Patterns of the sensory integration dysfunctions in South African children. *South African Journal of Occupational Therapy*, **44**(2), 2–6.

Van Jaarsveld, A., Venter, A., Joubert, A. & Van Vuuren, S. (2001a) The effect of a sensory integration-orientated stimulation programme on three- to five-year-old black pre-school children in semi-structured pre-school programmes in Mangaung, Bloemfontein. *The South African Journal of Occupational Therapy*, **31**(3), 9–13.

Van Jaarsveld, A., Venter, A., Joubert, A. & Van Vuuren, S. (2001b) The prevalence of sensory integration problems in three to five-year-old black pre-school children in semi-structural preschool programmes in Mangaung, Bloemfontein. *The South African Journal of Occupational Therapy*, **31**(2), 3–6.

Varney-Blackburn, J. (1985) Breakthrough! The reduction of self-injurious behaviour and other problems related to mental retardation and autistic behaviour in children. *South African Journal of Occupational Therapy*, **15**, 27–30.

Wilczynski, J., Habik, N. & Wypych, Z. (2018) The effects of sensory integration techniques on muscle tone in children after prenatal exposure to alcohol. *Journal of Education, Health and Sport*, **8**(8), 347–358. https://doi.org/10.5281/zenodo.1312425

Wilczynski, J. & Zawada, K. (2016) The impact of sensory integration therapy on gross motor function in children after prenatal exposure to alcohol. *Studia Medyczne*, **31**(1), 10–17. https://doi.org/10.5114/ms.2015.49947

Attention Deficit Hyperactive Disorder Through a Person's Life Span

Occupational Therapy to Enhance Executive and Social Functioning

CHAPTER 20

Ray Anne Cook[1] and Gina Rencken[2]

[1]South African Institute for Sensory Integration (SAISI), Cape Town, South Africa
[2]South African Institute for Sensory Integration (SAISI), University of KwaZulu-Natal (UKZN), KwaZulu-Natal, South Africa

KEY LEARNING POINTS

- An understanding of attention deficit hyperactivity disorder (ADHD) across the life span.

- Core symptoms of the disorder and diagnostic features.

- Major areas of dysfunction and the effect of ADHD on the person's occupational performance.

- The multidisciplinary treatment approach in the management of ADHD.

- Occupational therapy assessment and intervention through the life span.

INTRODUCTION

Attention Deficit Hyperactivity Disorder (ADHD) is a neuro-developmental disorder, diagnosed in childhood and often extending into later life phases. It is estimated that globally 5–11% of children under the age of 18 years have ADHD (Francés et al. 2022). The estimated prevalence in adults is 6.8% for symptomatic ADHD and 2.6% for persistent adult ADHD (Song et al. 2021). Occupational therapists are confronted by this disorder in clients across the paediatric, adolescent and adult populations. The impact of ADHD on participation in life is pervasive, and clients may experience challenges in participating in age-appropriate occupations, interaction in their environment or with personal factors, their performance patterns, performance skills as well as client factors (American Occupational Therapy Association [AOTA] 2020). There is no cure for ADHD, and the best results are achieved when each client is managed individually with a combination of pharmaceutical management, behaviour modification, psycho-education and therapeutic support as indicated (Barkley 2005; Wolraich et al. 2019).

ADHD has a high heritability, with specific genetic factors implicating dopamine pathways being identified in molecular genetic studies (Faraone et al. 2001). The genetic theory is supported by similarities in the symptoms experienced by the child with ADHD and close relatives who manifest the condition. Examples of symptoms noted in adults include restlessness, inattention and a low frustration tolerance. Studies on identical twins support the genetic link (Green & Chee 1997; Hunt et al. 2001; Strong & Flanagan 2005). Due to the genetic disposition of this disorder, it is important to include the family in the occupational therapy intervention, as structure and routine in the home will assist executive functioning (EF). The perpetuating cycle of disorganisation needs to be broken to empower the family members.

Crouch and Alers Occupational Therapy in Psychiatry and Mental Health, Sixth Edition.
Edited by Rosemary Crouch, Tania Buys, Enos Morankoana Ramano, Matty van Niekerk and Lisa Wegner.
© 2025 John Wiley & Sons Ltd. Published 2025 by John Wiley & Sons Ltd.

There are varying opinions as to the specific areas of the brain involved in ADHD, including reduced size of the frontal lobes, the basal ganglia, posterior cerebellar vermis and reticular formation (Castellanos & Swanson 2002; Dunn & Bennett 2002). With regard to processing differences, the frontal lobe has been identified as playing a key executive role in screening whether information is appropriate, prioritising and taking future implications into consideration before responding. In a child with ADHD, these steps seem to be omitted, resulting in impulsive responses without going through this executive filtering process (Green & Chee 1997). Some researchers report that ADHD is associated with differences in brain chemistry, hence the term neurobiological disorder (Green & Chee 1997; Silver 1999; Kutscher *et al.* 2005) Attention needs to be given to what this EF problem leads to in the occupational performance of the person in the short and long term, and the type of intervention required to improve occupational performance. This also supports the need for Ayres Sensory Integration® (ASI®) intervention, motor skill development and rhythmic training in the intervention protocol. The DSM-5 (American Psychiatric Association 2022) particularly relates to the occupational performance of the person in the long term into their adulthood.

ATTENTION DEFICIT HYPERACTIVE DISORDER CRITERIA (DSM-5-TR)

The Diagnostic Statistical Manual of Mental Disorders (American Psychiatric Association 2022) describes ADHD as a persistent pattern of inattention and/or hyperactivity-impulsivity interfering with development or function in social and academic activities or occupations. A cluster of symptoms of inattention and/or hyperactivity-impulsivity have to be present prior to the age of 12 years, in two or more settings (home, school, work, social situations or other activities), with clear evidence that these symptoms reduce the quality of functioning in the person's life. The severity of symptoms is further qualified as mild, moderate or severe (American Psychiatric Association 2022).

Symptoms of inattention include failing to pay close attention or making mistakes in work or activities, difficulty sustaining attention, not seeming to listen when spoken to directly, not following through on instructions and failing to finish work, difficulty organising tasks and activities, avoidance of tasks requiring sustained mental effort, losing things necessary for tasks, easily distractible and forgetful.

Symptoms of hyperactivity-impulsivity include fidgeting, leaving a seat when remaining in a seated position is expected (such as in a learning environment), running or climbing when this is inappropriate for the situation, being unable to play or engage in leisure tasks quietly, seeming constantly 'on the go', talking excessively, unable to wait a turn (in a conversation, or a queue) and interrupting others' games, activities or conversations.

ADHD, SENSORY INTEGRATION AND EXECUTIVE FUNCTION

Precipitating features such as Sensory Integrative Dysfunction or Difficulty (SID) and epigenetic events such as environmental triggers contribute to ADHD manifesting in the person experiencing difficulties with executive function (EF). The variation in prevalence between males and females is commonly accepted as being 2:1 in children, and 1.6:1 in adults (American Psychiatric Association 2022). Although the interventions are similar for the subtypes, the use of alerting, calming or organising techniques, especially those used from a sensory perspective, differs significantly for the subtypes. Table 20.1 highlights the features of ADHD and how they relate to other co-morbid conditions, especially SID and difficulties in EF, relevant across the life span.

Table 20.1 DSM-5 TR diagnostic criteria related to sensory integrative dysfunction/difficulty (SID) and executive function difficulties (EF).

Inattention

The person may be under-reactive (UR) to sensory input from their environment and require more sensory input than others to respond.

The sensory craver (SC) seeks the input, and if he/she does not obtain it, he/she is unable to attend to the task at hand. This person also often has poor sensory discrimination and perception.

A person who is over-reactive (OR) to sensory input may be distracted by the extraneous input and not available to attend to the task at hand.

DSM-5 TR symptoms	Sensory integration and executive functioning
a. Often fails to give close attention to details or makes careless mistakes in schoolwork, work or other activities	Under reactive (UR)
b. Often has difficulty sustaining attention in task or play activities	UR needs external sensory input to increase arousal levels.
	SC needs to be given the opportunity to get sensory input throughout the day.
	Poor praxis: difficulties thinking of ideas, planning, sequencing and executing play individually or with companions.
	EF – poor working memory
c. Often does not seem to listen when spoken to directly	UR to auditory input
	Poor listening (hearing may be normal)

Table 20.1 (*Continued*)

d. Often does not follow through on instructions and fails to finish schoolwork, chores or duties in the workplace (not due to oppositional behaviour or failure to understand instructions)	Poor praxis: may have difficulty in the motoric output of the task, sequencing of tasks, or difficulty in forming an idea of what and how to do the task. EF – difficulty with memory, planning/organising
e. Often has difficulty in organising tasks and activities	Poor praxis: may have difficulty in the motoric output of the task, sequencing of tasks, or difficulty in forming an idea of what and how to do the task. EF – planning/ difficulty organising tasks and activities
f. Often avoids, dislikes or is reluctant to engage in tasks that require sustained mental effort (such as schoolwork or homework)	OR avoids tasks requiring sensory input such as glue on hands UR or SC to sensory input EF – no interest, the task may be too repetitive or lack novelty
g. Often loses things necessary for tasks or activities (e.g. toys, school assignments, pencils, books or tools)	Poor praxis: may have difficulty in the motoric output of the task, sequencing of tasks, or difficulty in forming an idea of what and how to do the task. EF – poor working memory, inhibition, or difficulty in planning/organising
h. Is often easily distracted by extraneous stimuli	OR to sensory input (usually visual, auditory or tactile) or inhibition
i. Is often forgetful in daily activities	UR to environmental stimuli Praxis: difficulties with sequencing steps in a task or, temporal concepts (time based) EF – poor working memory and memory

Hyperactivity

The SC seeks sensory input at all costs

Poor ideation and praxis abilities may make the person appear very busy, but actually, they do not achieve much.

Impulsivity

Poor EF of inhibition

The person may present as over-reactive to sensory input (OR), a sensory craver (SC) or under-reactive to sensory input (UR).

Praxis difficulties: include ideation, motor planning and execution

DSM-5 TR symptoms	Sensory integration and executive functioning
a. Often fidgets with hands or feet or squirms in seat	SC seeks movement or tactile input. The person needs to move to increase their postural tone, so they tend to squirm in their seat. Anxiety
b. Often leaves seat in classroom or in other situations in which remaining seated is expected	SC seeks movement. Postural control
c. Often runs about or climbs excessively in situations in which it is inappropriate (in adolescents or adults, may be limited to subjective feelings of restlessness)	SC seeks movement and proprioceptive input Praxis: Poor ideation
d. Often has difficulty playing or engaging in leisure activities quietly	SC seeks movement, proprioceptive, auditory, visual and tactile input
e. Is often 'on the go' or often acts as if 'driven by a motor'	Praxis especially ideation, needs help to work out what to do
f. Often talks excessively	UR uses voice to increase the level of arousal OR to sound uses own voice to drown out other noises. EF – poor inhibition of thoughts, talks self through task May talk to energise their body or to decrease anxiety or auditory input
g. Often blurts out answers before questions have been completed	EF – poor inhibition
h. Often has difficulty awaiting turn	Praxis: sequencing tasks EF – poor inhibition
i. Often interrupts or intrudes on others (e.g. butts into conversations or games)	SC Praxis (difficulty in planning how to join a game) EF – poor inhibition

DIFFERENTIAL DIAGNOSIS AND CO-MORBID CONDITIONS WITH ADHD IN CHILDREN AND ADULTS

The occupational therapist will have important contributions to make in helping the medical practitioner make a diagnosis as a comprehensive and thorough examination is important. Information is required from various environments in which the person functions such as school, home or work.

ADHD is diagnosed by behavioural symptoms. The severity and combination of behaviours vary greatly in individuals, making diagnosis and treatment challenging. More than 50% of individuals diagnosed with ADHD have co-morbid conditions (Green & Chee 1997). Silver (1999) suggests that anxiety, depression and learning disabilities often cause the described behaviours of ADHD. The causes of the presenting behavioural problems need to be identified as not all people with these symptoms have ADHD. The various conditions or behaviours also differ at various stages of life and may resemble ADHD.

Besides the co-morbid conditions, other factors need to be considered that influence, or look similar, to ADHD. Medical conditions such as allergies, sensitivities, epilepsy, cerebral palsy, thyroid dysfunction and brain diseases may cloud the picture (Taylor 2001; Strong & Flanagan 2005; Erasmus 2009). Other factors mentioned even less frequently are sleep disorders (Taylor 2001; Strong & Flanagan 2005) and antisocial personality disorders (Strong & Flanagan 2005). Furman (2009) goes even further to state that problems such as hypervigilance due to fear or stress and abuse are not usually co-morbid but often present similarly. Therefore, careful diagnosis by a medical specialist is essential.

The co-occurrence of co-morbid disorders is further supported in the Buitelaar (1996) summary of a study done on the epidemiology of ADHD and not a tendency of high occurrence of co-morbid disorders (approximately 25%). ADHD is most commonly associated with (Cook 2011):

- Modulation disorders of anxiety, anger and mood (Silver 1999).
- Autistic Spectrum Disorder (ASD) and Pervasive Developmental Disorder (PDD) (Kutscher et al. 2005; Strong & Flanagan 2005).
- Obsessive–compulsive disorder (OCD) (Amen 2001; Strong & Flanagan 2005).
- Tourette's syndrome/tic disorder (Strong & Flanagan 2005). Amen (2001) notes that there is a strong connection between ADHD, Tourette's syndrome and OCD.
- Oppositional Defiant Disorder (ODD) (Strong & Flanagan 2005). Forty to sixty percent have ODD with ADHD (Sandberg 2002).
- Conduct disorder (Strong & Flanagan 2005; Erasmus 2009; Furman 2009; Timimi & Leo 2009).

- Anxiety disorders (Cooper & Ideus 1996; Strong & Flanagan 2005; Erasmus 2009; Furman 2009).
- Depressive disorders (Cooper & Ideus 1996; Green & Chee 1997; Silver 1999; Amen 2001; Sandberg & Barton 2002; Strong & Flanagan 2005).
- Bipolar disorder (Sandberg & Barton 2002; Strong & Flanagan 2005; Erasmus 2009).
- Motor coordination difficulties (Silver 1999; Taylor 2001). Developmental coordination disorder and developmental dyspraxia would also fall into this category.
- Specific learning disability (Hagermann et al. 2002; Strong & Flanagan 2005; Erasmus 2009). Silver (1999) discusses input, integration, memory and output disabilities as well as motor skills, but he tends to put emphasis on the visual and auditory systems. Amen (2001) notes that 40% also have learning/developmental problems. The child with learning problems is mentioned by Ayres (1972, 2005).
- Sensory Integrative Dysfunction or Difficulty (SID) (Ayers 1972, 2005; Silver 1999; Strong & Flanagan 2005). In discussing SID, Strong (Strong & Flanagan 2005) emphasises a central auditory processing disorder and visual processing disorder as being the main facets of SID. In a nationwide study in the United States, involving 2140 typically developing children, it was found that about 7.5% of them had SID and/or ADHD. On further investigation, it was found that in 60% of those cases, the children presented with both SID and ADHD (Miller 2006). This relationship between SID and ADHD is now a major focus of research in the United States. Furthermore, there is a significant difference between the physiology of a child with SID and one with ADHD (McIntosh et al. 1999; Mangeot et al. 2001; Miller et al. 2001).

ADHD THROUGH THE LIFE SPAN

There is no cure for ADHD, and symptoms or challenges in function are treated with a multi-modal approach of pharmaceutical management, behaviour modification, lifestyle adaptations, therapeutic input to address functional challenges and psycho-education (Barkley 2005; Wolraich et al. 2019). People with ADHD are at increased risk of challenging behaviour and participation in occupations, including substance abuse, increased accidents while driving, speeding and antisocial behaviour. ADHD in adolescents has been associated with 40% of teenage pregnancies, as well as increased school dropout (32–40% of children with ADHD) and a high rate of lifelong underachieving in work, relationships and personal management (Barkley et al. 2008).

At all times the person should be considered in terms of their personal factors, environment and occupations.

Evaluation is an ongoing procedure, and the following should be considered: suitability and affordability for the person or family, the life stage of the person and previous interventions. It should cover the basic components in the reason for referral and the presenting problems. There are a few components that should form part of the assessment battery, and the appropriate tools and areas of evaluation will change across the life span as development and maturation occur. These components are sensory processing, motor skills, rhythmicity, time management, behaviour rating scales for ADHD, executive function, and occupational profiling. The presenting problems may lead to further assessment as the person may have a diagnosed co-morbid condition or a differential diagnosis may still be required.

The following need to be considered when evaluating the person with ADHD (Cook 2013):

- ADHD subtype.

- Sensory integration evaluation.

- Executive functioning.

- Emotions such as anxiety and depression.

- Rhythm and timing and motor skills.

- Interactive metronome assessment.

- Age of the client and previous interventions.

As far as possible, the entire family must be included in the therapeutic process in order to improve occupational performance of the person with ADHD. It is quite often found that the home environment has no structure or routine because one of the parents has ADHD.

The person with ADHD should be carefully counselled about the condition to help them understand that it can be treated so that they can reach their true occupational performance potential, as modelled by many successful persons who struggle with the condition. There is a vital need to teach the person with ADHD to take responsibility for his/her condition and not blame the condition for unacceptable behaviour. It is important to remember that due to co-morbid conditions as well as environmental influences, each person requires an individualised plan of intervention, which suits his/her needs and beliefs, culture and values within the family and/or communal setting.

The treatment is multidimensional. Treatment by medication is important and differs from country to country. It also differs in the various developmental stages of the life span. It must be understood that treatment with stimulants may lead to drug abuse, but if the medication is used responsibly, this can be prevented. The person with ADHD who is on medication has less need to use other substances such as alcohol and/or other drugs such as cocaine in order to provide stimulation. A team approach from various professionals is required, and during the various stages of the life span of the person with ADHD, different team members will be involved. Team members may include family members, medical practitioners, psychologists, occupational therapists, physiotherapists and social workers.

A thorough knowledge of development is necessary so that the intervention is aimed at the age of the person and his/her needs at that stage of his/her life cycle. The main features of ADHD are still present at each stage but differ slightly (Martin 1998). The long-term emotional, social, educational and occupational implications of ADHD through the life span are profound and well documented as cited by Cermack (Hahn-Markowitz et al. 2011).

Chu and Reynolds (2007b) support the value of the occupational therapist's multifaceted role in the intervention of children and adults with ADHD. The intervention should consist of a combination of interventions that change sensory processing, enhance EF and develop self-control. It should also provide the surrounding family, friends, teachers, colleagues and caregivers with the tools and structure to support the person.

Intervention can be likened to a see-saw. Occupational therapists need to maintain a balance between restoring function by treating the underlying causes and increasing occupational performance in the person's current situation by imparting some skills and/or making adaptations.

Adults with ADHD think differently from other people but often are entrepreneurial in their thinking and can certainly apply their minds. As they do not focus on the mundane and do not complete and finalise activities, they will not succeed unless supported by a co-executor who is not patronising. In this way, many people with this condition have become very successful throughout the world in business ventures. The occupational therapist has this important fact in mind to assist in the forward planning for these people. A support system is of paramount importance. Often, accommodations are required in the workplace, and the person must be adequately informed through co-executing, life coaching and medical intervention as required. These are very important aspects related to the occupational performance of the person throughout the life span.

INFANTS

PRESENTATION OF ADHD IN INFANCY

Infants are not diagnosed with ADHD, but may show signs of the disorder. The developmental history from the mother will often reveal the baby was very active or very quiet in utero. A history of trauma prior to the pregnancy, such as a stillbirth of an infant preceding the 'rainbow baby' (a baby born after a miscarriage or stillbirth), where the mother has not completed mourning the loss, seems to be a robust predictor of possible ADHD caseness (Kadesjö et al. 2001).

Neonates show significantly more state organisation difficulties and neurodevelopmental immaturity measured with Brazelton's Neonatal Behavioral Assessment Scale (NBAS) (Auerbach et al. 2005). Correlations have been drawn between infant disorganised states, characterised by freezing, stilling and sudden interruptions or inhibitions of an intended action, and teacher-rated ADHD symptoms when formal schooling starts. These disorganised behaviours noted in infancy, may present as disruptions to the attentional system as the child grows.

As infants, they present as high-maintenance babies, are overly fussy, and may have colic, allergies (including atopic dermatitis), ear infections or difficulties with eating and sleeping. A concerning finding from a birth cohort study undertaken in Germany found that children with atopic dermatitis who were prescribed and used systemic antihistamines had a 47% increased risk for later ADHD. Equally concerning is that children without atopic dermatitis, but who were exposed to systemic antihistamines in infancy had a 35% increased risk for ADHD, suggesting that it may be an independent risk factor for ADHD development (Fuhrmann *et al.* 2020). Antihistamines, which cross the blood-brain barrier, are occasionally used when infants present with sleep disorders, and the resulting reduction of REM sleep may increase the risk for later ADHD development due to the effect on brain maturation (Church *et al.* 2010; Schnatschmidt & Schlarb 2018; Díaz-Román & Buela-Casal 2019), or may be a sign of underlying but as yet undiagnosed ADHD (Gregory *et al.* 2004).

Observable behavioural differences in activity level may be apparent and are predictive of ADHD traits in preschool (Goodwin *et al.* 2021). It is important to note that although infant activity level is a potential early marker, there are multiple developmental pathways that may lead to the ADHD phenotype being noted at preschool or school age (Nigg *et al.* 2004; Sonuga-Barke & Halperin 2010).

ASSESSMENT OF ADHD IN INFANCY

These infants are often referred to occupational therapy due to poor sleeping, fussy feeding or irritability and then diagnosed with sensory integration and self-regulation difficulties (DeGangi 2000; Williamson & Anzalone 2001). Frequently, they are either over-responsive or under-responsive to sensory input and have problems with self-regulation. In a multidimensional evaluation approach (Chu & Reynolds 2007a), the infant is considered in the context of his/her family environment, and the larger community including daycare, the family's religious gatherings and practices, and infant activity or stimulation groups if the infant participated in these with a parent or caregiver. The infant's relevant occupational performance in rest and sleep, play, feeding and eating and personal management needs, which are largely taken care of by others, need to be considered. Information can be gathered from parents and caregivers through interviews or developmental checklists and appropriate rating scales.

Collateral information may be sought, with permission, from the infant's paediatrician or family doctor, day care/child care provider and stimulation group facilitators as appropriate. The information gathered through interviews and collateral, will provide information on the person (the infant's activity level and temperament), the environment (how the infant responds to quiet or noisy environments, cluttered or minimalistic environments, textures in the environment, the presence of other infants, children and older people, the presence of animals, environmental temperature) and task performance (play, is the infant able to feed effectively, rest and sleep, clothing or nappy changes, bath routine and process).

The infant's strengths and challenges should be identified, as well as the level of environmental support needed, available and utilised by the infant and parent/caregiver.

Table 20.2 details the standardised and non-standardised assessment tools or questionnaires which should be considered in assessing infants where ADHD is suspected, as well as persons across their life span.

Table 20.2   Assessment tools for areas of function impacted by ADHD across the life span.

	Infancy	Preschool	Primary school	High school/ (Adolescence)	Adult/elderly
Sensory integration: modulation/ reactivity and perception	Infant/ Toddler Sensory Profile™ (Dunn 2002)	Sensory Profile™ (Dunn 1999)	Sensory Profile™	Adolescent/Adult sensory Profile™ (Brown & Dunn 2002)	Adolescent/Adult sensory Profile™
	Infant/Toddler Symptom Checklist (DeGangi 2000)	Sensory Profile™ School Companion (Dunn 2006)	Sensory Profile™ School Companion	Adult/Adolescent Sensory History (ASH) (May-Benson 2015)	Adult/Adolescent Sensory History (ASH)
	Sensory Profile™2 Home/community (Parham *et al.* 2013)	Sensory Profile™2 Home/school/ community	Sensory Profile™2 Home/school/ community	Sensory Profile™2 Home/school/ community	
	Neonatal Behavioural Assessment Scale (NBAS) (Brazelton & Nugent 1995)				
	De-Gangi Berk Test of Sensory Integration (DeGangi 1983)	Sensory Processing Measure (SPM) – Preschool (Parham *et al.* 2007)	Sensory Processing Measure (SPM) – Home (Parham *et al.* 2007)		
	Infant Toddler Symptom Checklist (DeGangi *et al.* 1995)	Sensory Processing Measure 2– SPM™ 2 Preschool	SPM™2 (home and school)		

Table 20.2   (*Continued*)

	Infancy	Preschool	Primary school	High school/ (Adolescence)	Adult/elderly
		Evaluation of Ayres Sensory Integration (EASI) (Mailloux *et al.* 2020)	EASI	EASI	EASI
Motor skills	Bayley Scales of Development (Bayley 2009)	Bayley Scales of Development			
	Peabody Developmental Motor Scales (PDMS-2) (Rhonda & Fewell 2000)	PDMS-2			
		Movement -ABC (M-ABC) (Henderson *et al.* 1992)	M-ABC	M-ABC	
		Bruininks-Osteresky Test of Motor Proficiency (BOT-2) (Bruininks & Bruininks 1978)	BOT-2	BOT-2	BOT-2
Rhythmicity			Interactive Metronome Assessment	Interactive Metronome Assessment	Interactive Metronome Assessment
Rating scales for ADHD			Conners Scale 3rd edition (teacher/parent forms), 6–18 years	Conners Scale (teacher/parent forms), 6–18 years	
			Conners Scale self-report forms, 8–18 years	Conners Scale self-report forms, 8–18 years	
			ADHD rating scale 5 for children and adolescents (ADHD-RS-V) (DuPaul *et al.* 2016)	ADHD rating scale 5 for children and adolescents (ADHD-RS-V)	Barkley Adult ADHD rating scale-IV (BAARS-IV)
Executive function		Behavior Rating Inventory of Executive Functioning (BRIEF) Preschool Version (home and school) (Gioia *et al.* 2003)	Behavior Rating Inventory of Executive Functioning (BRIEF) (home and school) (Gioia *et al.* 2000)	BRIEF (home and school)	BRIEF (self-rating for adults)

TREATMENT OF ADHD IN INFANCY

Treatment should focus on the occupational challenges that are experiences by the infant and his/her family. This may include personal hygiene (coping with bathing, toileting, brushing teeth), functional mobility, feeding, communication (verbal and nonverbal), physical activity, rest and sleep, play and interactions with family member, caregivers and friends (AOTA 2020).

Rhythmical movement or singing can be very effective. The use of ASI® (Ayres 1972, 2005) and DIR®/Floortime (Greenspan & Wieder 2006) is very valuable. The parents are encouraged to implement an intervention programme and routine that is tailor-made to the family.

The mother-infant dyad needs to be protected and nurtured in treating infants in the context of their family, and responsive caregiving, activities such as baby massage and developmentally appropriate play in this dyad, should be encouraged (Margalit & Klietman 2006; Perks *et al.* 2020; Finalyson *et al.* 2020).

PRESCHOOL

PRESENTATION OF ADHD IN PRESCHOOL

The mean onset of ADHD manifests in the preschool years, between the ages of three and four years; however, the diagnosis is challenging and many children with ADHD are overlooked at this stage as parents will say that 'he is just an active, busy little boy', and transient ADHD like symptoms are very common in this developmental stage (Gurevitz *et al.* 2014). Some are diagnosed during this stage, especially the hyperactive/impulsive type, as they are always active and in trouble. They are clumsy, crash into anything in their way and have little frustration tolerance. They may have difficulties with friendships in preschool due to poorer social functioning (Shephard *et al.* 2022). Preschool children with ADHD often present, and are referred to occupational therapy with difficulties in gross and fine motor coordination, sequencing, verbal and nonverbal working memory, challenging behaviour and self-regulation (Braaten & Rosén 2000; Gurevitz *et al.* 2014; Shephard *et al.* 2022).

ASSESSMENT OF ADHD IN PRESCHOOL

It is important to note that pre-schoolers with ADHD may be uncooperative in formal assessments, and a playful approach is needed (Gurevitz *et al.* 2014). The occupational therapy assessment should include motor skill development, sensory integration, executive function, play as well as a detailed history of sleep preparation and participation (Shephard *et al.* 2022; Dunn & Bennett 2002). Assessments may need to take place over a few sessions, and the parent/caregiver and teacher should be aware of this. A preschool visit is useful in observing the child's participation in ring-time and class activities (executive function, fine motor skills, sensory reactivity) as well as free play (gross and fine motor skills, social interaction, praxis, sensory reactivity). An in-depth assessment of sensory integration, as well as a parent and teacher rating scale of sensory processing and ADHD symptomatology is required. A referral to a paediatrician or paediatric specialist is an important part of the assessment to determine if there are differential diagnoses that may present in a similar manner and to check anthropometrics.

TREATMENT OF ADHD IN PRESCHOOL

The occupational therapist needs a thorough knowledge of sensory integration and ADHD. The use of rhythmical strategies relevant to this age, such as swinging and rhythmical games, should be incorporated. Attention should be given to executive functions and behavioural inhibition (for sensory and emotional reactivity) with the help of adults and in consultation with the occupational therapist. Gross and fine motor skills which are delayed should be treated through a playful approach in occupational therapy, as well as executive function and play participation.

PRIMARY SCHOOL CHILD

PRESENTATION OF ADHD IN PRIMARY SCHOOL

With the increase in school hours and more formal education, there are more demands on children with ADHD. They need to sit still, attend, inhibit behaviours, organise, socialise and cooperate for longer periods of time. They are often identified and referred for ADHD assessment at this age, especially for both subtypes. The inattentive type is also now more easily identified, especially if there is an experienced teacher who understands ADHD. Poor handwriting, difficulty working in a group and lack of task completion are some of the most common reasons for referral.

The children begin to participate in sports. There is another set of potential difficulties inherent in sports for the ADHD person to overcome, ranging from forgetting sports clothes to being out of place in the team and not focusing on the game. Homework can become a nightmare for the parent, especially when children know their spelling very well the night before but fail the spelling test the following day.

Disorganisation, fluctuating abilities and social rejection then lead to low self-esteem. ASI® therapy (Ayres 1972, 2005) is frequently used by the occupational therapist at this stage.

Child Symptoms

Child symptoms of ADHD are shown through their behaviour. Examples are as follows (Serfontein 1990; Green & Chee 1997; Cook 2013):

- Inattention.
- Failure to listen and follow instructions and poor short-term memory.
- Emotionally labile.
- Poor frustration tolerance.
- Low self-esteem.
- Difficulty following instructions and task completion.
- Impulsivity and act or speak without thinking.
- Poor inhibition of behaviour and act without thought of consequences.
- Overactivity. They are restless, fidgety and on the move.
- Insatiable and cannot wait for their needs to be met.
- Social clumsiness and poor peer relationships.
- Poor motor coordination and handwriting as they either rush a task or have poor motor skills.
- Poor sleeping patterns.
- Disorganised, losing belongings and forgetting school homework.
- Fluctuations in performance and moods, that is, have good and bad days/times.

ASSESSMENT OF ADHD IN PRIMARY SCHOOL

An in-depth evaluation is vital here, including motor skills, sensory integration, executive function, visual perceptual skills and occupational participation in education, play, social participation, rest and sleep and ADL. All underlying possibilities need to be taken into consideration before a diagnosis is made.

TREATMENT OF ADHD IN PRIMARY SCHOOL

The largest part of the child's day is taken up with participation in education and play/social participation. The child in primary school needs to be independent in ADLs including toileting, hygiene, feeding and dressing. Occupational therapy should address all underlying challenges identified in the assessment, and a particular focus may be on executive functions to enable adequate participation in educational activities. It is important for the occupational therapist to put attention on rhythmical training, executive functioning and occupational group therapy (through a combination of the Alert Programme [Williams & Shellenberg 1996] and social skills). Consultation with regard to a particular sport that the child is interested in and able to participate in is also necessary.

HIGH SCHOOL/UNIVERSITY

PRESENTATION OF ADHD IN HIGH SCHOOL/ UNIVERSITY

A change of schools from primary to high school can be a major hurdle for a child with ADHD. He/she is required to be even more organised and independent. The typical adolescent at this stage is going through major physiological, cognitive, behavioural and emotional changes. ADHD interferes with this 'mastery of adolescence' and adds much stress, as they are aware of their differences and difficulties and compare themselves to others as part of adolescent development. Unpleasant conflicts and non-compliance are common. Adolescents with ADHD self-report variability in positive affect, fear and distress when compared to neurotypical peers. This is associated with more internalising symptoms, such as anxiety, depression and social withdrawal, as they are very aware of their affective states. Parent reports of their adolescents with ADHD indicate the same variability being associated with poorer social functioning and externalising symptoms, such as impulsivity, inattention, rule-breaking and aggression (Breaux et al. 2020).

ASSESSMENT OF ADHD IN HIGH SCHOOL/ UNIVERSITY/TERTIARY EDUCATION

The evaluation needs to put special emphasis on handling the adolescent ADHD person and his/her occupational performance in the social, home and school environment. If the person is only diagnosed at this age, it often comes as a relief to him/her. The assessment should include self-report questionnaires of sensory processing, anxiety and ADHD rating. The occupational therapist should also assess executive functioning, visual perception, motor skills and sensory integration as indicated. This may be a time when concessions for handwriting speed and legibility need to be considered either by extra time on tests or examinations or the use of a computer for typing, and the appropriate assessment tools should be utilised.

TREATMENT OF ADHD IN HIGH SCHOOL/ UNIVERSITY/TERTIARY EDUCATION

The occupational therapist often does more consultation with regard to executive functioning, sensory processing and the optimal band of arousal with adolescents. Empowerment into understanding their sensory reactivity and measures to influence that are needed. Rhythmical training is used and then often linked to finding a sport in which the adolescent can participate. Executive function challenges and specifically the influence if these on study skills still need to be addressed (Miller & Hinshaw 2010).

ADULTHOOD

PRESENTATION OF ADHD IN ADULTHOOD

Many adults are only diagnosed when they take their child to the paediatrician for an evaluation for ADHD. The adults' occupational roles have now evolved to include having a job, providing for a family and being a spouse and a parent. These complexities and responsibilities make it so much more difficult for the adult to cope. The adult ADHD person may have now developed co-morbid condition such as anxiety and/or substance abuse, and it is often difficult to recognise the underlying ADHD which was there from the beginning.

Adult symptoms of ADHD constitute a lack of executive functioning, namely:

- Inattention and failure to listen.
- Hyperactivity which may relate to anxiety. In adults, it is often more in the mind than in the body, with inconsistent attention, distractibility and executive function deficits.
- Impulsivity with self-selected activity.
- Irritability and low frustration tolerance.
- Procrastination.
- Disorganised careless mistakes.
- Impaired planning.
- Mood instability which is very common.
- Loss of jobs.
- Money spending.
- Lack of focus.

- Often also have dyslexia and poor memory.

- There is a tendency to compensate for difficulties by utilising organisational, motoric, attentional, social, psycho-pharmacological strategies and supports.

- Driving is impulsive and irritable. Fast driving and road rage are a problem.

- The mind is always on 'fast forward' and the individual gets tired quickly,

ASSESSMENT OF ADHD IN ADULTHOOD

The evaluation must consider the influence that ADHD has on the relationships within the family, work and community. It is important to try to get the adult clients to commit to at least six sessions as they tend not to see the therapy through due to their difficulties in executive function and the lack of novelty in routine. Barkley *et al.* (2008) have led two major studies on ADHD in adults and have concluded the following: ADHD has an adverse effect on the life activities of the adult. The most serious areas affected are educational and occupational functioning. Money management, management of daily responsibilities, parenting, vehicle driving and health risks were also ranked among the most important (Barkley *et al.* 2008). Self-report questionnaires and rating scales are useful here, and often empowering. If underlying difficulties are noted, then an additional assessment such as the Evaluation of Ayres Sensory Integration (EASI), a driving test, or a physical and psychiatric functional capacity evaluation is needed.

TREATMENT OF ADHD IN ADULTHOOD

The most serious areas affected are vocational (employment) and social functioning. Money management, management of daily responsibilities, parenting, vehicle driving and health risks were also ranked among the most important (Barkley *et al.* 2008). Adults are often dissatisfied with standard treatment as they feel that their occupational and functional needs are not being adequately addressed. Occupational therapy is one part of the team involved in the treatment of adults with ADHD, with other members including the adult client's psychiatrist, psychologist, dietician and often a life coach or business coach (Adamou *et al.* 2016). From an Occupational Therapy perspective, emphasis should be placed on organising and adapting the physical and/or social environment to enable participation, promoting social awareness and interactions within occupations, and encouraging self-management of symptoms through strategies such as sensory regulation, stress management techniques and adaptations to routines (Adamou *et al.* 2021). Adults with ADHD, with their neurodiversity, think differently from other people but often are entrepreneurial and can certainly apply their minds when the challenge and environments are conducive to this. As they do not focus on the mundane and do not complete and finalise activities, they will not succeed unless supported by a co-executor who is not patronising. In this way, many people with this condition have become very successful throughout the world in business ventures. The occupational therapist has this important fact in mind to assist in the forward planning for these people. A support system is of paramount importance. Often, accommodations are required in the workplace, and the person must be adequately informed through co-executing, life coaching and medical intervention as required. These are very important aspects related to the occupational performance of the person throughout the life span.

ELDERLY

PRESENTATION OF ADHD IN THE ELDERLY

The clinical presentation of ADHD in the elderly population is still largely unknown, and many may have experienced a lifelong struggle due to their ADHD symptoms because they may never have had recognition of or support for their challenges earlier in life. Many of the behaviours and attentional challenges were ascribed to the child being disobedient or poorly disciplined (Kooij *et al.* 2019). Studies are showing that ADHD symptoms do progress into late adulthood, but there is a marked decrease in symptoms. ADHD-related attentional deficits may be overlaid by neurodegenerative processes, including Alzheimer's and Lewy Body dementia. Careful evaluation and diagnosis are important to distinguish between these shared symptoms (Altable & De la Serna 2020). Elderly adults with ADHD may experience difficulties in social functioning, as well as social participation due to inattention and impulsivity (Michielsen *et al.* 2015).

ASSESSMENT OF ADHD IN THE ELDERLY

The factors underlying the elderly person's functional challenges in occupation need to be assessed. Some people may still be working on a part-time or full-time basis, so executive functions underlying participation in employment may be required, as well as preparation and adjustment for the transition to retirement (AOTA 2020). For many, the main occupation is social interaction, and the psychosocial impact of ADHD, attentional difficulties, and impulsivity may influence this. Self-care, home management and health management (including nutrition and medication) may be assessed through questionnaires, rating scales or interviews.

TREATMENT OF ADHD IN THE ELDERLY

As with other age groups, a multi-modal approach is necessary, including psycho-education, medication for ADHD and co-morbid disorders, support groups, life coaching and/or cognitive behavioural therapy (CBT) (Kooij *et al.* 2019).

FEEDBACK AFTER OCCUPATIONAL THERAPY ASSESSMENT IN ADHD ACROSS THE LIFE SPAN

A feedback session needs to follow the initial assessment. If ADHD is diagnosed, then information regarding ADHD and other findings need to be discussed to inform and empower the person. Depending on his/her insight, discuss the holistic approach for the intervention and how it can be implemented across the life span of the ADHD person. Be careful not to overload the parent/person with information initially as it may be overwhelming. It is often more beneficial to set up another feedback session after about 6–10 sessions to discuss progress and goals and plan the long-term intervention strategies.

Table 20.3 is an example of a handout given to parents at the initial feedback of the assessment findings. It focuses on the occupational therapy challenges related to ADHD and includes possible areas that may be addressed in occupational therapy intervention. Information about other multi-modal aspects of treatment is needed to empower clients, parents or caregivers to make an informed decision about treatment approaches and referral to other professionals.

Table 20.3 Assessment feedback inventory.

Area	Date	Comment
Monitor for possible ADHD diagnosis and medical examination for a differential diagnoses and medication		
Homeopathy		
Supplements and toxin insulation nutrition		
Routine and structure – Methods to implement at home		
DIR floortime		
Sensory integration therapy and sensory diet		
Books to read and websites		
Occupational group therapy (Alert Programme, Zone of regulation, social skills and EF)		
Support groups		
Possible psychological intervention or assessment		
EF and methods		
Behaviour modification or CBT approach such as STAR programme		
Remedial therapy		
Teacher insight/schooling		
Workplace evaluation		
Rhythmical training or interactive metronome		
Listening programmes such as Tomatis or therapeutic listening		
Other		
Managing ADHD through the life span		

Source: Cook (2013)/M&K Publishing.

There is no specific order as the methods may be indicated at different developmental life stages.

The occupational performance of the person needs to be considered, which includes the home and community environments.

SPECIFIC OCCUPATIONAL THERAPY MODALITIES USEFUL IN THE TREATMENT OF ADHD ACROSS THE LIFE SPAN

There are many occupational therapy modalities or techniques that are part of the therapeutic toolbox in addressing functional and occupational challenges experienced by the person with ADHD. By using the Ecological Model of Sensory Modulation (Miller *et al.* 2001) to analyse strengths and weaknesses, the occupational therapist can also act as a consultant for occupations outside therapy, using clinical reasoning skills. Table 20.4 serves as a guide to assist interpretation of assessment results and intervention planning.

The following intervention techniques (among others) can be linked to the intervention of ADHD and will be discussed in more detail (Cook 2013):

- ASI® and sensory diets
- Auditory training
- Rhythmicity and timing
- Executive functioning
- Occupational group therapy such as social skills, Alert Programme (Williams & Shellenberg 1996) and organisational strategies

ASI® AND SENSORY DIETS: LINKING SENSORY PROCESSING AND ADHD

Sensory responses differ vastly, and there are physiological and behavioural differences between typically developing people, those with ADHD and those with sensory modulation disorder (SMD). This highlights the complexities in understanding the person with ADHD. Researchers have used either or both physiological measurements and behavioural measurements in studies on sensory processing and ADHD (Parush *et al.* 2007; Reynolds & Lane 2009; Cook 2011).

With sensory integration intervention, the regulation of attention is the most important factor, and the occupational therapist works at restoring regulation with the optimal band of engagement, thus enhancing the ability to attend to the task at hand (Anzalone & Lane 2012). This is done through ASI® (Ayres 1972, 2005) intervention and sensory diets which initially the caregiver implements and later the person does independently. The sensory diet is not a specific intervention technique. It is a strategy of developing an individualised home programme based on the concept that controlled sensory

Table 20.4 Analysis of interpretation to assist planning of intervention.

Internal dimensions		
	Strengths	Challenges
Sensory processing		
Emotion		
Attention		
Executive functioning		

Link these findings to the external dimensions to plan intervention, considering the problems interfering/preventing the person from functioning optimally

Problematic external dimensions					
	Internal demand	Task	Relationships	Environment	Culture
Sensory processing					
Emotion					
Attention					
Executive functioning					

Consider the strengths or supporting systems available in external dimensions

	Internal demand	Task	Relationships	Environment	Culture
Sensory processing					
Emotion					
Attention					
Executive functioning					

Intervention strategies to be implemented

	Task	Relationships	Environment	Culture
Home				
School/college/work				
Community				

Source: Adapted from Cook (2013); Schaaf and Smith Roley (2006).

input can affect functional abilities. It is initially provided by the caregiver/parent and is a bottom-up approach (Cook 2013).

AUDITORY TRAINING

Auditory training is indicated when parents and/or teacher report that the child is unable to listen, follow instructions, organise their desk or bag and do not register their name when they are called (in the absence if a hearing difficulty). Children with ADHD may be unable to focus, analyse or direct their listening, and when faced with a variety of sounds, will take them all in. They thus listen with distortion, find verbal instructions hard to comprehend, tire easily and are only able to listen for short periods of time. The goal of auditory training is to improve filtering of senses and information, enabling the child to select and maintain an external event or thought in his/her consciousness. Listening therapies have a very close link with the vestibular system, through shared fibres in the vestibulo-cochlear nerve. This connection facilitates a state of arousal and alertness that enables the nervous system to be receptive to information reaching it.

The activation of the vagal nerve is an essential part of auditory training through the Solisten™ programme developed by Dr Tomatis. The vagal nerve connects the ear to every organ in the body, and though Solisten™ is accessed via the tympanic membrane in the ear as well as bone conduction and vestibular connections. Auditory training has shown improvements in cognition, attention and behaviour in children with ADHD, independent of medication use.

RHYTHMICITY AND TIMING

The Interactive Metronome (Leisman & Melillo 2010) is an advanced brain-based rehabilitation assessment and treatment programme developed to improve the processing abilities that affect attention, motor planning and sequencing. This is accomplished by using innovative neuro-sensory and neuro-motor exercises developed to improve the brain's inherent ability to repair or remodel itself through a process called neuroplasticity. This then strengthens motor skill and many cognitive capacities such as planning organising and language. The Interactive Metronome programme provides a structured, goal-oriented process that challenges the patient to synchronise a range of hand and foot exercises to a precise computer-generated reference tone heard through headphones. The person attempts to match the rhythmic beat with repetitive motor actions. A patented audio or audio and visual guidance system provides immediate feedback measured in milliseconds, and a score is provided indicating timing accuracy.

When the Interactive Metronome is not possible, rhythmical activities using a metronome can be used. These activities may be clapping, rhythmical cursive writing or patterns, jumping and drumming on a large ball (Koomar *et al.* 2001).

The occupational therapist can assist with general organisational strategies. These strategies may be to break the task into smaller components to accomplish task satisfaction and allowing multiple sensory methods to be used (visual, auditory, tactile and movement) to complete the task. Practical organisational strategies may be to use a shelf next to a desk for books or stacking drawers for stationery. Visual organisers give practical reminders like colour-coding books and cue cards/checklists tied to sports/school bags with pictures of all items that need to be in the bag. Visual referencing for the sequencing of daily tasks/activities assists as time organisers that may be pictures stuck in sequence of execution on a Velcro board and removed after completion or a star chart with a visual reminder of the dressing sequence. Adolescents and adults may use a mobile phone for reminders (Cook 2013).

EXECUTIVE FUNCTIONING: LINKING ADHD, EXECUTIVE FUNCTION AND TECHNIQUES USED FOR TREATMENT

Executive functions consist of higher-order cognitive abilities, including working memory, planning and emotional regulation (Barkley 2005; Barkley *et al.* 2008), which have a major influence on occupational performance. Although SID may also lead to behaviours such as seen in poor executive function, it is the occupational therapist's clinical reasoning skills that will be the guide of when to use which frame of reference. When working on executive functions, the occupational therapist needs to evaluate which areas the person finds challenging and address them appropriately. Attention needs to be given to environmental modification to support poor executive function as well as strategies for the person to improve and overcome these difficulties. Various frames of references have been used effectively (Cook 2013).

It is important to link the executive skills required for the developmental level of the person, the age, and the appropriateness of the tasks performed. This gives an indication of which skill to work on next, together with analysing the underlying causes albeit executive function or even a SID (Cook 2013). Occupational therapists use various daily organisers or picture schedules to improve occupational performance. The person needs to be involved in the planning to increase intrinsic motivation. It is often useful to use these

cognitive strategies to improve the implementation of these techniques. Once again, the strengths and challenges relating to auditory or visual reminders should be considered. Including executive skills as an intervention on an environmental level will enhance success (Cook 2013). This requires close collaboration with the occupational therapist, family and school or work (Dawson & Guare 2010). Various methods may be used to develop executive skills and tailor-make an intervention for each individual. Organisational strategies can be implemented together with the four-quadrant model of facilitated learning (Greber & Ziviani 2010) and Cognitive Orientation to daily Occupational Performance (CO-OP) (Haertl 2010; Hahn-Markowitz *et al.* 2011) used as techniques. CO-OP is a client-centred, performance-based problem-solving acquisition through a process of strategy and guided discovery. Motor learning has a cognitive phase and then an associative and automatic phase. CO-OP has four major objectives, namely, skills acquisition, strategy use, generalization and transfer. There are four steps:

- Goal (what do I want to do)
- Plan (how am I going to do it)
- Do (carry out the plan)
- Check (how well did my plan work)

Persons with ADHD often have problems with time, punctuality and the concept of time. They try to do too much in too little time and then find it stressful to complete the tasks when they already have challenges completing tasks. Rhythmic games or tasks help to engender an intrinsic time frame, which is then integrated with praxis skills. Visual, somatosensory and auditory perception must be incorporated into the rhythmic sequences and graded from simple rhythm to more complex rhythm in terms of elements and variation of time. To improve rhythm and the control of the time factors (perception of time), improve the underlying problems, especially bilateral integration and praxis; improve the ability to do two actions simultaneously (bounce a ball regularly, then bounce the ball and jump, and lastly bounce the ball and clap hands); and work on sequences of movements, sequences of sounds and sequences of incidents (Cook 2013). The STAR Programme is designed to teach children aged 8–12 psychological techniques to improve self-control and prosocial competence. The program makes use of a child-centred approach and CBT principles. It focusses on attention skills, emotional control, problem-solving and interpersonal skills (Young 2017).

OCCUPATIONAL GROUP THERAPY

The child could join an 'Alert' group, or the occupational therapist would teach the person how to implement the 'Alert Programme' (Williams & Shellenberg 1996). The Alert Programme takes a simple metaphor of 'How does your engine run?' and relates it to the person's body. This relates to the revolutions (revs.) of the engine being high, medium or low. The Alert Programme is a specific technique using a cognitive approach, and the primary focus is to help children to learn to monitor, maintain and change their level of alertness so that it is appropriate to the situation or task. The Alert Programme is done in an occupational group therapy setting. Understanding of 'how the body runs' helps the person to modulate his/her arousal level to the optimal range/band for appropriate attention and concentration to participate in the activities of daily life.

The occupational therapist needs to play an overt role in supporting and developing social skills and interaction (Cosbey *et al.* 2010). ADHD often results in poor social skills, and children often benefit from group sessions to specifically address their behaviour with others. This can then be transferred to skills in the school/work or home environment. By combining the concepts of the Alert Programme (Williams & Shellenberg 1996) and social skills according to the needs of the group, success has been demonstrated.

Occupational group therapy is also recommended for adults diagnosed with ADHD. Techniques such as stress management (incorporating time management), assertiveness training and psycho-educational groups are valuable. Sharing in a group with fellow sufferers of ADHD can assist with acceptance and compliance with treatment.

ADHD AND SPORT OR EXERCISE

One of the best ways to reduce ADHD symptoms is to get adequate physical exercise. This can mean playing with friends, playing a sport or aerobic exercises. This is relevant for children and adults. Intense exercise increases the blood flow and the levels of endorphins (especially serotonin) and acetylcholine in the brain, both of which seem to alleviate the symptoms of ADHD (Strong & Flanagan 2005). Vestibular and proprioceptive inputs play a regulatory role for people with sensory integration problems, and there is also a very strong association between sensory integration disorders and ADHD (Miller 2006). If the occupational therapist does not spend enough time clinically choosing the most appropriate sport together with the person and working out strategies to overcome potential difficulties, the person may not want to play sport at all (Cook 2013).

Strong and Flanagan (2005) list many advantages of playing sport or taking exercise. Endorphins released by the body lift the mood and self-esteem is improved with success. Stress is also reduced either through relaxation or getting rid of pent-up emotions, this being especially evident in the hyperactive or sensory-seeking person. It develops coordination and often involves rhythmicity, especially repetitive sport like running or swimming. The muscles contract and squeeze out unwanted by-products such as lactic acids, and the skin's pores open and release body toxins (Strong & Flanagan 2005). Exercise is a body balance regulator, and deep pressure exercises like hugging, wrestling and heavy work are both calming and organising for the body. Passive watching television and playing computer games do not regulate a person's body as previously described regarding movement and heavy work. Stretch exercises also tend to relax the body.

Enjoyment of exercise as a child means participation in exercise as an adult. The factors needing consideration when choosing an exercise are related to age, physical health, fitness, sensory needs, interests and the person's temperament (Cook 2013):

- About 50% of ADHD children have good coordination. However, if they have coordination problems, then take care to ensure success and enjoyment.

- Poor concentration and 'distractibility' can cause problems in organised sports or exercise classes. Adaptive and organisational strategies become key concepts here.

- Position a daydreaming child in the middle of the field rather than as a goalie or on the wing. Playing a position that requires fuller attention and demands higher activity levels will better suit this child.

- Certain sports have many transitions and rule changes, which provide challenges for the ADHD child. Many winter sports, like hockey, change direction at half-time. It can be helpful if an adult (e.g. the teacher or coach) can stand nearby and warn the child of transitions and their implications.

- Sensory modulation is important to consider if the child is sensory under-responsive, sensory seeking or sensory over-responsive. Place a tactile-defensive child as goalie or on the wing, or in an altogether non-contact sport. The sensory-seeking child needs to be active with lots of sensory input, whereas the sensory under responsive child has the same needs as the daydreamer. Avoid rock climbing for the gravitationally insecure child.

- Consider the implications of dyspraxia on the planning involved when learning a new sport, especially with children with developmental coordination disorder. A sport with ball skills or dancing rhythm may be too challenging.

- Helper or scorer/umpire is an administrative role suitable if coordination is a problem.

- Cooperative interaction in organised sport demands social skills, which are often a challenge. Social skills are required of a team player. If this is a problem, then an individual sport should be recommended.

- Helpful criteria to consider are related to whether the exercise is self-regulatory, the endurance capacity, intensity of the exercise and whether it can be easily broken down into steps.

- *The fun factor:* ADHD people often lose interest once the novelty has worn off. Maintain the interest by rather running cross-country than around an athletics track. In the gym, use the buttons on the treadmill/walkers to give variety.

- *Convenience factor:* Proximity to home and fitting in with the family's schedule enhance maintaining the exercise. Consider the seasonality of the sport and replace it with regular ongoing exercise. Encourage flexibility between individual and team sports.

- *Timing factor:* The ADHD person needs to exercise at various times of the day, for instance, before homework so that she/he can settle down easier; strenuous exercise in morning or early afternoon and milder exercises like stretching or walking in the evening. Endurance of at least 30 minutes is needed for exercises to trigger the release of endorphins. Intensity gets the blood flowing and maximises the benefit.

- Grading needs to be gradual. Hyperactive people have a way of overdoing almost everything they attempt.

- Keep it simple. Avoid exercise that takes too much mental energy to figure out or that can be frustrating if done incorrectly. Match the level of the person's ability to the appropriate sport. Consider the after-effects of team losses. Exercise is important, but playing in a team or individual sport where losses become the norm can have a negative effect on the person's self-esteem and temperament. Meaning attribution of the exercise is important, so the competitive aspect needs to be evaluated. Consider the external motivation versus the intrinsic motivation required for the sport. The same sport may fall into any category depending on whether it involves a group and spectators (to motivate) and how much internal motivation is required in the training (Lawlis 2005).

CASE STUDY

Andrew was a baby loved by his family yet would only sleep for 20 minutes during the day. At night, he woke frequently. His mother could not calm him – she herself had ADHD and was overactive. Luckily, her husband was able to calm the baby and put him to sleep. Feeding was an issue and he would sometimes vomit and become carsick easily. He was very active and accident-prone. While an adorable child, 'meltdowns' were frequent. Big family/social gatherings often ended in tears as he would either do something unacceptable and embarrassing or have another meltdown. His mother resorted to taking medication so that she could put structure into her life and thus put it into his. However, the difficulties continued. At preschool Andrew screamed when his mother said goodbye and he refused to do drawings or formal activities. He hurt himself before the school concert to avoid participation, and he particularly hated the dressing up and face painting. He became increasingly frustrated and meltdowns grew more frequent. Allergies and croup often needed attention, and there was no answer for the weekly vomiting.

He was diagnosed with a Sensory Processing and Integration Deficit (SID) (somatodyspraxia and sensory defensiveness) and ADHD. Occupational therapy began with many suggestions and calming routines. His mother had to use a star reward chart to get structure and routine into his life, which got her wondering who was benefiting more – herself or Andrew. Sunday school at church only worked when she was with him, and he could wear his old clothes and no shoes. Short camping family weekends were his absolute favourite because there was no pressure to hold it all together. His mother would dread fetching him from school, not knowing if it had been a good or bad day. His school uniform was uncomfortable and scratchy, so morning routines were a nightmare and only worked if the suggested set routine and sensory diet were followed. Bright lights were best avoided; a long cuddle with deep pressure and drinking water out of a long straw worked wonders. Occupational therapy continued, but now remedial

therapy, eye exercises, diet changes with supplements, listening therapies and neuro-feedback therapy were added to the list of interventions. Allergies and croup continued to require attention. Exercises such as handwriting and cutting were big issues with adaptations needed. His mother helped him use a computer for projects. She visited the teacher frequently and consulted with the occupational therapist to make the necessary accommodations in the classroom. Sport caused more frustration and failure. Eventually, swimming (only breaststroke) was attempted successfully, with better results. The occupational therapist explained to him that by using resistance though the water, he could get the proprioceptive feedback. This success resulted in an increased motivation to participate in swimming.

Short periods of depression followed, and the exploration of medications continued in a bid to find the correct type and dosage. Social gatherings were a roller-coaster ride depending on the people present. His mother needed to let go of the apron strings, but the fear of Andrew going into depression always concerned her.

Andrew attended the 'Alert' occupational group therapy. He impulsively swung on the trapeze with another child and fell, making the group over-aroused. The occupational therapist remained calm, acknowledged his need for movement and structured the situation to explain about consequences of impulsive behaviour and 'how your engine runs' at that time. The discussion that followed gave suggestions for both external and internal preventative strategies.

Andrew found that new teachers, more subjects and moving from one classroom to the next without getting lost required effort. Extra time for examinations was introduced, and finally, a scribe was used in Andrew's final year of school. Social acceptance amongst Andrew's peers became more difficult, and his parents needed to think differently about societies and

(continued)

CASE STUDY   *(Continued)*

sports. The contact sport of rugby was chosen, and the Interactive Metronome programme made a difference to his rugby skills and concentration. When his position on the field was changed to flank, his participation improved as he was interacting with a more stationary ball in the scrum. Water skiing sports outside school provided very intense proprioceptive input.

Andrew is not an adult, but his mother is an adult – with ADHD. She had to work out ways in which to get routine into her life so that she could give her child routine and structure. She so easily got absorbed in her interests that her husband had to remind

her of her role as a parent. Her husband needed to curb her when she forgot and became over-aroused wanting to do reckless activities such as sandboarding. However, her regular workout at the gym helped her modulate her arousal levels. Her choice of work with children in paediatrics was a good fit. Her cupboards were all colour-coded so that the equipment is organised and replaced where it should be. At meetings and courses, she surrounded herself with colleagues who could 'hold her together'. Many times, she would use 'self-talk' reminding herself not to be so impulsive and to 'stop and think'.

CONCLUSION

It is not only the child/adolescent or the adult with ADHD that needs occupational therapy intervention; it is the person within his/her life span and his/her family and school/work interactions that need consideration. The dysfunctional executive functions throughout life have a debilitating effect on the person towards their family, friends and their school/work environment. Different frames of reference can be used, but the outcome needs to be focused on occupational performance competence within daily living. Self-esteem and self-worth need to be upheld for the person with ADHD, but an understanding of the challenges that are faced is needed also. The person's strengths need to be used to overcome his/her challenges so that he/she can take his/her rightful place in society and the community. There is a vital need to teach the person

with ADHD to take responsibility for the condition and not blame the condition for unacceptable behaviour.

QUESTIONS

1. Describe how ADHD presents over the life span.

2. What are the frames of reference that the occupational therapist should consider when working with a family with a person with ADHD?

3. How does executive function play a role in ADHD?

4. When treating a person with ADHD, why are the family, work and school environment so important?

5. Name and describe the factors which can facilitate a successful life for a person with ADHD.

REFERENCES

Adamou, M., Asherson, P., Arif, M. *et al* (2021) Recommendations for occupational therapy interventions for adults with ADHD: a consensus statement from the UK adult ADHD network. *BMC Psychiatry*, **21**, 72.

Adamou, M., Graham, K., MacKeith, J. *et al* (2016) Advancing services for adult ADHD: the development of the ADHD Star as a framework for multidisciplinary interventions. *BMC Health Services Research*, **16**, 632.

Altable, M. & De la Serna, J.M. (2020) *ADHD in Elderly Age*. DOI: 10.13140/RG.2.2.15353.49763.

Amen, D. (2001) *Healing ADD*, 1st edn. Berkley Book, New York.

American Occupational Therapy Association (AOTA) (2020) *Occupational therapy practice framework: domain et process*.

American Psychiatric Association (2022) *Diagnostic and Statistical Manual of Mental Disorders*, 5th edn, Text Revision. American Psychiatric Association, Washington, DC.

Anzalone, M. & Lane, S. (2012) Sensory processing disorders. In: S. Lane & A. Bundy (eds), *Kids Can Be Kids. A Childhood Occupations Approach*, pp. 437–459. F.A. Davis Company, Philadelphia.

Auerbach, J.G., Landau, R., Berger, A., Arbelle, S., Faroy, M. & Karplus, M. (2005) Neonatal behavior of infants at familial risk for ADHD. *Infant Behavior and Development*, **28(2)**, 220–224.

Ayres, J. (1972) *Sensory Integration and Learning Disorders,* 4th edn. Western Psychological Services, Los Angeles.

Ayres, J. (2005) *Sensory Integration and the Child*, 2nd edn. Western Psychological Services, Los Angeles.

Barkley, R. (2005) *Taking Charge of ADHD,* 2nd edn. The Guilford Press, New York.

Barkley, R., Murphy, K. & Fischer, M. (2008) *ADHD in Adults. What the Science Says,* 1st edn. The Guilford Press, New York.

Bayley, N. (2009) *Bayley-III: Bayley Scales of Infant and Toddler Development.* Giunti OS, Florence, Italy.

Breaux, R., Langberg, J.M., Swanson, C.S., Eadeh, H.M. & Becker, S.P. (2020) Variability in positive and negative affect among adolescents with and without ADHD: differential associations with functional outcomes. *Journal of Affective Disorders*, **274**, 500–507.

Braaten, E.B. & Rosén, L.A. (2000) Self-regulation of affect in attention deficit-hyperactivity disorder (ADHD) and non-ADHD boys: differences in empathic responding. *Journal of Consulting and Clinical Psychology*, **68**(**2**), 313.

Brazelton, T.B. & Nugent, J.K. (1995) *Neonatal Behavioral Assessment Scale* (No. 137). Cambridge University Press, Cambridge.

Brown, C. & Dunn, W. (2002) *Adolescent/Adult Sensory Profile*. Therapy Skill Builders, San Antonio.

Bruininks, R.H. & Bruininks, B.D. (1978) *Bruininks-Oseretsky test of motor proficiency*.

Buitelaar, J. (1996) Epidemiological aspects: what have we learnt over the last decade? In: S. Sandberg (ed), *Hyperactivity and Attention Disorders of Childhood,* pp. 30–63. Cambridge University Press, Cambridge.

Castellanos, F. & Swanson, J. (2002) Biological underpinnings of ADHD. In: S. Sandberg (ed), *Hyperactivity and Attention Disorders of Childhood,* pp. 336–366. Cambridge University Press, Cambridge.

Chu, S. & Reynolds, F. (2007a) Occupational therapy for children with attention deficit hyperactivity disorder (ADHD), part 1: a delineation model of practice. *British Journal of Occupational Therapy,* **70**(**9**), 372–381.

Chu, S. & Reynolds, F. (2007b) Occupational therapy for children with hyperactivity disorder (ADHD), part 2: a multicentre evaluation of an assessment and treatment package. *British Journal of Occupational Therapy,* **70**(**10**), 439–448.

Church, M.K., Maurer, M., Simons, F.E.R. *et al* (2010) Risk of first-generation H(1)-antihistamines: a GA(2)LEN position paper. *Allergy*, **65**(**4**), 459–466.

Cook, R.A. (2011) *Sensory Processing of Learners in the Western Cape Diagnosed with Attention-deficit/Hyperactivity Disorder*. Masters Dissertation, University of Stellenbosch, Stellenbosch.

Cook, R.A. (2013) *Occupational therapist handbook for ADHD-attention difficulties*. www.sensorykidzone.co.za ()

Cooper, P. & Ideus, C. (1996) *Attention Deficit/Hyperactivity Disorder: A Practical Guide for Teachers*. David Fulton, London.

Cosbey, J., Johnston, S. & Dunn, M.L. (2010) Sensory processing disorders and social participation. *American Journal of Occupational Therapy*, **64**(**3**), 462–473.

Dawson, P. & Guare, R. (2010) *Executive Skills in Children and Adolescents,* 2nd edn. The Guilford Press, New York.

DeGangi, G.A. (1983) *DeGangi-Berk test of sensory integration (TSI)*. Western Psychological Services, Los Angeles.

DeGangi, G., Poisson, S., Sickel, R. & Weiner, A. (1995) *Infant Toddler Symptom Checklist*. Therapy Skill Builders, San Antonio.

DeGangi, G. (2000) *Pediatric Disorders of Regulation in Affect and Behaviour,* 1st edn. Academic Press, London.

Díaz-Román, A. & Buela-Casal, G. (2019) Shorter REM latency in children with attention-deficit/hyperactivity disorder. *Psychiatry Research*, **278**, 188–193.

Dunn, W. (1999) *Sensory Profile User's Manual,* 1st edn. The Psychological Corp., San Antonio.

Dunn, W. (2002) *Infant/Toddler Sensory Profile,* 1st edn. The Psychological Corp., San Antonio.

Dunn, W. (2006) *Sensory Profile School Companion User's Manual*, 1st edn. The Psychological Corp., San Antonio.

Dunn, W. & Bennett, D. (2002) Patterns of sensory processing in children with attention-deficit hyperactive disorder. *Occupational Therapy Journal of Research,* **22**(**1**), 4–15.

DuPaul, G.J., Power, T.J., Anastopoulos, A.D. & Reid, R. (2016) *ADHD Rating Scale? 5 for Children and Adolescents: Checklists, Norms, and Clinical Interpretation*. Guilford Publications, New York.

Erasmus, J. (2009) Attention deficit hyperactivity disorder: the medical perspective. In: A. Decaires-Wagner & H. Picton (eds), *Teaching and ADHD in the Classroom*, pp. 2–10. Macmillan, Northlands.

Faraone, S.V., Doyle, A.E., Mick, E. & Biederman, J. (2001) Meta analysis of the association between the 7-repeat allele of the dopamine d4 receptor gene and attention deficit hyperactivity disorder. *Journal of the American Academy of Child & Adolescent Psychiatry*, **158**, 1052–1057.

Finlayson, F., Olsen, J., Dusing, S.C., Guzzetta, A., Eeles, A. & Spittle, A. (2020) Supporting play, exploration, and early development intervention (SPEEDI) for preterm infants: a feasibility randomised controlled trial in an Australian context. *Early Human Development*, **151**, 105172.

Francés, L., Quintero, J., Fernández, A. *et al* (2022) Current state of knowledge on the prevalence of neurodevelopmental disorders in childhood according to the DSM-5: a systematic review in accordance with the PRISMA criteria. *Child and Adolescent Psychiatry and Mental Health*, **16**, 27. https://doi.org/10.1186/s13034-022-00462-1

Fuhrmann, S., Tesch, F., Romanos, M., Abraham, S. & Schmitt, J. (2020) ADHD in school-age children is related to infant exposure to systemic H1-antihistamines. *Allergy*, **75**(**11**), 2956–2957.

Furman, L. (2009) ADHD: what do we really know? In: S. Timimi & J. Leo (eds), *Rethinking ADHD from Brain to Culture*, pp. 21–57. Palgrave Macmillan, New York.

Gioia, G.A., Isquith, P.K., Guy, S.C. & Kenworthy, L. (2000) *Behavior Rating Inventory of Executive Functioning*. Psychological Assessment Resources Inc, Lutz.

Gioia, G.A., Espy, K.A. & Isquith, P.K. (2003) *Behavior Rating Inventory of Executive Functioning Preschool Version*. Psychological Assessment Resources Inc., Lutz.

Greber, C. & Ziviani, J. (2010) A frame of reference to enhance teaching-learning: the four quadrant model of facilitated learning. In: P. Kramer & J. Hinojosa (eds), *Frames of Reference for Pediatric Occupational Therapy*, pp. 234–265. Lippincott Williams & Wilkins, Baltimore.

Green, C. & Chee, K. (1997). *Understanding ADHD: A Parent's Guide to Attention Deficit Hyperactivity Disorder in Children*. Random House.

Greenspan, S.I. & Wieder, S. (2006) *Engaging Autism*. Da Capo Press, Cambridge, MA.

Gregory, A.M., Eley, T.C., O'Connor, T.G. & Plomin, R. (2004) Etiologies of associations between childhood sleep and behavioral problems in a large twin sample. *Journal of the American Academy of Child & Adolescent Psychiatry*, **43**(**6**), 744–751.

Goodwin, A., Hendry, A., Mason, L. *et al* (2021) Behavioural measures of infant activity but not attention associate with later preschool ADHD traits. *Brain Sciences*, **11**(**5**), 524.

Gurevitz, M., Geva, R., Varon, M. & Leitner, Y. (2014) Early markers in infants and toddlers for development of ADHD. *Journal of Attention Disorders*, **18**(**1**), 14–22.

Haertl, K. (2010) A frame of reference to enhance childhood occupations: SCOPE-IT. In: P. Kramer & J. Hinojosa (eds), *Frames of Reference for*

Pediatric Occupational Therapy, pp. 266–305. Lippincott Williams & Wilkins, Baltimore.

Hagermann, E., Hay, D. & Levy, F. (2002) Cognitive aspects of learning. In: S. Sandberg (ed), *Hyperactivity and Attention Disorders of Children,* pp. 214–241. Cambridge University Press, Cambridge.

Hahn-Markowitz, J., Manor, I. & Maeir, A. (2011) Effectiveness of cognitive-functional (cog-fun) intervention with children with attention deficit hyperactivity disorder: a pilot study. *The American Journal of Occupational Therapy,* **65**(4), 384–392.

Henderson, S.E., Sugden, D. & Barnett, A.L. (1992) *Movement Assessment Battery for Children-2.* Research in Developmental Disabilities. Psychological Corporation, London.

Hunt, R., Paguin, A. & Payton, K. (2001) An update on assessment and treatment of complex attention-deficit hyperactivity disorder. *Pediatric Annual,* **30**(3), 162–172.

Kadesjö, C., Kadesjö, B., Hägglöf, B. & Gillberg, C. (2001) ADHD in Swedish 3- to 7-year-old children. *Journal of the American Academy of Child & Adolescent Psychiatry,* **40**, 1021–1028.

Kooij, J.S., Bijlenga, D. & Michielsen, M. (2019) Assessment and treatment of ADHD in people over 60. *The ADHD Report,* **27**(4), 1–7.

Koomar, J., Burpee, J.D., DeJean, V., Frick, S., Kawar, M.J. & Fischer, D.M. (2001) Theoretical and clinical perspectives on the interactive metronome: a view from occupational therapy practice. *The American Journal of Occupational Therapy,* **55**(2), 163–166.

Kutscher, M.L., Attwood, T. & Wolff, R.R. (2005) *Kids in the Syndrome Mix of ADHD, LD, Asperger's, Tourette's, Bipolar, and More!: The One Stop Guide for Parents, Teachers, and Other Professionals.* Jessica Kingsley Publishers, London, England, United Kingdom Philadelphia, Pennsylvania, United States.

Lawlis, F. 2005 *The ADD answer: How to help your child now.* Penguin.

Leisman, G. & Melillo, R. (2010) Effects of motor sequence training on attentional performance in ADHD children. *International Journal on Disability and Human Development,* **9**(4), 275–282. http://www.interactivemetronome.com/IMW/IMPublic/Research/Leisman-Melillo-ADHD-IM-IJDHD-Proofs.pdf (accessed on 31 January 2014)

Mailloux, Z., Parham, L.D. & Roley, S.S. (2020). *Evaluation in Ayres Sensory Integration® (EASI) test sheets and test manual* [Manuscript in preparation]. Collaborative for Leadership in Ayres Sensory Integration®.

Margalit, M. & Kleitman, T. (2006) Mothers' stress, resilience and early intervention. *European Journal of Special Needs Education,* **21**(3), 269–283.

Martin, G.L. (1998) *The Attention Deficit Child.* Chariot Victor Publishing, Colorado Springs. www.drgrantmartin.com/pdf/ADHD-glm-final.pdf (accessed on 17 March 2014)

Mangeot, S., Miller, L., Mcintosh, D. *et al* (2001) Sensory modulation dysfunction in children with attention-deficit-hyperactive disorder. *Developmental Medical Child Neurology,* **43**(6), 399–406.

May-Benson, T.A. (2015) *Adult/Adolescent Sensory History: User's Manual.* SPIRAL Foundation, Newton, MA.

McIntosh, D., Miller, L., Shyu, V. & Hagerman, R. (1999) Sensory-modulation disruption, electrodermal responses and functional behaviors. *Developmental Medical Child Neurology,* **41**(9), 608–615.

Michielsen, M., Comijs, H.C., Aartsen, M.J. *et al* (2015) The relationships between ADHD and social functioning and participation in older adults in a population-based study. *Journal of Attention Disorders,* **19**(5), 368–379.

Miller, L. (2006) *Sensational Kids,* 1st edn. Penguin Group, New York.

Miller, M. & Hinshaw, S.P. (2010). Does childhood executive function predict adolescent functional outcomes in girls with ADHD? *Journal of Abnormal Child Psychology,* **38**, 315–326.

Miller, L.J., Reisman, J.E., McIntosh, D.N. & Simon, J. (2001) An ecological model of sensory modulation. In: S. Smith Roley, I. Blanche & R. Schaaf (eds), *Understanding the Nature of Sensory Integration with Diverse Populations,* pp. 57–82. Therapy Skill Builders, San Antonio.

Nigg, J.T., Goldsmith, H.H. & Sachek, J. (2004) Temperament and attention deficit hyperactivity disorder: the development of a multiple pathway model. *Journal of Clinical Child and Adolescent Psychology,* **33**(1), 42–53.

Parham, D., Ecker, C., Kuhaneck, H. & Glennon, T. (2007) *Sensory Processing Measure.* Western Psychological Services, Los Angeles.

Parham, D.L., Ecker, C.L., Kuhaneck, H., Henry, D.A. & Glennon, T.J. (2013) *Sensory Processing Measure (SPM-2).* WPS, Torrance, CA.

Parush, S., Sohmer, H., Steinberg, A. & Kaitz, M. (2007) Somatosensory functioning in boys with ADHD and tactile defensiveness. *Physiological Behaviour,* **90**(4), 553–558.

Perks, L.M., Rencken, G. & Govender, P. (2020) Therapists' consensus on an infant massage programme for high-risk infants from resource constrained contexts: a Delphi study. *South African Journal of Occupational Therapy,* **50**(3), 72–82.

Reynolds, S. & Lane, S. (2009) Sensory over responsivity and anxiety in children with ADHD. *American Journal of Occupational Therapy,* **63**(4), 433–440.

Rhonda Folio, M. & Fewell, R.R. (2000) *Peabody Developmental Motor Scales,* 2nd edn.

Sandberg, S. (2002) Psychosocial contributions. In: S. Sandberg (ed), *Hyperactivity and Attention Disorders of Childhood,* 2nd edn, pp. 367–416. Cambridge University Press, Cambridge.

Sandberg, S. & Barton, J. (2002) Historical development. In: S. Sandberg (ed), *Hyperactivity and Attention Disorders of Childhood,* 2nd edn, pp. 1–29. Cambridge University Press, Cambridge.

Schaaf, R.C. & Smith Roley, S. (2006) *Sensory Integration: Applying Clinical Reasoning to Practice with Diverse Populations,* 1st edn. Pro-ed., Austin.

Schnatschmidt, M. & Schlarb, A. (2018) Sleep and mental disorders in childhood and adolescence. *Z Kinder Jugendpsychiatr Psychother,* **46**(5), 368–381.

Serfontein, G. (1990) *The Hidden Handicap.* Simon and Schuster, East Roseville.

Shephard, E., Zuccolo, P.F., Idrees, I. *et al* (2022) Systematic review and meta-analysis: the science of early-life precursors and interventions for attention-deficit/hyperactivity disorder. *Journal of the American Academy of Child & Adolescent Psychiatry,* **61**(2), 187–226.

Silver, L. (1999) *Attention-Deficit Hyperactive Disorder,* 2nd edn. American Psychiatric Press, Washington, DC.

Song, P., Zha, M., Yang, Q., Zhang, Y., Li, X. & Rudan, I. (2021) The prevalence of adult attention-deficit hyperactivity disorder: a global systematic review and meta-analysis. *Journal of Global Health,* **11**, 04009.

Sonuga-Barke, E.J.S. & Halperin, J.M. (2010) Developmental phenotypes and causal pathways in attention deficit/hyperactivity disorder: potential targets for early intervention? Developmental phenotypes and causal pathways in ADHD. *Journal of Child Psychology and Psychiatry*, **51**, 368–389.

Strong, J. & Flanagan, M. (2005) *AD/HD for Dummies*. Wiley, Hoboken.

Taylor, J. (2001) *Helping Your ADD Child*. Three Rivers Press, New York.

Timimi, S. & Leo, J. (2009) *Rethinking ADHD from Brain to Culture,* pp. 1–17. Palgrave Macmillan, New York.

Williams, M. & Shellenberg, S. (1996) *How Does Your Engine Run? A Leaders Guide to the Alert Programme for Self Regulation,* 1st edn. Therapy Works Inc., Albuquerque.

Williamson, G. & Anzalone, M. (2001) *Sensory Integration and Self-Regulation in Infants and Toddlers,* 1st edn. Zero to Three: National Centre for Infants, Toddlers and Families, Washington, DC.

Wolraich, M.L., Chan, E., Froehlich, T. *et al* (2019) ADHD diagnosis and treatment guidelines: a historical perspective. *Pediatrics*, **144**(**4**), e20191682.

Young, S. (2017) *Becoming a Star Detective: Your Detective's Notebook for Finding Clues to How You Feel*. Jessica Kingsley Publishers.

Trauma and Its Impact on Individuals and Collectives

CHAPTER 21

Minkateko Wicht[1] and Thuli Godfrey Mthembu[2]

[1]Private and Community Practice, Cape Town, South Africa
[2]Faculty of Community and Health Sciences, Department of Occupational Therapy, University of the Western Cape, Bellville, South Africa

KEY LEARNING POINTS

- Adverse childhood experiences.

- Understanding trauma and types of trauma.

- Signs and symptoms of trauma.

- The impact of trauma on the brain and body.

- Perspectives on historical trauma.

- Self-care by the occupational therapist.

- Trauma-informed approach.

- Occupational therapy intervention with individuals and collectives.

INTRODUCTION

. . .trauma [not only] affects individuals at the emotional, spiritual, intellectual, physical, and social domains . . . but also the family unit, the community collective, and the nation
(Mitchell *et al.* 2019, p. 83)

Understanding the complexity of trauma is crucial for occupational therapists as trauma has a powerful impact on healthy growth and development, and is part of everyone's lifespan (Alers 2014). Trauma can '. . . disrupt functioning of the body and mind, relationships . . . the sense of safety . . . and one's place in the world or that of the one's social group' (Gultekin *et al.* 2019, p. 711). It can negatively impact occupational performance in home, school and work settings (Alers 2014). Furthermore, the effects of trauma place a significant burden on people and communities and create challenges for social systems (Substance Abuse and Mental Health Services Administration [SAMHSA] 2014, p. 2). Thus, trauma needs to be viewed as a public health concern as it does not only impact individuals but collectives as well. In this chapter, a collective is considered a group of people, family, community, organisation or nation. They are a significant part of collaborative relationship-focused practice and occupational therapists are called upon '. . . to attend to the relational aspects of practice including the self, and the individuals, families, groups, communities, and populations who use occupational therapy services within the context of the social and structural factors that promote and constrain occupations' (Restall & Egan 2021, p. 227).

Occupational therapists are encouraged to open up alternative ways of thinking, reacting, and responding to the call for understanding the historical wounds and trauma that individuals and collectives grapple with as they engage in their multiple occupations (Behari-Leak 2019; Mthembu & Duncan 2021).

ADVERSE CHILDHOOD EXPERIENCES

While stress and adversity may be a normal, and even an essential part of human development, research shows that

Crouch and Alers Occupational Therapy in Psychiatry and Mental Health, Sixth Edition.
Edited by Rosemary Crouch, Tania Buys, Enos Morankoana Ramano, Matty van Niekerk and Lisa Wegner.
© 2025 John Wiley & Sons Ltd. Published 2025 by John Wiley & Sons Ltd.

'. . . exposure to frequent and prolonged adversity, especially in the absence of protective factors, can result in toxic stress . . .' (Centers for Disease Control (CDC) 2021, p. 3). The impact of toxic stress, particularly during childhood, can have long-lasting effects on educational and employment outcomes, increase prevalence of health-risk behaviours, increase susceptibility to physical and mental health diseases, and impact the formation of healthy stable relationships (CDC 2021).

The Adverse Childhood Experiences (ACEs) study, a ground-breaking study which surveyed 17000 adults in the United States of America between 1995 and 1997, investigated the impact of ACEs on adult physical and mental health outcomes and health-related behaviours (Felitti *et al.* 1998). An ACE is a potentially traumatic experience that occurs within the first 18 years of life (CDC 2019). The initial 10 items of ACEs, measured by the original ACE study, included physical or emotional abuse or neglect, sexual abuse, witnessing violence at home and enduring other forms of household dysfunction such as parental separation, living with a household member with a mental health disorder or having a household member imprisoned (Felitti *et al.* 1998; Felitti & Anda 2010; CDC 2019).

The original ACE study had several important findings (Felitti *et al.* 1998), which are continuously discussed in contemporary literature (Felitti & Anda 2010; Leitch 2017; Merrick *et al.* 2017; Fette *et al.* 2019; PACEs Connection 2022a). Firstly, experiences of childhood trauma were more common than previously thought, with two-thirds of adults having experienced at least one ACE and one in five adults reporting experiences of three or more ACES (Leitch 2017; Fette *et al.* 2019). Secondly, experiences of ACEs were associated with health-risk behaviours, chronic health conditions, mental illness, violence and victimisation, and premature death. The correlation was found to be in a dose-response pattern, meaning that as experiences of ACEs increased, so did the risk of experiencing poorer outcomes as adults (Leitch 2017; Merrick *et al.* 2017). Thirdly, adults with the highest ACE scores had a lower life expectancy (20 years or less) than those with lower ACE scores (Leitch 2017). Lastly, ACEs contribute to many health and social problems experienced within society (Felitti & Anda 2010; PACEs Connection 2022a). These findings not only revealed the high prevalence of ACEs in the American population but also that ACEs contribute to a high burden of disease.

Since the original ACE study, there has been growing research and use of the understanding of ACEs and their impact in both the Global North (Felitti & Anda 2010; Leitch 2017; Merrick *et al.* 2017; Illinois ACEs Response Collaborative 2019; Anda *et al.* 2020; Ellis *et al.* 2022; PACEs Connection 2022a) and the Global South (Manyema & Richter 2019; Naicker 2022; Amene *et al.* 2023). Notably, this has resulted in a shift to viewing trauma as a multi-sectoral public health issue and not merely the health sector's sole responsibility (SAMHSA 2014; Illinois ACEs Response Collaborative 2019). Interventions, at both an individual and collective level, are required across sectors. To overcome the impact of trauma, at a public health level, strategies grounded in trauma-informed approaches need to be aimed at preventing ACEs, providing appropriate interventions and creating contexts in which individuals, families and communities can thrive

(CDC 2021). Key to this shift is understanding the complexity of the layers of trauma.

LAYERS OF TRAUMA

While the traumas which are measured within ACEs have expanded beyond the initial ten items to include other potentially traumatic situations like bullying and homelessness (PACEs Connection 2022b), it has been acknowledged that toxic stress can also be caused by a broader range of experiences such as poverty, racism and community violence, which may contribute and compound adversities experienced by individuals and collectives (Illinois ACEs Response Collaborative 2019).

The analogy of a tree is helpful to occupational therapists in thinking about the complex layers of trauma. Looking at a tree, one sees only that which is above ground, that is trunk, branches and leaves, while the roots and below-surface soil are not visible. However, the health of a tree is dependent on its surrounding conditions and whether these are nurturing or harmful. As in Figure 21.1, the tree's leaves and branches represent the symptoms of ACEs. Upon assessment, the occupational therapist may only consider what is most visible, that is the impact of ACEs on occupational engagement and health and well-being. However, similar to assessing the tree's health, considering what is lying underneath, that is roots and soil, is necessary to better understand the nurturing and harmful conditions faced by clients in their various contexts. The roots of the tree represent the *adverse community environments* in which ACEs occur and the soil represents *adverse collective historical experiences* over generations (Illinois ACEs Response Collaborative 2019; Ellis *et al.* 2022). Roots and soil contexts have both a direct and indirect influence on human development, occupational engagement and health and well-being. By considering the role of people's contexts in contributing to trauma, occupational therapists can use their skills to support individuals, families and communities experiencing trauma to move from surviving to thriving within their contexts and to advocate for change at various levels of systems, thus mitigating the impacts of trauma and disrupting the intergenerational transmission of trauma (Illinois ACEs Response Collaborative 2019).

UNDERSTANDING TRAUMA

THE DSM-5-TR AND POST-TRAUMATIC STRESS DISORDER

The fifth edition of the Diagnostic and Statistical Manual of Mental Disorders (DSM-5) saw the removal of Post-traumatic Stress Disorder (PTSD) from the anxiety disorders group, in the DSM-IV, to a new diagnostic category, that is, trauma- and stressor-related disorders (APA 2013; Pai *et al.* 2017). A text-revision of the DSM-5 (DSM-5-TR) has since been published in 2022 (APA 2022). The DSM-5 and DSM-5-TR also moved to a nonaxial documentation of diagnosis (APA 2013; APA 2022). The use of the Global Assessment of Function (GAF), as part of

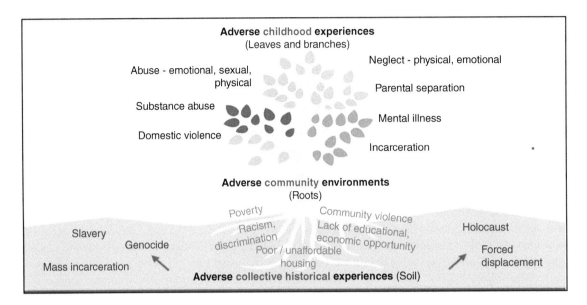

FIGURE 21.1 Trauma tree.

Source: The Illinois ACEs Response Collaborative 2019; Permission to use image granted. Image adapted by Stan Sonu, MD from Ellis & Dietz (2017).

the multiaxial classification of functioning in the DSM-IV was discontinued to shift to a disability assessment of function. The World Health Organization Disability Assessment Schedule (WHODAS.2.0) was adopted to assess clients' functioning amongst those with mental and health conditions (World Health Organization 2010; APA 2022). The WHODAS 2.0 is a 36-item outcome measure comprising six domains relevant in occupational therapy, namely, self-care, getting around, understanding and communicating, getting along with people, life activities (e.g. work and/or school activities), and participation in one's community/society.

For PTSD within the DSM-5-TR, criterion A requires the occurrence of or exposure to a traumatic event. It defines a traumatic event as '. . . exposure to actual or threatened death, serious injury, or sexual violence' (APA 2022, p. 301) and examples include exposure to war, physical assault, sexual violence and natural disasters. The traumatic event also needs to either be experienced directly or indirectly, witnessed in-person or by repeated or extreme exposure to aversive details of a traumatic event, for example, first responders, with further details being provided (Pai *et al.* 2017; APA 2022). Criteria B to E describe the symptoms of PTSD which need to be linked to trauma exposure and are grouped into symptoms relating to intrusion, avoidance, negative alterations in cognition and mood and alterations in arousal and reactivity (Pai *et al.* 2017; APA 2022). Furthermore, the disturbance should be present for more than a month (Criteria F) and cause distress or impairment in functioning (Criteria G) (Alers 2014; APA 2022). Lastly, there is an addition of a specifier to note dissociative features of depersonalization or derealisation as well as specific criteria for PTSD in children six years and younger (Alers 2014; Pai *et al.* 2017; APA 2022).

Often, trauma is considered in relation to PTSD; however, this chapter offers a broader understanding of trauma

beyond just that which is defined in the DSM-5-TR (APA 2022). Occupational therapists may work with individual and collective clients who have experienced various types of traumas (discussed below), but who may not necessarily meet the criteria for PTSD. Therefore, broadening the understanding of trauma, beyond PTSD, is necessary to adequately understand clients, their contexts and their occupational functioning and to support their healing (Kaminer *et al.* 2018).

TOWARDS A COMPREHENSIVE UNDERSTANDING OF TRAUMA

Trauma can be understood in terms of the *event,* the *experience* and the *effects* (SAMHSA 2014). Trauma results from an *event* that overwhelms an individual or collective's ability to cope and is harmful or threatening to their safety, lives, or health and well-being (SAMHSA 2014; American Occupational Therapy Association (AOTA) 2018). Events can include once-off incidents (e.g. rape or natural disaster); it can include cumulative, continuous or ongoing events (e.g. abuse, exposure to violence, or war); or it can include a set of circumstances (e.g. neglect, unemployment or poverty) (SAMHSA 2014; Fette *et al.* 2019; APA 2023). Recent literature introduced the idea of continuous traumatic stress, asserting that experiences of trauma are not only past events but can be ongoing conditions of living and anticipatory future events (Eagle & Kaminer 2013; Kaminer *et al.* 2018). Thus, it is important for practitioners to not only ask *what has happened to you* but also, *what is happening to you* and *what may happen to you?*

Secondly, turning to the *experience* of the event, trauma can be viewed as '. . . a subjective experience of violence, threat, loss, exclusion and powerlessness . . .' (R-Cubed 2016). Whether an event is experienced as traumatic or not is dependent on how the individual or group '. . . labels, assigns meaning to, and is disrupted physically and psychologically . . .' (SAMHSA 2014, p. 8). The variation in experience results from the impact of previous lived experiences, genetic makeup, trauma and attachment histories, sociocultural contexts and developmental stages (SAMHSA 2014; Payne *et al.* 2015). Payne *et al.* (2015) deepen the understanding of trauma as not only the subjective experience but what is specifically experienced in the nervous system and body, i.e. trauma is the physical and emotional response to an event (SAMHSA 2014).

Lastly, traumatic experiences can have a range of short- and long-term *effects*, which may be experienced immediately or with delayed onset and can impact peoples' physical, emotional, psychological and spiritual health as well as how they engage in their roles and routines and their occupational performance (SAMHSA 2014; AOTA 2018). Effects can include a range of physical or emotional responses. It can affect cognitive function, learning and behaviour, and influence emotional regulation. It impacts abilities to cope with daily stressors and build new and maintain existing relationships. Trauma can affect spiritual beliefs, the capacity for meaning-making and influence how individuals see themselves and their place in the world (SAMHSA 2014; R-Cubed 2016; Fette *et al.* 2019; APA 2023). Trauma can also increase rates of various health issues such as heart disease and autoimmune disorders and increase risk of engaging in health-risk behaviours (Fette *et al.* 2019).

UNDERSTANDING DIFFERENT TYPES OF TRAUMA

To uncover the complexity of traumatic experiences, the below classification aims to encompass the breadth of experiences and broaden the understanding of trauma beyond experiences of once-off events.

Types of Trauma

An **Acute Trauma** is sudden, unexpected and a once-off incident, e.g. death of a sibling, car accident or hijacking, but may have long-lasting effects (Alers 2014).

Complex Trauma is a prolonged repeated traumatic event and can be viewed as '. . . exposure to multiple, prolonged, or ongoing stressors' (Champagne 2011, p. CE1), for example, domestic violence or child abuse (Alers 2014). In complex cases, a relationship often exists between the victim and perpetrator. The victim is usually under the control of the perpetrator and often feels powerless to escape (Alers 2014). Complex trauma experienced during childhood can have detrimental effects on the child's development as it often occurs in the child's main support system, which should be nurturing and providing safety and security (Champagne 2011).

Developmental Trauma has recently been introduced to better understand the impact of prolonged abuse on children's development and functioning (van der Kolk 2005; Eagle & Kaminer 2013). According to van der Kolk (2005), PTSD does not adequately describe the pervasive impact of exposure to childhood trauma on the developing child. Thus, these children may be diagnosed with a range of co-morbid diagnoses such as conduct disorder or attention-deficit hyperactivity disorder (ADHD), while the impact of the causal factor, that is, childhood trauma, is missed (Van Der Kolk & D'Andrea 2010).

Collective Trauma occurs when a group of people, varying in size, experiences a traumatic event resulting in physical, emotional and/or psychological damage and pain. Depending on the event, the effects can be experienced across generations (Carra *et al.* 2019; Watson *et al.* 2020; Fortuna *et al.* 2022). When on a larger scale, the impact of collective traumas can result in social transformation as it can affect social processes, relationships, practices, institutions, capital and resources (Somasundaram 2011). Examples of collective traumas are the COVID-19 pandemic, war and natural disasters.

Historical Trauma is a collective experience of trauma inflicted upon a group of people with a particular shared identity, affiliation or circumstance and can occur over an extended period of time or across generations (Heart *et al.* 2011; Mohatt *et al.* 2014; Ehlers *et al.* 2022). The traumatic events create high levels of collective distress and include experiences of overwhelming physical and psychological violence, cultural dispossession, economic deprivation, displacement or segregation (Sotero 2006; Nutton & Fast 2015). Perpetrators of the events are usually not from the same group as victims and have purposeful and destructive intent (Evans-Campbell 2008; Bombay *et al.* 2014). Examples of historical trauma include Apartheid, Holocaust and Slavery.

Intergenerational Trauma refers to how trauma experienced within one generation, either individually or collectively, is transferred to the subsequent generation(s) and affects the functioning, health and well-being of the descendants (Barron & Abdallah 2015; Sangalang & Vang 2017; Jeyasundaram *et al.* 2020; Fortuna *et al.* 2022). The effects include distrust of self and others; feelings of fear, shame and humiliation; problematic family dynamics; increased levels of depressive and anxiety symptoms; low self-esteem; disconnection; loss of cultural values and practices; conflict; violence against self and others; risk-taking behaviours; and education and employment difficulties (Menzies 2019; Jeyasundaram *et al.* 2020).

Continuous Traumatic Stress (CTS) is experienced when individuals or groups are living in contexts with repeated present and ongoing exposure to threat and danger and where the anticipation of future threat and danger is realistic (Eagle & Kaminer 2013; Kaminer *et al.* 2018). Contexts of CTS may include conflict-affected areas such as war zones, chronic community violence or xenophobic contexts. Importantly, the trauma experienced with CTS is not in the past, but rather exists within the present and is anticipated in the future, impacting the way individuals and groups adapt to survive and cope in their contexts (Eagle & Kaminer 2013). CTS may result in individuals experiencing anticipatory anxiety, vulnerability, uncertainty and helplessness, and requires constant alertness and preparedness, which can impact daily routines and occupational patterns and put individuals at risk of other mental health disorders (Eagle & Kaminer 2013; Lahav 2020).

Vicarious trauma is '. . . considered the negative reactions that can develop among [professional's] as a result of their "empathetic engagement" with trauma victims . . .' (Burnett & Wahl 2015, p. 318). It is associated with cognitive, affective, and psychological effects, alterations of core beliefs and worldviews and the ability to maintain connections with self and others (Sprang *et al.* 2007; Burnett & Wahl 2015; Brend *et al.* 2020). Vicarious trauma can affect, for example, caregivers, healthcare workers, journalists or police (Alers 2014).

SIGNS AND SYMPTOMS OF TRAUMA

People can experience a number of signs and symptoms when faced with trauma. It is important to emphasise that these reactions are often 'normal reactions to abnormal events', and this insight needs to be conveyed in a warm, caring and sensitive way. The assessment by the occupational therapist is likely to reveal physical, cognitive, emotional, motivational, spiritual and behavioural signs as well as changes in occupational engagement. Signs and symptoms can vary according to age (Alers 2014).

- Physical signs may include headaches, backaches and stomach aches, sudden sweating and/or heart palpitations, changes in sleep, appetite and libido, constipation or diarrhoea, lowered immunity and hyper- or hypo-arousal (Snedden 2012; Alers 2014).

- Cognitive signs include poor problem-solving, decision-making, concentration and memory, confusion and disorientation, dissociation, intrusive images, nightmares, and rationalisation and/or minimisation of the experience (Snedden 2012; Alers 2014).

- Emotional signs include shock and disbelief, fear and anxiety, anger, guilt, grief and denial, irritability and emotional lability, emotional numbing and isolation, intrusive thoughts, loss of trust or self-esteem and an increased need to control everyday experiences (Snedden 2012; Alers 2014).

- Spiritual signs may include loss of hope, meaning and faith (Snedden 2012).

- Behavioural signs may include substance abuse, increased/decreased food intake, crying constantly or for no apparent reason, excessive checking of security, anger outbursts, social withdrawal and suspiciousness, avoidance of things associated with the trauma, self-blame or survivor's guilt, and difficulty trusting others (Alers 2014).

- Changes in occupational engagement may include '. . . disruption, loss and/or alienation from activities of daily living, leisure, school, work, social participation and valued life roles' (Snedden 2012, p. 27) as well as a diminished interest in activities that were once pleasurable (Alers 2014).

It is important to realise that the above signs and symptoms do not necessarily indicate psychopathology, yet as mental health professionals, occupational therapists need to be aware of the risk factors for the development of PTSD (Alers 2014; APA 2022). Referral to a psychologist or psychiatrist is very important in such cases (Alers 2014). Symptoms of PTSD are described in Criteria B – E in the DSM-5-TR (APA 2022).

THE IMPACT OF TRAUMA ON THE BRAIN AND BODY

As trauma can be considered an internal experience, understanding what happens in the brain and body is crucial. Contemporary literature supports the connection between trauma and the brain and body as '. . . it is widely acknowledged that the mind and body's responses to trauma are inseparable . . .' (O'Brien & Charura 2023, p. 2).

The Brain and Trauma

The effects of trauma on the brain are manifold and complex (Alers 2014; O'Brien & Charura 2023). Traumatic experiences, which fundamentally are a threat to safety, can have detrimental effects on the way the brain functions as '. . . the brain has developed with survival as its primary goal' (Benjamin & Fourie 2019, p. 279). The Triune Theory of the Brain (MacLean 1990) provides a simplification of the hierarchy of the brain by dividing it into three areas, namely, brainstem, limbic system and neocortex. While this theory has been critiqued for its compartmentalisation of the brain, it is helpful in making sense of the complexity of the impact of trauma on the brain (Benjamin & Fourie 2019).

The brainstem, or 'survival' brain, controls many of our vital bodily functions, which are critical for keeping us alive, such as breathing, heart rate and blood pressure. It is also involved with arousal and attention (Alers 2014; Benjamin & Fourie 2019).

The limbic system, or 'emotional' brain, is a complex integrated system and is the seat of survival instincts and reflexes including stress reflexes of fight, flight and freeze (Alers 2014). It regulates emotional experiences and responses (Benjamin & Fourie 2019) and to some extent the ability to control impulses to act out (Alers 2014). When a threat is detected in the environment, '. . . the amygdala alerts the hypothalamus, which activates the appropriate system to move the body into a heightened physiological arousal state' (Benjamin & Fourie 2019, p. 280). The amygdala and hippocampus are the structures involved in understanding traumatic memory (Alers 2014).

Lastly, the cortex, or 'thinking' brain, is involved in complex, cognitive processes such as problem solving, language and abstract thinking (Benjamin & Fourie 2019). It is also involved in memory and also performs sensory and motor functions, which regulate higher cognitive and emotional functions (Alers 2014).

The Body and Trauma

The autonomic nervous system (ANS) plays a vital role in our responses to trauma and comprises the parasympathetic and sympathetic nervous systems. The Polyvagal Theory (Porges 1995) describes how the body responds to threats of danger (Conroy & Perryman 2022). The vagus nerve carries information between the brain and specific parts of the body, such as digestive tract, lungs and heart, and is involved in functions such as speech and facial expressions (Physiopedia 2023). There are three branches of the vagus nerve responsible for the regulatory capacities of the body, namely, the parasympathetic ventral vagal system, the sympathetic nervous system, and the parasympathetic dorsal vagal system (Porges 1995). The different systems can be likened to traffic light colours. The green zone is represented by the parasympathetic ventral vagal system or the social engagement system. This is activated when one feels safe, calm and '. . . during safe social engagement and has a soothing effect on defensive responses of the sympathetic nervous system' (Conroy & Perryman 2022, p. 145). The orange zone is the sympathetic nervous system, or the fight or flight system. When the brain detects a threat, this system mobilises the body into action by either going into fight or flight responses. The parasympathetic dorsal vagal system, or the freeze response, is represented by the red zone and is activated when the body detects a '. . . life-threatening situation, increasing the pain threshold and minimizing other body movements' (Conroy & Perryman 2022, p. 144).

The Stress Response

The brain constantly receives information from the environment through the senses. When a real or perceived threat is detected, the stress response is activated. The brain sends signals to the body to releases hormones such as adrenaline and cortisol, through the hypothalamic-pituitary-adrenal axis and activates the 'survival mode' of fight, flight or freeze response (orange and red zones), depending on the severity of the threat (Benjamin & Fourie 2019; Conroy & Perryman 2022). This causes dysregulation in the ANS. Theoretically, once the danger is over, the brain and body should regulate to the green zone, or the parasympathetic ventral vagal system. However, for many individuals with high ACE scores or living in chronic states of stress and danger, their threat activation system does not have the opportunity to regulate, recover and return to a baseline physiological state of relaxation (Benjamin & Fourie 2019). They may therefore experience constant levels of either hyper-arousal, remaining alert and hypervigilant, despite the lack of apparent threat, or hypo-arousal where '. . . the body

becomes less responsive to emotionally salient stimuli' (Conroy & Perryman 2022, p. 144). Furthermore, when the fight, flight or freeze modes are activated, access to the thinking brain is limited as the cortex becomes '. . . turned down and less able to facilitate higher-order functions like problem solving . . . and logical thinking' (Benjamin & Fourie 2019, p. 281).

It is important to reiterate, that the stress response is a ***normal response to abnormal events.*** The brain and body work in tandem in response to threat and trauma and it is when the stress response is constantly activated and the nervous system is dysregulated that it becomes problematic to physical and mental health and impacts occupational functioning (Payne *et al.* 2015). As Porges (2022, p. 2) states '. . . when humans feel safe, their nervous systems support the homeostatic functions of health, growth, and restoration, while they simultaneously become accessible to others without feeling or expressing threat and vulnerability'.

ATTACHMENT THEORY

Attachment Theory is an important framework in considering styles of attachment of individuals with mental health problems (Alers 2014). Attachment behaviour is activated when a child seeks proximity to their caregiver due to being lost, frightened, injured, hungry or needing comfort (Alers 2014). Children develop different attachment patterns with different carers, but the attachment style between the child and their main carer will become the child's 'internal working model' and form the template for future relationships (Alers 2014). There are four attachment styles, namely, secure, insecure-avoidant, insecure-ambivalent and insecure-disorganised (Champagne 2011). Research suggests that '. . . forming healthy attachments early in life fosters a strong and positive sense of self-identity, clarity of boundaries between self and others, resiliency, and a general sense of wellbeing' (Champagne 2011, p. CE1). The importance of attachment styles is that the experiences of attachment and safety are laid down early in life and have a long-lasting effect (Alers 2014). Experiences of trauma can influence an individual's ability to build new relationships and maintain existing relationships. Thus, it is important for occupational therapists to consider attachment history and styles when working with clients who have experienced trauma (Champagne 2011).

PERSPECTIVES ON HISTORICAL TRAUMA

HISTORICAL TRAUMAS

Sotero's (2006) conceptual model of historical trauma could enable occupational therapists to enhance their efforts to address the traumas that families and communities experience where they live, work, play, and learn (Figure 21.2). It is

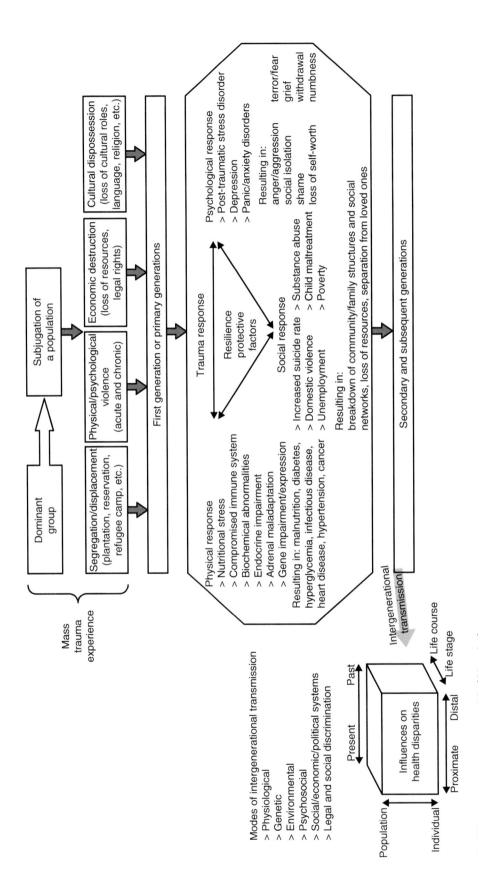

FIGURE 21.2 Conceptual model of historical trauma.
Source: Permission granted to reproduce: Sotero (2006).

crucial to demystify how poverty, inequality, unemployment, violence, crime, traumatic events, disasters and corruption influence families and communities' mental well-being, as highlighted in the Trauma tree (Alers 2008; Illinois ACEs Response Collaborative 2019; Ngcaweni 2018; Ellis *et al.* 2022). For instance, adversity emanating from massive group trauma experiences tends to perpetuate the vulnerability of young people not in education, employment or training (NEET), which results in the collective emotional and psychological wounding over the life span and across generations (Brave Heart 2003; Lawlor 2017; Chauke 2023). Occupational therapists should be aware of the masses' historical trauma responses (HTR) related to 'depression, self-destructive behaviour, suicidal thoughts and gestures, anxiety, low self-esteem, anger, and difficulty recognizing and expressing emotions' (Brave Heart 2003, p. 7).

There are still vestiges of racial discrimination and spatial segregation in housing, income inequality, and huge disparities that emanated from the apartheid era, still exist in the democratic era of South Africa (Alers 2008; Lawlor 2017; Basson & Wale 2019). The mass trauma experiences amongst the subjugated population involved segregation and displacement, physical and psychological violation, economic destruction, and cultural dispossession (Sotero 2006; Lawlor 2017). The government policies and legislatures restricted the population to exercise their human rights. Consequently, the existence of racism, discrimination, social and economic disadvantage influences the population, which is evident in families who are ripped apart and left with deep scars that affect their physical, material, and psychological components (Lawlor 2017; Basson & Wale 2019). For instance, the subjugated population 'witnessed great loss of life and endured brutality, starvation, and disease, many survivors are plagued with physical injuries, malnutrition, and high rates of infectious and chronic diseases' (Sotero 2006, p. 99). Furthermore, the primary generations' emotional and psychological responses originated from violence, stress, hardships, unresolved issues related to land, loss of kin and economic freedom. Hence, Sotero (2006) argues that trauma response amongst subjugated populations is visible in their 'PTSD, depression, self-destructive behaviors, severe anxiety, guilt, hostility, and chronic bereavement' (p. 99).

Primary generations tend to pass on their traumatic experiences to the secondary generations; they struggle to raise their offspring, which results in family dysfunction and disorders such as mental illness, depression, PTSD, substance abuse, gender-based violence and suicide (Sotero 2006). Similarly, engagement in occupations such as collective memory, storytelling and oral traditions of the population tend to perpetuate the historical trauma (Brave Heart 2003; Sotero 2006). For instance, the younger generations may inherit a loss of culture and language, discrimination, injustice, poverty and social inequality (Mthembu *et al.* 2023). This supports Fanon Frantz's perspective of the zone of nonbeing where poverty, inequalities, lack of resources, poor socio-economic status, lack of occupational opportunities for valued occupations, and the health disparities influence the well-being and quality of life of families (Sotero 2006; Ndlovu-Gatsheni 2020). However, some younger generations might attempt to break the cycle of intergenerational trauma inherited from their families and communities (Mthembu 2021; Mthembu *et al.* 2023).

Occupational disruptions emanating from trauma push families and communities 'to bounce back from the brink of despair, and to grow in the process while understanding the importance of the resiliency and protective factors that primary and secondary generations used to ameliorate the social problems' (Southwick & Charney 2012, p. 1). Similarly, survivors need to have the 'capacity to bend without breaking, to return to an original shape or condition' (Southwick & Charney 2012, p. 6). Occupational therapists can enable the survivors to 'successfully and creatively navigate and negotiate life stressors, challenging environments and difficult events, whereby changes and modifications to daily occupations and occupational participation are required' as part of their occupational resilience (Brown 2021, p. 104). Four capacities of resilience that people need to possess to deal with the problematic situations, which include absorptive, adaptive, anticipatory and transformative (Ziglio 2017; Savio 2023). Absorptive capacity is the survivors' need to cope with trauma and bounce back from adversities using skills, assets and resources available in their context. Adaptive capacity is the survivors' ability to respond to problematic situations, trauma, disturbances and shocks. Anticipatory capacity is survivors' ability to reduce disturbances and risks by means of proactive engagement in occupations to ameliorate vulnerability. Transformative capacity systems involve the ability to reconstruct existing policies and practices to address historical trauma, volatility, and insecurity. The survivors need capacities 'to do what they are required and have opportunity to do, to become who they have the potential to be' as part of occupational potential to regenerate, reintegrate, reorganise and rejuvenate their lives (Wicks 2005, p. 130; Savio 2023).

CASE STUDY 1   Legacies of Historical Trauma in the Marikana Massacre

---

The Marikana massacre is the killing of 34 miners by the South African Police Service on 16 August 2012, which took place in North-West Province (Alexander 2016). The law enforcement and policing systems are one of the most important pillars of a country to sustain not only the health and well-being of individuals and the community, but also to prevent or interrupt violence, injuries, and death (Bailey *et al.* 2022). However, the Marikana massacre is one of the modern traumas that highlighted existing brutal hegemony by law enforcement in the post-apartheid era. One of the mine-workers shared 'We are still oppressed and abused' (Alexander *et al.* 2012, p. 46; Alexander 2016). This brought memories of the 21 March 1960 Sharpeville massacre, where the law enforcement contributed to the death of 169 people during anti-pass campaigns in the era of the colonial apartheid systems (South African History Online 2023). Evans-Campbell (2008) elucidates that colonial trauma encompasses 'both historical and contemporary traumatic events that reflect colonial practices to colonise, subjugate, and perpetrate ethnocide and genocide' (p. 335). The economic inequalities influenced the collective well-being of the mine workers and their families, which resulted in limited opportunities to experience and express pleasure, purpose, and meaning in life through engagement in roles and accomplishment of occupations that are individually and/or collectively valuable for human development (Hammell 2017, p. 211). A lack of recreational facilities influenced the social health of the children, youth and adults in the community, which perpetuated young people's NEET status (Cairncross & Kisting 2016; Moleba 2016; Khuluvhe & Negogogo 2021).

Unmet well-being needs, such as lack of water, exposed the women in Marikana to sleep deprivation because they had to wake up in the early hours of the morning to get water for their families while they were still expected to prepare breakfast and other meals, which highlighted occupational imbalance due to being over-occupied (Benya 2015; Hocking 2017). However, the men experienced sleep deprivation because of retrenchments and loss of income, which influenced their mental health (Benya 2015; Cairncross & Kisting 2016). Therefore, families lacked engagement in a variety of occupations 'due to occupational patterns of being over or under-occupied, excessive work demands and enforced idleness' (Hocking 2017, p. 33).

Health disparities were evident in the community of Marikana because the women experienced a sense of isolation and discrimination, which is related to the silent or hidden inequalities that existed in the health care services. For instance, migrant women tend to struggle to access health services, as they are not fluent in the local language, seTswana (Benya 2015). The women's experiences provide evidence of occupational marginalisation, which refers to the 'discrimination of people by degraded occupational opportunities and resources that are less valued within a society' (Hocking 2017, p. 33). Communities were 'relocated at the last minute to barren sites and facilities much poorer than they had before' without 'refuse removal and adequate sewage systems' (Cairncross & Kisting 2016, p. 525).

Mineworkers experienced a sense of disempowerment, as they did 'not have power to take over or take any further steps' and they have been passed on social and financial inequalities to the young people, as a legacy of intergenerational poverty (Alexander *et al.* 2012, p. 113; Moleba 2016). Young people also had to live and deal with the death, pain and grief of losing their parents due to the massacre and injuries, which affected not only their quality of life and mental health but also their education (Moleba 2016). They also struggled to cope with a rapid transition to emerging adulthood; others dropped out of school after failing grades several times and some committed suicide because 'basic needs and wants appear impossible to attain or maintain' (Benya 2015; Moleba 2016; Cairncross & Kisting 2016; Hocking 2017, p. 33; Kros 2017; Shange 2019). Thus, the legacy of disempowerment indicates that women and young people were a more vulnerable population because the system perpetuated colonialism and enforced colonial powers, which are consistent with occupational apartheid (Mthembu 2021).

SPIRITUAL WOUNDING

Spiritual wounding has been an important concept in the literature that focuses on the human needs and well-being of the families and communities affected by poverty, unemployment as well as unhealthy environments, which supports Fanon Frantz's perspective of the zone of non-being (Ndlovu-Gatsheni 2020). In the zone of non-being, people in all stages are trapped between life and death, which indicates that they are not only experiencing existential despair but also pass on the psychological effects to their descendants through genes, as part of the legacies of social systems such as colonialism and apartheid (Gillson & Ross 2019; Ndlovu 2020; Avalos 2021). However, it should be noted that traumas happen in various contexts such as Marikana massacre, Rwandan genocide and George Floyd's death in the United States. In relation to the Marikana massacre, the younger generation inherited distress emanating from collective trauma (Moleba 2016). Consistent with Fanon's understanding of existential despair in the zone of non-being, the historical trauma in Marikana was passed on to the younger generation,

which resulted in some of them committing suicide. According to Ndlovu (2020), suicide is one of the universal phenomena that affects all humans. Regarding the Rwandan genocide, young and adult population were diagnosed with mental illnesses such as PTSD, which necessitated a comprehensive approach to their mental health (Kayiteshonga *et al.* 2022). On the other hand, the death of George Floyd on 25 May 2020 indicated that exposure to shared violence tends to influence the mental health of the population, which perpetuated the traumatic experiences and PTSD induced by racism and police brutality (Galovski *et al.* 2016; Williams *et al.* 2018; Eichstaedt *et al.* 2021). Therefore, spiritual wounding should be addressed by embracing interdependence and inclusivity, where people's humanity and dignity are valued, as part of *Ubuntu* to promote an ethos of care and respect for others and the importance of solidarity in the face of adversity. The healing process should promote engagement in 'occupations that contribute positively to their own well-being and the well-being of their communities' (Alers 2008; Hammell 2017, p. 209).

DECOLONIAL EPISTEMIC PERSPECTIVES OF HISTORICAL TRAUMA

In rethinking occupational therapy interventions for trauma and mental health conditions, occupational therapists should adopt the lens of a decolonial epistemic perspective to enhance their clinical reasoning and facilitate the healing process (Mignolo 2009). This perspective supports occupational therapists' actions to not only de-link from the status quo of Euro-centric biomedical models of diseases and symptomology but also embed decolonial approaches in healing the trauma (Mignolo 2009; Hammell 2021; Hunter & Pride 2021; Gautier *et al.* 2022). The occupational therapy profession has a number of problems such as the use of models and frameworks with missed or dismissed occupations and the promotion of independence rather than interdependence (Hammell 2021). Some examples of missed or dismissed occupations include connections with ancestors and ancestral lands, gods and spirits, cultures and nature (Hammell 2021). These actions have perpetuated injustices and vulnerabilities that exist among people living in environments affected by disasters, pandemics, and degradation (Hammell 2021). Practice perspectives need to shift through generative disruption whereby a variety of ways of thinking and doing occupational therapy are considered to conserve human dignity, a sense of life coherence and continuity (Galvaan & van der Merwe 2021; Hammell 2021). Therefore, occupational therapists need to de-link from the Eurocentric biomedical models that are not considering the needs of the racialised and colonised people and families, as it perpetuates oppressive patterns of coloniality of knowledge, power and being (Maldonado-Torres 2007; Mignolo 2009).

In dismantling oppressive patterns of coloniality of being, occupational therapists need to have a better understanding of the socio-historical traumas and events that are still evident in different contexts. It is evident that social suffering and wounds of racism have been passed on through the generations, which indicates that trauma is situated within places including homes, workplace, relationships and bodies (Eichstaedt *et al.* 2021; Mthembu 2021; Atallah *et al.* 2022). For instance, racism is one of the structurally violent actions that result in physical, mental and spiritual injuries amongst communities, which exacerbates colonial wounds, rage, grief, and humiliation (Eichstaedt *et al.* 2021; Atallah *et al.* 2022). The South African legacy of trauma indicates that the psychic wounds of the past are passed down to the young generations, as part of the multiple wound phenomenon (Ngcaweni 2018; Basson & Wale 2019). Cabrera (2003) propounds that trauma and pains not only influence individuals but also the collectives in the communities. It has been highlighted that communities exposed to the multiple wounded phenomenon tend to experience intergenerational trauma (Cabrera 2003; Ngcaweni 2018). Multiple wounding indicates that there is a need for collective healing from the pain and trauma inherited (Cabrera 2003; Ngcaweni 2018). Therefore, it indicates that there is a need for occupational therapists to ensure that the individuals and communities whose existence is questioned and insignificant should be attended to by adopting a decolonial attitude and love, which highlights the willingness to consider different perspectives (Maldonado-Torres 2017).

THE ROLE OF OCCUPATIONAL THERAPY

SELF-CARE BY THE OCCUPATIONAL THERAPIST: CARING FOR OURSELVES SO THAT WE CAN CARE FOR OTHERS

The impact of working with people who have experienced trauma and adversity must not be overlooked, as '. . .hearing stories of trauma may change the way the professional sees the world around them. . .' (Brend *et al.* 2020, p. 127). Compassion fatigue is the state of tension or exhaustion due to working with people in pain and is often seen as the cost of working in professions that require high levels of empathy and care (Alers 2014; Brend *et al.* 2020). Compassion fatigue can result in physical, emotional, cognitive, spiritual and behavioural symptoms, which in turn can affect relationships with self, colleagues and clients as well as the care which is provided (Alers 2014; Burnett & Wahl 2015; Sorenson *et al.* 2016).

Working with traumatised people requires a well-resourced and resilient occupational therapist to ensure that the impact of the work is well-managed and the health and well-being of the occupational therapist are prioritised (Alers 2014). While this is necessary to ensure delivery of a high-quality therapy, it is also important to ensure the longevity of services provided by the occupational therapist by mitigating the impacts of compassion fatigue and burnout.

Self-care is a critical strategy for the prevention of compassion fatigue amongst health care professionals (Sorenson *et al.* 2016). Occupational therapists are well equipped to assist clients with self-care plans and strategies, and thus using their own skills for themselves is needed. Consideration of one's self-care in terms of physical, emotional, relational, spiritual and intellectual health and well-being can be helpful. Self-care strategies can include eating a healthy diet, resting properly, regular movement or exercise; attending supervision or therapy sessions; journaling or mindfulness practices; continuous learning; engaging in spiritual practices; building a support system; regularly connecting with families, friends and colleagues. Additionally, engaging in activities that recharge oneself and setting clear and healthy boundaries is key to practicing self-care.

ADOPTING A TRAUMA-INFORMED APPROACH

In recognising that trauma is pervasive and permeates throughout various sectors in society, a trauma-informed approach (TIA) has been developed as a multilevel and multi-sectoral response to address trauma's detrimental impacts (SAMHSA 2014; Fette *et al.* 2019). TIA is an overarching framework and model of care which acknowledges that individuals, families and communities have been affected by trauma and organises its services to integrate this understanding into its interventions, programmes, policies and culture (Champagne 2011; Branson *et al.* 2017; Keeshin *et al.* 2021). Using a trauma-informed lens, requires practitioners to assume that their clients, colleagues and communities have experienced trauma and that this may shape their behaviours and occupational engagement. By doing so, practitioners are able to shift from asking 'what is wrong with you?' which can often pathologise and problematise someone's behaviour, to 'what happened to you?' which allows the practitioner to listen with empathy and understanding rather than judgement.

TIA can be applied at various levels, that is, individual, programme, organisational, community or system (Champine *et al.* 2019). The TIA recognises that it is not only up to practitioners who work with traumatised people in the health and social development sectors to address the impact of trauma, but rather that each and every person at various levels has a role to play. Furthermore, TIA needs to be applied across multiple areas of society, such as educational institutions and the criminal justice system. For example, all staff members, at a mental health care clinic, should be aware of the pervasiveness of trauma and how it impacts people. Trauma awareness will ensure that all interactions with clients, from the first contact a person has with the service, right up to the policies and high-level decision-making, is informed by a TIA and clients are not re-traumatised during their use of the services (Branson *et al.* 2017).

The Four 'R's of a Trauma-informed Approach

TIA has four key elements which individuals, teams, organisations or communities need to consider when becoming trauma-informed, namely *realise, recognise, respond* and *resist re-traumatisation* (SAMHSA 2014). These can be applied in different ways depending on the context.

Everybody in a team, organisation or community needs to *realise* the extent of trauma, its pervasiveness and how it affects individuals and collectives. Realisation includes understanding types of trauma, its impacts and building awareness of potential paths for recovery (SAMHSA 2014; Champine *et al.* 2019; Fette *et al.* 2019).

Everybody needs to be able to *recognise* trauma's effects on individuals and collectives from a micro- to macro-level. Recognition improves understanding of people and their contexts enabling practitioners to *respond* more appropriately to meet clients' needs (Champagne 2011; SAMHSA 2014; Champine *et al.* 2019; Fette *et al.* 2019).

TIA acknowledges that in the same way that trauma impacts us all differently, there are numerous ways to *respond to* and heal from trauma. As an overarching approach, TIA goes beyond interventions provided within biopsychosocial models of health to encompass a multitude of services, activities and processes addressing the impact of trauma at different levels. While trauma-specific interventions, which provide assessment, treatment or recovery services, form a key part of TIA, this approach recognises that not everybody may have access to or require such interventions (SAMHSA 2014). Ways of responding that go beyond the individual to be able to create systems

which are trauma-informed are encouraged. A TIA proposes the application of six principles (SAMHSA 2014):

1. Safety
2. Trustworthiness and transparency
3. Peer support
4. Collaboration and mutuality
5. Empowerment, voice and choice
6. Cultural, historical and gender issues

Responding may include ensuring physical and emotional safety and self-care practices; intentionally building trust, connection and belonging; fostering support and collaboration; empowering people and providing choice. Integration of knowledge about trauma needs to be fully integrated into the policies, procedures and practices (Branson *et al.* 2017; Champine *et al.* 2019; Fette *et al.* 2019).

TIA aims to *resist re-traumatisation* of clients, staff and organisations. Examining practices and procedures which may inadvertently re-traumatize people or create toxic environments is essential to preventing re-traumatisation. Awareness of potential triggers is critical to ensure that processes do not disrupt client's recovery journey (SAMHSA 2014). Awareness of one's self as the practitioner is critical and this may include '. . . knowing your own history and reactions, being aware of the potential for secondary trauma, and knowing how to care for yourself . . .' (Fette *et al.* 2019, p. CE3).

Occupational therapy's holistic understanding of the person, their contexts and occupations positions the profession in synergy with a TIA. Fette *et al.* (2019) discuss the application of TIA across occupational therapy settings to include, early childhood settings, school settings, primary care settings, psychiatric settings, residential settings, and community settings. Through applying TIA, occupational therapists can '. . . tak[e] a non-pathological view of the people [they] serve through respecting the person, seeing their humanity, and empathizing with their experiences with pain' (Fette *et al.* 2019, p. CE6). Utilising the TIA 4Rs and principles occupational therapists can assist trauma survivors across the life span to move from coping and surviving to thriving within their contexts.

OCCUPATIONAL THERAPY INTERVENTION

A systematic review and meta-analysis that assessed the prevalence and determinants of PTSD among road traffic accidents (RTA) raised concern about the needs of survivors of a motor vehicle accident (MVA) (Mekonnen *et al.* 2022). It is evident that many people who receive a life-threatening diagnosis and those who experience psychological problems are prone to suffer from PTSD. Therefore, occupational therapists need to provide effective intervention for those who are suffering from PTSD and lasting adverse effects on the functioning, mental, physical, social, emotional or spiritual well-being (SAMHSA 2014).

CASE STUDY 2 — Individual with PTSD

Mrs S Nyandeni is a 47-year-old widow who resides in a low-resource community. She was employed as an administrator at a car dealership for 15 years and travelled there by bus. On her way to work, she was severely injured after an motor vehicle accident, which resulted in an above-knee amputation (AKA). Due to her length of hospitalisation, she struggled to provide for her school-going children as she was the sole provider in the family. This influenced Mrs Nyandeni as she lacked social support, having nobody that she could confide in for assistance during the trying times. After she was discharged from the hospital, Mrs Nyandeni tended to experience negative emotions related to the traumatic event and stress. Later, it was noted that Mrs Nyandeni developed post-traumatic stress disorder and she lacked coping strategies and abilities to deal with the trauma and other stresses, which affected her recovery process. Therefore, occupational therapy intervention for Mrs Nyandeni to be effective should be guided by the assessments, plan, implementation and review phases, which are covered next (AOTA 2020).

Assessments

An assessment is a process whereby occupational therapists attempt to ascertain 'what the client wants and needs to do; determining what the client can do and has done; and identifying supports and barriers to health, well-being, and participation' (AOTA 2020). There are non-standardised and standardised assessments that the occupational therapists should conduct with the individuals or communities depending on the practice settings. Non-standardised assessments include clinical interviews and observations, which are used to evaluate how trauma affected the survivors' and their families' activities related to Basic Activities of Daily Living (BADL), Instrumental Activities of Daily Living (IDAL), play, leisure, education, work, rest and sleep, health management and social participation (AOTA 2020). Occupational therapists may evaluate and analyse the performance skills such as social interaction (AOTA 2020). These assessments are expected to highlight the enablers, activity limitations and restrictions that influence the survivors' occupational engagement.

Standardised assessments are used as outcome measures administered to obtain a baseline of the survivors' performance and to monitor intervention effectiveness, progress and guide clinical decision-making (Law et al. 1990). Occupational therapists may use the World Health Organisation Disability Assessment Schedule 2.0 (WHODAS 2) to assesses the influence of trauma across six domains, including understanding and communicating, getting around, self-care, getting along with people, life activities (i.e. household, work, and/or school activities), and participation in society (WHO 2010). For mental health, Beck Depression Inventory (BDI) is a standardised outcome measure that can be used for depression (Beck et al. 1988) and PCL5 is a measure used to assess the 20 DSM 5 symptoms of PTSD (Weathers et al. 2013; Torchalla et al. 2019; Kerr et al. 2020). Results from the non-standardised and standardised assessments are used to construct an occupational profile of the individuals or community but also gain insight into 'functional limitations, strengths, and client-centered goals, past and present functioning in activities and participation, family and/or socioeconomic challenges' in preparation for a holistic intervention plan (Torchalla et al. 2019, p. 390). Occupational therapists may also perform the functional capacity evaluation (FCE) to assess the occupational history, job demands and vocational status as well as possibilities to return to work for the people living with PTSD (McArthur et al. 2013; Torchalla et al. 2019, p. 390; Kerr et al. 2020, p. 479).

Harmonious and Therapeutic Relationship

In serving others, occupational therapists need to establish harmonious and therapeutic relationships with individuals and collectives, which is grounded in the Ubuntu African ethic philosophy that espouses respect for conflicts of interests, personhood and solidarity with others (Ewuoso et al. 2021; Tolosa-Merlos et al. 2023). The therapeutic relationship should be enacted in a safe environment that is conducive to exploration of difficult sensations, feelings, emotions, and thoughts, which is facilitated in respect of dignity and personhood (Champagne 2011, p. CE4; Kornhaber et al. 2016). Therapeutic interpersonal engagement between occupational therapists and survivors of trauma and their families should enable rapport, listening, empathy, relating as equals, compassion, genuineness, trust, time responsiveness, and unconditional positive regard (Lees et al. 2014). Occupational therapists should also be present in the individuals' healing journey and listen to their concerns. However, an occupational therapist's self-disclosure in sessions can be productive, counterproductive or irrelevant. Self-disclosure should be done for modelling, validating the individual's reality and moving past an impasse (Alers 2014). Self-disclosures should be brief, judicious and authentic. A thoughtful 'here and now' response from the occupational therapist in order to clarify the interactions that are taking place is often preferable and more appropriate (Alers 2014). Their feelings are of utmost importance, and they need to have an empathetic individual to listen to them attentively. However, they must be cautious of compassion fatigue and overcommitment, which result in exhaustion, anger and irritability, negative coping behaviours, such as substance use, absenteeism, and presenteeism (Bonsaksen *et al.* 2021). Presenteeism is perceived as a reduced work functioning due to alcohol consumption (Bonsaksen *et al.* 2021).

Interventions with Individuals

In occupational therapy practice, occupational therapists need to incorporate the principles of the TIA (SAMHSA 2014). Interventions should include occupational therapy for post-traumatic disorder (PTSD), regeneration and healing arch through occupations (Torchalla *et al.* 2019; Avalos 2021) and trauma-focused psychodrama (Giacomucci & Marquit 2020; Giacomucci *et al.* 2022).

Occupational Therapy Interventions for PTSD
It is evident that the lack of training and support for PTSD interventions in occupational therapy profession tend to affect therapists' confidence (Clarke 1999; Finch *et al.* 2020). However, occupational therapists may attempt to bridge the gap by using available evidence to guide their clinical decision-making and interventions (Lindström & Bernhardsson 2018). PTSD disconnects the mind, body and spirit (Althaver 2020) and interferes with occupational performance (Edgelow *et al.* 2019). Therefore, occupational therapists have insight into clients' occupational profiles; as a result, they can set goals, plan and implement interventions in collaboration with the clients and their families (Althaver 2020). Research has shown that occupational therapy intervention for people living with PTSD should focus on a variety of areas (Clarke 1999; Gerardi 2017). The areas include stress management (relaxation and anger management); social skills (effective verbal and non-verbal communication, assertiveness training and time management); cognitive skills (decision-making, problem-solving and coping skills) and healthy living skills (promoting a sense of well-being and physical health) (Clarke 1999, p. 137; Gerardi 2017, p. 76). These interventions will enable clients to maximise their adaptive behaviours and coping strategies (Clarke 1999; Britt *et al.* 2017). Occupational therapists may also focus on the different coping strategies such as problem-focused, emotion-focused, and avoidant coping (Britt *et al.* 2017; Althaver 2020). In problem-focused coping, occupational therapists should collaborate with the clients and their families to address environmental stressors (Britt *et al.* 2017). Regarding emotion-focused coping, occupational therapists need to enable clients to try to manage their emotions triggered by the environmental stressors (Britt *et al.* 2017). Concerning avoidant coping, occupational therapists may assist clients to avoid the environmental

stressors and emotions linked to the stressors (Britt *et al.* 2017). However, Althaver (2020) cautions that avoidance tends to influence clients' health outcomes. Therefore, it was suggested that proactive coping should be used in the treatment of tr,uma, which is perceived as a 'set of multidimensional and forward-looking strategies that integrates processes of personal quality of life management with those of self-regulatory goal attainment' (Zambianchi & Bitti 2014, p. 497).

Proactive coping strategies involve coping skills and symptoms training in enhancing personal skills needed for action areas that enable survivors to engage in occupational decision-making based on their occupational choices. This is imperative in occupational therapy practice because recognising signs and symptoms in clients, families, staff, and others involved in the system will assist in dealing with the circumstances. Therefore, occupational therapists should help individuals with PTSD to validate and normalise their emotions by accepting and tolerating emotional distress and unpleasant sensations (Gone 2009; Torchalla *et al.* 2019). It is important that occupational therapists should collaborate with the survivors in setting the plan of action by incorporating the zone of regulation to facilitate the healing process and connection with their emotions (Katz 2012; SAMHSA 2014). The Zone of Regulation provides survivors with opportunities to hone their self- and emotional-regulation skills so that they can move through four colour-code zones. In the red zone, survivors' emotions are so intense to the extent that they may feel out of control. In the yellow zone, survivors' emotions are less intense to the point that they cannot deal with their situations; however, they have some control. In the green zone, survivors are able to experience calmness and alertness, which enables them to engage in their multiple areas of occupation to promote their quality of life and well-being. However, the blue zone is perceived as a low state of alertness among survivors, which results in poor participation and completion of tasks. In transitioning between the zones, the survivors learn to employ their emotional and cognitive skills so that they may adjust when dealing with the environmental and social demands. Transitions within the zones may facilitate coping and adaptive strategies that the survivors need to deal with their emotions and live a healthy life (Crider *et al.* 2015). Therefore, occupational therapists contribute to the continuity of occupation that survivors may need to buffer the hardships associated with the transition within the zones. It is evident that the survivors might experience emotions such as frustration, confusion, fear, anxiety, and grief as they transition through the zones. Occupational therapists also design interventions to enable survivors to cultivate self-advocacy and regulation skills needed for the occupation of social participation with family, friends and communities in different zones.

CASE STUDY 3

In a 'youth at risk' group in Ivory Park, a densely populated area in the Gauteng province in South Africa, a male member's girlfriend passed away due to human immunodeficiency virus/acquired immunodeficiency syndrome (HIV/AIDS). Her parents had custody of their child, and as the father of the child, the male member was not allowed visiting rights. There were complex cultural issues involved, one being that the father needed to respect the girlfriend's parents and thus could not 'make demands of older people'. During psychodrama sessions facilitated by the occupational therapist, the man concretised his strengths, being able to role-play an interaction to externalise his righteous anger about the situation. Opportunity was created for him to psychodramatically discuss with his girlfriend in the 'here and now'. As a result, he was able to view the situation from a different perspective without shame or blame. By using the observing ego card, the occupational therapist created a space for the man to pick an animal card, object/scarf that represents his ego and then reverse roles to allow different perspectives while considering his rights as a father. With the support of other group members, he immediately depicted his strengths in his Trauma Survivor's Intrapsychic Role Atom (TSIRA) by constructing a cake box as an art project, which is considered as a soul portrait that was displayed in the therapy room (Giacomucci 2018). He asked if he could keep his personal strength scarf that had emerged from the drama for the following week. This personal strength was 'a good-enough father'. The support from the group was truly tangible and later resulted on to the father of the child approaching the girlfriend's parents for visitation rights in a culturally acceptable manner. He embraced the strength of a 'good-enough father', which led him to involve the elders of his family to communicate with the parents of his late girlfriend in an appropriate manner that showed respect (Alers 2014).

Regeneration and Healing Arc Through Occupations The aim of occupational therapy for survivors of trauma is to regenerate not only healthy human-to-human relationships but also healthy human-to-environment relationships, which supports engagement in occupations and activities (Dunn et al. 1994; Clarke 1999; Gerardi 2017; Edgelow et al. 2019). Therefore, occupational therapists need to promote health and well-being of people living with PTSD and psychological problems by providing opportunities for creative expression of emotions through engagement in goal-directed meaningful activities (Gerardi 2017; Edgelow et al. 2019). Evidence indicates that occupational therapists can provide effective intervention for individuals who are exposed to trauma and develop PTSD by focusing on their occupational roles, habits and routine (Gerardi 2017; Hammell 2017; Torchalla et al. 2019; Edgelow et al. 2019). The intervention should promote post-traumatic growth and resilience as well as the healthy lifestyle choices so that clients can transition through their challenges (Gerardi 2017). Occupational therapists can use strategies that enable the establishment of new skills and restore the skills that trauma survivors lost due to their life-threatening events. Additionally, occupational therapists may use an altered intervention strategy to plan change in a specific context where the survivors can perform different tasks related to multiple areas of occupation. The multiple areas of occupation not only limited to BADL, IADL, play, leisure, education, work, health management, rest and sleep, social participation but also self-care activities, contemplative, contributing, connecting, centering and creative occupations (Thibeault 2011; Torchalla et al. 2019; AOTA 2020). Occupational therapists have responsibilities to reactivate and reconnect survivors with healthy self-care activities such as regular exercises, relaxation, mindfulness practices, sleeping hygiene strategies and optimal nutrition (Torchalla et al. 2019). Consequently, survivors who engage in valued and meaningful activities may also foster a sense of normalcy and routine in their lives (Torchalla et al. 2019). By enabling the survivors' and communities' occupational potentials to engage in the multiple areas of occupation, occupational therapists will facilitate the healing process and promote recovery from trauma, which fosters empowerment. Occupations can be performed in a context that is made up of physical, temporal, social and cultural aspects. However, it needs to be noted that the contexts can be both enabling and restricting to the performance of the survivors of trauma.

Drawing upon the healing value of traditional cultural connections, occupational therapists may need to collaborate with other disciplines, community healthcare works, traditional leaders and faith-based organizations to address historical trauma and return survivors to their sense of identity and positive orientation in the universe (Avalos 2021). The healing arc that occupational therapy can take into consideration in treating trauma acknowledges individual, group and community levels (Avalos 2021). Everyone has a role to play in a TIA, as part of collaboration and mutuality (SAMHSA 2014), which is consistent with Hammell's (2017) explanation of well-being as the need:

> 'to experience a sense of belonging and connectedness to families, friends, and communities, and perhaps also to the natural world, to cultural and spiritual traditions, and to ancestors and ancestral lands, and the intrinsic need and responsibility to care for and contribute to the well-being of these others'. (p. 211)

Evidence suggests that traditional values and ceremonial life are among the most important factors for enhancing healthy relationships with one's self and social body as a whole (Gone 2009; Avalos 2021). The social body comprises 'the natural world and all living within it, human and other-than-human, such as plants and animals, but also one's ancestors' (Avalos 2021, p. 496). Considering the social body is significant for occupational therapists who provide trauma-informed intervention because they will need to avail a safe space for interpersonal interactions and promote a sense of safety (SAMHSA 2014). Occupational therapists may build therapeutic relationships with clients, families, staff and other stakeholders, which is governed by the principle of trustworthiness and transparency. It is for this reason that healing is a relational process that allows survivors to connect with others and their wounds and pain emanating from the exposure to trauma (Gone 2009; Avalos 2021). For instance, a discovery-oriented methodology such as that conducted by Gone (2009) has shown that meaning of healing from historical trauma involves 'emotional burdens, cathartic disclosure, self-as-project reflexivity, and impact of colonisation' (p. 755).

Trauma-focused Psychodrama Developments in mental health have heightened the need for occupational therapists to enhance their competencies and confidence in treating people with PTSD (Alers 2008; Finch *et al.* 2020). It has been reported that treatment modalities such as action methods, psychodrama, projective techniques and guided imagery are effective in aiding the trauma survivor to process the trauma material from the right brain and give accurate labelling, via the left brain (Hudgins 2002). For instance, psychodrama has been found to be effective in reducing the symptoms of PTSD (Alers 2008; Giacomucci & Marquit 2020; Giacomucci *et al.* 2022). Van der Kolk in Wylie (2004) explains that 'talk therapy' only accesses the left brain and that theatre work involves movement, thus integrating the left and right brain functions to access the trauma memories and make meaning of them (Alers 2014). Even though psychodrama is equally effective at reducing PTSD, occupational therapists need further training under supervision to enhance their competence in using the psychodynamic approaches.

Intervention with Collectives

There are processes used to address traumas and occupational injustices that influence groups and communities as collectives. Regarding occupational group therapy with a collective, occupational therapists have diverse skills and modalities to enable the trauma survivor to access or process trauma material, which is not accessed normally in traditional talk therapy due to Broca's area shutting down during the incident. The conceptual use of strengths and strength-building throughout the treatment is essential to promote self-affirmation.

The concept of the observing ego is effective in putting perspective on to the situation in the here and now and viewing the self with more clarity (Alers 2014). The facilitation of Yalom and Leszcz's (2005) curative factors (altruism, cohesion, universality, interpersonal learning input and output, guidance, catharsis, identification, family re-enactment, self-understanding, instillation of hope and existential) within the groups are the foundation and cornerstones of successful occupational group therapy with trauma survivors. It is imperative for the group therapist to facilitate universality, instillation of hope, cohesion and existential factors to get the desired outcomes with trauma survivors (Jelly Beanz Inc 2013; Alers 2014). Occupations are incorporated in occupation-focused group-work as both a means and an end in facilitating health, and promoting participation in meaningful life roles (Occupational Therapy Association South Africa 2014). Social participation with family, peers and community tends to be affected by the traumatic events; therefore, occupational therapists need to ensure that they address the survivors' social skills by using psychosocial interactive approach with activities to facilitate reconnections, interpersonal relationships, coping skills and a sense of belonging (Mthembu *et al.* 2017).

It is important to note that a traumatised community is '. . . more than a collection of traumatised individuals. Rather, they are communities that have a history of disenfranchisement and oppression and that disproportionately carry the burden of structural violence' (Illinois ACEs Response Collaborative 2019, p. 2). In responding to the community needs such as those highlighted in Case Study 1, occupational therapists need to shift to authentic connectedness with communities and create possibilities for enacting human occupation in an environment that is conducive (Galvaan 2021; Galvaan & van der Merwe 2021). Authentic connectedness will enable occupational therapists to collaborate with the community members for collective commitment to understanding the voices of those who were subjugated, ignored and made invisible by the social systems such as colonialism and apartheid (Mignolo 2007; Allegretti & Magalhães 2022). In doing praxis for addressing the colonial matrix of power to be and do, occupational therapists need to employ participatory action learning methodologies that are grounded in the decolonial perspectives (Galvaan 2021; Galvaan & van der Merve 2021). Occupational therapists may use Occupation-based Community Development (ObCD) as a framework developed by the University of Cape Town (Galvaan & Peters 2013). It is envisaged that ObCD could assist occupational therapists to address the traumas in communities.

Applying Trauma-informed Approaches to Collectives

Application of TIA within collectives like teams, organisations or communities necessitates a thorough knowledge of organisational and community development practice principles to ensure that the approach is appropriately embedded within the culture over time. The complex nature of trauma and its impacts on people and systems requires an interdisciplinary intervention to address the various facets, which may include organisational and community development practitioners, psychologists and occupational therapists. A partnership between the service provider and receiver is crucial to ensure co-created and co-designed processes, thus enabling ownership and agency.

As an emerging role for the profession, the occupational therapist brings valuable expertise to the interdisciplinary team, including a holistic understanding of people, impact of environments and contexts on occupational engagement, sensory processing and self-regulation skills, group work and facilitation skills, building safe and containing spaces, and use of occupations as a means and an end and community development practice and occupational justice.

An assessment process is important to understand what the main issues and generative themes are and to explore already existing trauma-informed practices. Through the use of the trauma-informed four 'R's

(SAMHSA 2014), processes can be facilitated with teams, whole organisations, or groups within communities. Enabling people to realise and recognise the effects of trauma allows people to understand their contexts and make sense of their own and others' reactions and responses. By exploring ways of responding, beyond only that of trauma-specific interventions, which are culturally driven, focused on strengthening human connections between people, enabling self- and co-regulation, addressing issues of safety, and reviewing policies, processes and procedures is key. Through application of TIA and self-care practices, re-traumatisation can be resisted. As issues of historical trauma are rarely apolitical, addressing issues of power within the contexts is also key to resisting re-traumatisation.

Interventions of this nature need to run over an extended period suchas one to three years, allowing clients time to process and integrate knowledge shared; to implement, evaluate and re-implement plans; access support; and make fundamental shifts in organisational cultures. Through committing to trauma-informed processes for collectives, the legacies of historical traumas which are experienced in our societies can be addressed.

| CASE STUDY 4 | Application of a Trauma-Informed Approach |

An occupational therapist was part of a team assisting a child and youth care centre[1] in South Africa to adopt a TIA. This proces ran over a period of two years and focused on interventions with the staff specifically. Staff comprised of the centre manager, social worker, programme manager, centre supervisor and child and youth care workers. Two needs were identified, namely to equip staff with an understanding of how social trauma[2] affects themselves and the young people in the centre and to equip staff with skills to implement a TIA in the centre.

The trauma-informed four R's were used to guide this specific intervention. Training took place to assist the staff to realise the extent of social trauma and recognise its effects on themselves and the young people. This was important as the staff and young people came from different backgrounds and had experienced varying levels of trauma during their lives. Collectively, they had also experienced high levels of stress during the COVID-19 pandemic, which resulted in the staff using strategies to 'cope' within their context. Training also looked at how to respond collectively and resist re-traumatization to create positive emotional climates and assist the centre to move out of 'survival' mode to being able to thrive within the challenging context. This included development of a trauma-informed plan for the centre, assisting the staff with self-care plans and self- and co-regulation strategies, reviewing the centre's high-stress times (within

a 24-h cycle) and implementing strategies to manage this, strengthening connection and belonging and addressing issues of power in the staff team.

Regular support processes, either group or one-on-one, were provided during implementation and included ongoing reflections and evaluations on progress. Workshops and sessions were participatory, experiential and used principles of adult education and popular education methodologies. The facilitators worked closely with the staff member leading the TIA intervention to ensure that the process was co-created. Where needed, staff were referred for additional therapeutic support.

Outcomes of the intervention included staff being better equipped to manage their stress levels and understand young people's behaviours and respond in trauma-informed ways; review of day-to-day processes and implementing strategies to mitigate high levels of stress in the centre; strengthening emotional safety and connection and belonging; implementation of regular staff check-ins, breaks and wellness days; using TIA principles in youth development; and restructuring of the management team.

---

[1] A child and youth care centre is a term used in South Africa for an orphanage.
[2] Social trauma includes historical, intergenerational and collective trauma.

CONCLUSION

Occupational therapists working in the trauma field have a role to play in promoting the health and well-being of mental health users. The evidence from this chapter rovides strategies for occupational therapists to promote the importance of occupation-based intervention when working with people in a holistic manner. This work contributes to existing knowledge of occupational therapy practice by providing effective trauma-informed interventions geared towards emotional, spiritual, physical, psychological and functional being of the individual as well as their families and communities. Therefore, occupational therapists need to be part of the interdisciplinary team that enables trauma survivors to reconnect with their lives. With confidence, experience and expertise, occupational therapists can take their rightful place in the treatment of trauma survivors at an individual and collective level TIA and principles should be integrated into occupational therapy intervention, which is grounded in a therapeutic relationship and engagement in occupations. The decolonial epistemic approach should be used to address the hegemonies that influence occupational engagement of the oppressed individuals and collectives.

QUESTIONS

1. Describe the importance of considering the root causes of ACEs.

2. What are the different types of trauma?

3. How can the conceptual model of historical trauma be used to address the influences on occupations?

4. How can compassion fatigue impact our work as occupational therapists?

5. Describe the our 'R's of a Trauma-informed Approach.

6. Which assessments should be in occupational therapy practice with trauma survivors?

7. Describe the Yalom curative fators that can be used in occupational group therapy.

8. What are the occupational science constructs that occupational therapists may adopt as part of their collective intervention?

ACKNOWLEDGEMENT

The authors would like to acknowledge the contributions of the late Vyvian Alers, who was the author of the chapter *Trauma and Its Effects on Children, Adolescents and Adults: The Role of the Occupational Therapist* in the fifth edition of this book. Sections from the previous chapter have been incorporated and referenced in the current chapter.

REFERENCES

Alers, V. (2008) The 20th Vona du Toit Memorial Lecture 2007: proposing the social atom of occupational therapy: dealing with trauma as part of an integrated inclusive intervention. *South African Journal of Occupational Therapy,* **38**(3), 3–10.

Alers, V. (2014) Trauma and its effects on children, adolescents and adults: the roles of the occupational therapist. In: R. Crouch & V. Alers (eds), *Occupational Therapy in Psychiatry and Mental Health,* 5th edn. pp. 337–355. Wiley, Hoboken.

Alexander, P., Lekgowa, T., Mmope, B., Sinwell, L. & Xezwi, B. (2012) *Marikana – A View from the Mountain and a Case to Answer.* Jacana Media, Johannesburg.

Alexander, P. (2016) Marikana commission of inquiry: From narratives towards history. *Journal of Southern African Studies,* **42**(5), 815–839. https://doi.org/10.1080/03057070.2016.1223477

Allegretti, M. & Magalhães, L. (2022) A mosaic of experiences and narratives about collective practices in occupational therapy: methodological considerations. *Cadernos Brasileiros de Terapia Ocupacional,* **30**, e3163. https://doi.org/10.1590/2526-8910.ctoAO2426316302

Althaver, M. (2020) *Treating Trauma: The Occupational Therapy Perspective.* Senior Honors Projects, Bridgewater College. https://digitalcommons .bridgewater.edu/cgi/viewcontent.cgi?article=1014&context=honors_ projects (accessed 20 May 2023)

Amene, E.W., Annor, F.B. & Gilbert, L.K. *et al* (2023) Prevalence of adverse childhood experiences in sub-Saharan Africa: a multi-county analysis of the violence against children and youth surveys (VACS). *Child Abuse & Neglect,* 106353. https://doi.org/10.1016/j. chiabu.2023.106353

American Occupational Therapy Association (2020) Occupational therapy practice framework: domain and process—fourth edition. *American Journal of Occupational Therapy,* **74** (**Supplement_2**), 7412410010p1–7412410010p87. https://doi.org/10.5014/ajot.2020.74S2001

American Occupational Therapy Association (AOTA) (2018) AOTA's societal statement on stress, trauma, and posttraumatic stress disorder. *American Journal of Occupational Therapy,* **72**, 1–3. https://doi .org/10.5014/ajot.2018.72S208

American Psychiatric Association (APA) (2013) *Diagnostic and Statistical Manual of Mental Disorders,* 5th edn. APA, Washington, DC.

American Psychiatric Association (APA) (2022) *Diagnostic and Statistical Manual of Mental Disorders,* 5th edn, text revision, APA, Washington, DC.

American Psychological Association (2023) *Trauma.* https://www.apa. org/topics/trauma#:~:text=Trauma%20is%20an%20emotional%20 response,symptoms%20like%20headaches%20or%20nausea (accessed 22 February 2023)

Anda, R.F., Porter, L.E. & Brown, D.W. (2020) Inside the adverse childhood experience score: strengths, limitations, and misapplications. *American Journal of Preventive Medicine*, **59**(2), 293–295. https://doi.org/10.1016/j.amepre.2020.01.009

Atallah, D.G., Dutta, U. & Masud, H.R. *et al* (2022) Transnational research collectives as "constellations of co-resistance": counter storytelling, interweaving struggles, and decolonial love. *Qualitative Inquiry*, **28**(6), 681–693. https://doi.org/10.1177/10778004211068202

Avalos, N. (2021) What does it mean to heal from historical trauma? *American Medical Associations Journal of Ethics*, **23**(6), E494–E498. https://doi.org/10.1001/amajethics.2021.494

Bailey, J.A., Jacoby, S.F., Hall, E.C., Khatri, U., Whitehorn, G. & Kaufman, E.J. (2022) Compounding trauma: the intersections of racism, law enforcement, and injury. *Current Trauma Reports*, **8**, 105–112. https://doi.org/10.1007/s40719-022-00231-7

Barron, I. & Abdallah, G. (2015) Intergenerational trauma in the occupied Palestinian territories: effect on children and promotion of healing. *Journal of Child & Adolescent Trauma*, **8**(2), 103–110. https://doi.org/10.1007/s40653-015-0046-z

Basson, A. & Wale, K. (2019cited 15 February 2023) *SA has a legacy of trauma, the mail & guardian*. https://mg.co.za/article/2019-09-20-00-sa-has-a-legacy-of-trauma/ (accessed 15 February 2023)

Beck, A.T., Steer, R.A. & Carbin, M.G. (1988) Psychometric properties of the beck depression inventory: twenty-five years of evaluation. *Clinical Psychology Review*, **8**(1), 77–100. https://doi.org/10.1016/0272-7358(88)90050-5

Behari-Leak, K. (2019) Decolonial turns, postcolonial shifts, and cultural connections: are we there yet? *English Academy Review*, **36**(1), 58–68. https://doi.org/10.1080/10131752.2019.1579881

Benjamin, L. & Fourie, M.M. (2019) The intergenerational effects of mass trauma in sculpting new perpetrators. In: S.C. Knittel & Z.J. Goldberg (eds), *The Routledge International Handbook of Perpetrator Studies*, pp. 276–286. Routledge eBooks.

Benya, A. (2015) The invisible hands: women in Marikana. *Review of African Political Economy*, **42**(146), 545–560. http://doi.org/10.1080/03056244.2015.1087394

Bombay, A., Matheson, K. & Anisman, H. (2014) The intergenerational effects of Indian residential schools: implications for the concept of historical trauma. *Transcultural Psychiatry*, **51**(3), 320–338. https://doi.org/10.1177/1363461513503380

Bonsaksen, T., Thørrisen, M.M., Skogen, J.C., Hesse, M. & Aas, R.W. (2021) Are demanding job situations associated with alcohol-related presenteeism?, the WIRUS-screening study. *International Journal Environmental Research Public Health*, **18**, 6169. https://doi.org/10.3390/ijerph18116169

Branson, C.E., Baetz, C.L., Horwitz, S.M. & Hoagwood, K.E. (2017) Trauma-informed juvenile justice systems: a systematic review of definitions and core components. *Psychological Trauma: Theory, Research, Practice, and Policy*, **9**(6), 635–646. https://doi.org/10.1037/tra0000255

Brave Heart, M. (2003) The historical trauma response among natives and its relationship with substance abuse: a lakota illustration. *Journal of Psychoactive Drugs*, **35**(1), 7–13. https://doi.org/10.1080/02791072.2003.10399988

Brend, D.M., Krane, J. & Saunders, S. (2020) Exposure to trauma in intimate partner violence human service work: a scoping review. *Traumatology*, **26**(1), 127–136. https://doi.org/10.1037/trm0000199

Britt, T.W., Adler, A.B., Sawhney, G. & Bliese, P.D. (2017) Coping strategies as moderators of the association between combat exposure and posttraumatic stress disorder symptoms. *Journal of Traumatic Stress*, **30**(5), 491–501. https://doi.org/10.1002/jts.22221

Brown, T. (2021) The response to COVID-19: occupational resilience and the resilience of daily occupations in action. *Australian Occupational Therapy Journal*, **68**(2), 103–105. https://doi.org/10.1111/1440-1630.12721

Burnett, H.J. & Wahl, K. (2015) The compassion fatigue and resilience connection: a survey of resilience, compassion fatigue, burnout, and compassion satisfaction among trauma responders. *International Journal of Emergency Mental Health*, **17**(1) https://doi.org/10.4172/1522-4821.1000165

Cabrera, M. (2003) *Living and surviving in a multiply wounded country. Paper presented at the University of Klagenfurt*. Klagenfurt. https://www.medico.de/download/report26/ps_cabrera_en.pdf (accessed 8 March 2023)

Cairncross, E. & Kisting, S. (2016) Platinum and gold mining in South Africa: the context of the Marikana massacre. *New Solutions: A Journal of Environmental and Occupational Policy*, **25**(4), 513–534. http://doi.org/10.1177/1048291115622027

Carra, K., Hyett, N., Kenny, A. & Curtin, M. (2019) Strengthening occupational therapy practice with communities after traumatic events. *British Journal of Occupational Therapy*, **82**(5), 316–319. https://doi.org/10.1177/0308022618795594

Centers for Disease Control and Prevention (CDC) (2019) *Preventing Adverse Childhood Experiences: Leveraging the Best Available Evidence*. National Center for Injury Prevention and Control, Centers for Disease Control and Prevention, Atlanta, GA.

Centers for Disease Control and Prevention (CDC) (2021) *Adverse Childhood Experiences Prevention Strategy*. National Center for Injury Prevention and Control, Centers for Disease Control and Prevention, Atlanta, GA.

Champagne, T. (2011) Attachment, trauma, and occupational therapy practice. *OT Practice*, **16**(5), CE1–CE8.

Champine, R.B., Lang, J.M., Nelson, A.M., Hanson, R.F. & Tebes, J.K. (2019) Systems measures of a trauma-informed approach: a systematic review. *American Journal of Community Psychology*, **64**(3–4), 418–437. https://doi.org/10.1002/ajcp.12388

Chauke, T.A. (2023) Strategies adopted by not in education, employment, or training youth in dealing with the psychological and emotional stress caused by COVID-19. *Progression*, **43**(2022), 15. https://doi.org/10.25159/2663-5895/11966

Clarke, C. (1999) Treating post-traumatic stress disorder: occupational therapist or counsellor. *British Journal of Occupational Therapy*, **62**(3), 136–138.

Conroy, J. & Perryman, K.L. (2022) Treating trauma with child-centered play therapy through the SECURE lens of polyvagal theory. *International Journal of Play Therapy*, **31**(3), 143–152. https://doi.org/10.1037/pla0000172

Crider, C., Calder, C.R., Bunting, K.L. & Forwell, S. (2015) An integrative review of occupational science and theoretical literature exploring transition. *Journal of Occupational Science*, **22**(3), 304–319. https://doi.org/10.1080/14427591.2014.922913

Dunn, W., Brown, C. & McGuigan, A. (1994) The ecology of human performance: a framework for considering the effect of context. *American Journal of Occupational Therapy*, **48**, 595–607. https://doi.org/10.5014/ajot.48.7.595

Eagle, G. & Kaminer, D. (2013) Continuous traumatic stress: expanding the lexicon of traumatic stress. *Peace and Conflict: Journal of Peace Psychology*, **19**(2), 85–99. https://doi.org/10.1037/a0032485

Edgelow, M.M., MacPherson, M.M., Arnaly, F., Tam-Seto, L. & Cramm, H.A. (2019) Occupational therapy and posttraumatic stress disorder: a scoping review. *Canadian Journal of Occupational Therapy*, **86**(2), 148–157. https://doi.org/10.1177/0008417419831438

Ehlers, C.L., Yehuda, R., Gilder, D.A., Bernert, R. & Karriker-Jaffe, K.J. (2022) Trauma, historical trauma, PTSD and suicide in an American Indian community sample. *Journal of Psychiatric Research*, **156**, 214–220. https://doi.org/10.1016/j.jpsychires.2022.10.012

Eichstaedt, J.C., Sherman, G.T., Giorgi, S., Roberts, S.O., Reynolds, M.E., Ungar, L.H. & Guntuku, S.C. (2021) The emotional and mental health impact of the murder of George Floyd on the US population. *Proceedings of the National Academy of Sciences of the United States of America*, **118**(39), e2109139118. https://doi.org/10.1073/pnas.2109139118

Ellis, W.R. & Dietz, W.H. (2017) A new framework for addressing adverse childhood and community experiences: the building community resilience model. *Academic Pediatrics*, **17**(7), S86–S93. https://doi.org/10.1016/j.acap.2016.12.011

Ellis, W.E., Dietz, W.H. & Chen, K.-L. (2022) Community resilience: a dynamic model for public health 3.0. *Journal of Public Health Management and Practice*, **28** (**Supplement 1**), S18–S26. https://doi.org/10.1097/phh.0000000000001413

Evans-Campbell T. (2008) Historical trauma in American Indian/Native Alaska communities: a multilevel framework for exploring impacts on individuals, families, and communities. *Journal of Interpersonal Violence*, **23**(3), 316–338. https://doi.org/10.1177/0886260507312290

Ewuoso, C., Fayemi, A.K. & Aramesh, K. (2021) *Ubuntu* ethics and moral problems in traditional bone-healing. *Journal of Global Health Reports*, **5**, e2021032. https://doi.org/10.29392/001c.21958

Felitti, V.J. & Anda, R.F. (2010) *The Relationship of Adverse Childhood Experiences to Adult Medical Disease, Psychiatric Disorders and Sexual Behavior: Implications for Healthcare*. Cambridge University Press eBooks, 77–87. https://doi.org/10.1017/cbo9780511777042.010

Felitti, V.J., Anda, R.F. & Nordenberg, D. *et al* (1998) Relationship of childhood abuse and household dysfunction to many of the leading causes of death in adults: the adverse childhood experiences (ACE) study. *American Journal of Preventive Medicine*, **14**(4), 245–258.

Fette, C., Lambdin-Pattavina, C. & Weaver, L.L. (2019) *Understanding and Applying Trauma-Informed Approaches Across Occupational Therapy Settings. AOTA Continuing Education Article, CE1-9.*

Finch, J., Ford, C., Lombardo, C. & Meiser-Stedman, R. (2020) A survey of evidence-based practice, training, supervision and clinician confidence relating to post-traumatic stress disorder (PTSD) therapies in UK child and adolescent mental health professionals. *European Journal of Psychotraumatology*, **11**(1), 1815281. https://doi.org/10.1080/20008198.2020.181528

Fortuna, L.R., Tobón, A.L., Anglero, Y.L., Postlethwaite, A., Porche, M.V. & Rothe, E.M. (2022) Focusing on racial, historical and intergenerational trauma, and resilience. *Child and Adolescent Psychiatric Clinics of North America*, **31**(2), 237–250. https://doi.org/10.1016/j.chc.2021.11.004

Galovski, T.E., Peterson, Z.A., Beagley, M.C., Strasshofer, D.R., Held, P. & Fletcher, T.D. (2016) Exposure to violence during Ferguson protests: mental health effects for law enforcement and community members. *Journal of Traumatic Stress*, **29**, 283–292.

Galvaan, R. (2021) Generative disruption through occupational science: enacting possibilities for deep human connection. *Journal of Occupational Science*, **28**(1), 6–18. https://doi.org/10.1080/14427591.2020.1818276

Galvaan, R. & Peters, L. (2013) *Occupation-based community development framework*. https://vula.uct.ac.za/access/content/group/9c29ba04-blee-49b9-8c85-9a468b556ce2/OBCDF/index.html (accessed 23 February 2018)

Galvaan, R. & van der Merwe, T.R. (2021) Re-orienting occupational therapy: embracing generative disruption and revisiting a posture that acknowledges human dignity. *South African Journal of Occupational Therapy*, **51**(2), 99–103. https://dx.doi.org/10.17159/2310-3833/2021/vol51n2a13

Gautier, L., Karambé, Y., Dossou, J. & Samb, O.M. (2022) Rethinking development interventions through the lens of decoloniality in sub-Saharan Africa: the case of global health. *Global Public Health*, **17** 2, 180–193, https://doi.org/10.1080/17441692.2020.1858134

Gerardi, S.M. (2017) *Development of a consensus-based occupational therapy treatment for veterans with combat-related posttraumatic stress disorders: a Delphi study*. PhD Thesis, Texas Woman's University. https://twu-ir.tdl.org/bitstream/handle/11274/9382/2017Gerardi.pdf?sequence=1&isAllowed=y (accessed 20 May 2023)

Giacomucci, S. (2018) Trauma survivor's inner role atom: a clinical map for posttraumatic growth. *The Journal of Psychodrama Sociometry, and Group Psychotherapy, 66*(1), 115–129. https://doi.org/10.12926/18-00006.1

Giacomucci, S. & Marquit, J. (2020) The effectiveness of trauma-focused psychodrama in the treatment of PTSD in inpatient substance abuse treatment. *Frontiers in Psychology*, **11**, 896. https://doi.org/10.3389/fpsyg.2020.00896

Giacomucci, S., Marquit, J., Walsh, K.M. & Saccarelli, R. (2022) A mixed-methods study on psychodrama treatment for PTSD and depression in inpatient substance use treatment: a comparison of outcomes pre-pandemic and during Covid-19. *The Arts in Psychotherapy*, **81**, 101971, https://doi.org/10.1016/j.aip.2022.101971

Gillson, S.L. & Ross, D.A. (2019) From generation to generation: rethinking "soul wounds" and historical trauma. *Biological Psychiatry*, **86**(7), e19–e20. https://doi.org/10.1016/j.biopsych.2019.07.033

Gone, J.P. (2009) A community-based treatment for Native American historical trauma: prospects for evidence-based practice. *Journal of Consulting and Clinical Psychology*, **77**(4), 751–762. https://doi.org/10.1037/a0015390

Gultekin, L., Kusunoki, Y., Sinko, L. *et al* (2019) The eco-social trauma intervention model. *Public Health Nursing (Boston, Mass.)*, **36**(5), 709–715. https://doi.org/10.1111/phn.12619

Hammell, K.W. (2017) Opportunities for well-being: the right to occupational engagement. *Canadian Journal of Occupational Therapy*, **84**(4–5), 209–222. https://doi.org/10.1177/0008417417734831

Hammell, K.W. (2021) Building back better: imagining an occupational therapy for a post-COVID-19 world. *Australian Occupational Therapy Journal*, **68**(5), 444–453. https://doi.org/10.1111/1440-1630.12760

Heart, M.Y.H.B., Chase, J., Elkins, J. & Altschul, D.B. (2011) Historical trauma among indigenous peoples of the Americas: concepts, research, and clinical considerations. *Journal of Psychoactive Drugs*, **43**(4), 282–290. https://doi.org/10.1080/02791072.2011.628913

Hocking, C. (2017) Occupational justice as social justice: the moral claim for inclusion. *Journal of Occupational Science,* **24**(1), 29–42. https://doi.org/10.1080/14427591.2017.1294016

Hudgins, K.M. (2002) *Experiential Treatment for P.T.S.D. The Therapeutic Spiral Model,* p. 224. Springer Publishing Co, New York.

Hunter, C. & Pride, T. (2021) Critiquing the Canadian model of client-centered enablement (CMCE) for indigenous contexts. *Canadian Journal of Occupational Therapy, Revue Canadienne D'ergotherapie,* **88**(4), 329–339. https://doi.org/10.1177/00084174211042960

Illinois ACEs Response Collaborative (2019) *Widening the lens on ACEs: the role of community in trauma, resilience, and thriving.* 1–5. https://hmprg.org/wp-content/uploads/2019/02/Role-of-Community-in-Trauma-Resilience-and-Healing.pdf (accessed 28 March 2023)

Jelly Beanz Inc (2013) *Seminar on anxiety, depression and PTSD in children and adolescents, Pretoria.* http://www.jellybeanz.org.za/ (accessed 31 January 2014)

Jeyasundaram, J., Cao, L.Y.D. & Trentham, B. (2020) Experiences of inter-generational trauma in second-generation refugees: healing through occupation. *Canadian Journal of Occupational Therapy,* **87**(5), 412–422. https://doi.org/10.1177/0008417420968684

Kaminer, D., Eagle, G. & Crawford-Browne, S. (2018) Continuous traumatic stress as a mental and physical health challenge: case studies from South Africa. *Journal of Health Psychology,* **23**(8), 1038–1049. https://doi.org/10.1177/1359105316642831

Katz, M. (2012) *The zones of regulation: a curriculum designed to foster self-regulation and emotional control. Practice,* pp. 7–8.

Kayiteshonga, Y., Sezibera, V., Mugabo, L. & Iyamuremye, J.D. (2022) Prevalence of mental disorders, associated comorbidities, health care knowledge and service utilisation in Rwanda – towards a blueprint for promoting mental health care services in low- and middle-income countries? *BMC Public Health,* **22**, 1858. https://doi.org/10.1186/s12889-022-14165-x

Keeshin, B.R., Bryant, B. & Gargaro, E.R. (2021) Emotional dysregulation. *Child and Adolescent Psychiatric Clinics of North America,* **30**(2), 375–387. https://doi.org/10.1016/j.chc.2020.10.007

Kerr, N.C., Ashby, S., Gerardi, S.M. & Lane, S.J. (2020) Occupational therapy for military personnel and military veterans experiencing post-traumatic stress disorder: a scoping review. *Australian Occupational Therapy Journal,* **67**, 479–497. https://doi.org/10.1111/1440-1630.12684

Khuluvhe, M. & Negogogo, V. (2021) *Fact Sheet on NEETs (Persons who are not in employment, education or training).* The Department of Higher Education and Training, Pretoria. https://www.dhet.gov.za/Planning%20Monitoring%20and%20Evaluation%20Coordination/Fact%20Sheet%20on%20NEET%20-%202021.pdf (accessed 18 April 2023)

Kornhaber, R., Walsh, K., Duff, J. & Walker, K. (2016) Enhancing adult therapeutic interpersonal relationships in the acute health care setting: an integrative review. *Journal of Multidisciplinary Healthcare,* **9**, 537–546. https://doi.org/10.2147/JMDH.S116957

Kros, C. (2017) We do not want the commission to allow the families to disappear into thin air: a consideration of widows' testimonies at the truth and reconciliation commission and the Farlam (Marikana) commission. *Psychology in Society,* **55**, 38–60. http://dx.doi.org/10.17159/2309-8708/2017/n55a4

Lahav, Y. (2020) Psychological distress related to COVID-19 – the contribution of continuous traumatic stress. *Journal of Affective Disorders,* **277**, 129–137. https://doi.org/10.1016/j.jad.2020.07.141

Law, M., Baptiste, S., McColl, M., Opzoomer, A., Polatajko, H. & Pollock, N. (1990) The Canadian occupational performance measure: an outcome measure for occupational therapy. *Canadian Journal of Occupational Therapy,* **57**(2), 82–87. https://doi.org/10.1177/000841749005700207

Lawlor, L. (2017) Armed response: an unfortunate legacy of apartheid. *Journal of Comparative Urban Law and Policy,* **1**(1), Article 12. https://readingroom.law.gsu.edu/jculp/vol1/iss1/12 (accessed 30 March 2023)

Lees, D., Procter, N. & Fassett, D. (2014) Therapeutic engagement between consumers in suicidal crisis and mental health nurses. *International Journal of Mental Health Nursing,* **23**(4), 306–315. https://doi.org/10.1111/inm.12061

Leitch, L. (2017) Action steps using ACEs and trauma-informed care: a resilience model. *Health & Justice,* **5**(5). https://doi.org/10.1186/s40352-017-0050-5

Lindström, A.C. & Bernhardsson, S. (2018) Evidence-based practice in primary care occupational therapy: a cross-sectional survey in Sweden. *Occupational Therapy International,* **2018**, 5376764. https://doi.org/10.1155/2018/5376764

MacLean, P. (1990) *The Triune Brain in Evolution: Role in Paleocerebral Functions.* Plenum Press, New York.

Maldonado-Torres, N. (2007) On the coloniality of being. *Cultural Studies,* **21**(2–3), 240–270. https://doi.org/10.1080/09502380601162548

Maldonado-Torres, N. (2017) Frantz Fanon and the decolonial turn in psychology: from modern/colonial methods to the decolonial attitude. *South African Journal of Psychology,* **47**(4), 432–441. https://doi.org/10.1177/0081246317737918

Manyema, M. & Richter, L.M. (2019) Adverse childhood experiences: prevalence and associated factors among South African young adults. *Heliyon,* **5**(12), e03003. https://doi.org/10.1016/j.heliyon.2019.e03003

McArthur, J., Tran, B.J & Roberts, St. (2013) Occupational therapy interventions for individuals with posttraumatic stress disorder returning to work: a systematic review. *Mental Health,* **2**. https://scholarworks.gvsu.edu/ot_mental_health/2 (accessed 3 March 2023)

Mekonnen, N., Duko, B., Kercho, M.W. & Bedaso, A. (2022) PTSD among road traffic accident survivors in africa: A systematic review and meta-analysis. *Heliyon,* **8**(11), e11539. https://doi.org/10.1016/j.heliyon.2022.e11539

Menzies, K. (2019) Understanding the Australian aboriginal experience of collective, historical and intergenerational trauma. *International Social Work,* **62**(6), 1522–1534. https://doi.org/10.1177/0020872819870585

Merrick, M.T., Ports, K.A., Ford, D.C., Afifi, T.O., Gershoff, E.T. & Grogan-Kaylord, A. (2017) Unpacking the impact of adverse childhood experiences on adult mental health. *Child Abuse & Neglect,* **69**, 10–19. https://doi.org/10.1016/j.chiabu.2017.03.016

Mignolo, W.D. (2007) Delinking: the rhetoric of modernity, the logic of coloniality and the grammar of decoloniality. *Cultural Studies,* **21**(2–3), 449–514. https://doi.org/10.1080/09502380601162647

Mignolo, W.D. (2009) Epistemic disobedience, independent thought and decolonial freedom. *Theory, Culture & Society,* **26**(7–8), 159–181. https://doi.org/10.1177/0263276409349275

Mitchell, T. Arseneau, C. & Thomas, D. (2019) Colonial trauma: complex, continuous, collective, cumulative and compounding effects on the health of Indigenous peoples in Canada and beyond. *International Journal of Indigenous Health,* **14**(2), 74–94. https://doi.org/10.32799/ijih.v14i2.32251

Mohatt, N.V., Thompson, A.B., Thai, N.D. & Tebesa, J.K. (2014) Historical trauma as public narrative: a conceptual review of how history impacts present-day health. *Social Science & Medicine*, **106**, 128–136. https://doi.org/10.1016/j.socscimed.2014.01.043

Moleba, E. (2016) *Marikana youth: (re)telling stories of ourselves and our place. Masters in Diversity Studies*. University of the Witwatersrand, Johannesburg, South Africa. https://wiredspace.wits.ac.za/server/api/core/bitstreams/4ca78c7d-0be4-4b29-8180-27f7a827d4a2/content (accessed 10 April 2022)

Mthembu, T.G. (2021) A commentary of occupational justice and occupation-based community development frameworks for social transformation: the Marikana event. *South African Journal of Occupational Therapy*, **51**(**1**), 72–75. https://dx.doi.org/10.17159/2310-3833/2021a10

Mthembu, T.G. & Duncan, M. (2021) An African philosophy of personhood in southern occupational therapy. In: S. Taff (ed), *Philosophy and Occupational Therapy: Informing Education, Research, and Practice*, pp. 111–126. Slack, Thorofare, New Jersey.

Mthembu, T.G., Havenga, K., Julius, W.A., Mdawira, T.I. & Oliver, K. (2023) Decolonial turn of human occupation through the voices of young people regarding occupational legacy. *South Africa Journal of Occupation Journal*, **53**(**2**), 43–54.

Mthembu, T.G., Wegner, L. & Roman, N.V. (2017) Exploring occupational therapy students' perceptions of spirituality in occupational therapy groups: a qualitative study. *Occupational Therapy in Mental Health*, **33**(**2**), 141–167. https://doi.org/10.1080/0164212X.2016.1245595

Naicker, S. (2022) '*How violence and adversity undermine human development*' institute for security studies policy brief. http://issafrica.s3.amazonaws.com/site/uploads/pb-174.pdf (accessed 5 October 2023)

Ndlovu, S. (2020) Race and the coloniality of being: the concept of alienation in the existential thought of Frantz Fanon. *Journal of Eastern Caribbean Studies*, **45**(**1**), 1–16.

Ndlovu-Gatsheni, S.J. (2020) Geopolitics of power and knowledge in the COVID-19 pandemic: decolonial reflections on a global crisis. *Journal of Developing Societies*, **36**(**4**), 366–389. https://doi.org/10.1177/0169796X20963252

Ngcaweni, W. (2018) *Trauma and unhealed scars of South Africa*. https://sascenarios2030.co.za/2018/10/23/trauma-and-unhealed-scars-of-south-africa-by-wandile-ngcaweni/ (accessed 26 March 2023)

Nutton, J. & Fast, E. (2015) Historical trauma, substance use, and indigenous peoples: seven generations of harm from a 'Big Event'. *Substance Use & Misuse*, **50**(**7**), 839–847. https://doi.org/10.3109/10826084.2015.1018755

O'Brien, C.V. & Charura, D. (2023) Refugees, asylum seekers, and practitioners' perspectives of embodied trauma: a comprehensive scoping review. *Psychological Trauma: Theory, Research, Practice, and Policy*, **15**(**7**), 1115–1127. https://doi.org/10.1037/tra0001342

Occupational Therapy Association South Africa. (2014) Position statement on therapeutic group-work in occupational therapy. *South African Journal of Occupational Therapy*, **44**(**3**), 43–44.

PACEs Connection (2022a) *Understanding ACEs*. https://www.pacesconnection.com/ws/Handouts_UnderstandingACEs_EN.pdf (accessed on 25 March 2023)

PACEs Connection (2022b) *Three realms of ACEs*. https://www.pacesconnection.com/ws/Handouts_3RealmsACEs_EN.pdf (accessed 25 March 2023)

Pai, A., Suris, A.M. & North, C.S. (2017) Posttraumatic stress disorder in the DSM-5: controversy, change, and conceptual considerations. *Behavioral Sciences*, **7**(**1**), 1–7. https://doi.org/10.3390/bs7010007

Payne, P.R., Levine, P. & Crane-Godreau, M.A. (2015) Somatic experiencing: using interoception and proprioception as core elements of trauma therapy. *Frontiers in Psychology*, **6**, 93. https://doi.org/10.3389/fpsyg.2015.00093

Physiopedia (2023) *Vagus nerve*. https://www.physio-pedia.com/Vagus_Nerve (accessed 26 March 2023)

Porges, S.W. (1995) Orienting in a defensive world: mammalian modifications of our evolutionary heritage. A polyvagal theory. *Psychophysiology*, **32**(**4**), 301–318.

Porges, S.W. (2022) Polyvagal theory: a science of safety. *Frontiers in Integrative Neuroscience*, **16**, 27. https://doi.org/10.3389/fnint.2022.871227

R-Cubed (2016) *Intergenerational trauma is individual and collective*. https://r-cubed.co/ (accessed 26 February 2023)

Restall, G.J. & Egan, M.Y. (2021) Collaborative relationship-focused occupational therapy: evolving lexicon and practice. *Canadian Journal of Occupational Therapy*, **88**(**3**), 220–230. https://doi.org/10.1177/00084174211022889

Sangalang, C.C. & Vang, C. (2017) Intergenerational trauma in refugee families: a systematic review. *Journal of Immigrant and Minority Health*, **19**(**3**), 745–754. https://doi.org/10.1007/s10903-016-0499-7

Savio, D. (2023) *Psycho-spiritual counselling to enhance resiliency as transformative education: an auto/ethnographic inquiry of the interface between spirituality and positive psychology*. PhD Thesis, Edith Cowan University, Australia.

Shange, N. (2019) *Marikana children' still battling with wounds from the 2012 massacre*. https://www.sowetanlive.co.za. (accessed 20 April 2019)

Snedden, D. (2012) Enhancing practice: mental health trauma-informed practice: an emerging role of occupational therapy. *OT Now*, **14**(**6**), 26–28.

Somasundaram, D. (2011) 'Collective Trauma'. In: Bhugra, D. & Gupta, S. (eds), *Migration and Mental Health*. Cambridge University Press, 149–158. https://doi.org/10.1017/cbo9780511760990.014

Sorenson, C., Bolick, B., Wright, K. & Hamilton, R. (2016) Understanding compassion fatigue in healthcare providers: a review of current literature. *Journal of Nursing Scholarship*, **48**(**5**), 456–465. https://doi.org/10.1111/jnu.12229

Sotero, M. (2006) A conceptual model of historical trauma: implications for public health practice and research. *Journal of Health Disparities Research and Practice*, **1**(**1**), 93–108.

South African History Online (2023) *Sharpeville massacre, 21 March 1960*. https://www.sahistory.org.za/article/sharpeville-massacre-21-march-1960 (accessed 31 May 2023)

Southwick, S.M. & Charney, D.S. (2012) *Resilience: The Science of Mastering Life's Greatest Challenges*. Cambridge University Press, Cambridge.

Sprang, G., Clark, J.H. & Whitt-Woosley, A. (2007) Compassion fatigue, compassion satisfaction, and burnout: factors impacting a professional's quality of life. *Journal of Loss & Trauma*, **12**(**3**), 259–280. https://doi.org/10.1080/15325020701238093

Substance Abuse and Mental Health Services Administration (SAMHSA) (2014) *SAMHSA's Concept of Trauma and Guidance for a Trauma-Informed Approach*. HHS Publication No. (SMA) 14-4884. Substance Abuse and Mental Health Services Administration, Rockville, Maryland.

Thibeault, R. (2011) Occupational gifts. In: M.A. McColl (eds), *Spirituality and Occupational Therapy,* 2nd edn. pp. 111–120. CAOT Publications.

Tolosa-Merlos, D., Moreno-Poyato, A.R. & González-Palau, F. *et al* (2023) Exploring the therapeutic relationship through the reflective practice of nurses in acute mental health units: a qualitative study. *Journal of Clinical Nursing,* **32,** 253–263. https://doi.org/10.1111/jocn.16223

Torchalla, I., Killoran, J., Fisher, D. & Mahen, M. (2019) Trauma-focused treatment for individuals with posttraumatic disorder: the role of occupational therapy. *Occupational Therapy in Mental Health,* **35**(**4**), 386–406. https://doi.org/10.1080/0164212X.2018.1510800

Van der Kolk, B. A. (2005) Developmental trauma disorder: toward a rational diagnosis for children with complex trauma histories. *Psychiatric Annals,* **35**(**5**), 401–408. https://doi.org/10.3928/00485713-20050501-06

Van Der Kolk, B.A. & D'Andrea, W. (2010) *Towards a Developmental Trauma Disorder Diagnosis for Childhood Interpersonal Trauma, Cambridge University Press eBooks.* Cambridge University Press, 57–68. https://doi.org/10.1017/cbo9780511777042.008

Watson, M.F., Bacigalupe, G., Daneshpour, M., Han, W-J. & Parra-Cardona, R. (2020) COVID-19 interconnectedness: health inequity, the climate crisis, and collective trauma. *Family Process,* **59**(**3**), 832–846. https://doi.org/10.1111/famp.12572

Weathers, F.W., Litz, B.T., Keane, T.M., Palmieri, P.A., Marx, B.P. & Schnurr, P.P. (2013) *The PTSD checklist for DSM-5 (PCL-5) – standard [measurement instrument].* https://www.ptsd.va.gov/ (accessed 27 May 2023)

Wicks, A. (2005) Understanding occupational potential. *Journal of Occupational Science,* **12**(**3**), 130–139. https://doi.org/10.1080/14427591.2005.9686556

Williams, M.T., Metzgerm, I.W., Leins, C. & DeLapp, C. (2018) Assessing racial trauma within a DSM-5 framework: the UConn racial/ethnic stress & trauma survey. *Practice Innovation (Washington DC),* **3,** 242–260.

World Health Organisation (2010) *Measuring Health and Disability: Manual for WHO Disability Assessment Schedule (WHODAS 2.0).* In: T.B. Üstün, N. Kostanjsek, S. Chatterji & J. Rehm (eds), World Health Organization, Geneva.

Wylie, M.S. (2004) The limits of talk Bessel van der Kolk wants to transform the treatment of trauma. *Psychotherapy Networker,* **28**(**1**), 30–41.

Yalom, I.D. & Leszcz, M. (2005) *The theory and practice of group psychotherapy.* 5. New York, Basic Books.

Zambianchi, M. & Bitti, P.E.R. (2014) The role of proactive coping strategies, time perspective, perceived efficacy on affect regulation, divergent thinking and family communication in promoting social wellbeing in emerging adulthood. *Social Indicators Research,* **116**(**2**), 493–507. http://www.jstor.org/stable/24720857 (accessed 7 July 2023)

Ziglio, E. (2017) *Strengthening Resilience: A Priority Shared by Health 2020 and the Sustainable Development Goals.* WHO Regional Office for Europe. https://www.euro.who.int/__data/assets/pdf_file/0005/351284/resilience-report-20171004-h1635.pdf (accessed 15 June 2023)

CHAPTER 22

Occupational Therapy for Persons with Anxiety Disorders

Elvin Williams[1] and Shanay Davidson[2]

[1]Division of Occupational Therapy and Arts Therapies, School of Health Sciences, Queen Margaret University, Edinburgh, Scotland

[2]Western Cape Department of Health, Valkenberg Hospital, Cape Town, South Africa

KEY LEARNING POINTS

- Identify the impact of anxiety disorders on occupational engagement.

- Understand occupational therapy processes within a recovery-oriented mental health care framework.

- Identify appropriate theoretical models, practice frameworks and principles for guiding interventions in occupational therapy.

- Develop critical thinking for integrated and recovery-orientated practice within varied practice contexts.

'There is hope, even when your brain tells you there isn't'.

— John Green

INTRODUCTION

People who are clinically anxious often report feeling overwhelmed by a sense of impending doom and an inability to control their thoughts and emotions. This can manifest as physical symptoms such as rapid heartbeat, sweating, trembling and muscle tension, as well as psychological symptoms such as excessive worrying, fear and avoidance of certain situations or activities (Daviu *et al.* 2019).

In the 2004 South African Stress and Health (SASH) study, which is a seminal piece of research conducted in South Africa, Herman *et al.* (2009) concluded that anxiety disorders were the most prevalent mental disorders experienced by South Africans, both in terms of lifetime prevalence and over a 12-month period. Earlier data from the SASH study showed a significant prevalence of trauma in South Africa, with approximately 75% of South Africans having experienced at least one traumatic event and 55.6% experiencing multiple

traumatic events (Williams *et al.* 2007). These findings are significant as research shows that witnessing trauma and other chronic adverse events can deleteriously impact mental health and well-being, particularly anxiety and depression (Atwoli *et al.* 2015).

Occupational therapists, therefore, play a crucial role in helping persons with anxiety disorders manage their anxiety and create enabling environments that facilitate engagement in occupations that promote health and well-being.

THE DIAGNOSTIC CRITERIA AND CLINICAL PRESENTATION

Anxiety is a normal, subjective, human emotion that is experienced by everyone at some point in their lives. Differentiating between normal anxiety, which serves as a motivator for adaptation and action, and clinical anxiety, which induces distress and impairs functioning, is challenging. However, when anxiety becomes excessive and persistent and interferes with daily functioning, it can be classified as an anxiety disorder. It is important to acknowledge that anxiety disorders are not

Crouch and Alers Occupational Therapy in Psychiatry and Mental Health, Sixth Edition.
Edited by Rosemary Crouch, Tania Buys, Enos Morankoana Ramano, Matty van Niekerk and Lisa Wegner.
© 2025 John Wiley & Sons Ltd. Published 2025 by John Wiley & Sons Ltd.

limited to any gender, culture or age group and are diagnosed in children as young as two to three years of age and in the elderly.

The Diagnostic and Statistical Manual of Mental Disorders, Fifth Edition, Text Revision (DSM-5-TR) (American Psychiatric Association 2022) is currently used to diagnose and classify mental disorders, such as anxiety disorders. Figure 22.1 illustrates the criteria used by the DSM-5-TR (American Psychiatric Association 2022), to objectively determine the presence of generalised anxiety disorder, in a variety of clinical settings.

THE IMPACT ON OCCUPATIONAL ENGAGEMENT

Studies have shown that a range of environmental, psychological and biological factors may play a role in the development and maintenance of anxiety disorders (Chorpita *et al.* 1996; Smoller *et al.* 2009; Bantjes *et al.* 2019). By acknowledging the complex interplay between these factors, which may manifest as psychiatric signs and symptoms of anxiety, the occupational therapist can gain valuable insights into a person's internal world, emotional distress, coping mechanisms and inherent strengths. In addition, the individual's life history, and occupational narrative may offer clues about three possible factors contributing to clinical anxiety:

1. *Precipitating factors*: What traumatic or trigger event(s) happened recently or in the distant past has set the anxiety response in motion? Did the loss of functioning trigger further distress and if so, how?

2. *Perpetuating factors*: What perpetuates the experience of anxiety? What personal, social and/or occupational circumstances or risks prevent the person from overcoming anxiety?

3. *Predisposing factors*: What made the person vulnerable in the first place? Which personal or environmental factors inclined the person towards an anxiety response?

The ability to engage in meaningful and fulfilling daily activities, including what people want to do and need to do, is considered essential to health and well-being and is a central tenet of the occupational therapy profession. Enduring anxiety and stress can lead to occupational disruption and have a deleterious impact on the occupational being's[1] (Yerxa 1990; Clark 1997) ability to perform and fulfil various tasks, and activities associated with roles such as being a parent, worker, scholar, friend and citizen.

To assist in understanding the occupational implications of anxiety disorders, the following analytical frameworks can be utilised:

- Bio-psycho-social and occupational performance taxonomy (Stein & Cutler 2002)

- An occupational perspective of health (Wilcock & Hocking 2015)

- International Classification of Functioning, Disability and Health (ICF) (World Health Organization 2001)

- DSM-5-TR (American Psychiatric Association 2022)

Duncan and Prowse (2014) provided an integrated analysis of the frameworks above and delineated six domains for the systematic identification of potential occupational implications of mental health disorders. According to Duncan and Prowse (2014), these domains operate in a bidirectional manner, with individual strengths, vulnerabilities and illness narratives being unique and multifaceted. Their integrated analysis of the frameworks is depicted in Table 22.1. Duncan and Prowse (2014) further assert that it is critical to interpret each domain considering the cultural diversity and indigenous health practices of the person, group or community. These cultural considerations are essential for improving mental health outcomes and reducing health disparities in marginalised and underserved populations (Chowdhary *et al.* 2014; World Health Organization 2022).

THE ROLE OF OCCUPATIONAL THERAPY

The occupational therapist follows the occupational therapy process to address the occupational challenges associated with anxiety disorders. The occupational therapy process is a complex, iterative and reflective one, encompassing several cycles of problem identification and solution generation with a central emphasis on occupation (Law *et al.* 1996; American Occupational Therapy Association 2020). The process involves a collaborative and person-centred approach to care that is sensitive to the occupational needs and aspirations of the occupational being, as well as the contextual factors that shape their engagement in daily activities (World Federation of Occupational Therapists 2012).

According to Duncan and Prowse (2014), once the prioritised occupational needs have been determined, a comprehensive occupation-focussed plan may focus on the following objectives:

- 'Promote mental health, well-being and quality of life;

- Prevent relapse or features of the disorder from developing into a chronic illness;

- Remediate performance component impairments associated with the disorder;

---

[1] The authors have deliberately chosen to use the term occupational being (Yerxa, 1990; Clark, 1997) to contest the use of the term patient or client, which often problematises the experience of mental health distress as primarily located within the person. By using the term occupational being, the authors acknowledge the complexities of the person and the interacting systems that may contribute to the varying manifestations of anxiety.

A. Excessive anxiety and worry (apprehensive expectation), occurring more days than not for at least six months, about a number of events or activities (such as work or school performance)

B. The individual finds it difficult to control the worry.

C. The anxiety and worry are associated with three (or more) of the following six symptoms (with at least some symptoms having been present for more days than not for the past six months):
   Note: Only one item required in children.
   1. Restlessness, feeling keyed up or on edge.
   2. Being easily fatigued. 3. Difficulty concentrating or mind going blank. 4. Irritability. 5. Muscle tension. 6. Sleep disturbance (difficulty falling or staying asleep, or restless, unsatisfying sleep).

D. The anxiety, worry, or physical symptoms cause clinically significant distress or impairment in social, occupational, or other important areas of functioning.

E. The disturbance is not attributable to the physiological effects of a substance (e.g. a drug of abuse, a medication) or another medical condition (e.g. hyperthyroidism).

F. The disturbance is not better explained by another medical disorder (e.g. anxiety or worry about having panic attacks in panic disorder, negative evaluation in social anxiety disorder [social phobia], contamination or other obsessions in obsessive-compulsive disorder, separation from attachment figures in separation anxiety disorder, reminders of traumatic events in posttraumatic stress disorder, gaining weight in anorexia nervosa, physical complaints in somatic symptom disorder, perceived appearance flaws in body dysmorphic disorder, having a serious illness in illness anxiety disorder, or the content of delusional beliefs in schizophrenia or delusional disorder).

FIGURE 22.1 The Diagnostic and Statistical Manual of Mental Disorders DSM-5-TR diagnostic criteria for generalised anxiety disorder Source: American Psychiatric Association (2022).

- Rehabilitate occupational performance dysfunctions stemming from the disorder;

- Develop occupationally enriched contexts that provide opportunities for self-determination, social inclusion and participation' (Duncan & Prowse 2014, p. 374).

The various phases of the occupational therapy process are discussed below.

ASSESSMENT: UNCOVERING THE OCCUPATIONAL NEEDS AND ABILITIES

The process of uncovering the needs and abilities of the occupational being usually begins at the initial phase of the occupational therapy process and must be part of the ongoing interactions with the occupational being. This phase involves building a therapeutic relationship with the occupational being to understand their experiences of anxiety and its impact on their occupational lives. It is important that this therapeutic relationship is built on principles of person-centredness, enablement and empowerment.

The assessment phase is focused on establishing the need for occupational therapy; what the occupational being wants and needs to do; determining what the occupational being can do and has done; and identifying what might help or hinder their health, well-being and participation. The type and focus of the assessment will differ depending on the service context; however, all assessments should be geared towards collaboratively uncovering the complex and multifaceted needs of the occupational being. In addition, the process

of uncovering the occupational needs and abilities of the occupational being must be supported by the occupational therapist's theoretical model of practice, which will be discussed later.

Below are examples of methods used to collaboratively uncover the needs and abilities of the occupational being.

OBSERVATIONS

The occupational therapist employs all five senses to observe and interpret both verbal and non-verbal cues in various structured and unstructured settings. This process is critical to inform the occupational therapist's clinical reasoning and subsequent interventions. In addition, astute knowledge of the signs and symptoms associated with different mental disorders is essential for interpreting objective clinical observations. This knowledge base informs the occupational therapist's understanding of the underlying condition and its impact on occupational performance and engagement. It also informs differential diagnoses, directs what further assessments can be undertaken, and guides the selection of evidence-based interventions (American Psychiatric Association 2022). Through activity and occupation analysis, structured, purposeful and culturally relevant activities, such as preparing a meal, gardening, or participating in a creative art group, serve as a useful means of observation for the occupational therapist and the occupational being to collaboratively identify functional limitations during the assessment process. In addition, unstructured environments, such as the home, school setting and work, can be leveraged to observe and

Table 22.1 Integrated analysis of main occupational challenges for the occupational being with anxiety.

Domain 1 Occupational risks	Domain 2 Experiencing anxiety	Domain 3 Performance component impairments	Domain 4 Occupational performance limitations	Domain 5 Participation restrictions	Domain 6 Occupational consequences
Life events	'I'm lethargic'	Cognitive	Self-maintenance	Microsystem	Occupational imbalance
Poor role modelling of adaptive occupational performance	'I do everything in a rush because I am so jittery'	Poor concentration	Excessive sweating causing body odour	For example, implications of living in a crowded informal dwelling or in a children's home	Restricted engagement in occupations that meet physical, social, mental or rest needs
Trauma leading to learnt helplessness or underdeveloped agency	'I'm always tired and nauseous'	Forgetfulness	Bitten nails and skin		
	'The constant headaches get me down'	Indecisive	Chapped, dry and irritated hands and skin from repetitive washing/eczema		Insufficient time for a range of fulfilling occupations, for example, worker role overload leads to burnout
	'I'm losing it, feeling out of control, like I'm going crazy'	Poor problem-solving			
		Distorted, irrational ideas	Gum lesions from excessive teeth cleaning/grinding		
	'Something dreadful is going to happen; I expect disaster any moment'	Obsessions	Bald patches or unkempt appearance from hair pulling		
	'My vision is blurred; things change size'	Self-critical thoughts			
	'My heart beats very fast and I feel like fainting; sometimes I do'				
	'A suffocating and choking feeling in my throat . . . like I can die'				
	'It's like ants crawling over my hands, like pins and needles'				
	'Worry, worry, worry . . . that's all I do; in fact it stops me doing anything else'				
	'I go hysterical; I panic just thinking of . . .' (phobia)				
	'It's like a movie in my mind; I experience flashes of it over and over'				
	'I'm on edge, hyper-alert, irritable and ready to blow up'				
	'I check and recheck, over and over; checking takes over my life'				
	'My nose is so hideous; I can't stop looking at it'				

(continued)

Table 22.1 (*Continued*)

Domain 1 Occupational risks	Domain 2 Experiencing anxiety	Domain 3 Performance component impairments	Domain 4 Occupational performance limitations	Domain 5 Participation restrictions	Domain 6 Occupational consequences
Natural environment Exposure to pollutants that decrease resilience of body and mind		Conative Excessive drive Restless, jittery Lethargy Demotivation	Temporality Disorganised habit patterns and routines result in untidy or dirty living/working space Poor time management, for example, compulsive cleaning, therefore neglects other tasks	Mesosystem For example, social anxiety reinforced by overprotectiveness of parent/partner Family adjust their lifestyle around illness behaviour of person leading to resentment or co-dependency Domestic abuse	Occupational deprivation Illness behaviour keeps person from using or enjoying life opportunities Reduced occupational engagement leads to sensory deprivation or repetitive compulsions lead to sensory overload that in turn exacerbates anxiety symptoms
Temporal environment Income and structural poverty: lack of financial/practical means to do occupations of choice Too few or too many opportunities/choices leading to occupational boredom or overload		Affective Low self-esteem Irritability Mood swings Aggression Depression	Productivity Over-conscientious or avoidant: creates tension at work Perfectionism leads to work overload and 'burnout' Work habits decline as worry or phobias increase Unable to meet deadlines/commitment, for example, compulsions waste time	Exosystem Patterns of avoidance leading to withdrawal from formal and informal social structures Refuses social invitations Restricts lifestyle to cope with or focus on symptoms Work support structures take strain	Occupational alienation Illness behaviour estranges anxious person from the mainstream of society, disconnected from social networks
Sociocultural environment Cultural values and indigenous practices such as gender roles that regulate occupational choice, for example, stressors of an arranged marriage or adult circumcision Social isolation due to decline of nuclear family and social networks, for example, being a refugee Anti-occupations such as crime-related activities Changing patterns of work, for example, migrant labour, unemployment or executive burnout		Behavioural Substance abuse Sleeping problems Accident prone Loss of libido Altered eating patterns Social withdrawal Physical High blood pressure and tachycardia Migraine Stomach ulcers Dyspnoea or choking feeling Frequency of urination Skin rashes Diarrhoea or irritable Bowl	Leisure/play/creativity and spirituality Reduced pleasure and self-efficacy in previously valued hobbies and interests Boredom or frenetic participation with little restfulness and mindfulness	Macrosystem Inadequate reasonable accommodation policies in the workplace Inadequate mental health support services Civil unrest and high crime create enduring stress	

mutually recognise occupational performance issues. Finally, observational assessments, such as the Assessment of Motor and Process Skills (AMPS) (Fisher & Jones 2014), are additionally valuable for evaluating the occupational performance quality of individuals' activities of daily living (ADL) within their natural environments.

INTERVIEWS

Interviewing is a dynamic and adaptable approach to gathering information, which can be conducted formally or informally, or while the individual is engaged in an occupation. This process normally consists of a purposeful dialogue where the occupational therapist and occupational being work in partnership to uncover the barriers and facilitators to participation. The occupational therapist uses a mental state examination to guide the interview process and to gain insights into the occupational being's sense of efficacy, self-determination, values, interests and spirituality. As a result, interviewing based on the mental state examination can be a valuable tool for occupational therapists to develop a deeper understanding of the occupational being with anxiety and to begin the process of co-producing potential goals to support health and well-being.

General types of interviews that may be used in practice can be classified as open-ended or unstructured, structured or semi-structured. Examples of these interviews used in occupational therapy practice are provided in Table 22.2.

Table 22.2   General types of interviews.

Open-ended or unstructured	Structured	Semi-structured
	• Functional Independence Measure (FIM)™ (Uniform Data System for Medical Rehabilitation 2009) • McGill Pain Questionnaire (Melzack 1975)	• The Canadian Occupational Performance Measure (COPM) (Law *et al.* 1990) • Occupational Circumstances Assessment Interview and Rating Scale (OCAIRS) (Kirsty Forsyth & Model of Human Occupation Clearinghouse 2005) • Occupational Performance History Interview – II (OPHI-II) (Kielhofner & University of Illinois at Chicago. Model Of Human Occupation Clearinghouse 2004) • The Worker Role Interview (WRI (version 10.0) (Braveman *et al.* 2005)

LIFE HISTORIES

Life histories are a powerful tool for occupational therapists to gain a comprehensive understanding of an individual as an occupational being. According to Llewellyn *et al.* (1999), life histories provide a means of comprehending the significance of life events within overlapping contexts of time and space. This perspective enables occupational therapists to gain insights into an individual's development, including how early experiences may have influenced later life, how occupational transitions were negotiated, and how occupational identities are shaped. Additionally, life histories can reveal future goals, hopes and aspirations, providing a life span perspective on individuals that can inform the occupational therapist's interventions and support a person-centred approach to care.

NARRATIVES

Narratives, also known as storytelling (Cole & Knowles 2001), can be a powerful means of communication in occupational therapy, by allowing the occupational being to focus on retelling their stories and constructing meaning, rather than focusing on their pathologies. By listening empathically and allowing the occupational being to reflect and express themselves freely, the occupational therapist can assist the individual with anxiety to re-construct or rediscover their sense of self, whilst allowing the focus to be redirected from the anxiety itself (Bonsall 2011).

MEASUREMENT

Occupational therapists use standardised assessment tools and outcome measures to gather objective information about anxiety-related problems and their impact on occupational performance and engagement. These tools provide a baseline for setting recovery goals, monitoring progress and identifying the outcomes of occupational therapy interventions. The following are examples of standardised assessment measures that can be used:

- The Canadian Occupational Performance Measure (COPM) (Law *et al.* 1990)

- The Model of Human Occupation Screening Tool (MOHO-ST) (Parkinson *et al.* 2006)

- World Health Organisation Disability Assessment Schedule 2.0 (WHODAS 2.0) (World Health Organization 2010)

- Depression Anxiety Stress Scale-21 (DASS21) (Lovibond & Lovibond 1995; Henry & Crawford 2005)

- The Hospital Anxiety and Depression Scale (HADS) (Zigmond & Snaith 1983; Stern 2014)

It is important to emphasise that before selecting a standardised assessment or outcome measure, the occupational therapist must consider the following:

* Its suitability for the context of the occupational being and service

* The occupational being's perception of success, their personal goals, and its congruence with the selected measurement

* The specific purpose of the tool in relation to the diagnosis of anxiety

* The presence of detailed guidance on the administration and interpretation of results

* Literature investigating the psychometric properties of the standardised assessment or outcome measure (e.g. reliability and validity).

OBTAINING COLLATERAL INFORMATION

The process of obtaining and exchanging collateral information from, and with, significant others and healthcare professionals is an integral part of occupational therapy practice. The Occupational Therapy Practice Framework: Domain and Process, Fourth Edition (OTPF–4) (American Occupational Therapy Association 2020) highlights the importance of collecting information from multiple sources such as family members, caregivers, employers and healthcare professionals to comprehensively understand the occupational being's occupational performance issues. The OTPF-4 also highlights the significance of interprofessional collaboration and communication for providing person-centred care. Occupational therapists therefore frequently consult and collaborate with family members, caregivers and members of the multi-disciplinary team etc. to obtain and share relevant information pertaining to the occupational being.

SOCIAL PRESCRIBING AND RESOURCE MAPPING

Social prescribing is a person-centred approach to healthcare that normally takes place within the community and encourages the occupational being to identify their needs and generate personal solutions to address the identified occupational challenges (Vidovic *et al.* 2021). The process of identifying needs and personal solution generation provides the occupational being with the skills and resources needed to improve their overall health and well-being. In practice, this method can be used in conjunction with resource mapping. Mapping of the occupational being's resources involves creating a graphical depiction of social connections and identifying locations or establishments within the community that offer opportunities to engage in meaningful and purposeful occupations. Crane and Mooney's (2005) community resource mapping toolkit can assist occupational therapists in identifying and utilizing resources within the community, such as peer support groups, community agencies, work or skills groups, religious organizations etc. that can assist in promoting participation in valued occupations and ultimately enhancing the occupational being's overall well-being.

In addition to identifying available resources within the community, by using social prescribing and resource mapping, the occupational therapist can identify various occupational risk factors such as occupational deprivation, imbalance, alienation and marginalization that may contribute to the development, or exacerbation, of the anxiety disorder (and other mental health conditions).

PRIORITISING OCCUPATIONAL NEEDS AND CO-CREATING PERSON-CENTRED GOALS

The process of identifying, prioritising and co-creating occupation-centred goals for the occupational being with anxiety should be guided by the values of person-centredness. McCormack *et al.* (2020) identify the following seven core values of person-centred practice that are relevant to the occupational process and to working with persons with an anxiety disorder:

* Respect for personhood

* Being authentic

* Sharing autonomy

* Showing respect for, and active engagement with, a person's individual abilities, preferences, lifestyles and goals

* Demonstrating mutual respect and understanding

* Therapeutically caring

* Committed to healthfulness as process and outcome.

Occupational therapists use the information gathered during the assessment phase, alongside occupational therapy practice models, to carefully co-create person- occupation-centred goals. These goals aim to address the prioritised occupational needs of the occupational being and are informed by the following:

* The nature of the occupational being – is this an individual, group or population that may benefit from the occupational therapy intervention?

* The practice or service context – government agency; non-government organisation; private; acute; sub-acute; chronic, in-patient or out-patient etc.

* The acute nature of the anxiety experience and the stage of recovery – is this an acute episode or part of an ongoing experience of anxiety?

* The focus of the occupational therapy intervention.

* The available resources for the occupational being and the occupational therapist – what are the social, financial and human resources available to support the co-creation of the person and occupation-centred goals?

THE OCCUPATIONAL THERAPY INTERVENTION

The intervention process can be divided into three phases: (i) intervention planning, (ii) intervention implementation and (iii) intervention review (American Occupational Therapy Association 2020). The occupational therapist integrates information from the assessment phase with sound theory, models of practice and evidence-based guidelines to direct their clinical and professional reasoning throughout the process. It is important to emphasise that these three phases are iterative and must be continuously reviewed, with the occupational being and their context always held at the centre of the process. The three phases are discussed below.

Intervention Planning

The occupational therapist working within an acute setting often focuses on remediating performance component deficits, using individual and/or group sessions, with a focus on clinical recovery, discharge preparation, community re-integration or relapse prevention. In contrast, an occupational therapist working within a community setting might focus on personal recovery, primary prevention of mental health distress in the context of addressing broader social determinants of health, addressing participation restrictions, or by working at a systems or policy level to advocate for social inclusion, health and well-being. Regardless of the service or practice context, the occupational therapist must ensure that occupation is at the core of the intervention planning process and supported by contextually relevant occupational therapy practice models and frameworks. The following are examples of occupational therapy practice models and frameworks that can be used when working in the area of anxiety disorders:

- The Vona du Toit Model of Creative Ability (Van der Reyden *et al.* 2019)

- The Model of Human Occupation (Kielhofner & Burke 1980; Forsyth 2021)

- The Person-Environment-Occupation Model (Law *et al.* 1996)

- The Person-Environment-Occupation-Performance Model (Baum *et al.* 2021)

- The Canadian Model of Occupational Performance and Engagement (CMOP-E) (Polatajko & Davis 2021)

- The Kawa Model (Iwama *et al.* 2009; Lim & Iwama 2021)

- The Ecology of Human Performance Framework (EHP) (Dunn *et al.* 1994)

- The Participatory Occupational Justice Framework (POJF) (Whiteford & Townsend 2011).

In addition to the above occupational therapy practice models and frameworks, the following theories can be used to address specific performance component deficits related to anxiety disorders:

- Behavioural (Stein 1983) and cognitive-behavioural theories (Duncan & Fletcher-Shaw 2021)

- Psychodynamic and psychoanalytic theories (Nicholls *et al.* 2012).

Whilst the above-mentioned models and theories are useful in grounding occupational therapy intervention planning and implementation, it is important to exercise caution when applying Western models and theories to explain the origins of anxiety in non-Western cultures. As demonstrated in the study by Beshai *et al.* (2023), cultural and indigenous explanations of anxiety are critical in developing and implementing interventions that are authentic, culturally sensitive and person-centred.

Intervention Implementation

Intervention implementation refers to the execution of the occupational therapy intervention plan. The implementation of occupational therapy interventions can address specific or multiple performance component deficits, one or more occupations, or the varied contexts in which occupation occurs and which either supports the occupational being, or places them at risk of mental health distress.

The implementation of the occupational therapy intervention can occur at an individual, group, or population level and may consist of the following types of interventions depicted in Figure 22.2 (American Occupational Therapy Association 2020).

The various approaches to interventions that may be applicable to the occupational being presenting with an anxiety disorder are presented in Figure 22.3 (American Occupational Therapy Association 2020).

The occupational therapy intervention implementation will be discussed in relation to the six domains presented in the integrated analysis depicted in Table 22.1, by Duncan and Prowse (2014).

Domain 1: Reducing Occupational Risks Chronic adversity, poverty, violence, climate change, pandemics such as COVID-19, terrorism, war, displacement and trauma have been associated with life span physical health challenges and mental health disorders, such as anxiety (Nelson *et al.* 2020; King 2021). Occupational therapists, therefore, aim to address the various contextual barriers that could induce or exacerbate an anxiety disorder. Domain 6 provides examples of prevention and promotion strategies employed by occupational therapists. In addition to these, opportunities for income generation and entrepreneurial initiatives to enhance economic participation, as well as education on climate change and the prevention of chronic diseases of lifestyle can effectively support the well-being of individuals with anxiety and reduce risks for the development of other serious health conditions.

Domain 2: Learning to Cope with Anxiety The occupational therapist enables the occupational being who experiences anxiety to uncover their strengths and abilities, cope with their personal

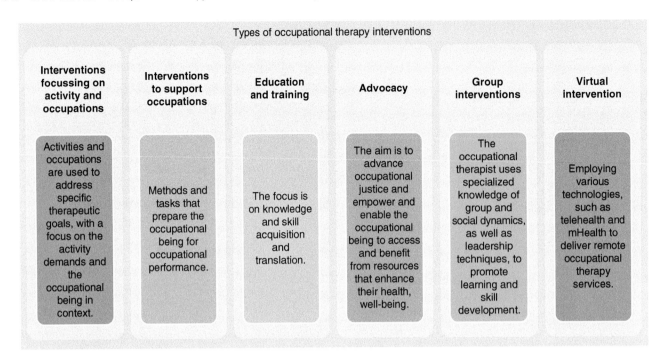

FIGURE 22.2 Types of occupational therapy interventions.

Create and promote mental health (health promotion)	Establish and restore (remediate and restoration)	Maintenance	Modify (compensate; accommodate; adapt)	Prevention
Aimed at enhancing mental health and promoting health, well-being, and participation in health-enriching occupations. Interventions could be geared towards addressing social determinants of health at a population or systems level.	Aimed at restoring occupational performance deficits. E.g. improving concentration and attention, emotional insight or judgment, etc.	To provide support to the occupational being to preserve skills, knowledge and insights that will enable continued engagement in health-enriching occupations.	Revising the activity demands or context in which occupations occur.	To prevent the occurrence of mental health distress or preventing the evolution of barriers to performance in context. E.g., psycho-education and raising awareness about stress and anxiety; education about the positive impact of participation in occupations on mental health; etc.

Types of occupational therapy interventions

FIGURE 22.3 Occupational therapy approaches.

challenges in identifying and managing their anxiety, and ultimately live a fulfilled life. Occupational therapists do this by recommending various self-help tools and peer support that can be useful in coping with an anxiety disorder. These resources can:

- Create a sense of community and empowerment among those with similar lived experiences relating to their anxiety.

- Allow for the sharing of information and the development of alternative coping strategies and self-efficacy.

- Galvanise collective support and personal agency to advocate for the rights of persons with mental health conditions.

- Enable the improvement of mental health services, through participation in research, policy development and review.

There are a variety of self-help tools and resources that can be accessed via the internet and via the occupational being's community. The occupational therapist must ensure that there is due consideration for the occupational being's developmental stage, access to digital and material resources (e.g. finance to access data to retrieve information from the internet, or to access transport to attend support groups), and digital and mental health literacy.

Domain 3: Treating Anxiety-related Performance Component Impairments The presence of clinical anxiety and distress can lead to impairments in cognitive, affective, behavioural and physical performance components, which conversely, can hinder the occupational being's occupational performance and engagement.

THERAPEUTIC STRATEGIES FOR MANAGING PERFORMANCE COMPONENT IMPAIRMENTS

MANAGING A PANIC ATTACK

Inexplicably and without an identifiable stressor or trigger, the occupational being may experience a strong sense of apprehension and impending doom characteristic of a panic attack. Physical symptoms such as dizziness, palpitations, nausea, tingling sensations in the hands, feet and mouth, as well as chest tightness, can accompany these attacks. Those experiencing a panic attack may respond with a fright or flight reaction and may believe that their symptoms are indicative of a severe medical condition such as heart disease or an impending mental breakdown. If a panic episode occurs during a therapy session, the occupational therapist should:

- Model calm, empathic behaviour and provide reassurance that the wave of panic will subside. You may say: '*It seems that you are experiencing a panic attack. I want you to know that I am here with you and that what you are experiencing is temporary. Let's try taking slow, smooth, and gentle breaths to help you to gain control and relax*'.

- Advise the person to place their hands over their mouth, limiting the amount of air from outside entering the lungs. This should be done for a few minutes until the carbon dioxide level in the body reduces and breathing subdues.

- Encourage the occupational being not to leave the therapy session, emphasising that they have the ability to control their panic reaction.

- After the incident has passed, review it with the occupational being to manage any fears and develop practical coping strategies (see below) for future panic attacks.

- Document the incident in the medical record and report it to the rest of the multi-disciplinary team.

USING CHANGE MODALITIES

- *Anxiety and stress management training:* Cognitive-behavioural therapy is the most widely researched treatment approach for persons with anxiety and appears to be both efficacious and effective in the treatment of anxiety disor-

ders (Kaczkurkin & Foa 2015; Carpenter *et al.* 2018). Occupational therapists integrate cognitive behavioural techniques with an astute focus on occupation, to help the occupational being understand their destructive or intrusive thoughts, behaviours, emotions and physiological responses to anxiety and how to manage them to mitigate the negative impact on occupational performance and engagement.

- *Relaxation therapy:* Evidence suggests that progressive relaxation is successful in reducing the symptoms of anxiety (Manzoni *et al.* 2008; Ranjita & Saranda 2014). Mentalization and mindfulness techniques have also been found useful in helping the occupational being cope with stress and anxiety (Desrosiers *et al.* 2013; Rodrigues *et al.* 2017).

- *Occupational group therapy:* According to Cole (2023), group interventions in occupational therapy have the potential to maximise the therapeutic power of social learning and emotional support provided by member interactions. By using occupational therapy practice models (e.g. The Vona du Toit Model of Creative Ability [Van der Reyden *et al.* 2019]), together with Yalom's therapeutic group factors (Yalom & Leszcz 2005), the occupational therapist can implement occupation-centred groups to enable functional skills for managing anxiety. In a study conducted by Tokolahi *et al.* (2013), an occupation-based group intervention was implemented to address anxiety symptoms in children between the ages of 10 and 14 years. The results of the study indicated that the intervention was both acceptable and beneficial, leading to a reduction in parent-rated and clinician-rated symptoms of anxiety and an increase in overall functioning. The purpose of the group was to focus on developmentally appropriate occupations to teach cognitive, behavioural and functional skills, such as activity scheduling and graded occupational engagement, to mitigate impairments in functioning associated with anxiety, such as school refusal or excessive participation in ritualistic occupations. The use of art and music may also be incorporated into occupational group therapy.

- *Social skills training:* Dysfunctional interpersonal skills, as observed with persons with anxiety, may lead to feelings of worthlessness and further exacerbate their anxiety symptoms. Social skills training is a therapeutic intervention that aims to improve interpersonal abilities through various techniques, including role-playing, mirroring, modelling, feedback and repetition. The process of social skills training allows individuals to build their confidence in social situations, ultimately reducing their anxiety levels (Beidel *et al.* 2014; Olivares-Olivares *et al.* 2019).

- *Role play:* Simulated enactment of stressful situations in controlled environments enables the occupational being to transfer stress and anxiety management skills to everyday occupations. Behavioural modification methods that can be employed during simulated problem scenarios include modelling, role reversal, doubling and role rehearsal (Abeditehrani *et al.* 2021).

- *Psycho-education:* Psycho-education involves the delivery of up-to-date, evidence-based and relevant information regarding the occupational being's diagnosis and treatment plan. For individuals with anxiety disorders, psycho-education can provide specific information on the recognition and management of the symptoms, as well as general guidance on how to live with the anxiety disorder. This may include promoting a healthy lifestyle, problem-solving, communication skills training, identifying stressors at home or in the workplace, peer support groups and educating family members and primary caregivers on the condition and its management. Psycho-educational interventions combine elements of cognitive-behavioural therapy, group therapy and education so that the occupational being and family can work collaboratively with mental health professionals to achieve better outcomes (Motlova *et al.* 2017).

- *Activity participation:* When feeling distressed, the occupational being may not consider participating in activities as important to their immediate needs, health and well-being. As such, it is crucial for occupational therapists to highlight the significance of activities in addressing performance-related issues, improving self-confidence, enhancing life skills and promoting self-awareness.

ACTIVITY PRESENTATION

- Clarify and communicate activity requirements in a detailed and concise manner, focusing on one task at a time and repeating instructions as necessary to accommodate difficulties with concentration and attention.

- Model a calm, solution-oriented and rational approach to problem-solving, serving as an example for the person with anxiety to emulate.

- Acknowledge and address stress-related physical sensations, emotional reactions and tense behaviour that may arise during the activity, and guide the person to apply self-help techniques such as thought-stopping or controlled breathing to manage them effectively.

- Teach the person with anxiety to be mindful of their self-talk and to take control over negative thoughts and behaviours through cognitive restructuring, empowering them to improve their coping skills and emotional well-being.

- Encourage the person with anxiety to practice relaxation techniques in real-life situations, either during individual or group therapy sessions, to develop a habitual relaxation response and reduce anxiety levels.

CRITERIA FOR SELECTING ACTIVITIES

- Allows for redirection of their attention away from their symptoms and from ruminating negative thoughts.

- Encourages communication and positive responses from others.

- Creates opportunities to practice anxiety and stress management techniques in real-life situations.

- Activities should remain unaffected by acute anxiety symptoms such as tremors, sweating or blurred vision.

- Use specific and concrete information to encourage the person to engage in logical thinking and effective decision-making.

- Encourage the occupational being with anxiety to explore the meaning behind their symptoms through creative outlets such as art, music and drama in group therapy sessions. Close collaboration with mental health team members, particularly the individual psychologist, is recommended for the effective implementation of these techniques.

- To maximise therapeutic benefits, it is essential to consider factors such as gender, culture and other intersections that may influence the occupational being's experience.

Domain 4: Overcoming Occupational Performance Limitations

Performance component deficits that persist over time can significantly impact occupational performance across all areas. The following interventions relate to the relevant occupational performance areas:

- *Self-care:* excessive sweating, bowel movements, salivation and poor diet can hinder hygiene and grooming. Psycho-education is recommended to address these challenges.

- *Nutrition and eating habits:* providing contextually relevant information about healthy eating habits, and exploring the connection between one's eating habits, daily routine and the impact on anxiety levels can offer valuable insights. Facilitating access to a qualified dietitian who can provide personalised guidance is also useful. In addition, encouraging individuals to engage in self-help groups can also be advantageous, as it fosters a supportive environment for shared experiences and knowledge exchange.

- *Sleep and rest:* facilitating the acquisition of self-management skills, such as sleep hygiene, is important. For instance, providing guidance on the importance of maintaining a consistent sleep schedule, creating a conducive sleep environment and practicing relaxation techniques before bed can help improve sleep quality and overall well-being. Moreover, advising on seeking medical assistance, such as consulting a sleep specialist or discussing sleep concerns with their healthcare provider, can ensure they receive the necessary support and guidance for addressing underlying sleep disorders or issues.

- *Leisure and socialisation:* encouraging individuals to reconnect with past hobbies or discover new ones can offer a healthy outlet for managing anxiety and fostering a sense of fulfilment. Moreover, suggesting alternative activities that align with their interests and abilities can expand their options for engaging in meaningful and enjoyable occupations. Furthermore, informing individuals about community resources, such as local clubs, groups or organisations that cater to their specific interests, can help them connect with like-minded individuals and access additional support and opportunities for personal growth.

- *Exercise:* promote physical fitness to manage symptoms and reduce distress. Incorporating a variety of activities, such as yoga, Pilates and aerobics can be useful.

- *Productivity:* develop goal-oriented productivity skills, information on worker rights and income generation strategies.

- *Spirituality:* encouraging engagement in activities that nurture spiritual well-being can provide a sense of inner peace and help redirect their focus away from distressing thoughts. For example, suggesting practices such as meditation, prayer, mindfulness exercises or engaging in nature walks can provide opportunities to cultivate a deeper connection with themselves and their surroundings. By incorporating contextually relevant spiritual activities into their daily routine, individuals can create a space for reflection, connection and relaxation.

Domain 5: Addressing Participation Restrictions

The ICF (WHO 2001, p. 112) defines participation restrictions as 'problems an individual may experience in involvement in life situations or the "lived experience" of people in the actual context in which they live and conduct their lives. The context here refers to all aspects of the physical, social and attitudinal world'.

The occupational being with anxiety disorder may face participation restrictions in major areas of life, such as education, employment and community activities, due to unaccommodating services and negative attitudes from others. The illness behaviour associated with these disorders can be internally regulated by the individual and, if necessary, accommodated externally by the contexts in which they live, work and play. Examples of specific interventions are provided below:

- *Education:* Reasonable accommodations during exams (e.g. extra time during and in preparation for tests/exams; recorded presentations as opposed to in-person viva voces etc.)

- *Productivity:* Supported employment, adjustments to work schedules or productivity outputs; awareness raising workshops etc.

Domain 6: Overcoming Occupational Consequences

Occupational risk factors, such as occupational imbalance, deprivation and alienation (Wilcock & Hocking 2015) may lead to or cause mental illness. The occupational therapist uses the Participatory Occupational Justice Framework (POJF) (Whiteford & Townsend 2011) to address occupational injustices, by not just working with the occupational being with anxiety, but also through working collaboratively at a group and population level, to address the socio-cultural and socio-political factors impacting mental health.

INTERVENTION REVIEW

Continuous and collaborative reviewing and evaluation of the intervention process will ensure the effectiveness of the intervention plan and attainment of the co-created, occupation-centred outcomes. It is important for the occupational therapist to review the intervention plan in relation to the occupational being's recovery and changing occupational needs, particularly in the context of recovery-orientated care and community integration.

CASE STUDIES

CASE STUDY 1

Mandy is a 33-year-old law enforcement officer working in a crime-riddled and impoverished area of Johannesburg, South Africa. She has been part of this law enforcement unit for the past five years. She is a single mother to her son, who is 10 years old. She lives with her ageing mother and younger brother. She recently experienced a traumatic home invasion where her family home was ransacked while they were locked in the bathroom. Since the incident, she has had difficulty returning to work, and she has withdrawn from friends and colleagues. She has been experiencing frequent headaches and nausea. She is not sleeping well and has frequent stomach upsets. She has had difficulty engaging with her son and assisting him with his schoolwork as she usually does. She spends a significant amount of time watching the cameras and security beams in the house and regularly checking and updating the neighbourhood crime-group online. She frequently checks that the doors and windows are locked. She used to regularly go for hikes and exercise; however, she has not been doing either.

Her employer has referred her to an employee wellness programme where there is an occupational therapist. According to Mandy, she had a difficult upbringing, her parents used to fight frequently, and her father would often express his anger physically. He would habitually use alcohol and leave the home

for extended time periods. Her parents separated when she was 16 years old, and she has had very little contact with her father since then. She says that after the separation, her mother had a 'breakdown' and was put on medication to 'relax' her. Mandy does not know whether her mother was formally diagnosed with a mental illness, and they do not talk about these difficult times. Her mother continued to work after the separation; however, Mandy describes knowing that the family was experiencing financial pressure. The family is religious, and, throughout their difficulties, have attended their local church. Mandy states that she feels disconnected from her church and her fellow members.

QUESTIONS:

- What contribution can occupational therapy make towards the mental health of individuals such as Mandy?

- What occupational domains will you address with Mandy? Why and how?

- Discuss the pre-disposing, precipitating and perpetuating factors that influence the manifestation of Mandy's anxiety.

CASE STUDY 2

Alex is a 20-year-old second-year university student. He expresses that lately he has felt like he 'is going mad'. He feels anxious most of the time. The problem started when he entered university. Despite wanting to be part of the university, he feels as if he is unable to cope, noting that he most likely will 'flunk' (fail) the year. Alex worries that he has made the wrong decision in studying engineering and feels that his family would be disappointed if he changes his study choice. He is sleeping badly and has persistent worries about his situation and his future. He describes himself as someone who cannot relax. He has been spending much of his time in his apartment playing games and rarely attends classes. He has avoided reaching out to the academic staff in an attempt to salvage the year. Alex has always been described as quiet and shy and has very few friends. When he meets new people, he worries about what they think of him and usually avoids making new friends. One of his professors suggests he join an outpatient programme at a private clinic that involves group therapy.

At the groups, he meets the following:

Peter, a 25-year-old editor, who has been diagnosed with social anxiety disorder three years ago. He is comfortable with his family; however, his worst fear is public speaking. He has recently been promoted and as part of his new job needs to do regular presentations. This makes him incredibly anxious. He has struggled with anxiety for a number of years anticipating that he will embarrass or humiliate himself whenever he has to talk in public.

Phumza is also a member of the group. She is 51 years old and works as a secretary at a primary school. She presents with bizarre movements of her face and hands including rolling eyes, protruding tongue and wringing gesticulations. She witnessed the gruesome murder of her uncle, with whom she had a close relationship, three months previously. She now ruminates about ways in which she could have prevented his death. She feels compelled to perform these movements to appease the ancestors whom she says spoke to her through the cow that was slaughtered at his funeral. Phumza lives with six other people in a small shack in an informal settlement that is renowned for crime, violence and poverty.

QUESTIONS:

- In which ways do Alex's, Peter and Phumza's occupational choices, interests and needs differ and which types of occupational intervention strategies will be best suited for each of them?

- Which occupational risk factors rendered Phumza vulnerable and what may the occupational consequences be should she not receive mental health intervention?

- How would you consider Phumza's culture in uncovering her occupational needs?

- Discuss how you would go about developing an occupational group program for Alex, Peter and Phumza. Include the change modalities that you would consider.

CONCLUSION

There is a need for collaborative, person and occupation-centred approaches when working with persons with anxiety disorders. The occupational implications of anxiety disorders, along with proposed interventions, are presented. The importance of working at an individual, group and population level when working with persons with anxiety disorders is emphasised.

REFERENCES

Abeditehrani, H., Dijk, C., Neyshabouri, M.D. & Arntz, A. (2021) Beneficial effects of role reversal in comparison to role-playing on negative cognitions about other's judgments for social anxiety disorder. *Journal of Behavior Therapy and Experimental Psychiatry*, 70, 101599. https://doi.org/10.1016/j.jbtep.2020.101599

American Occupational Therapy Association (2020) Occupational therapy practice framework: domain and process. *American Journal of Occupational Therapy*, [online] 74(4), 7412410010p1–7412410010p87. https://doi.org/10.5014/ajot.2020.74s2001

American Psychiatric Association (2022) *Diagnostic and Statistical Manual of Mental Disorders*, 5th edn. American Psychiatric Association, Washington, DC.

Atwoli, L., Platt, J., Williams, D.R., Stein, D.J. & Koenen, K.C. (2015) Association between witnessing traumatic events and psychopathology in the South African stress and health study. *Social Psychiatry and Psychiatric Epidemiology*, 50(8), 1235–1242. https://doi.org/10.1007/s00127-015-1046-x

Bantjes, J., Lochner, C., Saal, W. *et al* (2019) Prevalence and sociodemographic correlates of common mental disorders among first-year university students in post-apartheid South Africa: implications for a public mental health approach to student wellness. *BMC Public Health*, 19(1), 922. https://doi.org/10.1186/s12889-019-7218-y

Baum, C.M., Bass, J.D. & Christiansen, C.H. (2021) The person-environment-occupation-performance model. In: E. Duncan (ed), *Foundations for Practice in Occupational Therapy*, 6th edn, pp. 87–95. Elsevier, Edinburgh.

Beidel, D.C., Alfano, C.A., Kofler, M.J., Rao, P.A., Scharfstein, L. & Wong Sarver, N. (2014) The impact of social skills training for social anxiety disorder: a randomized controlled trial. *Journal of Anxiety Disorders*, 28(8), 908–918. https://doi.org/10.1016/j.janxdis.2014.09.016

Beshai, S., Desjarlais, S.M. & Green, G. (2023) Perspectives of indigenous university students in Canada on mindfulness-based interventions and their adaptation to reduce depression and anxiety symptoms. *Mindfulness*, 14, 538–553. https://doi.org/10.1007/s12671-023-02087-7

Bonsall, A. (2011) An examination of the pairing between narrative and occupational science. *Scandinavian Journal of Occupational Therapy*, **19**(1), 92–103. https://doi.org/10.3109/11038128.2011.552119

Braveman B., Robson M., Velozo C. *et al* (2005) *The Worker Role Interview (WRI) (Version 10.0)*. Model of Human Occupation Clearinghouse, University of Illinois at Chicago, Chicago.

Carpenter, J.K., Andrews, L.A., Witcraft, S.M., Powers, M.B., Smits, J.A.J. & Hofmann, S.G. (2018) Cognitive behavioral therapy for anxiety and related disorders: a meta-analysis of randomized placebo-controlled trials. *Depression and Anxiety*, **35**(6), 502–514. https://doi.org/10.1002/da.22728

Chorpita, B.F., Albano, A.M. & Barlow, D.H. (1996) Cognitive processing in children: relation to anxiety and family influences. *Journal of Clinical Child Psychology*, **25**(2), 170–176. https://doi.org/10.1207/s15374424jccp2502_5

Chowdhary, N., Jotheeswaran, A.T., Nadkarni, A. *et al* (2014) The methods and outcomes of cultural adaptations of psychological treatments for depressive disorders: a systematic review. *Psychological Medicine*, **44**(6), 1131–1146. https://doi.org/10.1017/S0033291713001785

Clark, F. (1997) Reflections on the human as an occupational being: biological need, tempo and temporality. *Journal of Occupational Science*, **4**(3), 86–92. https://doi.org/10.1080/14427591.1997.9686424

Cole, A.L. & Knowles, J.G. (2001) *Lives in Context: The Art of Life History Research*. Altamira Press, Walnut Creek, California.

Cole, M. (2023) Client-centred groups. In: W. Bryant, J. Fieldhouse & N. Plastow (eds), *Creek's Occupational Therapy and Mental Health*, 6th edn, pp. 257–277. Elsevier, Glasgow.

Crane, K. & Mooney, M. (2005) *Essential Tools — Community Resource Mapping. Improving Secondary Education and Transition for Youth with Disabilities*. ICI Publications, Minneapolis. Community Resource Mapping [online]. http://www.ncset.org/publications/essentialtools/mapping/NCSET_EssentialTools_ResourceMapping.pdf (accessed on 12 February 2023)

Daviu, N., Bruchas, M.R., Moghaddam, B., Sandi, C. & Beyeler, A. (2019) Neurobiological links between stress and anxiety. *Neurobiology of Stress*, **11**(1), 100191. https://doi.org/10.1016/j.ynstr.2019.100191

Desrosiers, A., Klemanski, D.H. & Nolen-Hoeksema, S. (2013) Mapping mindfulness facets onto dimensions of anxiety and depression. *Behavior Therapy*, **44**(3), 373–384. https://doi.org/10.1016/j.beth.2013.02.001

Duncan, E. & Fletcher-Shaw, S. (2021) The cognitive behavioural frame of reference. In: E. Duncan (ed), *Foundations for Therapy*, 6th edn, pp. 141–151. Elsevier, Edinburgh.

Duncan, M. & Prowse, C. (2014) Occupational therapy for anxiety, somatic and stressor-related disorders. In: V. Alers (ed), *Occupational Therapy in Psychiatry and Mental Health*, 5th edn, pp. 368–388. Wiley-Blackwell, London.

Dunn, W., Brown, C. & McGuigan, A. (1994) The ecology of human performance: a framework for considering the effect of context. *American Journal of Occupational Therapy*, **48**(7), 595–607. https://doi.org/10.5014/ajot.48.7.595

Fisher, A.G. & Jones, K.B. (2014) *Assessment of Motor and Process Skills. Volume 2: User Manual*. Three Star Press, Inc., Fort Collins, Colorado.

Forsyth, K. (2021) The model of human occupation: embracing the complexity of occupation by integrating theory into practice and practice into theory. In: E. Duncan (ed), *Foundations for Practice in Occupational Therapy*, 6th edn, pp. 46–74. Elsevier, Edinburgh.

Henry, J.D. & Crawford, J.R. (2005) The short-form version of the Depression Anxiety Stress Scales (DASS-21): construct validity and normative data in a large non-clinical sample. *The British Journal of Clinical Psychology*, **44**(2), 227–239. https://doi.org/10.1348/014466505X29657

Herman, A.A., Stein, D.J., Seedat, S., Heeringa, S.G., Moomal, H. & Williams, D.R. (2009) The South African Stress and Health (SASH) study: 12-month and lifetime prevalence of common mental disorders. *South African Medical Journal*, **99**(5), 339–344.

Iwama, M.K., Thomson, N.A. & Macdonald, R.M. (2009) The Kawa model: the power of culturally responsive occupational therapy. *Disability and Rehabilitation*, **31**(14), 1125–1135. https://doi.org/10.1080/09638280902773711

Kaczkurkin, A. & Foa, E. (2015) Cognitive-behavioral therapy for anxiety disorders: an update on the empirical evidence. *Dialogues in Clinical Neuroscience*, **17**(3), 337–346. https://doi.org/10.31887/dcns.2015.17.3/akaczkurkin

Kielhofner, G. & University of Illinois at Chicago. Model of Human Occupation Clearinghouse (2004) *A User's Manual for the Occupational Performance History Interview (Version 2.1) OPHI-II*. The Model of Human Occupation Clearinghouse, Department of Occupational Therapy, University Of Illinois at Chicago, Chicago.

Kielhofner, G. & Burke, J.P. (1980) A model of human occupation, part 1. Conceptual framework and content. *American Journal of Occupational Therapy*, **34**(9), 572–581. https://doi.org/10.5014/ajot.34.9.572

King, A.R. (2021) Childhood adversity links to self-reported mood, anxiety, and stress-related disorders. *Journal of Affective Disorders*, **292**, 623–632. https://doi.org/10.1016/j.jad.2021.05.112

Kirsty Forsyth & Model of Human Occupation Clearinghouse (2005) *A User's Manual for the Occupational Circumstances Assessment Interview and Rating Scale (Version 4.0) OCAIRS*. Model of Human Occupation Clearinghouse, Department of Occupational Therapy, College of Applied Health Sciences, University of Illinois at Chicago, Chicago.

Law, M., Baptiste, S., McColl, M., Opzoomer, A., Polatajko, H. & Pollock, N. (1990) The Canadian occupational performance measure: an outcome measure for occupational therapy. *Canadian Journal of Occupational Therapy*, **57**(2), 82–87.

Law, M., Cooper, B., Strong, S., Stewart, D., Rigby, P. & Letts, L. (1996) The person-environment-occupation model: a transactive approach to occupational performance. *Canadian Journal of Occupational Therapy*, **63**(1), 9–23. https://doi.org/10.1177/000841749606300103

Llewellyn, G., Sullivan, G. & Minichiello, V. (1999) Sampling in qualitative research. In: V. Minichiello, G. Sullivan, K. Greenwood & R. Axford (eds), *Handbook of Research Methods in Health Sciences*, pp. 173–201. Addison-Wesley, Sydney.

Lim, K.H. & Iwama, M. (2021) The Kawa (river) model. In: E. Duncan (ed), *Foundations for Practice in Occupational Therapy*, 6th edn, pp. 111–126. Elsevier, Edinburgh.

Lovibond, S.H. & Lovibond, P.F. (1995) *Manual for the Depression Anxiety Stress Scales*, 2nd edn. Psychology Foundation of Australia, Sydney, NSW.

Manzoni, G.M., Pagnini, F., Castelnuovo, G. & Molinari, E. (2008) Relaxation training for anxiety: a ten-years systematic review with meta-analysis. *BMC Psychiatry*, **8**(1), 41. https://doi.org/10.1186/1471-244x-8-41

McCormack, B., McCance, T. & Martin, S. (2020) What is person-centredness? In: B. McCormack, T. McCance, C. Bulley, D. Brown, A. McMillan & S. Martin (eds), *Fundamentals of Person-centred Healthcare*. Wiley-Blackwell, Oxford.

Melzack, R. (1975) The McGill pain questionnaire: major properties and scoring methods. *Pain*, **1**(**3**), 277–299.

Motlova, L.B., Balon, R., Beresin, E.V. *et al* (2017) Psychoeducation as an opportunity for patients, psychiatrists, and psychiatric educators: why do we ignore it? *Academic Psychiatry*, **41**(**4**), 447–451. https://doi .org/10.1007/s40596-017-0728-y

Nelson, C.A., Bhutta, Z.A., Burke Harris, N., Danese, A. & Samara, M. (2020) Adversity in childhood is linked to mental and physical health throughout life. *BMJ*, **371**. https://doi.org/10.1136/bmj.m3048

Nicholls, L., Cunningham-Piergrossi, J., de Sena-Gibertoni, C. & Daniel, M. (2012) *Psychoanalytic Thinking in Occupational Therapy*. John Wiley & Sons, West Sussex, UK.

Olivares-Olivares, P.J., Ortiz-González, P.F. & Olivares, J. (2019) Role of social skills training in adolescents with social anxiety disorder. *International Journal of Clinical and Health Psychology*, **19**(**1**), 41–48. https://doi.org/10.1016/j.ijchp.2018.11.002

Parkinson, S., Forsyth, K., Kielhofner, G. & Model of Human Occupation Clearinghouse and University of Illinois at Chicago, Department of Occupational Therapy (2006) *A User's Manual for Model of Human Occupation Screening Tool (MOHOST)*. Model of Human Occupation Clearinghouse, Department of Occupational Therapy, College of Applied Health Sciences, University of Illinois at Chicago, Chicago.

Polatajko, H.J. & Davis, J.A. (2021) Canadian model of occupational performance and engagement (CMOP-E): a tool to support occupation-centred practice. In: E. Duncan (ed), *Foundations for Practice in Occupational Therapy*, 6th edn, pp. 75–86. Elsevier, Edinburgh.

Ranjita, L. & Saranda, N. (2014) Progressive muscle relaxation therapy in anxiety: a neurophysiological study. *IOSR Journal of Dental and Medical Sciences*, **13**(**2**), 25–28. https://doi.org/10.9790/0853-13212528

Rodrigues, M.F., Nardi, A.E. & Levitan, M. (2017) Mindfulness in mood and anxiety disorders: a review of the literature. *Trends in Psychiatry and Psychotherapy*, **39**(**3**), 207–215. https://doi.org/10.1590/ 2237-6089-2016-0051

Smoller, J.W., Block, S.R. & Young, M.M. (2009) Genetics of anxiety disorders: the complex road from DSM to DNA. *Depression and Anxiety*, **26**(**11**), 965–975. https://doi.org/10.1002/da.20623

Stein, F. (1983) A current review of the behavioral frame of reference and its application to occupational therapy. *Occupational Therapy in Mental Health*, **2**(**4**), 35–62. https://doi.org/10.1300/j004v02n04_03

Stein, F. & Cutler, S.K. (2002) *Psychosocial Occupational Therapy*. Singular Publishing Group, Albany, New York.

Stern, A.F. (2014) The hospital anxiety and depression scale. *Occupational Medicine*, **64**(**5**), 393–394. https://doi.org/10.1093/occmed/kqu024

Tokolahi, E., Em-Chhour, C., Barkwill, L. & Stanley, S. (2013) An occupation-based group for children with anxiety. *British Journal of Occupational Therapy*, **76**(**1**), 31–36. https://doi.org/10.4276/0308022 13x13576469254694

Uniform Data System for Medical Rehabilitation (2009) *The FIM System® Clinical Guide, Version 5.2*. UDSMR, Buffalo.

Van der Reyden, D., Casteleijn, D., Sherwood, W. & de Witt, P. (eds) (2019) *The Vona du Toit Model of Creative Ability: Origins, Constructs, Principles and Application in Occupational Therapy*. The Vona and Marie Du Toit Foundation, Pretoria.

Vidovic, D., Reinhardt, G.Y. & Hammerton, C. (2021) Can social prescribing foster individual and community well-being? A systematic review of the evidence. *International Journal of Environmental Research and Public Health*, **18**(**10**), 5276. https://doi.org/10.3390/ ijerph18105276

Whiteford, G. & Townsend, E. (2011) Participatory occupational justice framework (POJF) 2010: enabling occupational participation and inclusion. In: N. Pollard & D. Sakellariou (eds), *Occupational Therapies Without Borders, Volume 2*, pp. 65–84. Elsevier, Edinburgh.

Wilcock, A.A. & Hocking, C. (2015) *An Occupational Perspective of Health*, 3rd edn. Slack Incorporated, Thorofare, New Jersey.

World Federation of Occupational Therapists (2012) *About occupational therapy* [online]. WFOT. https://wfot.org/about/about-occupational-therapy (accessed 10 April 2023)

Williams, S.L., Williams, D.R., Stein, D.J., Seedat, S., Jackson, P.B. & Moomal, H. (2007) Multiple traumatic events and psychological distress: the South Africa stress and health study. *Journal of Traumatic Stress*, **20**(**5**), 845–855. https://doi.org/10.1002/jts .20252

World Health Organization (2001) *International Classification of Functioning, Disability and Health*. World Health Organization, Geneva.

World Health Organization (2010). Measuring health and disability: Manual for WHO Disability Assessment Schedule (WHODAS 2.0). [online] Geneva: World Health Organization. Available at: https:// www.who.int/publications/i/item/measuring-health-and-disability -manual-for-who-disability-assessment-schedule-(-whodas-2.0) (accessed 10 April 2023)

World Health Organization (2022) *Mental health* [online]. World Health Organization. https://www.who.int/news-room/fact-sheets/ detail/mental-health-strengthening-our-response (accessed on 10 April 2023)

Yalom, I.D. & Leszcz, M. (2005) *The Theory and Practice of Group Psychotherapy*. 5th edn. Basic Books, New York.

Yerxa, E. (1990) An introduction to occupational science, a foundation for occupational therapy in the 21st century. *Occupational Therapy in Health Care*, **6**(**4**), 1–17. https://doi.org/10.1300/j003v06n04_04

Zigmond, A.S. & Snaith, R.P. (1983) The hospital anxiety and depression scale. *Acta Psychiatrica Scandinavica*, **67**(**6**), 361–370. https://doi .org/10.1111/j.1600-0447.1983.tb09716.x

Occupational Therapy for Individuals with Depressive Disorders and Bipolar Disorders

CHAPTER 23

Enos Morankoana Ramano and Mpho Sylvia Ramano

Occupational Therapy Private Practitioner, Soweto, Gauteng, South Africa

KEY LEARNING POINTS

- Overview of depressive disorders and bipolar disorders.

- Impact of depressive disorders and bipolar disorders on functioning and participation.

- Occupational therapy evaluation methods of depressive disorders and bipolar disorders.

- Specific interventions used for depressive disorders and bipolar disorders.

- Advocacy and case management.

INTRODUCTION

Depressive disorders and bipolar disorders are clinical conditions that share the essential features of a disturbance in mood that is not due to any other mental or physical disorder, medication or substance abuse. Mood is 'a pervasive and sustained emotion or feeling tone that is experienced internally and that influences a person's behaviour and colours his or her perception of being in the world' (Sadock *et al.* 2015, p. 347).

The distinction between depressive disorders and bipolar disorders lies in the type, intensity and duration of the symptoms; the amount of distress they cause to the individual and those around them; and the extent to which the symptoms affect functioning and participation in everyday life. The difference between the two disorders is the issues of duration, timing or presumed aetiology (APA 2022). The signs and symptoms of depressive disorders and bipolar disorders include changes in mood, cognitive abilities, speech, activity levels and vegetative functions (e.g. sleep, appetite, sexual activity and other biological rhythms) (Sadock *et al.* 2015).

The individual's behaviour and functioning are best understood, assessed and addressed in occupational therapy by taking into consideration the participation demands of their environment. What people are able to do every day and how they go about performing their various life tasks and activities depends as much on their mental and physical state as it does on the environments in which they live, work, play and socialize (Duncan & Prowse 2014). For example, poverty, poor living conditions, violence and unemployment require particular forms of coping strategies and adaptation. Occupational therapy intervention must therefore be adjusted with due consideration of the setting within which the service is rendered. An overview of the aetiology, signs and symptoms of depressive disorders and bipolar disorders follows in the next section.

DEPRESSIVE DISORDER

Depressive disorders include disruptive mood dysregulation disorder, major depressive disorder (MDD) (including major depressive episode), persistent depressive disorder (dysthymia), premenstrual dysphoric disorder, substance/medication-induced depressive disorder, depressive disorder due to

Crouch and Alers Occupational Therapy in Psychiatry and Mental Health, Sixth Edition.
Edited by Rosemary Crouch, Tania Buys, Enos Morankoana Ramano, Matty van Niekerk and Lisa Wegner.
© 2025 John Wiley & Sons Ltd. Published 2025 by John Wiley & Sons Ltd.

another medical condition, other specified depressive disorder and unspecified depressive disorder. The common feature of all of these disorders is the presence of sadness, emptiness or irritability, accompanied by somatic and cognitive changes that significantly affect the individual's capacity to function (APA 2022; Morrison 2023). The criteria for depressive disorders should include at least two of the following conditions: lack of appetite or overeating, insomnia or hypersomnia, fatigue, low self-esteem, difficulty concentrating or indecision, and hopelessness (APA 2022). Depressive disorders cause significant distress and impairment in social, academic, vocational or other important areas of functioning.

For the detailed discussion of the depressive disorders and bipolar disorders, it is advisable for the reader to refer to DSM-5-TR and related editions for a detailed explanation of depressive disorders and bipolar disorders (APA 2022).

DISRUPTIVE MOOD DYSREGULATION DISORDER

Disruptive mood dysregulation disorder presents with frequent outbursts of temper, which typically occur in response to low frustration tolerance over a period lasting at least one year with no more than a three-month period without outbursts (APA 2022; Morrison 2023). On average, the outbursts occur three or more times weekly, and the individual is chronically irritable and angry. The age onset of disruptive mood dysregulation disorder is before 10 years, and diagnosis is made between ages (6 and 18) years (APA 2022). Diagnosis specifies the presentation of persistent irritability and frequent episodes of extreme uncontrolled behaviour for children up to 12 years of age (APA 2022).

These children have difficulty succeeding in school and are often unable to participate in the activities typically enjoyed by healthy children; their family life is severely disrupted by their outbursts and irritability; and they have trouble initiating or sustaining friendships (APA 2022; Morrison 2023).

PERSISTENT DEPRESSIVE DISORDER (DYSTHYMIA)

Persistent depressive disorder or dysthymia is a disorder of mood that occurs for most of the day and persists for at least two years in adults (one year in children) (Sadock *et al.* 2015; APA 2022; Morrison 2023). Individuals whose symptoms meet MDD criteria for two years should be given a diagnosis of persistent depressive disorder as well as MDD.

MAJOR DEPRESSIVE DISORDERS

MDD is a mood disorder that is characterized by (i) episodes of a depressed mood and (ii) a decreased interest or pleasure in doing activities (APA 2013). An episode must last for at least two weeks (Sadock *et al.* 2015). The individuals with MDD may experience single or recurrent episodes of significant and persistent performance component impairments (insomnia, anhedonia and loss of libido), emotional disturbances (sadness, emptiness and hopelessness) and occupational performance dysfunction (decreased productivity at work, inability to socialise and restricted participation in valued activities) (Woo *et al.* 2016; Pan *et al.* 2019;

Lachaine *et al.* 2020). While the causes of MDDs are unknown, the complex interaction of multiple factors such as genetic transmission, biochemical imbalance, temperament, emotional trauma and adverse socio-environmental conditions are considered to play a role (Sadock *et al.* 2015).

Affected individuals report a deep sense of despair and hopelessness beyond their normal emotional experience. These feelings may lead some depressed individuals to become withdrawn and passive, while others may become irritable and agitated. While some forms of depression may lead to delusional or suicidal thoughts, a depressed individual's cognition is usually marked by distortions in ways of explaining things, self-evaluations and information processing. The depressed individual's thoughts are dominated by a view of self as worthless, the world as bleak and the future as hopeless. Through this negative view of the world, they distort experiences and display information processing errors such as overgeneralising and making predictions of poor outcomes (Duncan & Prowse 2014). They exaggerate the implications of minor life events, blaming themselves when things go wrong. No matter how bright the day is, how many goals are accomplished or how many compliments are received, the individual tends to find a flaw or a reason for self-criticism (Duncan & Prowse 2014). Depressive thinking has a self-sustaining, self-defeating quality that curtails role functioning and occupational performance.

MDD is classified according to severity, determined by the number of symptoms present. It can be classified as mild, moderate and severe. MDD has different forms such as adjustment disorder with depressed mood, dysthymia, major depression with melancholia, major depression with psychosis, peri-partum depression, atypical depression and masked depression (Sadock *et al.* 2015).

MDDs are viewed as the common cold of mental health problems due to the prevalence (Kandhakatla *et al.* 2018) and are expected to be a leading burden of disease by 2030 (Wolmarans & Brand 2016; Osuch & Marais 2017). It affects 8–15% of the population globally and one out of ten people in South Africa (Stander *et al.* 2016; Wolmarans & Brand 2016). Females are more vulnerable to develop major depression than males with a twofold greater prevalence due to hormonal differences, as well as childbirth and social conditions related to women's roles and stressors (Sadock *et al.* 2015). Although depression is three times more common in relatives, many professionals do not follow the 'genetic' school of thought. They believe that the intergenerational presence of depression within families is the result of 'a learnt pattern of behaviour' in which unhealthy coping mechanisms are used to resolve life stressors. Irrespective of its causes, MDD can be a debilitating mental illness that causes considerable distress and impairment in all areas of functioning (Bains & Abdijadid 2023), which includes their declining work performance, absenteeism and presenteeism (Talatala *et al.* 2020).

PSYCHIATRIC TREATMENT

Treatment of depressive disorders is aimed at reducing depressive symptoms. The absence or near absence of depressive symptoms indicates effectiveness of the treatment (Cameron *et al.* 2014; Novick *et al.* 2017). A combination of medication, psychotherapy, social intervention and occupational therapy is indicated. Anti-depressive medication, prescribed by a medical practitioner, includes tricyclic, serotonin norepinephrine reuptake inhibitors, selective serotonin reuptake inhibitors, monoamine oxidase inhibitors and many other classes of antidepressants. Electroconvulsive therapy (ECT) may be used for those who do not respond to antidepressant medication or as an adjunct to available medical treatments. Other psychiatric treatments for depressive disorders besides pharmacological treatments are vagal nerve stimulation, transcranial magnetic stimulation, phototherapy and ketamine (Sadock *et al.* 2015). Occupational therapists should familiarise themselves with the effects and side effects of different types of medication because this information is addressed during psycho-education sessions aimed at strengthening adherence to medication regimes and equipping clients with coping skills.

PSYCHOTHERAPY

Various types of short-term psychotherapy (cognitive therapy, interpersonal therapy, behavioural therapy, psychoanalytically oriented psychotherapy and dynamic therapy) are suggested for the treatment of MDDs (Sadock *et al.* 2015). Psychological treatment for MDD includes cognitive behavioural therapy, behavioural activation therapy, problem-solving therapy, interpersonal therapy, social skills training and family therapy (Cuijpers *et al.* 2011). Psychotherapy may focus on behavioural and cognitive behavioural change, adjusting the individual's self-concept and increasing their emotional insight into the maladaptive use of defence mechanisms.

SOCIAL INTERVENTIONS

Social interventions may address family and other significant relationships as well as ameliorate housing, economic, legal, environmental, educational and other social stressors. The social worker and other team members may be part of offering individualised social interventions.

OCCUPATIONAL THERAPY

The signs and symptoms of depressive disorders have an impact on functioning, which is the focal domain for occupational therapy interventions. These are discussed later in the chapter. The signs and symptoms are grouped into mood, cognition, motor activity and physical impairments, while the functional consequences (activity limitations and participation restrictions) are discussed under occupations as defined by the Occupational Therapy Practice Framework in the Fourth Edition (American Occupational Therapy Association [AOTA] 2020). Table 23.1 summarises some of the most prominent impairment specifiers (signs and symptoms) and functional consequences of depressive disorders.

Table 23.1 Signs and symptoms of major depressive disorder and the functional consequences.

Signs and symptoms	Functional consequences
Mood	**Activities of daily living and instrumental activities of daily living**
Low mood	
Anhedonia	Lack of interest, low energy levels and fatigue result in neglect of self, poor grooming, staying in bed the whole day, living and/or working area left untidy. Changes in sexual functioning such as decreased libido.
Irritability	
Anger	
Hopelessness	
Lack of interest	
Irritability	
Aggression	**Health management**
Feelings of guilt	Appetite changes affect the loss or gain of body weight.
Anxiety	
Low self-esteem	**Rest and sleep**
Cognition	Sleeping patterns and rest are affected due to insomnia. Fatigue has a negative impact on engagement in all occupations. Some experience excessive sleep, which affects their engagement in daily activities.
Impaired attention and concentration	
Indecisiveness	
Impaired short-term memory	
Impaired problem-solving skills	**Education and/or work**
Impulsivity	The cognitive impairments, lack of motivation and lack of interest result in poor productivity presenteeism (lost productivity), and absenteeism. Low self-esteem is worsened by lack of self-efficacy and competence. With low self-esteem, they withdraw from engaging in occupations creating a vicious cycle.
Impaired executive function	
Thought	
Excessive worrying	
Suicidal thoughts, ideation and or attempts	
Motor activity/ conation	
Low motivation	**Play and/or leisure**
Low energy levels	Play and leisure tend to be neglected causing occupational imbalance.
Extreme fatigue	
Psychomotor retardation	
Low psychological endurance	**Social participation**
Physical	Social withdrawal and impairments in mood affect social participation negatively as the depressed person does not want to be around people.
Headaches	
Muscle tension (neck, shoulder and back pains)	
Appetite changes	

BIPOLAR DISORDER

Bipolar disorder is a serious mental disorder that can become chronic. It is associated with marked reduction in functioning and well-being and is considered a major public mental health problem (Anyayo & Ashaba 2021). It affects roughly one percent of the global population (Biazus *et al.* 2023). Most individuals with bipolar disorder might eventually develop general disability thereby contributing to the public mental health burden of the disease (Miziou *et al.* 2015). Bipolar disorder is characterised by manic episodes, hypomanic episodes and major depressive episodes alternating with periods of remission of symptoms and euthymia (Koene *et al.* 2022). The manic episode has an abnormal and persistently elevated, expansive or irritable and high-spirited mood lasting for at least one week or less (Sadock *et al.* 2015). The hypomanic episode has an elevated, irritable and high-spirited mood that is less severe than a manic episode and lasts for four to five days (Sadock *et al.* 2015). A major depressive episode presents with a depressed mood and a loss of interest or pleasure for a period of two weeks (Sadock *et al.* 2015).

Individuals with bipolar disorder will experience a swing from one affective state to the other in terms of the duration, timing, depth and type of mood change. Although there is a significant genetic component to bipolar disorder, some kind of stress usually triggers the onset of a discernible mood change.

Bipolar disorder is one of the most incapacitating diseases among the youth and working-age adults and it is associated with reduced productivity levels, functional and social impairments and premature mortality (Biazus *et al.* 2023). Individuals who are diagnosed with bipolar disorder at a young age tend to have longer durations and recurrent mood episodes, psychosis, lingering residual symptoms, higher number of hospitalisation and co-occurring substance use disorders. Affected individuals have enduring psychosocial dysfunction, inconsistency in educational and vocational pursuits and repeated disruption of interpersonal engagements (Levy & Manove 2012).

Bipolar disorder can be classified into bipolar I disorder, bipolar II disorder, cyclothymic disorder, bipolar and related disorder due to medical condition and substance/ medication-induced bipolar (Sadock *et al.* 2015).

BIPOLAR II DISORDER

Bipolar II disorder has clinical features similar to those of MDD with hypomanic episode (Sadock *et al.* 2015). The diagnostic criteria of bipolar II disorder specify the severity, frequency and duration of hypomanic symptoms present during an episode that lasts for at least four days (Sadock *et al.* 2015). The individuals with hypomania experience a sense of well-being and increased productivity that may mask more serious aspects of the illness such as irritability, argumentativeness, insomnia, poor judgement and engaging in high-risk behaviours such as casual sexual encounters or making irrational business decisions. Hypomanic symptoms can adversely affect the individual's social life, family life and employment if the illness is not medically managed.

BIPOLAR I DISORDER

The individuals with bipolar I disorder may experience single manic episodes or recurrent episodes (Sadock *et al.* 2015; APA 2022). During an extreme state of excitation, the manic person is clearly psychotic and does not understand the

consequences of their expansive behaviour. They become preoccupied with religious, political, financial, sexual or persecutory ideas (Sadock *et al.* 2015). The manic episodes are more common in men while women present with a mixed picture of rapid cycles of mania and depression (Sadock *et al.* 2015). Bipolar I disorder is mostly found amongst the higher-income group. It is more common in divorced and single persons. Bipolar 1 disorder causes psychosocial morbidity that can affect the individuals' marriage, children, occupation and other aspects of life (Zarate *et al.* 2000). The individuals with bipolar 1 disorder have a high relapse rate of 50% in the first five months and 80–90% within 18 months (APA 2022). Individuals with bipolar 1 disorder frequently show a comorbidity of substance use and/or anxiety disorder.

CYCLOTHYMIC DISORDER

Cyclothymic disorder is usually diagnosed in individuals who experience at least two years (one year for children and adolescents) of both hypomanic and depressive periods without ever fulfilling the criteria for an episode of mania, hypomania or major depression (APA 2022; Morrison 2023). The hypomanic symptoms are of insufficient number, severity, pervasiveness, or duration to meet full criteria for a hypomanic episode, and the depressive symptoms are of insufficient number, severity, pervasiveness or duration to meet full criteria for a major depressive episode (APA 2022; Morrison 2023). Some of the individuals may function particularly well during some of the periods of hypomania, over the prolonged course of the disorder. The individuals with cyclothymic disorder present with clinically significant distress or impairment in social, occupational, or other important areas of functioning (APA 2022).

SUBSTANCE/MEDICATION-INDUCED BIPOLAR AND RELATED DISORDER

Some prescribed medications, substances of abuse and several medical conditions can be associated with mania, resulting in the diagnosis of substance/medication-induced bipolar and related disorder (APA 2022). A key exception to the diagnosis of substance/medication-induced bipolar and related disorder is the case of hypomania or mania that occurs with the use of antidepressant medication or other treatments and persists beyond the physiological effects of the medication. Similarly, individuals with apparent ECT-induced manic or hypomanic episodes that persist beyond the physiological effects of the treatment are diagnosed with bipolar disorder, not substance/ medication-induced bipolar-related disorder.

TREATMENT

Similar to depressive disorders, medication is the most effective approach for attaining a stable mood and restoring the functioning of persons diagnosed with bipolar disorder (Goodwin *et al.* 2016). Medication includes mood stabilisers such as sodium valproate, lithium and carbamazepine. The most effective pharmacological treatment is a combination of sodium valproate and lithium. Antipsychotic medication is highly effective in treating bipolar disorder, especially second-generation antipsychotics such as risperidone, quetiapine, olanzapine, aripiprazole and ziprasidone, which can be used on their own or in combination with other medications. Benzodiazepines can also be highly effective in the short term. Some of the medications may produce unpleasant side effects such as weight gain, which may lead to premature mortality, owing partly to cardiovascular disease (Goodwin et al. 2016). The majority of the medication has not been tested in pregnancy; therefore, it must be used with caution. Mood stabilisers (such as sodium valproate, lithium and carbamazepine) are known to be highly teratogenic (may cause congenital disorders in the developing embryo or foetus) and should not be used in pregnancy; they must be used with contraception in females of child-bearing age. Individuals with bipolar disorder are at substantially increased risks of self-harm, suicide, victimisation, violence and criminality (Goodwin et al. 2016). Weight gain and other relevant risk factors should be observed and reported to the treating team (Goodwin et al. 2016). Full functional recovery seldom occurs within 12 weeks following the remission of mood symptoms (Goodwin et al. 2016).

PSYCHOTHERAPY

Psychological interventions appear to be more successful with Individuals early in their illness course (Goodwin et al. 2016). There is very little evidence of efficacy of psychological treatments (for example, family-focused therapy, cognitive behaviour therapy, interpersonal social rhythm therapy) alone without pharmacotherapy in the treatment of acute bipolar disorder (Goodwin et al. 2016). The key ingredients of all psychotherapies for bipolar disorder (including psycho-education) are to: (i) monitor moods and early warning signs, (ii) recognise and manage stress triggers and interpersonal conflicts, (iii) develop relapse prevention plans, (iv) stabilise sleep/wake rhythms and daily routines, (v) encourage medication adherence, (vi) reduce self-stigmatization and (vii) reduce alcohol or drug use (including caffeine in sensitive individuals) (Goodwin et al. 2016). The involvement of carers/family is highlighted in family-focused treatment.

PSYCHO-EDUCATION

Psycho-education for both the individual and the family is likely to promote compliance with medication and encourage consistent use of self-help methods. It is important to address individuals' poor insight, the seriousness of the illness, the risk of relapse and the benefit of therapeutic engagement (Goodwin et al. 2016). Psycho-education may include information on the physiology of the disorder, identification of relapse risk factors and strategies for coping with the side effects of medication and lifestyle adjustments to manage stressors.

FAMILY INTERVENTION

The standard family intervention for individuals with bipolar disorders should include psycho-education focusing on the knowledge of the illness, skills training in communication and problem-solving, support and self-care training for the family or caregivers (Miziou et al. 2015). The Individuals, family members, caregivers and significant others should be educated on how to recognise emerging symptoms of manic or depressive episodes so that early intervention can be requested when needed (Goodwin et al. 2016).

OCCUPATIONAL THERAPY

A manic state is characterised by elated or irritable mood for four days or more. Quality of life tends to be reduced, functioning is impaired and social disruptions experienced during the manic phase of the illness. Furthermore, individuals with bipolar disorder experience cognitive impairments which persist to periods of euthymia (normal, stable mood) (Levy & Manove 2012). Table 23.2 summarises the typical impairments and functional consequences (activity limitations and participation restrictions) of mania, which are the focal domains for occupational therapy interventions.

EVALUATION

Evaluation is the gathering of information and its interpretation in order to plan for intervention and review intervention effectively (Schell & Gillen 2019). According to the Occupational Therapy Practice Framework, Fourth Edition (OTPFT 4), evaluation should include the Occupational Profile and Analysis of Occupational Performance (AOTA 2020). There are various methods that are used during evaluation of individuals and these can either be standardised (formal methods) and/or non-standardised (informal methods).

STANDARDISED METHODS

The occupational therapist usually selects standardised methods that are criterion or norm-referenced and that are considered excellent in terms of safety, utility, validity and reliability (Ramano & Buys 2018). It must be noted that some individuals with mental illness live in underdeveloped environments whereby some standardised methods may need to be adapted to suit the context and its utility, validity and reliability may be compromised.

Some of the standardised methods that can be used to augment the mental state examination include self-report questionnaires (Hospital Anxiety and Depression Scale, Hamilton Depression Inventory, Patient Health Questionnaire), norm-referenced tools (Bay Area Functional Performance Evaluation-Revised, Rivermead-Behavioural Memory Test, Trail Making A and B, Mini-Mental Status Examination, Montreal Cognitive Assessment) and criterion-referenced tools (Thurstone, Valpar

Table 23.2 Signs, symptoms and functional consequences of mania and hypomania.

Hypomania/mania	Functional consequences
Mood Euphoric, irritability, low frustration tolerance, labile affect, anger and hostility.	**Activities of daily living and instrumental activities of daily living** Grooming is usually overdone, makeup is thickly applied and extravagant, bright coloured clothing, lots of jewellery. Poor financial management due to impulsive spending.
Speech Loud, rapid/ pressurized, incoherent.	**Health management** Lack of inhibition and increased sexual activity expose client to possible sexually transmitted infections. Reckless use of substances (drugs, caffeine and alcohol).
Thought Flight of ideas, delusions of grandeur, racing thoughts, tangential and circumstantial.	**Rest and sleep** Lack of sleep, lack of rest due to hyperactivity. Stressors that lead to reduced sleep may contribute to relapses.
Motor activity/ conation Hyperactivity, restlessness and psychomotor agitation.	**Education and/or work** Distractibility, poor concentration and flight of ideas result in incomplete tasks, trying new things and quickly losing interest in them and leaving them incomplete.
Impulse control Increased sexual activity, impulsive spending and lack of inhibition.	Starts projects or makes promises impulsively with little foresight into feasibility or long-term implications. There is also difficulty with job retention and problems at work such as reduced productivity with poor quality due to errors, absenteeism, underemployment (low-skill and low-income).
Cognition Distractibility. Impaired sustained attention span. Impaired concentration. Impaired short-term memory. Impaired problem-solving skills. Impaired executive function.	**Play and/or leisure** Impulsive involvement in creative activities and new hobbies that get abandoned. **Social participation** Poor social skills and poor social judgement. Unable to identify and respond to social cues (verbal and nonverbal cues). Expansive and intrusive interpersonal relationships create tension in social contexts. Overfamiliar with strangers.

Component Work Sample number 6) (Ramano & Buys 2018; Schell & Gillen 2019; AOTA 2020). Performance Assessment of Self-Care Skills (PASS), Assessment of Motor and Process Skills (AMPS) and Kohlman Evaluation of Living Skills (KELS) might be used to assess individuals' activities of daily living and instrumental activities of daily living (Schell & Gillen 2019).

NON-STANDARDISED METHODS

The non-standardised evaluation methods include clinical interviews (structured, unstructured and or semi-structured interviews), clinical observations of mental state, collateral sources such as team members, family members and employers (with due attention to informed), and observations of the individual's participation in structured and unstructured activities (Schell & Gillen 2019; AOTA 2020).

INTERVIEW

Unstructured interviews occur informally when the occupational therapists engage the client in casual conversation as and when the opportunity arises to make a therapeutic connection. Structured and semi-structured interview guidelines that might assist with formal information gathering include the following: the Occupational Self-Assessment (Baron *et al.* 2002), Occupational Performance History Interview II (OPHI-II) (Kielhofner *et al.* 2004) and the Canadian Occupational Performance Measure (COPM) (Law *et al.* 2005). The occupational therapist may need to adapt the items in these guidelines to match the socio-economic and cultural context of the interviewee (Duncan & Prowse 2014).

The occupational therapy interview assists in the initial phase of assessment (Schell & Gillen 2019). During the interview, the occupational therapist obtains the individual's particulars and pertinent background history such as previous illness and treatment, relationships, education, occupational history, occupational profile, occupational environments and current occupational performance. Note that other team members also interview the individual and that his or her admission folder is likely to contain information pertinent to the provision of integrated, multi-professional care. The occupational therapy interview should focus on information about the psychosocial stressors of the individuals' feelings and related behaviours that affect role performance and how impairments in body structures and functions contribute to activity limitations and participation restrictions. Interview also assists in the development of a therapeutic relationship, rapport and negotiating the individuals' recovery goals (Schell & Gillen 2019).

Since individuals share their feelings and life stories during interview, the occupational therapist needs to remain trustworthy by treating their information with respect and the confidentiality it deserves (Duncan & Prowse 2014). In lieu of an interview, the occupational therapist may ask the individual to write their life story or an essay about themselves (Duncan & Prowse 2014).

OBSERVATIONS

Observation is an important occupational therapist skill that involves noting, recording, interpreting and validating an individual's mental well-being and capabilities (Bryant *et al.* 2014). Observation during activity participation is useful in assessing the impact of a mood disorder on an individual's functioning (Duncan & Prowse 2014). The individual can be observed alone (during interview or activity participation) or in a group in the presence of others. Individual observation can happen in structured and unstructured environments to assess the individual's mental state including its impact on physical appearance, verbal and non-verbal communication skills (e.g. facial expression and body language), quality of self-care, task execution and participation in various activities. Observing an individual in a group can assist to assess their interaction and social behaviour towards others.

COLLATERAL INFORMATION

Collateral information may only be obtained with informed consent from the individual or legal guardian. It may be obtained from the professional mental health team, family members, friends, employers and colleagues to gain further valuable information and understanding about the impact of the mood disorder on the functioning of the individual. Collateral information might be used to corroborate or augment the information provided by the individuals seeking help (Duncan & Prowse 2014).

Activity Participation Individuals may be engaged in structured and unstructured activities by an occupational therapist to observe their ability to follow instructions, motivation and interest to initiate and complete activities. During task execution, the occupational therapist could observe the individuals' ability to plan and organise a task, cognitive abilities that include attention span (focused, selective, shifting and sustained), decision-making, judgement, memory, emotional regulation and frustration tolerance, facial expression, handling of materials and tools, accuracy, and ability to complete tasks. At the end of the activity participation, the occupational therapist will observe the individuals' ability to evaluate their task performance, ability to self-correct, number of errors and the quality of the end product. During activity participation and other observations, the occupational therapist might be able to establish the individual's level of creative ability according to the Vona du Toit Model of Creative Ability (VdTMoCA), which includes their level of motivation and level of action (du Toit 2009; van der Reyden et al. 2019).

Occupational Therapy Domains

The occupational therapy practice framework explains the domains that might need to be assessed by the occupational therapist while using standardised and non-standardised methods (AOTA 2020). The occupational therapist may need to perform a comprehensive psychiatric evaluation as stated in the Diagnostic Statistical Manual (DSM-5-TR), which includes specific mental functions (thought process, cognition, mood and affect, insight, psychomotor activity and visual-perceptual abilities) and global mental functions (orientation, sleeping patterns, energy levels, drive and endurance). The domains that an occupational therapist may need to assess include client factors (body functions, body structures, values, beliefs and spirituality), performance skills (motor skills, process skills and social interaction skills),

performance patterns (habits, routines, roles and rituals), occupations (activities of daily living, leisure participation and interest, socialisation and work), and context (personal factors and environmental factors (AOTA 2020).

Occupation therapists use relevant cognitive assessment tools such as the Montreal Cognitive Assessment (MOCA) (Julayanont et al. 2012) to determine the cognitive functioning of individuals with depressive disorders and bipolar disorders. Executive dysfunction in bipolar disorders predicts poorer academic performance, worse vocational outcomes, reduced social adjustments and diminished quality of life (Zarate et al. 2000; Levy & Manove 2012).

The occupational therapy evaluation is aimed at identifying impairments in body functions and structures, their severity and how they impact the occupational performance of the individuals in different contexts. Objective information during the evaluation provides both the occupational therapist and the individuals concerned with a baseline from which to identify recovery goals and ways of addressing the practical challenges of 'doing' daily life.

INTERVENTION

Various interventions are used in occupational therapy with the aim of preventing performance difficulties, promoting healthy participation and reducing the impact of impairment and disability on daily life (AOTA 2020). The occupational therapist should use appropriate intervention strategies such as health promotion, remediation/restoration, maintenance, compensation or adaptation and disability prevention (AOTA 2020). The occupational therapy intervention should be designed to establish, modify, and or maintain performance, prevent disability and promote health and wellness in daily occupations (AOTA 2020). Occupational therapists can use activity analysis, activity adaptations, compensatory strategies, environmental modifications to foster occupational performance and to empower individuals (AOTA 2020). In order to maximise the intervention, the occupational therapist may need to grade it. Factors to be considered when grading the intervention are the number of activity steps, the complexity of the activity, the way of presenting the activity, the duration of the activity, the handling principles and the therapist profile.

Furthermore, occupational therapists provide either individual and/or group intervention to increase the individuals' participation in occupations such as activities of daily living, instrumental activities of daily living, leisure, rest and sleep, health management, education, work and social participation (AOTA 2020). The occupational therapy intervention should empower individuals to be able to engage in day-to-day activities and enhance their well-being, lifestyle adjustment and participation in the community.

Holistic management of individuals with depressive disorders and bipolar disorders includes leisure participation and enhancement (recreation, sports and games), expressive groups, vocational guidance, work assessment, readiness and supported employment, stress management and creative pursuits. The occupational therapy interventions that are commonly used for the management of depressive disorders and bipolar disorders are psychosocial, psycho-educational, cognitive and leisure/exercise interventions (Rocamora-Montenegro *et al.* 2021).

PSYCHOSOCIAL INTERVENTION

Psychosocial intervention is aimed at improving mental state, functioning in life roles including occupational balance and reintegration (personal care, learning, social and work). Psychosocial interventions are efficacious at an early stage of bipolar disorder (Miziou *et al.* 2015). Psychosocial interventions need to be sensitive to cognitive impairments and residual symptoms of MDD and bipolar disorder (Levy & Manove 2012). Psychosocial intervention can be offered in an individual therapy session but mostly it is offered in a group therapy session.

The choice of group therapy is its encouragement for group interaction, feedback and facilitation of Yalom and Leszcz therapeutic factors (Yalom & Leszcz 2020) as discussed in Chapter 7. Occupational group therapy promotes personal growth because it encourages social interaction with people who face similar life challenges in a supportive and containing environment (Crouch 2021). In many cases, the person with a mood disorder will have felt 'alone' or that 'no-one understands how I feel'. By participating in occupational therapy group, they start to feel less alone and realise that there are many others who have similar feelings and challenges (Ramano *et al.* 2021). Although their circumstances may differ, group members are able to connect with one another on an emotional level. Experiential learning in groups leads to shifts in motivation, self-esteem and belief in self, all of which empower members to regain control over their lives. Groups foster altruism, which helps some individuals with depressive disorders and bipolar disorders to move beyond egocentric thinking and self-centred behaviour.

The occupational therapy group should be client centred and the occupational therapist should show respect, empathy, acceptance and support to the individuals (Caruso *et al.* 2013). The occupational therapist should not group severely depressed individuals together as it may affect the characteristics of the group and create a stifling atmosphere. Different types of occupational therapy groups (refer to Chapter 7), each drawing on different frames of reference and group theory, will be discussed below.

Life Skills Groups

The goal of life skills groups is to equip individuals with effective and healthy coping skills necessary for optimal functioning (Cole 2012, 2019). Life skills sessions impart knowledge, promote insight and provide opportunity to train, practise and plan for challenging life situations. Life skills promote individuals' physical, mental and emotional well-being and competence. Group members share their own experiences as this produces a rich source of learning. They learn the skill of identifying problems and assets and systematically working towards practical solutions (Ebersohn & Eloff 2003). Some of the topics covered may include stress management, anger management, time management, sleep hygiene, assertiveness, healthy eating, conflict resolution, goal setting, money management/budgeting, problem-solving and balanced living. Relaxation therapy should be avoided with individuals who are severely depressed or manic.

The cognitive behavioural frame of reference is used during life skills group sessions to individuals to problem-solve their current needs and to modify dysfunctional behaviours and/or distorted thinking (Cole 2019; Cole & Tufano 2019). The cognitive behavioural frame of reference can be used to challenge distorted thoughts by allowing individuals to acknowledge irrational ideas and negative thoughts. It can also be used during assertiveness, mindfulness and coping skills training and role play (Cole & Tufano 2019; AOTA 2020).

Dialectical behaviour therapy (DBT) is a modified type of cognitive behavioural therapy. It teaches individuals with depressive disorders and bipolar disorders to develop healthy ways of coping with stress, regulating emotions and developing healthy ways to relate with others. There are four core skills that are taught while using DBT, which are mindfulness, distress tolerance, emotional regulation and interpersonal skills (Gillespie *et al.* 2022).

When occupational therapists target life skills (e.g. financial management, education, community mobility, health maintenance and leisure engagement), well-being and quality of life are improved through independent functioning and community reintegration in and outside of work environments (DeAngelis *et al.* 2019).

Expressive Groups

The goal is to promote emotional insight by allowing members to express feelings, discuss recent experiences needing to be processed for their recovery, as well as reflect on their life and relationships with others (Becker & Duncan 2005). These groups provide an open and unstructured space for interpersonal interaction and feedback in an environment that is non-threatening, containing and confidential and promotes sharing. These groups may make use of evocative techniques such as projective art, psychodrama and growth games as the means through which members can process the dynamics of their behaviour.

A psychoanalytic/psychodynamic approach may inform the therapist's thinking in these groups (Nicholls *et al.* 2012). Projective techniques are activities that help group members to express emotions and communication such as painting, drawing, collage, free clay modelling, sculpture, music, movement or musical expression, poetry, creative writing, empty chair, journaling and psychodrama (Cole 2019; Cole & Tufano 2019). Psychodrama and projective techniques should be avoided with individuals who are severely depressed or manic.

A mood disorder can leave the person in a negative cycle of feeling guilty, unworthy and unable. By adopting a reality focus, the occupational therapist prevents the individual from taking on a 'sick role' and wallowing in a sense of helplessness. The occupational therapist guides the individuals in identifying how their feelings sabotage health-promoting occupational performance and encourages constructive thinking as the basis for the agency. Combining unconditional acceptance with confrontation of the consequences of maladaptive behaviours, the occupational therapist guides and affirms the individual's efforts in working towards recovery and well-being. By so doing, the occupational therapist encourages self-awareness through reality testing and feedback from others (Cole & Tufano 2019).

Activity-based Groups

Concrete products or tangible activities or practical tasks are executed during activity groups. Some of the activity groups may require some creativity, and task concept. The activity groups may assist the individuals to be distracted from negative thoughts, relax, learn a new skill or leisure opportunity, encourage self-expression and affirm their creativity. Group members in an activity group work towards a common goal in the 'here and now', that is, on the 'doing' and the 'being' in action as a means for clarifying feelings, motives, needs and response patterns. Interest in activities is enhanced when the person experiences a 'just right challenge' and a sense of anticipation and enjoyment when engaging in a task.

In a qualitative study by Ramano et al. (2021), the individuals who were diagnosed with MDDs participated in activities in the occupational therapy activity-based group and they shared that they experienced feelings of happiness, pleasure and laughter and inner fulfilment through task satisfaction. Furthermore, they reported that activities provided healing and wellness and improved their self-confidence to feel strong enough to face life problems and the world (Ramano et al. 2021).

During the activity groups, the occupational therapist must adopt an affirmative approach to ensure that the activities offer a motivating and supporting therapeutic effect to the person's successful doing.

PSYCHO-EDUCATIONAL INTERVENTIONS

The objective of psycho-educational intervention is to improve disease management as insight training is done with the individuals using education and training as the type of occupational therapy intervention (AOTA 2020). Insight training includes imparting information regarding diagnosis, the signs and symptoms, medication compliance and the importance of relapse prevention. Psycho-educational interventions aiming at relapse prevention are found to be effective as bipolar disorder can increase the stress level of individuals (Levy & Manove 2012; Miziou et al. 2015). While it is necessary for MDD, it is far more important for bipolar disorder due to its high relapse rate of about 50% in the first five months and 80–90% within the first 18 months. Psycho-education empowers, and provides skills and information to individuals. Self-stigma, public stigma and discrimination remain the major obstacles for psychological growth of individuals with bipolar disorders (Michalak et al. 2007; Levy & Manove 2012; Talatala et al. 2020). Therefore, psycho-education should be extended to the family and employers. A range of frames of reference and group theories are used in individuals' education (Dreeben 2010).

The goal of psycho-educational groups is to increase the individuals' understanding of their illness and how to self-manage it as they share their experiences within the occupational therapy group. Where indicated, risks and treatment options are explored with due recognition of the interface between traditional (cultural) and medical interventions. The person's strengths, resources and coping skills are reinforced in order to prevent relapse and to promote active involvement in the plan of care. These sessions are also used to increase adherence to medication and treatment regimes, leading to a more efficient and cost-effective health care delivery service.

Symptom Management

As part of health management, occupational therapists assist individuals with symptom management by teaching techniques to manage side effects of medications, memory strategies, and relaxation techniques (AOTA 2020). Sleep disruption is often the final common pathway triggering manic episodes and is also associated with depression. Therefore, the individuals should be encouraged to participate in daily activities or the group programme while in the ward (Goodwin et al. 2016). Occupational therapy will guide the person towards occupations that affirm self-esteem and enable emotions to be expressed in ways that promote a positive sense of identity, purpose and belonging.

Occupational therapy interventions are found to have medium effect in improving occupational performance and small effect on improving well-being (Ikiugu et al. 2017). Ikiugu et al. (2017) in their meta-analysis further reported that occupational therapy interventions improve mental health symptoms and occupations such as home management and maintenance, parenting, work and social participation. The interventions are based on theoretical frameworks such as the Canadian Model of Occupational Performance and Engagement (CMOP-E), Cognitive Disabilities (CD) model, Model of Human Occupation (MOHO), Client centred model, Psychodynamic theoretical conceptual practice model and Occupational Adaptation (OA) (Ikiugu et al. 2017).

Ramano et al. (2021) in their study found that activities assist with symptom reduction of individuals who are diagnosed with MDD. Occupational therapy activities improved their mood and regained their self-esteem (Ramano et al. 2021). Therefore, the occupational therapist should engage individuals with depressed mood in carefully graded activities to stimulate enjoyment, improve their mood and self-esteem and expression of emotions. The activities used should be flopproof or guarantee an element of success. Activities such as sports and leisure should also be introduced as they stimulate enjoyment.

COGNITIVE INTERVENTION

Cognitive occupational therapy intervention is when meaningful and purposeful occupations are used to improve the cognitive abilities of an individual. MDD and bipolar disorder result in impairments in cognition and executive functions, which in turn affects functional participation. Cognitive intervention is intended to improve cognitive functioning and processing strategies of individuals with depressive disorders and bipolar disorders.

Cognitive Remediation

Cognitive remediation has been proven to be successful with depressive disorders and bipolar individuals as an emerging non-pharmaceutical option to improve cognitive performance (Levy & Manove 2012). Cognitive remediation improves judgement, decision-making, working memory and psychosocial functioning while reducing disability.

Cognitive Rehabilitation

Cognitive rehabilitative interventions are effective at later stages of intervention as they are used to retrain previously learned skills and they teach compensatory strategies (Miziou et al. 2015). The two approaches used in cognitive rehabilitation are restorative and compensatory (AOTA 2020). Examples of cognitive rehabilitation activities for individuals with depressive disorders and bipolar disorders are memory games, problem-solving games and mental activities.

Occupational therapists incorporate cognitive rehabilitation, cognitive remediation/stimulation and cognitive training into cognitive intervention. Social skills, life skills, neurocognitive interventions coupled with vocational, social and IADL training were found to be effective in enhancing executive functioning and healthy routines for individuals with depressive disorders and bipolar disorders (Ikiugu et al. 2017).

LEISURE ACTIVITIES

Leisure activities can address motor activity and cognitive difficulties by using sports and table games. For individuals with MDD, exercise will be more upbeat in order to energise them as they present with psychomotor retardation and depressed mood. With bipolar disorder, the focus is more on calming exercises to reduce hyperactivity and elated mood.

The neurophysiological approach is beneficial with individuals who suffer from MDD as it encourages large arm movements, psychomotor activation, physical activity, sunlight, diaphragmatic breathing and tactile stimulation. The use of the neurophysiological approach advises on the use of outdoor and indoor sport to improve the mood of individuals with MDDs. Cardiovascular activities also increase more circulation of blood and increase oxygen to the brain, which also helps in improving the mood of individuals with MDD. While treating individuals with bipolar I disorder, the occupational should not overtire them and strenuous physical activities should be avoided.

INTERVENTION INTO WORK

Symptoms of depressive disorders and bipolar disorders are associated with reduced work quality and output and increased interpersonal problems with colleagues at work (Michalak et al. 2007). Rates of employment are low amongst individuals with bipolar disorders (Michalak et al. 2007). Furthermore, individuals with bipolar disorders undergo occupational loss (loss of job prospect, loss of time at work, financial loss and loss of identity) (Michalak et al. 2007).

Work focussed intervention provided as part of usual therapy or by an occupational therapist with advanced experience in vocational rehabilitation assists individuals to find and maintain competitive employment and to overcome barriers that affect their participation in the workplace (Rocamora-Montenegro et al. 2021).

Client-centred

Vocational intervention employs a client-centred approach as there is consultation and collaboration with the individual to devise a work readiness, return-to-work or a supported employment plan. Other client-centred approaches may be facilitated through vocational counselling to eliminate recurring symptoms and empower individuals (Levy & Manove 2012).

Being client-centred involves working with understanding, empathy and validating the individuals' unique circumstances. The occupational therapist should be ethical, reality-focused and solution-orientated during vocational intervention. Furthermore, the occupational therapist should be mindful of their professional boundaries, limitations and recognise that the individual is ultimately responsible for his/her own decisions and healing process. An individual with mania is likely to have few internal boundaries. The occupational therapist therefore needs to be consistent and clear in the external boundaries that are set, using the client-centred relationship to model appropriate social behaviour.

Currently, there are limited treatment options that address work deficits (prevocational skills and vocational skills) for individuals with bipolar disorders (Goodwin et al. 2016). There is a need for more effective work interventions specifically designed for bipolar disorders and MDDs (Goodwin et al. 2016). There are limited studies aimed at identifying predictors of poor employment outcome for bipolar disorders (Goodwin *et al.* 2016). Earlier return to work is suggested for bipolar disorders as it provides individuals with a structured schedule and a greater chance for support from both co-workers and supervisors (Priebe *et al.* 1998). Individuals with bipolar disorders experience substantial difficulty getting along with co-workers and supervisors due to their clinical symptoms (Goodwin *et al.* 2016). Therefore, vocational interventions should include vocational rehabilitation groups that focus on social skills, conflict resolutions, conflict management, setting boundaries and communication skills.

Cognitive Work Hardening

Cognitive work hardening assists individuals with depression and bipolar disorders to attain their goals and succeed in their preparation for return-to-work. The focus of cognitive work hardening is on the workplace and the skills required (mental and physical) by the individual to be effective at work (Wisenthal & Krupa 2013). Life coaching including strategies for mental health promotion through occupation is likely to strengthen the individual's capacity for productive participation in life roles.

Reasonable Accommodation

The occupational therapist may suggest reasonable accommodation for individuals with depressive disorders and bipolar disorders such as suggesting flexibility in their work schedule (working flexi-time or working from home) to encourage a normal sleep-wake cycle and reducing their workload (Michalak *et al.* 2007). The legislation promoting the implementation of reasonable accommodations or work place adaptations may be considered to allow the individuals to continue working and to meet their productivity standards.

Incapacity

The occupational therapist may suggest temporary incapacity (which is provided for under Code of Good Practice: Dismissal (CGP:D) contained as Schedule 8 of the Labour Relations Act No 66 of 1995) for the individuals with depressive disorders and bipolar disorders from their work settings while they are still symptomatic with poor work habits and poor vocational skills (Labour Relations Act No 66 of 1995; Michalak *et al.* 2007).

Advocacy Care Efforts

Advocacy uses client-centred approach as it involves both the therapist and the individual with mood disorder. Its main objective is to bring about change in the individuals' environment in order to ensure occupational engagement, which in turn improves quality of life. The occupational therapist will advocate for the work needs of individuals. Furthermore, the occupational therapist should act as an advocate for the individual and back up their negotiations with relevant legislation appropriate to each country. These may include legislation affecting working conditions, health and safety regulations, wellness in the workplace and work place adaptations (Modise *et al.* 2014; Ramano & Buys 2018).

Case Management

Case management is a collaborative supported employment process that assesses, plans, implements, coordinates, monitors and evaluates options and services to meet the health needs of an individual through communication and available resources to promote cost-effective outcomes (Schell & Gillen 2019). It is used during an extended period of absence from work or a high rate of absence from work due to illness. It helps to facilitate return-to-work for employees with mental illness. The occupational therapist is expected to develop an intervention care plan, reskilling/retraining and liaise with the employer of individuals with depressive disorders and bipolar disorders to aid in reintegration back into the workplace (Chimara *et al.* 2022).

The case manager, who is an occupational therapist, assesses the needs of individuals with depressive disorders and bipolar disorders, develops their care plan, arranges suitable care in the workplace and constantly keeps contact with the individual and involved stakeholders (Dieterich *et al.* 2017). Case management and occupational therapy are compatible in both philosophy and practice as they both use client-centred and holistic approach (Dieterich *et al.* 2017). An occupational therapist as a case manager focuses beyond services provided in the hospital and assists the individual with depressive disorders and bipolar disorders to achieve optimum participation during and after incapacity (Dieterich *et al.* 2017).

OUTCOMES

An outcome measure is used to evaluate the intervention that is being provided to the individuals, to capture change over time in order to trace improvement in performance skills, client factors, contexts and individuals' ability to engage in desired occupations (Gateley & Borcherding 2016; AOTA 2020). The outcome measure should be valid, reliable and sensitive to change in the individuals' occupational performance as it measures intervention progress (AOTA 2020). The outcomes in occupational therapy should be measured with the same methods used at evaluation compared with the individual's status at discharge or transition (AOTA 2020: 26). Examples of outcome measures are Assessment of Motor and Process Skills (AMPS), Canadian Occupational Performance Measure (COPM) and Kohlman Evaluation of Living Skills (KELS) (Schell & Gillen 2019).

Outcomes targeted in occupational therapy for individuals with depressive disorders and bipolar disorders can be occupational performance, role competence, health and wellness, and occupational justice (AOTA 2020).

| CASE STUDY 1 | Mrs M, Who Is Diagnosed with Major Depressive Disorder |

MRS M BACKGROUND

Mrs M is 52 years old. She has been married for 20 years. She is the mother of two boys who are both teenagers in grades 12 and 10, respectively. Her boys avoid assisting with household chores and she has to perform the tasks alone. Her husband runs a taxi business but does not contribute financially to the household. She takes all the financial responsibility of the household and she has a lot of debts including loans and owing people at work.

She is a grade three educator at a primary school. She has been working as an educator for 25 years. She is the Head of Department (HOD) of home languages for the foundation phase. As an HOD, the expected maximum number of learners in a class should be 33 including administrative duties. She teaches a class of 65 learners. When other HODs in foundation phase are absent, she is expected to perform their duties. She is also expected to act as a deputy principal when the deputy principal is absent and still teach and head her department. The principal is also dependent on her because of her vast knowledge and experience in education and administration. She is extremely overloaded and she has to work long hours. She also takes work home most of the time.

A mother of one of her learners came to their school to complain to the principal about Mrs M's misconduct of ill-treating her daughter in class. A meeting was held between the principal, the mother and Mrs M; however, Mrs M felt that the principal took the side of the parent and did not listen to her side of the story. She felt bullied, betrayed, unsupported and victimised by the principal.

She is currently anxious about returning to work as she finds the workplace to be unsupportive and she is confused about how she is going to handle the learner in her class. She is angry with the principal because she feels the principal over-burdens her and does not support or protect her. She noticed her reduced motivation to work, declining work performance and being unable to meet her deadlines. She is not interested to return to her workplace.

Another role she has is being a member of the Mothers' Union at the Anglican church. However, lately, she has been unable to participate in Mothers' Union activities and she sometimes misses church services, as she is trying to catch up on her job responsibilities that are left behind.

Mrs M was admitted to a mental healthcare facility by the treating psychiatrist, who diagnosed her with major depressive disorder. Her clinical presentation on admission includes feelings of sadness, anger and frustration, constant worrying, persistent headaches, back pains, crying, mixed insomnia, forgetfulness, lack of interest in her daily activities, social withdrawal as she locks herself in the house, fatigue, and feelings of helplessness and hopelessness.

The treating psychiatrist prescribed antidepressants, sleeping medications and analgesics. In addition, she referred Mrs M to the clinical psychologist, social worker and occupational therapist for interdisciplinary team intervention.

EVALUATION

Mrs M had her first contact with the occupational therapist who did the evaluation using non-standardised methods (interview, observations, collateral information, activity participation) and standardised measures (Patient Health Questionnaire [PHQ-9], Montreal Cognitive Assessment [MOCA], Bay Area of Functional Performance-Revised [BaFPE-R], Burnout questionnaire). During the clinical interview, the occupational therapist obtained Mrs M's occupational history, occupational profile, psychosocial stressors and client factors. Mrs M was further observed during activity participation and standardised measures.

Her assessment findings were as follows:

Client factors affected are body functions (depressed mood, anxiety, high level of anger, restricted affect, low motivation, lack of interest, social withdrawal, lack of assertiveness skills, poor memory, poor planning and organisation, poor attention and ability to concentrate, poor decision-making, poor problem-solving) and values, beliefs and spirituality (unable to participate in Mothers Union activities and attend church services).

The standardised measures were used to triangulate the therapists' findings. Mrs M scores were:

- PHQ-9 scored 23 (20–27 is severe depression)

- MOCA scored 21/30 and average is 26/30 (impaired cognitive ability)

- Burnout questionnaire scored 118 (91 up is a dangerous level of burnout)

- BaFPE-R she scored below average on cognition (memory, planning and organisation and attention), performance (task completion, speed and quality) and affective (depressed mood).

Occupations affected are IADLs (financial management, neglects her home as she struggles to execute her household chores), rest and sleep (insomnia and working long hours), sexual activity (low libido and loss of interest in her relationship with her husband), work (inability to handle the learner in her class, low work motivation, poor work performance), leisure and social participation (unable to participate in Mothers' Union activities and attend church services) and poor work-life balance. She neglects her roles as mother and wife.

Her psychosocial stressors are marital problems, financial strain, high workload (occupational overload) and working long hours.

Her self-management skills show that she is non-assertive and struggles to set boundaries since she is a pleaser and associates her behaviour with her spiritual role as a Christian.

According to the Vona du Toit Model of Creative Ability, Mrs M is on the level of self-presentation, patient-directed phase.

INTERVENTION

Mrs M attended a comprehensive full-day multidisciplinary group programme. The occupational therapy group programme focused on life skills groups (assertiveness, boundaries, coping with stress in the workplace and work-life balance), socio-emotional and support groups (collage of my life story, self-awareness and creative drawing) and leisure groups (30 seconds and finger board).

Individual sessions with the occupational therapist focused on (1) symptom management by involving her in arts and crafts activities to affirm her self-worth and positive feelings about self and life, (2) life skills (financial management, delegation of responsibilities as part of carry-over and reinforcement of assertiveness skills and boundaries that she learned in the group) and (3) cognitive remediation (activities that simulate her cognitive requirements as an educator were chosen and graded by complexity and duration).

A client-centred approach was employed during vocational intervention, which included vocational counselling and guidance, reasonable accommodation and advocacy. The occupational therapist contacted collateral sources (the principal) for collateral information and to negotiate preparation for Mrs M return to work with reasonable accommodations to enable her to meet her key job functions.

Mrs M showed good response to intervention with good vocational prognosis. Her scores prior to discharge from hospital were as follows:

- PHQ-9 scored 8 (5–9 is mild depression)
- MOCA scored 28/30 (normal cognitive ability with some improvements)

After advocating to the principal, the occupational therapist compiled a progress report. Mrs M returned to work one week post-discharge. She will be reviewed two weeks after returning to work to assess whether the occupational therapy recommendations were implemented.

CASE STUDY 2 — Cindy, Who Is Diagnosed with Bipolar I Disorder

CINDY'S HISTORY

Cindy is 52 years old. She is the only child. She speaks Setswana. She was born and grew up in Soweto. Her parents were not married. Her father is still alive and they do not have a relationship. Her mother died in the year 2002. She was raised by her 96-year-old grandmother, who died from a heart attack on 1 February 2023.

She got married in 2003 and divorced in 2005. They had two daughters, aged 20 years and 18 years. Her 20-year-old daughter is struggling to be admitted at the university where Cindy is employed. Her 18-year-old daughter is in grade 12. Her ex-husband is currently unemployed and financially unsupportive. Cindy reports that her ex-husband has never been financially supportive. They used to fight a lot during their marriage as he was unreasonable and he did not want her to spoil herself like, buying clothes. Cindy reports that she does not have a boyfriend currently and she feels lonely. She reports that her intimate relationships with other partners after her divorce usually last for less than six months because of her lack of interest and mistrust in men.

Cindy is a Christian and currently studying theology at Bible school. She is currently unhappy with her fathers' family as they told her that she needs to consult traditional healer as she might be having a calling to train as a sangoma (traditional healer). She believes that she has a gift to become a pastor and to heal people in a Christian way. She is even convinced that God speaks to her and He gives her messages about our country and presidents. She reports that her paternal failure wants to destroy her and see her as a failure, which is why they are referring her to traditional healers. They want to stop her spiritual gift from God.

Cindy has two certificates in management and a bachelors' degree in administration. She is employed as a senior faculty officer at a university in Gauteng. She joined the university on 1 June 2005. Her job responsibility involves assisting the post-graduate students and academic staff.

On 12 February 2023, Cindy was admitted to a psychiatric facility with a history of being talkative, singing, preaching and praying for everyone in the house. Her energy levels were high and she reported that she did not sleep or go to work for the past three days as she was talking to God. She is angry with her 20-year-old daughter, who forcefully brought her to the psychiatric facility. Her treating psychiatrist diagnosed her with Bipolar Disorder I (BDI), complicated bereavement and work-related stress. Her treating psychiatrist referred her to consult with the social worker, clinical psychologist and occupational therapist.

EVALUATION

The occupational therapist had a session with Cindy for clinical interview and building a therapeutic relationship. The occupational therapist used a semi-structured interview which allowed Cindy to narrate her story. Standardised (MOCA, BaFPE-R, Burnout questionnaire) and non-standardised (observation, clinical interview, activity participation) methods were used to assess Cindy. Below is a summary of occupational therapists' findings.

Roles: single mother and worker role
Rituals: Christian
Interests: enjoys sewing and knitting, using her computer or cell phone
Habits: Non-smoker and non-alcohol drinker

Cindy reported her **issues** as follows:

- Death of her grandmother on the 1 February 2023
- Unsupportive father (ex-husband) of her two daughters

(Continued)

CASE 2   *(Continued)*

- Serious financial problems

- Work-related problems (declining work performance, unable to meet deadlines and conflicting relationship with the head of department)

Clinical picture during interview and observations:

- *Mood:* Irritable mood and elevated mood

- *Affect:* Labile affect

- *Speech:* Pressure of speech and over-inclusive

- *Form of thought:* Flight of ideas

- *Content of thought:* Religiosity, grandiosity and persecutory delusions

- *Motor activity/conation:* Hyperactivity and high energy levels

- *Impulse control:* Lack of inhibition and impulsive spending

- *Rest and sleep:* Mixed insomnia

- *Behaviour:* Aggression and low frustration tolerance

- *Cognition:* Impaired concentration, impaired concrete-decision making, impaired executive functioning

- *Physical:* Body pains

Activity of daily living (ADL):

Her self-care was overdone with extravagant make-up, lipsticks and dressed professionally in bright clothes and high-heeled shoes.

Instrumental activities of daily living: She reported poor financial management and an inability to budget. She reported that she spends most of her time buying clothes. She even renovated her grandmothers' house in December 2022 without proper planning and the project could not be completed. During collateral information with her daughter, she informed the occupational therapist that Cindy does not sleep at night. Cindy would clean the house at night and start praying afterwards. She does not cook anymore.

Work:

Cindy is employed as a senior faculty officer since 1 June 2005. She reported a declining work performance due to arriving late at work and she is unable to complete her duties. Her job is too much and it frustrates as she does not know where to start. Her manager worsens the situation as she makes unnecessary demands and she is always on her case. '. . . I feel micromanaged . . .' She further reported that she is expected to manage three other faculty officers and her responsibilities are overwhelming her. The occupational therapist contacted Cindy's employer (boss and human resource) for collateral information and to notify them about Cindy's admission. It is clear that Cindy presents with poor work habits and poor vocational skills.

Socialisation:

Cindy was overfamiliar with the occupational therapist with poor social skills. She was unable to read the non-verbal cues from the occupational therapist. She informed the occupational therapist that everyone is her friend at work and home. '. . . they are all my friends . . . I preach and pray for them . . .' She would buy things for people and give them some of her clothes.

Leisure participation:

She does not engage in leisure due to high workload. She is always using her laptop when she is at home. She reports that she has to catch-up with her incomplete work.

Task performance: leatherwork (making a keyholder). Materials (leather, leather tool, scissor, ring, glue, sponge, hammer and revolving punch).

During activity participation, Cindy needed demonstrated instructions with repetitions. She was impulsive and attempted the task with poor task comprehension. The instructions had to be repeated again to assist Cindy in understanding the expectations from her. She executed the task very haphazardly with poor handling of the tools and materials with poor accuracy when cutting the leather. She did not pay attention to details. She did not follow a logical sequence and she showed impaired task planning and organisation. She showed no delay of gratification with impaired concrete decision-making, inattention and low frustration tolerance. She requested a lot of assistance from the occupational therapist due to her feelings of insecurity and inadequacy. She needed a lot of affirmation from the therapist as she was struggling with the task. She was talkative and easily distracted, which affected her poor performance. She became frustrated and left the task incomplete asking the occupational therapist to do it. '. . . you can't do it as well . . . otherwise, do it yourself . . . this thing [task] is impossible . . .' She shows poor task completion and she was unable to self-correct due to her poor task evaluation. Her quality of endproduct was poor due to her incomplete task and high number of errors.

Standardised measures:

The standardised measures that were used to triangulate the therapists' findings were Montreal Cognitive Assessment (MOCA), Burnout questionnaire, and Bay Area of Functional Performance-Revised (BaFPE-R). Her scores were:

MOCA scored 18/30 and average is 26/30 (impaired cognitive ability).

Burnout questionnaire scored 123 (91 up is a dangerous level of burnout).

BaFPE-R she scored below average on cognition (memory, planning and organisation, and attention), performance (task completion, efficiency and errors) and affective (manic and frustration tolerance).

INTERVENTION

The occupational therapist formulated an intervention plan for Cindy with clear objectives, aim and goals. Cindy attended a two-week occupational therapy group programme and individual occupational therapy sessions on a daily basis while she was treated in-hospital.

Hospital Group Program:

She attended a comprehensive full day multidisciplinary group programme. The occupational therapy group programme focused on activity-based groups (beadwork making a bracelet/necklace, painting jewellery box, cardmaking for feedback, fabric painting, candle making and flower arrangement), life skills groups (assertiveness, boundaries, emotional blackmail, coping with stress in the workplace and financial management), socio-emotional and support groups (coping with loss), psycho-education (insight on condition and medication) and leisure groups (30 seconds). During occupational therapy groups, the occupational therapist constantly followed the group procedure, used Yalom therapeutic factors, psychosocial interactive approach and the principles of Vona du Toit Model of Creative Ability.

The occupational therapist ensured that the groups were concrete and activity-based during week one. Educational and socio-emotional groups were introduced in week two.

Hospital Individual Sessions:

Cindy attended ten individual occupational therapy sessions over a period of two weeks. She was initially seen for 45 minutes in week 1 and 60 minutes in week 2. In week 1, the occupational therapist followed the principles of Vona du Toit Model of Creative Ability while using the activities. The activities that were used during the sessions were word search, scratch paper, looming (making a beanie) and mosaic angel in remembrance of her deceased granny. Some of the activities had to be carried over to the next day.

In week 2, the occupational therapist commenced with psycho-education to reinforce insight to her condition and the importance of compliancy with medication. Cindy was calmer and cooperative. She continued to have pressure of speech and some religiosity. Other sessions that followed included financial management and budgeting, bereavement sessions coping with work stress and vocational counselling.

Prior to discharge, Cindy was not ready to return to work.

OUTPATIENT FOLLOW-UP

She was reviewed after two weeks for a functional capacity evaluation. An occupational therapy report was compiled for Cindy to take a copy to her psychiatrist and the employer. She was booked off work for three months of temporary incapacity leave.

She attended two sessions of occupational therapy per month for a period of three months while she was on incapacity leave. The sessions focused on cognitive remediation, psycho-education, bereavement occupational therapy sessions (mosaic angel, reminiscence session and journaling), empowerment, vocational counselling session on work habits and to prepare her to return to work. On reassessment, she scored as follows:

MOCA scored 29/30 and average is 26/30 (no cognitive impairment).

BaFPE-R: she scored average on cognition, performance and affective functioning. She shows marked improvement compared to her admission to the hospital.

CASE MANAGEMENT

The occupational therapist became a case manager for Cindy and liaised with Cindy's manager and Human Resource manager (HR). When Cindy was ready to return to work, the occupational therapist wrote a follow-up letter requesting the HR to mediate between Cindy and her boss in order to create a harmonious work environment. Furthermore, the occupational therapist recommended reasonable accommodations as guided by the employment equity act 55 of 1998. The reasonable accommodations included requesting restructuring her job so that her non-essential functions are re-assigned when she is adjusting at work. The rest of the functions were added monthly over a period of three months. Cindy was reviewed by her occupational therapist once a month after she returned to work for three months and she adjusted well to her job functions. There was circulatory follow-up feedback between the occupational therapist, manager and HR. She was compliant with her medication and her children were happy with her progress and good response to team intervention. Her 20-year-old daughter reported that Cindy has started to cook, knit clothes and enjoy looming, sleeps well at night and no longer preaches or shouts at them. Cindy reported that she is trying to be disciplined and committed with regards to the budget that she compiled while in the hospital. She is relating well with her manager and she finds her team to be cooperative. Cindy was discharged from occupational therapy as she showed a good outcome to intervention.

QUESTIONS

1. Explain the steps that you would follow to provide a comprehensive occupational therapy assessment of an individual who is diagnosed with bipolar II disorder.

2. Discuss the psychosocial intervention that you will offer for individuals with depressive disorders and bipolar disorders. Explain how you will grade your intervention.

3. Compare the intervention for individuals who are newly diagnosed with major depressive disorder and bipolar I disorder (manic episode).

4. Explain your case management plan in facilitating the return to work for Cindy, who is diagnosed with bipolar I disorder (BDI) and she has been on temporary incapacity leave for a period of three months (as discussed in Case 2).

REFERENCES

American Occupational Therapy Association (AOTA) (2020) Occupational therapy practice framework: domain and process. 4th edn. *The American Journal of Occupational Therapy*, **74 (Supplement 2)**, 1–87.

American Psychiatric Association (APA) (2013) *Diagnostic and Statistical Manual of Mental Disorders*, 5th edn. American Psychiatric Association, Washington, DC.

American Psychiatric Association (APA) (2022) *Diagnostic and Statistical Manual of Mental Disorders: DSM-5-TR*, 5th edn. *American Psychiatric Association*, Washington, DC.

Anyayo, L. & Ashaba, S. (2021) Health-related quality of life among patients with bipolar disorder in rural southwestern Uganda: a hospital based cross sectional study. *Health and Quality of Life Outcomes*, **19**, 84. https://doi.org/10.1186/s12955-021-01729-5

Bains, N. & Abdijadid, S. (2023) *Major Depressive Disorder*. National Library of Medicine

Baron, K., Kielhofner, G., Iyenger, A., Goldhammer, V. & Wolenski, J. (2002) *The Occupational Self-Assessment (OSA) (Version 2.0)*. Model of Human Occupation Clearinghouse, Department of Occupational Therapy, College of Applied Health Sciences, University of Illinois at Chicago, Chicago.

Becker, L. & Duncan, M. (2005) Thinking about groups. In: L. Becker (ed), *Working with Groups*, pp. 25–32. Oxford University Press, Cape Town.

Biazus, T.B., Beraldi, G.H. & Tokeshi, L. *et al* (2023) All-cause and cause-specific mortality among people with bipolar disorder: a large-scale systematic review and meta-analysis. *Molecular Psychiatry*, **28**, 1–17.

Bryant, W., Fieldhouse, J. & Bannigan, K. (2014) *Creek's Occupational Therapy and Mental Health*, 5th edn. Churchill Livingston Elsevier, China.

Cameron, C., Habert, J., Anand, L. & Furtado, M. (2014) Optimizing the management of depression: primary care experience. *Psychiatry Research*, **220**, S45–S57.

Caruso, R., Grassi, L. & Biancosino, B. *et al* (2013) Exploration and experiences in therapeutic groups for patients with severe mental illness: development of the Ferrara group experiences scale (FE-GES). *BioMed Central Psychiatry*, **13(242)**, 1–9.

Chimara, M., van Biljon, H. & van Niekerk, L. (2022) Scoping review exploring vocational rehabilitation intervention for mental health service users with chronic illness in low-income to upper—middle-income countries. *Biomedical Journal*, **12**, e05921, 1–13.

Cole, M. (2012) *Group Dynamics in Occupational Therapy: The Theoretical Basis and Practice Application of Group Intervention*. SLACK Inc, Thorofare, New Jersey.

Cole, M. (2019) *Group Dynamics in Occupational Therapy: The Theoretical Basis and Practice Application of Group Intervention*, 2nd edn. SLACK Inc, Thorofare, New Jersey.

Cole, M.B. & Tufano, R. (2019) *Applied Theories in Occupational Therapy: A Practical Approach*, 2nd edn. Slack Publishing.

Crouch, R. (2021) *Occupational Group Therapy*. Wiley Blackwell, Oxford.

Cuijpers, P., Clignet, F., van Meijel, B., van Straten, A., Li, J. & Anderson, G. (2011) Psychological treatment of depression in inpatients: a systematic review and meta-analysis. *Clinical Psychology Review*, **31**, 353–360.

DeAngelis, T., Mollo, K., Giordano, C., Scotten, M. & Fecondo, B. (2019) Occupational therapy programming facilitates goal attainment in a community work rehabilitation setting. *Journal of Psychosocial Rehabilitation Mental Health*, **6**, 107–115.

Dieterich M., Irving C.B., Bergman H., Khokhar M.A., Park B., Marshall M. (2017) Intensive case management for severe mental illness. *Cochrane Database Systematic Reviews*, **1**, CD007906.

Dreeben, O. (2010) *Patient Education in Rehabilitation*. Jones and Bartlett Publishers, Sudbury.

Du Toit, V. (2009) *Patient Volition and Action in Occupational Therapy*, 4th Revised edn. The Vona & Marie du Toit Foundation, South Africa.

Duncan, M. & Prowse, C. (2014) Occupational therapy with mood disorders. In: R.B. Crouch & V.M. Alers (eds), *Occupational Therapy in Psychiatry and Mental Health*, 5th edn. John Wiley and Sons LTD, United Kingdom.

Ebersohn, L. & Eloff, I. (2003) *Life Skills and Assets*. Van Schaik, Pretoria.

Gateley, C. & Borcherding, S. (2016) *Documentation Manual for Occupational Therapy: Writing SOAP Notes*, 4th edn. SLACK Incorporated.

Gillespie, C., Murphy, M., Kells, M. & Flynn D. (2022) Individuals who report having benefitted from dialectical behaviour therapy (DBT): a qualitative exploration of processes and experience at long-term follow-up. *Borderline Personality Disorder and Emotional Dysregulation*, **9(8)**, 1–14.

Goodwin, G.M., Haddad, P.M. & Ferrier, I.N. *et al* (2016) Evidence-based guidelines for treating bipolar disorder: revised third edition. The British Association for Psychopharmacology. *Journal of Psychopharmacology*, **30(6)**, 495–553. https://doi.org/10.1177/0269881116636545

Ikiugu, M.S., Nissen, R.M., Bellar, C., Maassen, A. & Van Peursem, K. (2017) Clinical effectiveness of occupational therapy in mental health: meta-analysis. *The American Journal of Occupational Therapy*, **71(5)**, 1–9.

Julayanont, P., Phillips, N., Chertkow, H. & Nareddine, Z.S. (2012) The Montreal Cognitive Assessment (MoCA): concept and clinical review. In: A.J. Larner (ed), *Cognitive Screening Instruments: A Practical Approach*, 111–152. Springer-Verlag.

Kandhakatla, R., Yarra, R., Pallepati, A. & Patra, S. (2018) Depression – a common cold of mental disorders. *Alzheimer's, Dementia & Cognitive Neurology*, **124(1)**. https://doi.org/10.15761/ADCN.1000124

Kielhofner, G., Mallinson, T., Crawford, D., Nowak, M., Rigby, M. & Henry, A. (2004) *Users Manual for the OPHI-II. Version 2.1.* Model of Human Occupation Clearinghouse, University of Illinois, Chicago.

Koene, J., Zyto, S., van der Stel, J. *et al* (2022) The relations between executive functions and occupational functioning in individuals with bipolar disorder: a scoping review. *International Journal of Bipolar Disorders*, **10(8)**, 1–25.

Labour Relations Act 1995 *Republic of South Africa government gazette, notice 66 of 1995*. Vol 366: No. 16861. Pretoria: Government Printers.

Lachaine J., Beauchemin C. & Bibeau J. *et al* (2020) Canadian economic impact of improved workplace productivity in patients with major depressive disorder treated with vortioxetine. *CNS Spectrums*, **25(3)**, 372–379.

Law, M.C., Baptiste, S., Carswell, A., Mccoll, M.A., Polatajko, H. & Pollock, N. (2005) *Canadian Occupational Performance Measure Manual (COPM),* 4th edn. SLACK Inc, Thorofare, New Jersey.

Levy, B. & Manove, E. (2012) Functional outcome in bipolar disorders: the big picture. *Depression Research and Treatment,* **2012,** 1–12.

Michalak, E.E., Yatham, L.N., Maxwell, V., Hale, S. & Lam, R.W. (2007) The impact of bipolar disorder upon work functioning: a qualitative analysis. *Bipolar Disorders,* **9,** 126–143.

Miziou, S., Tsitsipa, E. & Moysidou, S. *et al* (2015) Psychosocial treatment and interventions for bipolar disorder: a systematic review. *Annals of General Psychiatry,* **14(19),** 1–11.

Modise J.R., Olivier M.P. & Miruka O. (2014) Reasonable accommodation for people with disabilities in the labour market. *Mediterranean Journal of Social Sciences,* **5(4),** 578–588. https://doi.org/10.5901/mjss.2014.v5n4p578

Morrison, J. (2023) *DSM—5-TR Made Easy: The Clinician's Guide to Diagnosis.* The Guilford Press, New York.

Nicholls, L., Cunningham-Piergrossi, J., DE Sena-Giberton, C. & Daniel, M. (2012) *Psychoanalytic Thinking in Occupational Therapy.* Wiley-Blackwell, Chichester.

Novick, D., Montgomery, W., Vorstenbosch, E., Moneta, M.V., Dueñas, H. & Haro J.M. (2017) Recovery in patients with major depressive disorder: results of a 6-month, multinational, observational study. *Patient Preference and Adherence,* **11,** 1859.

Osuch, E. & Marais, A. (2017) The pharmacological management of depression- update. *South African Family Practice,* **59(1),** 6–16.

Pan, Z., Park, C., Brietzke, E. *et al* (2019) Cognitive impairment in major depressive disorder. *CNS Spectrums,* **24(1),** 22–29.

Priebe, S., Warner, R., Hubschmid, T. & Eckle, I. (1998) Employment, attitudes towards work, and quality of life among people with schizophrenia in three countries. *Schozophrenia Bulletin,* **24(3),** 469–477.

Ramano, E. & Buys, T. (2018) Occupational therapists' views and perceptions of functional capacity evaluations of employees suffering from major depressive disorders. *South African Journal of Occupational Therapy,* **48(1),** 9–15.

Ramano, E.M., de Beer, M. & Roos, J.L. (2021) The perceptions of adult psychiatric inpatients with major depressive disorder towards occupational therapy activity-based groups. *South African Journal of Psychiatry,* **27,** 1–8.

Rocamora-Montenegro, M., Compan-Gabucio, L. & de la Hera, M.G. (2021) Occupational therapy interventions for adults with severe mental illness: scoping review. *British Medical Journal,* **11(10),** e47467.

Sadock, B.J., Sadock, V.A. & Ruiz P. (2015) *Synopsis of Psychiatry: Behavioral Sciences, Clinical Psychiatry.* Wolters Kluwer.

Schell, B.A.B. & Gillen, G. (2019) *Willard and Spackman's Occupational Therapy,* 13th edn. Wolters Kluwer, Philadelphia.

Stander, M.P., Korb, F.A., de Necker, M., de Beer, J.C., Miller-Johnson, H.E. & Moont, R. (2016) Depression and the impact on productivity in the workplace: findings from a South African survey on depression in the workplace. *Journal of Depression and Anxiety,* 1–8.

Talatala, M., Ramano, E. & Chiliza, B. (2020) Reducing psychosocial disability for persons with severe mental illness in South Africa. *South African Health Review,* 11–18.

Van der Reyden, D., Casteleijn, D., Sherwood, W. & de Witt, P. (2019) *VdTMoCa The Vona du Toit Model of Creative Ability: Origins, Constructs, Principles and Application in Occupational Therapy.* Softcover published, South Africa.

Wisenthal, A. & Krupa, T. (2013) Cognitive work hardening. A return-to-work intervention for people with depression. *Work,* **45(4),** 423–430. https://doi.org/10.3233/WOR-131635

Wolmarans, D.W. & Brand, S.J., (2016) Mind your state: insights into antidepressant non-adherence. *South African Family Practice,* **58(4),** 5–8.

Woo, Y.S., Rosenblat, J.D., Kakar, R., Bahk, W.M. & McIntyre R.S. (2016) Cognitive deficits as a mediator of poor occupational function in remitted major depressive disorder patients. *Clinical Psychopharmacology and Neuroscience,* **14(1),** 1–16. https://doi.org/10.9758/cpn.2016.14.1.1

Yalom, I.D. & Leszcz, M. (2020) *The Theory and Practice of Group Psychotherapy,* 5th edn. Cambridge, Basic Books.

Zarate, C.A., Tohen, M., Land, P.H.M. & Cavanagh, S. (2000) Functional impairment and cognition in bipolar disorder. *Psychiatric Quarterly,* **(71)4,** 309–329.

CHAPTER 24

Maternal Mental Health Concerns as a Priority in Occupational Therapy

Gina Rencken[1], Pragashnie Govender[1] and Stephanie Redinger[2]

[1]University of KwaZulu Natal, Durban, South Africa
[2]DSI-NRF Centre of Excellence in Human Development, University of the Witwatersrand, Johannesburg, South Africa

KEY LEARNING POINTS

- Maternal mental health is an area of growing concern and priority worldwide.

- Pregnancy and the postnatal period are times of high psychopathological risk.

- Occupational therapists can influence the developmental trajectory and quality of life of the parent/s and the child/ren through careful and appropriate assessment and tailored intervention.

- Occupational therapists are suitably positioned given their holistic approach and focus on fulfilling roles rather than managing individual symptoms of disease.

INTRODUCTION

MATERNAL MENTAL HEALTH IS A GLOBAL PRIORITY

Pregnancy is a time of tremendous change and adjustment for women, their partners and families. This adjustment is made more difficult when pregnancies are higher risk, unplanned, unsupported or occur under stressful conditions. Approximately one in three women experience mental health problems during the perinatal period (Howard *et al.* 2014; Gelaye *et al.* 2016). The World Health Organisation (WHO) defines maternal mental health as 'a state of well-being in which a mother realises her own abilities, can cope with the normal stresses of life, can work productively and fruitfully, and is able to make a contribution to her community' (Herrman & Swartz 2007). Non-psychotic maternal mental health disorders affect the way the mother thinks, feels or behaves, without the presence of psychosis. They are often less severe but include symptoms like excessive worrying, trouble sleeping, lack of energy, irritability, restlessness, difficulty concentrating, feelings of worthlessness, social isolation and possibly suicidal thoughts, which impact her ability to function in the occupation of motherhood (Howard *et al.* 2014).

High rates of maternal mental health disorders are not surprising given the multitude of physical, hormonal, emotional and sometimes relational changes occurring during the perinatal period (Hanlon *et al.* 2014). Recent studies have shown that dynamic and functional changes occur in the brain during pregnancy. Synaptic pruning reorganises neural connections to disregard irrelevant synapses and make processing critical information more effective, allowing a new mother to respond to the needs of her baby (Sakai 2020). The body and brain are preparing for the occupation of mothering. The physical changes of pregnancy and the postnatal period may be met with significant emotional challenges, struggles with bonding, a lack of sleep or difficulties with feeding. For some women, this period also triggers distress linked to other major life events, such as adverse childhood events or bereavement in early pregnancy (Buehler *et al.* 2022).

A series of studies have demonstrated that the influence of pregnancy related-mental health problems from conception up to one year after birth in low-to-middle-income countries differs from high-income countries (HIC) (Bertolote 2008; Hendrix *et al.*

Crouch and Alers Occupational Therapy in Psychiatry and Mental Health, Sixth Edition.
Edited by Rosemary Crouch, Tania Buys, Enos Morankoana Ramano, Matty van Niekerk and Lisa Wegner.
© 2025 John Wiley & Sons Ltd. Published 2025 by John Wiley & Sons Ltd.

2022; Benarous *et al.* 2023). In lower-resourced settings, perinatal mental health disorders are of particular public health concern given that women face multiple adversities from disease, poverty and stressed social environments, making pregnancy a particularly stressful and vulnerable period (Mendenhall *et al.* 2017). Despite being relatively common, very few healthcare systems, especially those in lower-resourced settings, include routine screening for, and access to, care for maternal mental health disorders (Rahman *et al.* 2013). Maternal mental health is however an area of growing concern and priority worldwide, with policies and programmes implemented in HIC, including the United States, the United Kingdom and Australia (Sepulveda 2019). Recent studies have also looked at maternal mental health difficulties and the influence on attachment to the infant, including studies on the global prevalence and risks associated with increased maternal mental health difficulties throughout the antenatal and postnatal period (Benarous *et al.* 2023; Kerker *et al.* 2023; Parcesepe *et al.* 2023; Thsehla *et al.* 2023). Although low- and middle-income countries (LMIC) share the concern, there are additional barriers to developing and implementing policies due to a lack of specialists to address these concerns (Pitchik *et al.* 2020). In South Africa, the National Department of Health is currently developing guidelines for maternal mental health care.

While it is possible for an array of disorders to be diagnosed during the perinatal period, the most common are non-psychotic mental disorders (Figure 24.1) (Howard *et al.* 2014). Support measures should be considered for women during pregnancy or the perinatal period to guarantee mental health for this at-risk population with regard to screening, identification and appropriate treatment (Hessami *et al.* 2022). It is important to note that mental health difficulties experienced in pregnancy and the postnatal period may be under-reported, as society views this distress as detrimental to motherhood, and the stigma attached is significant (Perfetti *et al.* 2004). Postpartum depression is evident in 100–150 mothers per 1000 births and is one of the most common postpartum psychiatric disorders (Issac *et al.* 2021). Up to 20% of perinatal women are affected with depression, where anxiety is prevalent in 25% of mothers during their third trimester and 15% during their postpartum period. These statistics are even higher for mothers of low socioeconomic status (Kerker *et al.* 2023). In recent reports, LMIC show increases in postpartum prevalence in mothers at an estimated 22% (Issac *et al.* 2021; Benarous *et al.* 2023).

DEPRESSION

Depression during pregnancy and the postpartum period is a significant concern, with high prevalence rates globally, including in South Africa. Depression is the most commonly occurring psychiatric condition among women of childbearing age. Perinatal depression prevalence rates globally have been reported as 9–21% in developed countries and 19.8–38.5% in developing countries, including South Africa (O'Hara & Wisner 2014; Biaggi *et al.* 2016; Redinger *et al.* 2020). A recent study in South Africa highlighted prevalence rates as high as 72% two days following the delivery of healthy singleton infants (Rencken *et al.* 2022).

During pregnancy, depression has been associated with adverse pregnancy outcomes such as miscarriage, preterm labour, low birth weight and intrauterine growth restriction (Govender *et al.* 2020). It can also contribute to significantly higher rates of injuries, malnutrition, diarrhoea and asthma (Pierce *et al.* 2020).

In the postpartum period, depression can have a profound effect on the mother-infant relationship. It can impair mother-infant bonding, hinder infant weight gain and affect cognitive and motor development in infancy. Furthermore, it is associated with more severe outcomes such as depression in infants, child abuse, child neglect, maternal substance abuse and self-harm (Pitchik *et al.* 2020; Govender *et al.* 2020).

Given the significant challenges posed by depression during pregnancy and the postpartum period, it is crucial to prioritise the identification and treatment of this condition.

ANXIETY

Anxiety disorders during pregnancy and postpartum can have a significant impact on a mother's well-being and daily functioning. Generalised anxiety disorder is the most commonly diagnosed disorder in the perinatal period, whilst postpartum anxiety is also prevalent usually in the first year after giving birth (Vismara 2017). It is important to note that anxiety disorders often co-occur with depression.

Prevalence rates of around 13% are reported in both developed and developing countries, with a significant comorbid occurrence of depression (Biaggi *et al.* 2016; Dennis *et al.* 2017). Pregnant and postpartum women are at a higher risk of obsessive-compulsive disorder particularly with intrusive thoughts related to harm towards the infant (Russell *et al.* 2013).

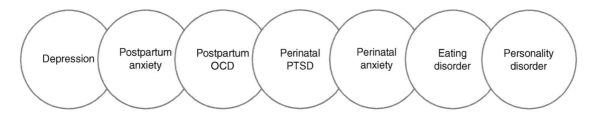

FIGURE 24.1 Antenatal and postnatal non-psychotic maternal mental health disorders.
Source: Adapted from Howard *et al.* (2014).

POST-TRAUMATIC STRESS DISORDER

Post-traumatic stress disorder (PTSD) often co-occurs with depression and can be characterised by various signs and symptoms. Perinatal PTSD may occur in mothers who have had traumatic births with adverse events. These events can either affect the mother's health or that of their child. Some examples of such events include amniotic fluid embolism, haemorrhage or pulmonary embolism (Pizur-Barnekow *et al.* 2014). Postpartum PTSD can be characterised by fear, a loss of control, a sense of helplessness, avoidance, hyper-arousal and re-experience of the traumatic event. The prevalence of postpartum PTSD varies between HIC and LMIC. Rates in high-income countries are typically around 1–2%, whilst LMIC show a higher prevalence of 5–9% when considering women with a history of a traumatic birth experience.

EATING DISORDERS

The course and trajectory of eating disorders during the perinatal period are complex. Factors such as disordered eating, body changes during pregnancy and increased stress and anxiety can all contribute to the onset or re-occurrence of eating disorders. Women may already engage in disordered eating before they become pregnant, and this group may have an increased rate of fertility problems and difficulty conceiving without assistance (Janas-Kozik *et al.* 2021). Pregnancy may also be a particularly sensitive time due to shape and body weight changes and increases in stress and anxiety. This may lead to the onset of an eating disorder or for the re-occurrence of disordered eating such as restriction, binging or purging (Abrahams *et al.* 2018). While some studies suggest a decrease in disordered eating symptoms during pregnancy, there may be an increase in symptoms in the postnatal period, given the pressure to confirm to a perceived ideal postpartum body type (Abrahams *et al.* 2018; Janas-Kozik *et al.* 2021). The impact of eating disorders during the perinatal period can also disrupt various occupations association with motherhood, such as rest and sleep, meal preparation and feeding, health management and work that accompany the transition to motherhood and caring for an infant. Women with a history of eating disorders are also vulnerable to the development of postnatal depression, even in the absence of an active eating disorder (Micali *et al.* 2011).

PSYCHOSIS

Psychosis may occur during pregnancy or after the birth of the baby. During pregnancy, non-organic psychosis may occur due to medication for pre-existing conditions that was stopped for the duration of the pregnancy, or may be related to pre-existing bipolar or cycloid disorders. Organic psychosis is rare in pregnancy, and resolves with adequate medical management. In labour and delivery, organic psychosis may be related to eclamptic and epileptic psychosis, or a bipolar psychosis, which can have devastating effects such as auto-caesarean or suicidality at the height of pain in labour. Neonaticide is a risk factor when the pregnancy is concealed. In the postpartum period, organic psychosis may develop shortly after birth, although this is rare. Causes include infective delirium, eclampsia, central venous thrombosis, hypopituitarism, water intoxication and substance withdrawal. The incidence of psychosis in the first few weeks after birth is more common and is usually related to bipolar/cycloid disorders or due to hormonal changes with the occurrence of the first postpartum menses or weaning from breastfeeding. If psychosis does occur, a heightened alert during future pregnancies is needed (Brockington *et al.* 2017).

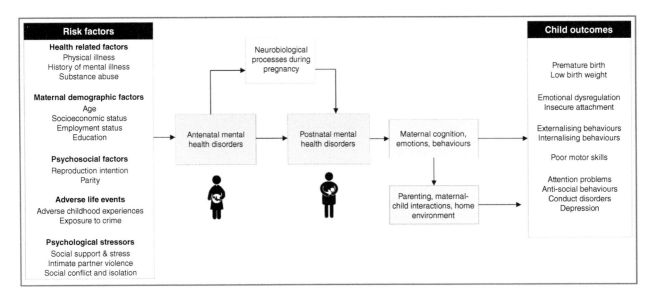

FIGURE 24.2 Risk factors for maternal health disorders and child outcomes.
Source: Adapted from Redinger (2021).

RISK FACTORS FOR MATERNAL MENTAL HEALTH DISORDERS

It is important to recognise the various risks to maternal mental health to provide appropriate support and interventions (Figure 24.2). Some of the identified personal factors include maternal age, maternal health (including HIV status), alcohol or drug consumption during pregnancy, planned or unplanned pregnancy, socio-economic factors, previous mental health challenges, pregnancy-related complications, mode of delivery and relationship status (Biaggi *et al.* 2016; Herba *et al.* 2016; Rencken *et al.* 2022). Environmental factors that contribute to maternal mental health include aspects such as food insecurity (including hunger and undernutrition), social stigma, partner support, social support, intimate partner violence and access to health facilities (Biaggi *et al.* 2016; Herba *et al.* 2016; Rencken *et al.* 2022). Occupational factors such as the transition to motherhood, social isolation, changes or loss of educational pursuits or employment adding to economic disempowerment, can also impact maternal health (Biaggi *et al.* 2016; Herba *et al.* 2016; Rencken *et al.* 2022). By understanding these risks, healthcare professionals can provide targeted interventions and support to help mitigate the negative effects and promote well-being of both the mother and the infant.

COVID AND MATERNAL MENTAL HEALTH

The COVID-19 pandemic has had a significant influence on pregnant women and their mental health. At the height of the pandemic, pregnant women were exposed to restrictions on gatherings, activities and community engagement, changes in medical care and limited social support. Moreover, healthcare institutions placed little emphasis on screening maternal mental health challenges and their infant's developmental outcomes, whilst the significant risk to the well-being of infants due to separation caused by isolation measures was a concern (Davenport *et al.* 2020). These factors contributed globally to women experiencing increased anxiety, depression and stress (Tomfohr-Madsen *et al.* 2021; Hessami *et al.* 2022; Kerker *et al.* 2023; Parcesepe *et al.* 2023). Prior to the pandemic (before 2020), postpartum depression had a prevalence ranging from between 6.5% and 25.8%; however, more recent studies have reported an increased prevalence of postpartum depression in mothers during the pandemic, ranging from 32.6% to 34% (Adrianto *et al.* 2022; Chen *et al.* 2022).

Pregnant women also reported decreased participation in physical activity, which has led to a decrease in the physiological and mood-enhancing benefits of physical activity (Hessami *et al.* 2022). The isolation measures acted as situational stress factors and caused widespread psychological stress on the populations globally (Choi *et al.* 2020). Furthermore, the perinatal care during the early months of the pandemic was viewed as highly disrupted.

During the perinatal period, the mother must have a partner or supporting person present throughout labour to help manage anxiety and facilitate skin-to-skin contact between the caregivers and their newborns (Hendrix *et al.* 2022). These aspects have, however, significantly been impacted by the social distancing protocols set during the pandemic (Hendrix *et al.*, 2022; Benarous *et al.* 2023). Prenatal and postnatal care delivery was modified to reduce the risks of contracting the virus. Due to social-isolation measures, there was reduced social support during these services and delivery (Almeida *et al.* 2020; Dib *et al.* 2020; Villar *et al.* 2021). Mothers had significantly decreased opportunities for in-person healthcare and support.

ADOLESCENT MOTHERS

Adolescent mothers face several challenges, particularly in terms of their educational engagement in the form of schooling, and have an increased risk for non-completion of schooling ('dropping out'), lowered chance of economic success related to this, as well as social stigma (Nkani 2012; Brandon *et al.* 2013; Cook & Cameron 2015). Adolescent pregnancies are also high risk, with potential adverse outcomes for both the mother and the baby, such as low birth weight and foetal growth restrictions being a concern (Traisrisilp *et al.* 2015; Wells & Thompson 2016). Their infants are also at risk of medical complications such as malnourishment, developmental delays and learning difficulties (Wells & Thompson 2016). Return to schooling for an adolescent mother after the birth of their child is challenging, especially if they do not have assistance with childcare responsibilities. This is specifically related to late nights tending to her infant, balancing time between infant care and school tasks, and keeping up to date with infant vaccinations and wellness checks (Wells & Thompson 2016), which can make it difficult to focus on education. Adolescent mothers are three times more likely to experience postpartum depression, and this is likely to last longer too (Boath *et al.* 2013). This is an additional barrier to returning to school. The timing of the return to school can vary, with some returning soon after discharge and others waiting until the following academic year. The decision is also influenced by factors such as ongoing examinations and the school principal's approval. It has been noted that some mothers return to school and then proceed to drop-out at a later stage, approximately six months after their return. Children of teenage mothers may tend to live in single-parent and poorer socio-economic environments, which can be linked to a higher rate of behavioural and mental issues (Goossens *et al.* 2015). Children born to adolescents are more at risk for health difficulties and may experience lowered cognitive development, intellectual and developmental delays, poor educational outcomes and are notably at risk for becoming adolescent parents themselves (Goossens *et al.* 2015).

CONSEQUENCES OF PERINATAL MATERNAL MENTAL HEALTH DISORDERS AND THE EFFECT ON THE CHILD

Maternal mental health disorders can have negative consequences for the affected woman, her child and her family. For example, antenatal depression and anxiety have been found to be associated with increased substance and tobacco use in pregnancy, lower compliance with antenatal care, lower health behaviours (such as attending antenatal care visits) and thoughts of self-harm (Grote *et al.* 2010; Grigoriadis *et al.* 2013; Ding *et al.* 2014). Disorders arising in the antenatal period, such as antenatal depression and antenatal anxiety, and a previous history of depression are also one of the strongest predictors of mental health disorders in the postnatal period (Milgrom *et al.* 2008). Besides the negative impact of maternal mental health disorders on a mother herself, there is research which shows that antenatal depression is associated with negative birth outcomes and negative outcomes later in the child's life, such as cognitive and behavioural difficulties (Stein *et al.* 2014; Accortt *et al.* 2015; Herba *et al.* 2016).

There is a growing body of evidence which shows that perinatal mental health disorders are associated with a wide range of negative outcomes on children's well-being and development. Assessment tools which can be used to identify sensory processing and neurobehavioural concerns in all children (infants to adolescents) are presented in Table 24.1. For most disorders, the mechanism by which risk is transmitted is complex, for example antenatal disorders often continue after birth and it is therefore difficult to determine the contribution of the antenatal or postnatal exposure. The effects of poor maternal mental health on children can vary depending on factors such as the severity or chronicity of the mother's mental health problems, and whether she has other comorbidities.

It must be remembered that the consequences on the child are not inevitable. Early identification and intervention, along with providing support and treatment for the mother's mental health, can help mitigate the potential negative impact on children and promote their well-being and development. Below we described some of the potential effects that perinatal maternal mental health disorders can have on the child.

ADVERSE BIRTH OUTCOMES

Antenatal depression and anxiety have been shown to be associated with premature deliveries (<37 weeks). Eating disorders in pregnancy are associated with preterm births, low birth weight, lower Appearance, Pulse, Grimace response, aCtivity and Respiration (APGAR) scores and higher rates of perinatal mortality (Janas-Kozik *et al.* 2021).

EMOTIONAL AND BEHAVIOURAL DIFFICULTIES

Children of mothers with poor mental health may be at higher risk of experiencing emotional and behavioural difficulties themselves. They may exhibit symptoms of anxiety, depression, aggression or withdrawal. The unstable emotional environment created by the mother's mental health struggles can impact the child's emotional regulation and contribute to the development of psychosocial problems. PTSD is associated with poor self-regulation in the child during the toddler years (Dvir *et al.* 2014).

Table 24.1 Assessment tools for identifying effects on the child.

Scale	Detail	Age range	Format
Sensory processing measure[a]	Provides a complete picture of children's sensory processing difficulties at school and at home.	SPM-P extends the popular SPM down to age 2, making early intervention possible	Parent and/or teacher rating scale; additional rating sheets completed by other school personnel for SPM; Parent and preschool teach or daycare provider for SPM-P
Sensory profile™ 2[b]	A family of assessments providing standardised tools to help evaluate a child's sensory processing patterns in the context of home, school and community-based activities.	Birth – 14:11 years	Standardised forms completed by caregivers and teachers to assess children' sensory processing patterns
De Gangi infant/toddler symptom checklist[c]	Checklist to assist clinicians in early identification of sensory and regulatory disorders in children	7–30 months old	Administered by a trained examiner
Neonatal behavioural assessment scale (NBAS)	An assessment of the neurobehavioral functioning of the infant in the domains of autonomic stability, regulation of state, motor skills and social interaction	0–6 weeks	Administered by a trained examiner

[a]Parham *et al.* (2007).
[b]Dunn (2014).
[c]De Gangi (2000).

ATTACHMENT PROBLEMS

Poor maternal health in the postnatal period can interfere with the formation of a secure attachment between the mother and child. The evidence suggests that mothers with depression, anxiety and personality disorders struggle to respond appropriately to their child's cues and to provide consistent emotional support (Lazarus *et al.* 2014). This can disrupt the development of a secure attachment, leading to potential long-term consequences for the child's emotional well-being and relationships.

COGNITIVE AND ACADEMIC OUTCOMES

The evidence for a relationship between maternal mental health and child cognition is strongest for maternal depression and anxiety; however, these are the two disorders which have been most widely studied (Gentile 2017). Studies have shown that children of mothers with depression or other mental health problems may have lower cognitive abilities, including difficulties with attention, memory and problem-solving skills (Evans *et al.* 2007; Manikkam & Burns 2012). These challenges can then have implications for their educational attainment and overall cognitive functioning.

SOCIAL AND INTERPERSONAL DIFFICULTIES

Children of mothers with poor mental health may experience challenges in their social interactions and relationships. They may have difficulties forming and maintaining friendships, exhibit social withdrawal or struggle with social skills (Ogundele 2018). The instability and emotional distress in the family environment can impact the child's social development and ability to navigate social situations effectively.

MATERNAL MENTAL HEALTH AND OCCUPATIONAL THERAPY

Occupational therapists assess and manage clients holistically within their cultural and environmental context. They have a window of opportunity in the life phase of the pregnant and postpartum mother where they can influence the developmental trajectory and quality of life of the parent/s and the child/ren through careful and appropriate assessment and tailored intervention. From a mental health perspective, this may include providing resources and support to address mental health concerns raised by the pregnant or postpartum mother or identified by a service provider (Sepulveda 2019).

ASSESSMENT AND DIAGNOSTIC TOOLS

Specific assessment tools for maternal mental health concerns are freely available, primarily as self-report questionnaires in English, with permission for use granted by the publishers. These tools have been used in many studies globally and show good sensitivity and specificity when compared to gold standard measures such as *The Diagnostic and Statistical Manual of Mental Disorders*, Fifth Edition (DSM-5) diagnostic interviews. Most of these have been validated in other languages and have shown good reliability (Table 24.2).

OCCUPATIONAL THERAPY INTERVENTION

Occupational therapy provides a distinct perspective and contribution to promoting the health and participation of persons, groups and populations through engagement in occupation (2020). Occupational therapists have the privilege of working with persons across the life span, and maternal mental health can influence the occupational performance of the mother, the infant and the family structure. Mothers and infants are interconnected, and establishing a secure mother-infant bond is essential to the child's developmental trajectory throughout their life (Sepulveda 2019). The correlation between a child's developmental delay and a mother's mental health, specifically with depression and anxiety, leads to challenges where the mother is not able to provide the necessary support for a child who has additional challenges and requires extra support and care (Reynolds *et al.* 2012). As an added factor, developmental delays may contribute to parental stress and depression (Barba-Müller *et al.* 2019). Occupational therapists assess and manage their clients holistically, in the context of their environment and with attention to them as individuals. Occupational therapists consider the interaction in the mother-baby dyad in their environment (domestic, societal, cultural and institutional), along with the personal factors of the mother and baby, in individual and shared occupations (including feeding, sleeping, resting, playing, socialising, education and communication to foster physical, social and emotional development) (Law *et al.* 1996).

USING OCCUPATION IN TREATMENT OF MATERNAL MENTAL HEALTH DIFFICULTIES

ACTIVITIES OF DAILY LIVING (ADL)

Activities of daily living (ADL) in motherhood include any activities orientated toward the mother taking care of her own body, which are completed routinely. Activities such as bathing, showering, toileting and hygiene, grooming, dressing, eating and sexual activity are included here (2020). In the transition to motherhood and the postpartum period, the mother's self-care is often not considered a priority and overlooked with the demands of caring for an infant (Briltz 2019), with healthcare for mother's post-childbirth focused on the health of their infant (George 2011). For example it is important to empower the mother in ways so that she can manage to shower or bath regularly without worrying about her baby crying or something happening to him/her, either by having

Table 24.2 Assessment tools for maternal mental health.

Scale	Detail	Items	Response and interpretation	Symptoms assessed
Edinburgh Postnatal Depression Scale (EPDS)[a]	• A tool that assists health professionals in screening for depressive symptoms among perinatal women. • Measured as a response to symptoms over the last 7 days.	10 items	Likert scale ranging from 0 (not at all) to 3 (all the time). A score of 0–30 is possible. Scores at or above 10/30 indicate depression. Specific attention is on the question of thoughts of self-harm.	• Mood reactivity • Anhedonia • Self-blame • Anxious • Feelings of panic • Coping ability • Difficulty in sleeping • Feelings of sadness • Crying episodes • Self-harm
Patient health questionnaire-9 items (PHQ-9)[b]	• A tool for assessing major depressive disorder in primary care settings. • It is based on the DSM-IV for diagnosis of major depressive disorder. • An adolescent version is also available.	9 items	Likert scale ranging from 0 (not at all) to 3 (nearly every day) If there are at least 4 items indicated with a frequency of '2: more than half the days' or '3: nearly every day' (including Questions #1 and #2), consider a depressive disorder. Add scores to determine severity.	• Anhedonia • Low mood and hopelessness • Insomnia or hypersomnia • Fatigue • Poor appetite or Hyperphagia • Poor self-esteem • Lack of concentration • Psychomotor retardation or agitation • Suicidal ideation/self-harm
Whooley questions[c]	Two item screeners for perinatal depression recommended by the National Institute of Healthcare Excellence in the UK, for use in busier settings.	2 items	Dichotomous (Yes/No)	• Depressed/hopeless • Anhedonia
The Kessler Psychological Distress Scale (K10)[d]	The measure can be used as a brief screen to identify levels of psychological distress over the past 4 weeks.	10 items	Five-level response scale (5 = all of the time, 1 = none of the time). Scores of the 10 items are summed, yielding a minimum score of 10 and a maximum score of 50. Low scores indicate low levels of psychological distress and high scores indicate high levels of psychological distress.	• Fatigue • Nervousness • Unable to calm down • Hopelessness • Restlessness or fidgetiness • Psychomotor agitation • Depression • Psychological exertion • Anhedonia • Worthlessness
Generalised Anxiety Scale-2 (GAD-2)[e]	The Generalised Anxiety Scale, GAD-2, is a 2-item form of the GAD-7, measured in response to symptoms over the last 2 weeks.	2 items	Score of 0–3 on each of the 2 questions. A score of 3 points is the preferred cut-off for identifying possible cases and in which further diagnostic evaluation for generalised anxiety disorder is warranted.	• Feeling nervous, anxious or on edge • Inability to stop or control worrying

(continued)

Table 24.2 (*Continued*)

Scale	Detail	Items	Response and interpretation	Symptoms assessed
DSM-5-TR self-rated level 1 cross-cutting symptom measure[f]	Self- or informant-rated measure that assesses mental health domains that are important across psychiatric diagnoses. It is intended to help clinicians identify additional areas of inquiry that may have a significant impact on the individual's treatment and prognosis. Rights granted: This measure can be reproduced without permission by researchers and by clinicians for use with their patients.		This adult version of the measure consists of 23 questions that assess 13 psychiatric domains, including depression, anger, mania, anxiety, somatic symptoms, suicidal ideation, psychosis, sleep problems, memory, repetitive thoughts and behaviours, dissociation, personality functioning and substance use. Each item inquires about how much (or how often) the individual has been bothered by the specific symptom during the past 2 weeks.	Each item on the measure is rated on a 5-point scale (0 = none or not at all; 1 = slight or rare, less than a day or two; 2 = mild or several days; 3 = moderate or more than half the days; and 4 = severe or nearly every day). The score on each item within a domain should be reviewed. Because additional inquiry is based on the highest score on any item within a domain, the clinician is asked to indicate that score in the 'Highest Domain Score' column. A rating of mild (i.e. 2) or greater on any item within a domain (except for substance use, suicidal ideation and psychosis) may serve as a guide for additional inquiry and follow-up to determine if a more detailed assessment for that domain is necessary. For substance use, suicidal ideation and psychosis, a rating of slight (i.e. 1) or greater on any item within the domain may serve as a guide for additional inquiry and follow-up to determine if a more detailed assessment is needed.
Sensory profile (Brown & Dunn (2002)	Self-rated scale describing response to sensory input in Taste/Smell, Movement, Visual, Touch, Activity Level and Auditory systems.	60	Likert scale from 1 to 5 (almost never – almost always)	

[a]https://www.fresno.ucsf.edu/pediatrics/downloads/edinburghscale.pdf OR https://perinatology.com/calculators/Edinburgh%20Depression%20Scale.htm.

[b]https://med.stanford.edu/fastlab/research/imapp/msrs/_jcr_content/main/accordion/accordion_content3/download_256324296/file.res/PHQ9%20id%20date%2008.03.pdfhttps://www2.gov.bc.ca/assets/gov/health/practitioner-pro/bc-guidelines/depression_patient_health_questionnaire.pdf.

[c]https://whooleyquestions.ucsf.edu/.

[d]https://www.worksafe.qld.gov.au/__data/assets/pdf_file/0010/22240/kessler-psychological-distress-scale-k101.pdf.

[e]https://www.aacap.org/App_Themes/AACAP/docs/member_resources/toolbox_for_clinical_practice_and_outcomes/symptoms/GLAD-PC_PHQ-9.pdfhttps://www.hiv.uw.edu/page/mental-health-screening/gad-2.

[f]https://www.psychiatry.org/File%20Library/Psychiatrists/Practice/DSM/APA_DSM5_Level-1-Measure-Adult.pdf#:~:text=The%20DSM-5%20Level%201%20Cross-Cutting%20Symptom%20Measure%20is,significant%20impact%20on%20the%20individual%E2%80%99s%20treatment%20and%20prognosis.

the baby safely contained in the bathroom where they can see each other (e.g. in a supported seat or a carry-cot), or by taking the opportunity to perform these tasks when there is a responsible caregiver or partner present to watch the baby.

Sexual activity is an important ADL, enabling the expression of affection and the experience of pleasure (2020). In the postpartum period, if maternal mental health concerns such as depression arise, spouses or partners may become depressed and discourse may increase (George 2011). 'Date nights' after the birth of a baby often switch from experiences outside the home to staying in, possibly watching television, as mothers report nervousness in taking their baby out in public, risking them getting sick (Briltz 2019). On the more sinister side of sexual activity, intimate partner violence has a negative effect on sexual health and participation in this ADL (Nwafor *et al.* 2023).

INSTRUMENTAL ACTIVITIES OF DAILY LIVING (IADL)

Instrumental activities of daily living (IADL) include any activities undertaken to support daily life in the home and community, such as care for others, child rearing, communication management, driving and community mobility, financial management, safety and emergency maintenance and meal preparation and clean-up (2020). New mothers' lives are often dominated by obligatory responsibilities and occupations geared towards childcare, household management and work participation (Horne *et al.* 2005). Mothers may have to find a balance between maintaining a household, maintaining employment and caring for older children or other family members. Treatment and temporary compensatory measures for executive function difficulties to manage this may be needed, such as using organisers which are regularly referred to as scheduling tasks, setting auditory reminders and asking for written instructions. The mother can be guided into the resumption of family-centred routines, or the establishment of new routines, including breastfeeding and establishing a sleep routine with the new baby (Abrahams *et al.* 2018).

Financial management in budgeting for nappies, vaccinations and formula (if needed), as well as paediatrician or well-baby clinic visits can be addressed. For mothers who are paying for private services as well as mothers who access free vaccination services and well-baby checks: scheduling, planning and transport or community mobility challenges may need to be overcome. Many babies have regular checkups, depending on their medical needs and mothers may need help scheduling and keeping track of all these commitments. Safety and emergency management can be addressed by having emergency numbers in an easily accessible place, as well as ensuring that the mother knows what to do in the case of common emergencies. Depressed mothers are less likely to remember and follow safety precautions, including safe sleep positions, 'baby-proofing' and reacting appropriately in an emergency (Balbierz *et al.* 2015). While the teaching of first-aid is out of the scope of occupational therapy, mothers can be encouraged to attend courses and appropriate resources supplied or access facilitated.

HEALTH MANAGEMENT

These are activities which relate to the development, management and maintenance of health and wellness routines (2020). Physical activity, maintaining strength, postural alignment and ergonomics when picking up and handling the baby (especially after a physically traumatic birth or a caesarean section where healing needs to occur) is essential in preventing strain and injury. Medication management to continue with postpartum vitamins, as well as any pharmacological management for mental health difficulties can be addressed as part of setting up and maintaining a routine of health maintenance. Encouraging physical exercise when it is safe to do so is a protective factor against the development of postpartum depression, and improves mental and self-perceived physical health (George 2011). The occupational therapist can facilitate participation in activities that the mother and baby can do together to promote bonding and attachment. Client-centred occupational participation is key, and the mother and infant should experience enjoyment and comfort in these activities through intentional activity choices which are enjoyable to both. This may include walking with the infant in a carrier, participation in a mother–infant gentle exercise class or spending time in a safe outside area. Occupational therapists are well-trained in psychosocial techniques and can facilitate anxiety management and relaxation techniques as needed.

Depressed mothers, or those with eating disorders that resurface in the postpartum period may have difficulty accessing nutritious foods and preparing meals. Maintaining an adequate nutritional status to continue breastfeeding, or safely preparing formula and then later appropriate infant meals may be a challenge and increase anxiety levels. Mothers may need visual schedules for this, as well as relaxation techniques to decrease their anxiety.

REST AND SLEEP

Sleep is an occupational need and has a pervasive effect on the person's ability to effectively participate in other occupations and experience quality of life (Tester & Foss 2017). Adequate, restorative sleep improves emotional well-being. Interventions include participation in physical activity, modification of the sleep environment, sleep hygiene and ergonomics (Tester & Foss 2017). Adjustment to the family routine and a shift in home maintenance or work responsibilities may allow the mother to rest while the baby is sleeping during the day.

WORK AND/OR EDUCATION

Mothers who are employed may have varying amounts of maternity leave, depending on their conditions of employment. Having a baby is an occupational disruption to this aspect of a mother's life and may be met with mixed feelings. Mothers who are self-employed may need assistance and coaching in developing and maintaining a balance between the tasks and responsibilities in their roles as a mother and as a breadwinner. Childcare plans for return to work and establishment of the work-baby-life routine after maternity leave are important, paying attention to aspects such as time management and maintaining breastmilk supply (if needed) through regular pumping and safe storage of breastmilk. Adolescent mothers may wish to return to school after the birth of their baby and need additional support in navigating this, with emphasis on their executive function skills.

PLAY

Maternal mental health difficulties interfere with the mother's ability to bond with her infant and negatively influence the infant's behaviour (Stein *et al.* 2014). Difficult infant temperament may exacerbate maternal depression and anxiety, setting up a vicious circle of reactions. Addressing co-occupations, responsive caregiving and age-appropriate play in co-occupations can promote mother–infant bonding. The success in infant play and responsiveness to their mother can also promote mental health (Briltz 2019). To improve bonding, at-risk mothers (with mental health difficulties) could be facilitated to adopt joint attention, play to support their infant's development on a cognitive, motor, neurological and social-emotional level (Winston & Chicot 2016).

LEISURE AND SOCIAL PARTICIPATION

Social support, optimism and situations where there is minimal stress decrease the risk for developing postpartum depression (George 2011). Participation in mother–infant groups, where play and joint attention are facilitated and mothers can feel less isolated in their journey, as well as develop realistic expectations of motherhood are helpful. A mother who presents with significant depression and/ or anxiety may not feel safe in these groups until individual therapy has been done for a while and she is feeling less vulnerable and likely to be judged (George 2011). There is an inevitable change in relationships with friends and family members after the birth of a baby, and even more so when the mother is experiencing mental health difficulties. Often, friendships established before pregnancy and birth become non-existent. This may leave the mother feeling overwhelmed, unsupported and isolated, adding to her mental health burden. In this case, a safe, supported easing into homogenous groups (like mother–infant stimulation groups) is required in a scaffolded manner after individual psychosocial therapy and treatment of other underlying factors.

PHYSICAL HEALTH OUTCOMES

Maternal mental health problems can also influence a child's physical health. The consequences appear to be most serious for perinatal eating disorders and child outcomes. Disordered eating during pregnancy has also been shown to result in nutritional deficits and alterations in hormonal pathways that may cause neurocognitive delays or foetal disabilities (Sebastiani *et al.* 2020).

CASE STUDY   Supporting Maternal Mental Health and Infant Care

Alice is a 27-year-old primiparous mother, who gave birth to a baby girl six weeks ago. She is married, and lives with her husband in a three-bedroom suburban townhouse, where one of the rooms has been decorated and set up as a nursery for the baby. Alice has a high school qualification, and prior to her delivery, was working as a personal assistant. They have comprehensive medical aid, due to her husband's job as a new car salesman for a luxury brand. They do not have any family living close by, and his job requires occasional travel. Alice has a group of mom-friends from the ante-natal classes they attended in preparation for the birth. Alice had wanted an unmedicated natural delivery but had to have an emergency caesarean section due to her labour not progressing adequately and concern about foetal distress. Alice is experiencing the transition to motherhood as more challenging than she had anticipated. She is having difficulty breastfeeding, but firmly believes 'breast is best' and will not consider an alternative. Her baby is not sleeping as well as anticipated, and frequently wakes at night, taking a long time to settle again. In addition, the baby has colic, and presents with the classic pattern of excessive crying between 4 p.m. and 7 p.m. daily, which upsets Alice terribly, and resulting in her becoming irritable and tired. Alice's husband is an involved father and adores his daughter. He however is finding the lack of sleep tough. Alice follows a rigid schedule of tracking feeds (including time on each breast), sleep time and nappy quality and quantity. She weighs the baby weekly at the well-baby facility at the hospital she delivered in and keeps track of this too. Alice has not been sleeping well, has not been eating properly (she reports that she does not have time to make meals for herself and that she is always busy with the baby and her needs) and is feeling isolated and tearful. She is due to return to work after four months of maternity leave, as the current economic climate necessitates this.

Alice took her baby to her paediatrician for her six-week immunisations and check-up and raised her concerns about her 'poor sleep'. The paediatrician has referred Alice to occupational therapy to assist with this.

OCCUPATIONAL THERAPY ASSESSMENT

Alice completed the Edinburgh Postnatal Depression Scale (EPDS) and the Generalised Anxiety Disorder 2-item (GAD-2) as part of the holistic assessment of the mother-infant dyad with Alice and her baby. She scored 12 on the EPDS, indicating clinically significant symptoms of postpartum depression and six on the GAD, indicating significant symptoms of anxiety. As the primary referral was for difficulties sleeping and the baby not settling, a sensory profile (SP 2) was done on the baby as well as Alice. Informal assessments through an interview and observations gave information about Alice's daily routine, her interests, support structure, perceived challenges and occupational performance. The baby' SP indicates that she is more sensitive to sensory input than typical babies of her age. Alice's SP shows a similar pattern of sensitivity, with auditory processing being particularly problematic. Alice reports that she regulates by walking and dancing. There is a match in sensory profiles between Alice and her baby.

OCCUPATIONAL THERAPY GOALS AND INTERVENTION

1. *Physical recovery: Support the patient's physical rehabilitation post-caesarean section.* Alice was guided through gentle post-caesarean exercises and mobility routines – including ergonomic factors such as bending from her knees, rolling to her side before getting out of bed, baby

wearing in a comfortable, ergonomic carrier, respecting her pain threshold and medication appropriately for this (as directed by her doctor). Alice was encouraged to go for walks with her mom friends from antenatal classes, with her baby in a pram or while baby wearing. She was also encouraged and shown how to dance with her baby in a carrier, which facilitated bonding, as well as provided them both with the vestibular and proprioceptive input they required to regulate their sensory systems.

2. *Emotional well-being: Provide coping strategies for maternal anxiety and emotional challenges.* Alice was educated about mindfulness techniques, and a few were explored to find a good fit for her. She was encouraged to see her doctor for an evaluation of medication – but declined this as she wants to continue breastfeeding. Alice was guided through evaluating her daily routine and responsibilities – seeing what can be passed on to someone else, or which items can take a lower priority to ease the mental load on her.

3. *Breastfeeding support: Offer guidance and techniques to address breastfeeding difficulties and concerns.* Alice was referred to a lactation consultant to address correct latching. Environmental modifications were suggested and implemented, including a comfortable chair with adequate ergonomic support to ease the strain on her body, as well as having carbohydrate-rich snacks and hydration easily available. A drinking vessel with a sealed lid and straw was placed next to the chair, containing either water or an appropriate breastfeeding hydration drink (this could not spill and mess and was easy to pick up and sip from while feeding), as well as a plate of bite-size snacks (which would not mess or fall on the baby, and which could easily be managed with one hand). Alice was encouraged not to scroll on her phone while feeding, or to be too concerned about time on each breast – and educated in reading her baby's cues instead. Social touch during feeding was encouraged to facilitate bonding, as well as soothe both Alice and her baby. Alice was concerned about being bored while she is 'just sitting feeding', and was encouraged to listen to music, podcasts or audiobooks during day time feeds. Suggested podcasts could be on topics of mindfulness, relaxation or infant development.

4. *Routine flexibility: Help create a flexible routine that accommodates the baby's needs.* Alice was educated in reading her baby's cues, instead of sticking to a rigid routine. She was encouraged to try baby wearing and allow her baby to sleep in this position while she was having a walk with friends. A collaborative discussion was held regarding aspects of home maintenance which could be 'outsourced' to others such as employment of domestic help for cleaning tasks was explored, as well

as breaking up these tasks into short, manageable 5–10 minutes tasks that could be done when the baby was sleeping. Online shopping and delivery of groceries were considered and implemented as an occasional assistance when Alice felt like she was not able to get to the shops to do this herself. A list of ready-to-eat, healthy snacks that support breastfeeding was included in her shopping list, as well as some ready meals. Alice was also encouraged to nap with the baby at one nap time during the day, and to include either baby dancing or a walk outside (weather permitting) daily. Alice was guided into generating many of these ideas in a collaborative manner and evaluating if they could work in her life, or if she was willing to try them.

5. *Infant sleep: Provide strategies for improving the baby's sleep patterns.* Alice was educated about biologically normal infant sleep to ease her anxiety about this. Baby wearing and contact napping were encouraged, as the proximity between the mother and baby is soothing to the baby and facilitate a smoother transition to sleep. Sensory strategies such as adapting sound levels and lighting in the home in the afternoons to facilitate a gentle transition into sleep and biological circadian rhythms were implemented. Alice's diet was assessed to look for food and drink, which could be triggers to disruptive sleep as they are being passed through breastmilk, including caffeine and foods which exacerbate colic. Alice was taught to read her baby' cues and to respect these when she was signalling a need to sleep. During awake times, Alice was encouraged to play with her baby and transition her through arousal states, instead of sticking rigidly to a schedule. Alice was taught how to do baby massage, which she did at night after her baby had been bathed and before her final feed before bedtime. This soothed and relaxed the baby, as well as facilitated bonding in the mother-infant dyad. The dyad enjoyed the massage, and often did an extra session in the morning too.

6. *Parenting support:* Alice was encouraged to 'tag team' with her husband in the late afternoons and early evenings, so that both parents could have time to bond and play with the baby, while the other parent prepared a meal for them. Part of this was to ensure that both parents were on the same page regarding soothing techniques and sensory strategies for the baby, to lay the foundation for a smooth transition to sleep later on.

7. *Nutrition and self-care: Encourage proper nutrition and self-care for the mother.*

Follow up: Continuous assessment and checking in with Alice and the baby, with an adjustment to goals and treatment intervention as necessary. A short report (with consent) was sent to the paediatrician on the progress of the mother–infant dyad.

CONCLUSION

Maternal mental health is an important field where occupational therapists can deliver a much-needed service as part of a multi-disciplinary team. The prevalence of maternal mental health difficulties, especially anxiety and depression, has increased significantly over the time of the COVID-19 pandemic, and we are yet to see the effect on mothers, and infants born during that time, as they traverse the life span. Occupational therapy intervention can serve as a protective factor to infant and child development and mental health. Pregnant and postpartum mothers should be routinely screened and monitored for mental health difficulties, and not rely exclusively on self-identification and health-seeking to access help.

QUESTIONS

1. What non-psychotic maternal mental health disorders can be identified?

2. What assessments can be routinely used in antenatal clinics and at postpartum check-ups to identify maternal mental health difficulties?

3. What are the risk factors for the development of maternal mental health difficulties?

4. What are protective factors in maternal mental health?

REFERENCES

Abrahams, Z., Lund, C., Field, S. & Honikman, S. (2018) Factors associated with household food insecurity and depression in pregnant South African women from a low socio-economic setting: a cross-sectional study. *Social Psychiatry and Psychiatric Epidemiology, 53*, 363–372.

Accortt, E.E., Cheadle, A.C.D. & Dunkel Schetter, C. (2015) Prenatal depression and adverse birth outcomes: an updated systematic review. *Maternal and Child Health Journal, 19*, 1306–1337.

Adrianto, N., Caesarlia, J. & Pajala, F.B. (2022) Depression in pregnant and postpartum women during COVID-19 pandemic: systematic review and meta-analysis. *Obstetrics & Gynecology Science, 65*(4), 287.

Almeida, M., Shrestha, A.D., Stojanac, D. & Miller, L.J. (2020) The impact of the COVID-19 pandemic on women's mental health. *Archives of Women's Mental Health, 23*, 741–748.

Balbierz, A., Bodnar-Deren, S., Wang, J.J. & Howell, E.A. (2015) Maternal depressive symptoms and parenting practices 3-months postpartum. *Maternal and Child Health Journal, 19*, 1212–1219.

Barba-Müller, E., Craddock, S., Carmona, S. & Hoekzema, E. (2019) Brain plasticity in pregnancy and the postpartum period: links to maternal caregiving and mental health. *Archives of Women's Mental Health, 22*, 289–299.

Benarous, X., Brocheton, C., Bonnay, C., et al (2023). Postpartum maternal anxiety and depression during COVID-19 pandemic: Rates, risk factors and relations with maternal bonding. *Neuropsychiatrie de l'Enfance et de l'Adolescence, 71*(1), pp. 44-51.

Bertolote, J. (2008) The roots of the concept of mental health. *World psychiatry, 7*(2), 113.

Biaggi, A., Conroy, S., Pawlby, S. & Pariante, C.M. (2016) Identifying the women at risk of antenatal anxiety and depression: a systematic review. *Journal of Affective Disorders, 191*, 62–77.

Boath, E.H., Henshaw, C. & Bradley, E. (2013) Meeting the challenges of teenage mothers with postpartum depression: overcoming stigma through support. *Journal of Reproductive and Infant Psychology, 31*, 352–369.

Boop, C, Cahill, S.M. & Davis, C. et al. (2020) Occupational therapy practice framework: domain and process—fourth edition. *The American Journal of Occupational Therapy, 74*(S2), 1–85.

Brandon, N., Hofmeyr, C. & Lam, D. (2013) Progress through school and the determinants of school dropout in South Africa. *Development Southern Africa*, 106–126.

Briltz, V. (2019) *Occupational therapy's role in maternal mental health within transition from NICU to home.* Doctoral Thesis, University of St Augustine for Health Sciences, St. Augustine, Florida.

Brockington, I., Butterworth, R. & Glangeaud-Freudenthal, N. (2017) An international position paper on mother-infant (perinatal) mental health, with guidelines for clinical practice. *Archives of Women's Mental Health, 20*, 113–120.

Brown, C. & Dunn, W. (2002) *Adolescent/Adult Sensory Profile.* Therapy Skill Builders, San Antonio.

Buehler, C., Girod, S.A., Leerkes, E.M., Bailes, L., Shriver, L.H. & Wideman, L. (2022) Women's social well-being during pregnancy: adverse childhood experiences and recent life events. *Womens Health Reports, 3*, 582–592.

Chen, J., Zhang, S.X., Yin, A. & Yáñez, J.A. (2022) Mental health symptoms during the COVID-19 pandemic in developing countries: a systematic review and meta-analysis. *Journal of global health, 12*.

Choi, K.R., Records, K., Low, L.K. et al (2020) Promotion of maternal–infant mental health and trauma-informed care during the COVID-19 pandemic. *Journal of Obstetric, Gynecologic & Neonatal Nursing, 49*(5), 409–415.

Cook, S.M. & Cameron, S.T. (2015) Social issues of teenage pregnancies. *Obstetrics, Gynaecology and Reproductive Medicine, 25*, 243–248.

Davenport, M.H., Meyer, S., Meah, V.L., Strynadka, M.C. & Khurana, R. (2020) Moms are not OK: COVID-19 and maternal mental health. *Frontiers in Global Women's Health, 1*, 561147.

DeGangi, G., Poisson, S. & DeGangi, G. (2000) Infant–toddler symptom checklist: long version. Pediatric disorders of regulation in affect and behavior: a therapist's guide to assessment and treatment, 335–340.

Dennis, C.-L., Falah-Hassani, K. & Shiri, R. 2017 Prevalence of antenatal and postnatal anxiety: systematic review and meta-analysis. *The British Journal of Psychiatry, 210*, 315–323.

Dib, S., Rougeaux, E., Vázquez, A., Wells, J. & Fewtrell, M. (2020) The impact of the COVID-19 lockdown on maternal mental health and coping in the UK: data from the COVID-19 New Mum Study. *MedRxiv*, 2020-08.

Ding, X.-X., Wu, Y.-L., Xu, S.-J. et al (2014) Maternal anxiety during pregnancy and adverse birth outcomes: a systematic review and meta-analysis of prospective cohort studies. *Journal of Affective Disorders, 159*, 103–110.

Dunn, W. (2014) *Sensory Profile 2. User's manual.* Pearson, Bloomington, Minnesota.

Dvir, Y., Ford, J.D., Hill, M. & Frazier, J.A. (2014) Childhood maltreatment, emotional dysregulation, and psychiatric comorbidities. *Harvard Review of Psychiatry*, 22(3), 149–161. https://doi.org/10.1097/HRP.0000000000000014

Evans, J., Heron, J., Patel, P.R. & Wiles, N. (2007) Depressive symptoms during pregnancy and low birth weight at term. *British Journal of Psychiatry*, 191, 84–85.

Gelaye, B., Rondon, M.B., Araya, R. & Williams, M.A. (2016) Epidemiology of maternal depression, risk factors, and child outcomes in low-income and middle-income countries. *The Lancet Psychiatry*, 3, 973–982.

Gentile, S. (2017) Untreated depression during pregnancy: short- and long-term effects in offspring. A systematic review. *Neuroscience*, 342, 154–166.

George, M. (2011) *Proposed role for occupational therapy to serve new mothers.* Emerging Practice CATs. Paper, 10.

Goossens G., Kadji C., Delvenne V. (2015). Teenage pregnancy: a psychopathological risk for mothers and babies? *Psychiatria Danubina* 27(Suppl 1), S499-S503. PMID: 26417827.

Govender, D., Naidoo, S. & Taylor, M. (2020) Antenatal and postpartum depression: prevalence and associated risk factors among adolescents' in KwaZulu-Natal, South Africa. *Depression Research and Treatment*, 2020, 5364521.

Grigoriadis, S., Vonderporten, E.H., Mamisashvili, L. *et al* (2013) The impact of maternal depression during pregnancy on perinatal outcomes: a systematic review and meta-analysis. *The Journal of Clinical Psychiatry*, 74, 321–341.

Grote, N.K., Bridge, J.A., Gavin, A.R., Melville, J.L., Iyengar, S. & Katon, W.J. (2010) A meta-analysis of depression during pregnancy and the risk of preterm birth, low birth weight, and intrauterine growth restriction. *Archives of General Psychiatry*, 67, 1012–1024.

Hanlon, C., Luitel, N.P., Kathree, T. *et al* (2014) Challenges and opportunities for implementing integrated mental health care: a district level situation analysis from five low-and middle-income countries. *PLoS One*, 9, e88437.

Hendrix, C.L., Werchan, D., Lenniger, C. *et al* (2022) Geotemporal analysis of perinatal care changes and maternal mental health: an example from the COVID-19 pandemic. *Archives of Women's Mental Health*, 25(5), 943–956.

Herba, C.M., Glover, V., Ramchandani, P.G. & Rondon, M.B. (2016) Maternal depression and mental health in early childhood: an examination of underlying mechanisms in low-income and middle-income countries. *The Lancet Psychiatry*, 3, 983–992.

Herrman, H. & Swartz, L. (2007) Comment: promotion of mental health in poorly resourced countries. *Lancet*, 370, 1195–1197.

Hessami, K., Romanelli, C., Chiurazzi, M. & Cozzolino, M. (2022) COVID-19 pandemic and maternal mental health: a systematic review and meta-analysis. *The Journal of Maternal-Fetal & Neonatal Medicine*, 35, 4014–4021.

Horne, J., Corr, S. & Earle, S. (2005) Becoming a mother: occupational change in first time motherhood. *Journal of Occupational Science*, 12, 176–183.

Howard, L.M., Molyneaux, E., Dennis, C.-L., Rochat, T., Stein, A. & Milgrom, J. (2014) Non-psychotic mental disorders in the perinatal period. *The Lancet*, 384, 1775–1788.

Issac, A., Krishnan, N., VR, V., VR, R., Jacob, J., & Stephen, S. (2021). Postpartum depression amidst COVID-19 pandemic: What further could be done? *Asian Journal of Psychiatry*, 63, 102759. https://doi.org/10.1016/j.ajp.2021.102759

Janas-Kozik, M., Żmijowska, A., Zasada, I. *et al* (2021) Systematic review of literature on eating disorders during pregnancy—risk and consequences for mother and child. *Frontiers in Psychiatry*, 12, 777529.

Kerker, B.D., Willheim, E. & Weis, J.R. (2023) The COVID-19 pandemic: implications for maternal mental health and early childhood development. *American Journal of Health Promotion*, 37(2), 265–269.

Law, M., Cooper, B., Strong, S., Stewart, D., Rigby, P. & Letts, L. (1996) The person-environment-occupation model: a transactive approach to occupational performance. *Canadian Journal of Occupational Therapy*, 63, 9–23.

Lazarus, S.A., Cheavens, J.S. Festa, F. & Rosenthal, M.Z. (2014) Interpersonal functioning in borderline personality disorder: a systematic review of behavioral and laboratory-based assessments. *Clinical Psychology Review*, 34(3), 193–205.

Manikkam, L., Burns, J.K. (2012) Antenatal depression and its risk factors: an urban prevalence study in KwaZulu-Natal. *South African Medical Journal*, 102(12), 940–944.

Mendenhall, E., Kohrt, B.A., Norris, S.A., Ndetei, D. & Prabhakaran, D. (2017) Non-communicable disease syndemics: poverty, depression, and diabetes among low-income populations. *The Lancet*, 389, 951–963.

Micali, N., Simonoff, E. & Treasure, J. (2011) Pregnancy and post-partum depression and anxiety in a longitudinal general population cohort: the effect of eating disorders and past depression. *Journal of Affective Disorders*, 131, 150–157.

Milgrom, J., Gemmill, A.W., Bilszta, J.L. *et al* (2008) Antenatal risk factors for postnatal depression: a large prospective study. *Journal of Affective Disorders*, 108, 147–157.

Nkani, F. (2012) *An Ethnographic Study of Teenage Pregnancy: Femininities and Motherhood among Pregnant Teenagers and Teenage at School in Inanda.* Thesis, University of KwaZulu-Natal, Edgewood.

Nwafor, J.A., Chamdimba, E., Ajayi, A.I. *et al* (2023) Correlates of intimate partner violence among pregnant and parenting adolescents: a cross-sectional household survey in Blantyre District, Malawi. *Reproductive Health*, 20, 60.

Ogundele, M.O. (2018) Behavioural and emotional disorders in childhood: a brief overview for paediatricians. *World Journal of Clinical Pediatrics*, 7(1), 9–26. https://doi.org/10.5409/wjcp.v7.i1.9

O'Hara, M.W. & Wisner, K.L. (2014) Perinatal mental illness: definition, description and aetiology. *Best Practice & Research Clinical Obstetrics & Gynaecology*, 28, 3–12.

Parcesepe, A.M., Filiatreau, L.M., Gomez, A. *et al* (2023) Coping strategies and symptoms of mental health disorders among people with HIV initiating HIV care in Cameroon. *AIDS and Behavior*, 27(7), 2360–2369.

Parham, L.D., Ecker, C., Kuhaneck, H.M., Henry, D.A. & Glennon, T.J. (2007) *Sensory Processing Measure (SPM): Manual.* Western Psychological Services

Perfetti, J., Clark, R. & Fillmore, C.-M. (2004) Postpartum depression: identification, screening, and treatment. *WMJ-MADISON*, 103, 56–63.

Pierce, M., Hope, H.F., Kolade, A. *et al* (2020) Effects of parental mental illness on children's physical health: systematic review and meta-analysis. *British Journal of Psychiatry*, 217, 354–363.

Pitchik, H.O., Chung, E.O. & Fernald, L.C. (2020) Cross-cultural research on child development and maternal mental health in low-and middle-income countries. *Current Opinion in Behavioral Sciences*, **36,** 90–97.

Pizur-Barnekow, K., Kamp, K. & Cashin, S. (2014) An investigation of maternal play styles during the co-occupation of maternal-infant play. *Journal of Occupational Science*, **21**, 202–209.

Rahman, A., Fisher, J., Bower, P. *et al* (2013) Interventions for common perinatal mental disorders in women in low-and middle-income countries: a systematic review and meta-analysis. *Bulletin of the World Health Organization*, **91**, 593–601I.

Redinger, S. (2021) *A longitudinal study of antenatal depression and anxiety in urban Black South Africans*. University of the Witwatersrand.

Redinger, S., Pearson, R.M., Houle, B., Norris, S.A. & Rochat, T.J. (2020) Antenatal depression and anxiety across pregnancy in urban South Africa. *Journal of Affective Disorders*, **277**, 296–305.

Rencken, G., Govender, P. & Uys, C.J.E. (2022) Maternal mental health and caregiver competence of HIV-positive and negative women caring for their singleton newborns in KwaZulu-Natal Province, South Africa. *South African Medical Journal*, **112**, 494–501.

Reynolds, K.A., Sontag-Padilla, L.M., Schake, P., Hawk, J. & Schultz, D. (2012) Enhancing cross-system collaboration for caregivers at risk for depression. *Translational Behavioral Medicine*, **2**, 510–515.

Russell, E.J., Fawcett, J.M. & Mazmanian, D. (2013) Risk of obsessive-compulsive disorder in pregnant and postpartum women: a meta-analysis. *The Journal of Clinical Psychiatry*, **74**, 18438.

Sakai, J. (2020) How synaptic pruning shapes neural wiring during development and, possibly, in disease. *Proceedings of the National Academy of Sciences*, **117**, 16096–16099.

Sebastiani, G., Andreu-Fernández, V., Herranz Barbero, A. *et al* (2020) Eating disorders during gestation: implications for mother's health, fetal outcomes, and epigenetic changes. *Frontiers in Pediatrics*, **8**, 587.

Sepulveda, A. (2019) A call to action: addressing maternal mental health in pediatric occupational therapy practice. *Annals of International Occupational Therapy*, **2**, 195–200.

Stein, A., Pearson, R.M., Goodman, S.H. *et al* (2014) Effects of perinatal mental disorders on the fetus and child. *The Lancet,* **384**, 1800–1819.

Tester, N.J. & Foss, J.J. (2017) Sleep as an occupational need. *The American Journal of Occupational Therapy*, **72**, 7201347010p1–7201347010p4.

Thsehla, E., Balusik, A., Boachie, M.K. *et al* (2023) Indirect effects of COVID-19 on maternal and child health in South Africa. *Global Health Action*, **16**(1), 2153442.

Tomfohr-Madsen, L.M., Racine, N., Giesbrecht, G.F., Lebel, C. & Madigan, S. (2021) Depression and anxiety in pregnancy during COVID-19: a rapid review and meta-analysis. *Psychiatry Research*, **300**, 113912.

Traisrisilp, K., Jaiprom, J., Luewan, S. & Tongsong, T. (2015) Pregnancy outcomes among mothers aged 15 years or less. *The Journal or Obstetrics and Gynaecology Research*, **41**, 1726–1731.

Villar, J., Ariff, S., Gunier, R. B., *et al* (2021). Maternal and Neonatal Morbidity and Mortality among Pregnant Women with and without COVID-19 Infection: The INTERCOVID Multinational Cohort Study. *JAMA Pediatrics*, ***175***(8), 817–826. https://doi.org/10.1001/jamapediatrics.2021.1050

Vismara, L. (2017) Perspectives on perinatal stressful and traumatic experiences. *European Journal of Trauma & Dissociation*, **1**, 111–120.

Wells, R.A. & Thompson, B. (2016) Strategies for supporting teenage mothers. *Young Exceptional Children*, **7**(3), 20–27.

Winston, R. & Chicot, R. (2016) The importance of early bonding on the long-term mental health and resilience of children. *London Journal of Primary Care*, **8**, 12–14.

CHAPTER 25

The Assessment and Treatment of Eating Disorders in Occupational Therapy

Karlien Terblanche

Occupational Therapy, University of Stellenbosch, Cape Town, South Africa

KEY LEARNING POINTS

- Changing trends in populations among whom eating disorders are prevalent.

- Physical and psychiatric co-morbidities.

- The unique contributions of occupational therapy in the assessment of eating disorders.

- Treatment of clients with eating disorders; relevant theoretical models, occupational therapy intervention and levels of care.

INTRODUCTION

Food profoundly influences daily occupations, extending beyond its nutritional significance. Food and the occupation of preparing and consuming meals serve as a fundamental pillar of many cultural activities, fostering community connections, participation in religious gatherings, social events and emotional regulation. Difficulties in managing food intake can lead to considerable distress and significantly impair occupational functioning. As eating disorders affect occupations pivotal not only to physical, but also mental and social well-being, occupational therapists can bring a unique lens through which to view these disorders. This chapter explores the unique role of occupational therapy in the assessment and treatment of eating disorders.

Eating disorders are serious and chronic mental illnesses that affect all aspects of the afflicted person's life. *The Diagnostic and Statistical Manual of Mental Disorders*, Fifth Edition (DSM-5) categorises these disorders as feeding and eating disorders '. . . characterised by persistent disturbances, in eating or eating-related behaviour that results in the altered consumption or absorption of food and that significantly impairs physical health or psychosocial functioning' (American Psychiatric Association 2013, p. 329). Body image disturbances often accompany eating disorders (American Psychiatric Association 2013; Boland *et al.* 2021).

Eating disorders are complex illnesses, influenced by genetics, environmental and psychological factors (Frank 2015; Latzer & Stein 2016; Iannatonne *et al.* 2022). Females have an average risk of developing anorexia nervosa between 0.3% and 1% with a higher risk for bulimia nervosa, around 1.5% (Preti *et al.* 2009). Younger individuals are increasingly at risk, with over 22% of adolescents reporting disordered eating symptoms (López-Gil *et al.* 2023). Individuals with eating disorders possess an exceptionally high mortality rate due to a combination of suicide and physical complications resulting from their disordered eating behaviours (Corcos *et al.* 2002; Sachs *et al.* 2016; Smith *et al.* 2018; Goldstein & Gvion 2019). Suicide is especially common among clients with anorexia nervosa, but elevated among clients with bulimia nervosa and other specified feeding and eating disorders (OSFED) as well (Arcelus *et al.* 2011).

Crouch and Alers Occupational Therapy in Psychiatry and Mental Health, Sixth Edition.
Edited by Rosemary Crouch, Tania Buys, Enos Morankoana Ramano, Matty van Niekerk and Lisa Wegner.
© 2025 John Wiley & Sons Ltd. Published 2025 by John Wiley & Sons Ltd.

The eating disorders landscape has expanded in recent years, revealing that they are not, as previously thought, limited mainly to Caucasian females in their late teens and early twenties, but also affect younger children, older individuals, persons from all ethnicities and individuals across the gender spectrum (Swanson *et al.* 2011; American Psychiatric Association 2013; Boland *et al.* 2021). A 2023 systematic review shows that the proportion of individuals with eating disorders increases as average body mass index (BMI) increases (López Gil *et al.* 2023). Eating disorder treatment lacks diversity in specific interventions for minority groups, older adults and gender non-conforming individuals, leading to under-representation and challenges in access to care, diagnosis and risk management (Flores *et al.* 2022). Early intervention is crucial for treatment and prevention of eating disorders and thus occupational therapists need to be aware of the diversity within the presentation of clients with eating disorders.

In a weight-centric society, eating disorders are often missed or misdiagnosed by health professionals (American Psychiatric Association 2013; Boland *et al.* 2021). Clients may initially present with a range of symptoms before being diagnosed with an eating disorder. There is a common misconception that individuals must have an abnormal BMI, but in reality, the majority of individuals with eating disorders present within the 'normal' weight range as defined by the BMI (Nuttall 2015). This can lead to difficulty accessing appropriate treatment due to weight stigma and shame. The severity of an eating disorder cannot be determined by an individual's weight, and more research is needed to understand body diversity in eating disorders (Garber *et al.* 2019).

Risk factors for eating disorder include psychological, environmental and genetic factors (Culbert *et al.* 2015; Boland *et al.* 2021; Iannatonne *et al.* 2022).

These can include:

- Cultural and media representation of the ideal body (Culbert *et al.* 2015).

- Exposure to restrictive diets at an early age by primary caregivers and peer groups (Boland *et al.* 2021).

- A parent suffering from an eating disorder or modelling disordered eating (Boland *et al.* 2021).

- Personality traits such as perfectionism, obsession, neuroticism, impulsivity and cognitive inflexibility (Culbert *et al.* 2015; Zipfel *et al.* 2015).

- Early participation in body-focused activities like modelling or certain weight-centric sports like ballet, gymnastics, boxing and wrestling (American Psychiatric Association 2013; Boland *et al.* 2021).

- Sexual, emotional and physical abuse (Sanci *et al.* 2008; Boland *et al.* 2021).

- Family factors like difficult relationships, marital strain, disorganised or rigid upbringing, poor boundaries and hostile inter-personal dynamics (Boland *et al.* 2021).

- Peer pressure, teasing and bullying (Lie *et al.* 2019).

- Co-morbid mental health conditions like mood disorders and anxiety disorders (Boland *et al.* 2021).

- Dopamine and epigenetic factors (Culbert *et al.* 2015; Boland *et al.* 2021).

The acronym LGBTQIA+ refers to people who identify as lesbian, gay, bisexual, transgender, queer/questioning, intersex, asexual/ally, with the + symbolising the inclusion of other diverse sexual orientations, gender identities and expressions that may not be explicitly mentioned in the acronym. It recognises the evolving and diverse nature of LGBTQIA+ persons. Persons who identify as LGBTQIA+ historically have been under-represented in the eating disorder literature. Clinicians working with eating disorders must consider unique lived experiences and risk factors related to the relationship between body, sexuality, gender identity and body image in this population group (Jordan 2023). This group is highlighted, as they experience a significantly higher incidence of eating disorders in comparison to the general population (Nagata *et al.* 2020), particularly transgender and non-binary individuals, who have a 53.3% lifetime prevalence of disordered eating (Uniacke *et al.* 2021). This is astonishingly high in comparison to the 8.4% lifetime risk for cis-gender women and 2.2% lifetime risk for cis-gender men (Galmiche *et al.* 2019). A 2018 survey of 1305 self-identified LGBTQIA+ youth between the ages of 13 and 24 years residing in the United States found that 54% of participants had an eating disorder, and 88% of those diagnosed had considered suicide (The Trevor Project 2019).

Unique risk factors for the development of eating disorders in this group include:

- Fear of rejection, stigmatisation, discrimination and bullying due to nonconforming gender identity and sexual orientation (Brewster *et al.* 2019; Parker & Harriger 2020; Nagata *et al.* 2020).

- Individuals in this group are impacted by internalised messages regarding body norms, gender expression, identity as well as pressure to conform to conventional appearance ideals within normative gender roles (Brewster *et al.* 2019; Parker & Harriger 2020; Jordan 2023).

- Standard childhood growth charts are developed according to sex, which limits their accuracy when used with transgender youth (Nagata *et al.* 2020).

- Higher levels of violence and post-traumatic stress disorder within this population group (Brewster *et al.* 2019).

- Transgender youth particularly may experience dissonance between their external appearance and internal experience of their bodies, known as gender dysphoria (Brewster *et al.* 2019).

Specific barriers to access to treatment that this group experience include:

- Symptoms of eating disorders being missed due to puberty blockers or hormone treatment in transgender clients (The Trevor Project 2019).

- Experiences that do not promote inclusivity in accessing treatment, such as the absence of gender-neutral bathrooms or not asking for preferred pronouns on an intake form (The Trevor Project 2019; White *et al.* 2022; National Eating Disorders Association 2022).

- Healthcare providers may miss the presence of eating disorders in clients whose physical presentation does not fit their preconceived idea of how someone with an eating disorder should appear (Parker & Harriger 2020; White *et al.* 2022).

- Discrimination by staff or other clients in inpatient facilities such as refusal to treat such clients, or microaggressions like refusal to use the correct pronouns (The Trevor Project 2019; Parker & Harriger 2020; White *et al.* 2022; National Eating Disorders Association 2022).

- Lack of support from friends or family may prevent individuals in this population from accessing treatment. They may feel overwhelmed with having to explain themselves to others and may not believe their own symptoms are real or indicative of an eating disorder (The Trevor Project 2019; Parker & Harriger 2020; White *et al.* 2022; National Eating Disorders Association 2022).

As the understanding of the relationship between eating disorders and gender identity continues to evolve, it is important for clinicians to educate themselves on the norms, unique challenges and preferred vocabulary when treating LGBTQIA+ clients.

DIAGNOSTIC CRITERIA: FEEDING AND EATING DISORDERS

Eating behaviours exist on a spectrum, from ease of eating, to an eating disorder, with disordered eating in the middle, as illustrated in Figure 25.1. Eating with ease means being comfortable with food and eating with flexibility and variety, responding to hunger cues and social/environmental demands. Disordered eating involves anxiety around food, arbitrary rules, inadequate nutrition, or fear, guilt and loss of control. Eating disorders are extreme cases, meeting DSM-5 criteria. While not all individuals with disordered eating will develop an eating disorder, disordered eating is a risk factor and should always be taken seriously (Pennesi & Wade 2016).

This chapter describes the most common eating disorders an occupational therapist in this field may encounter, namely, anorexia nervosa, bulimia nervosa, binge eating disorder and OSFED, as can be seen in Table 25.1. For detailed diagnostic criteria, please refer to authoritative psychiatry textbooks.

CO-MORBIDITY

Psychiatric co-morbidity is common in eating disorders, with a significant proportion of individuals experiencing a co-occurring psychiatric condition at some point in their illness. The likelihood of co-morbidity is estimated at 55–95% (Hudson *et al.* 2007; Udo & Grilo 2018). Anorexia nervosa is associated with particularly high rates of co-morbidity, with between 71 and 100% of individuals experiencing at least three or more co-morbid psychiatric conditions (Boland *et al.* 2021). Depression is present in 65% of cases of anorexia nervosa, social phobia in 35% and obsessive-compulsive disorder in 25% (Boland *et al.* 2021). Given the high prevalence of psychiatric co-morbidity and increased

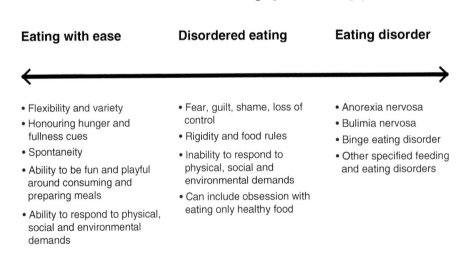

FIGURE 25.1 An illustration of the spectrum of eating behaviours ranging from eating with ease to eating disorders.
Source: author.

Table 25.1   Most common eating disorders.

	Anorexia nervosa (AN)	Bulimia nervosa (BN)	Binge eating disorder (BED)	Other specified feeding and eating disorders (OSFED)
Description	An eating disorder characterised by food intake restriction, resulting in weight-loss beyond the normal BMI category. It involves severe preoccupation with one's body shape and size (American Psychiatric Association 2013).	An eating disorder characterised by excessive food consumption and compensatory measures to eliminate excess calories, posing a threat to overall well-being (American Psychiatric Association 2013). Those with BN often have a preoccupation with body shape and weight, similar to anorexia nervosa (American Psychiatric Association 2013).	An eating disorder that involves consuming more food than similar people under comparable circumstances, without compensatory behaviours like in bulimia nervosa (American Psychiatric Association 2013). Binges cause numbness to satiety cues and feelings of losing control, followed by guilt and shame (American Psychiatric Association 2013). Binges often occur alone at odd hours, like eating leftovers in secret (American Psychiatric Association 2013). BED is linked to difficulty regulating emotions, and treatment should include behavioural and emotional aspects.	An eating disorder that causes clinically significant distress or impairment in social, occupational or other important areas of functioning (American Psychiatric Association 2013). It does not meet the full criteria for AN, BN or BED and cannot be better described by another physical or psychiatric disorder (American Psychiatric Association 2013).
Sub-types	Restrictive sub-type: Those with the restricting subtype place severe restrictions on the amount and type of food they eat during the last three months. Binge-purge sub-type: In addition to restricting food intake, those with this subtype also regularly engage in binge eating or purging behaviours, such as self-induced vomiting or misuse of laxatives or diuretics, or both binge eating and purging, during the last three months. (American Psychiatric Association 2013, p. 338)	Purging sub-type: During the current episode, the person has regularly engaged in self-induced vomiting or the misuse of laxatives, diuretics, or enemas. Non-purging sub-type: During the current episode, the person has used inappropriate compensatory behaviours, such as fasting or excessive exercise, but has not regularly engaged in self-induced vomiting or the misuse of laxatives, diuretics, or enemas. (American Psychiatric Association 2013, p. 351)		

(continued)

Table 25.1 *(Continued)*

	Anorexia nervosa (AN)	Bulimia nervosa (BN)	Binge eating disorder (BED)	Other specified feeding and eating disorders (OSFED)
Important development from DSM-IV TR to DSM-5-TR	The DSM-5 does not require the absence of three consecutive menstrual cycles, but it is still recommended to ask female clients about their menstrual cycles.		There is no mention of weight or appearance in the diagnostic criteria for BED. This diagnosis can be considered even when a client does not present overweight.	Previously known as EDNOS (eating disorders not otherwise specified) in the DSM-4 (American Psychiatric Association 2000), which was a broad classification eating and feeding challenges that did not fit the criteria of AN, BN or BED. However, grouping clients with varying symptoms together created difficulties in specific intervention and research. There also existed a misconception that EDNOS was less severe than the other eating disorders. The DSM-5 (American Psychiatric Association 2013) changed the category to OSFED to provide more specificity in the diagnostic criteria

Three other eating and feeding disorders that fall outside the scope of this textbook are described in the DSM-5 (American Psychiatric Association 2013):

- Persistent Eating of Nonnutritive Substances (PICA) is a disorder characterised by the persistent consumption of non-food substances such as dirt, clay, chalk, hair or other objects that lack nutritional value.

- Rumination disorder, where one regurgitates, re-chews then swallow or spits out their food.

- ARFID (Avoidant/Restrictive Food Intake Disorder), where one avoids certain foods or eats in a restrictive manner, related to the sensory characteristics of food. Clients on the autistic spectrum often experience this disorder due to sensory dysregulation.

mortality rates, treating eating disorders without addressing co-morbid psychiatric conditions is insufficient. Table 25.2 expands on co-morbid psychiatric conditions associated with eating disorders.

Eating disorders have a wide range of medical complications affecting multiple body systems. Individuals with eating disorders may present to various health professionals before getting a correct diagnosis of an eating disorder as the cause of their symptoms. Medical complications can cause damage in almost all of the bodily systems including the immune system, cardiovascular system, endocrine system, reproductive system, integumentary system, renal/urinary system, respiratory system, nervous system and musculoskeletal system (Boland *et al.* 2021; Hambleton *et al.* 2022). This highlights the importance of teamwork. Clients often need to be assessed by a psychiatrist, general practitioner and/or physician as part of the team.

Vignette 1: An Illustration of the Function of Eating Disorders Through an Outpatient Group Session

Sofia, aged 28 years, was part of an outpatient eating disorder programme. The programme consisted of two groups, twice a week. The occupational therapist facilitated the psycho-educational groups consisting of the following topics: understanding eating disorders, personality style and defence mechanisms, body image, emotional regulation, anxiety management and the road to recovery. A clinical psychologist facilitated the second weekly group, designed to provide a supportive environment for participants to explore emotions and interpersonal dynamics. This group focused on emerging themes, including but not limited to identity, relationships, emotional management, self-esteem, body imagine and the individuals' relationship with food.

Sofia was diagnosed with bulimia nervosa at the age of 12 years, but had started engaging in disordered eating behaviours from as young as 9 years. She began ballet classes at the age of 6 years, encouraged by her mother who was a professional ballet dancer. Sofia was a natural dancer, and eventually also became a professional ballet dancer, but was impacted by the demands of this profession from a young age. At the age of 9 years, she was encouraged by her mother, dance teacher and others in the profession to lose weight, as this would improve her performance. Bingeing and purging became an eventual solution to a problem she was faced with: how do I excel at my career by decreasing my weight, and still enjoy the experiences and socialisation around food? Sofia received positive feedback and a lot of affirmation for her weight loss from authority figures like her mother and ballet coach. A direct link was created between losing weight, performing better and feeling like those around her loved and accepted her more.

In one of the groups Sofia shared the following: 'I don't know how to value myself outside of dancing. I had to keep doing well. I couldn't perform if my body wasn't tiny. People also loved me when I was thin. Everyone wanted to be like me. Giving up my eating disorder means giving up my career, which is giving up who I am. Every day I think of this: who am I without my dancing? I don't know how to be myself. I get up in the morning thinking – who am I really?'

As occupational therapists, we view all occupations through the lens of function. It is important to explore the function of eating disorder behaviours in our eating disorder clients. As illustrated in Vignette 1, individuals engaging in behaviours such as restriction, bingeing, purging and other eating disorder behaviours do so as a solution to a problem. The function of these behaviours may be distress tolerance, an attempt at control when life feels out of control, dissociating from the body under traumatic circumstances, social inclusion and acceptance and identity formation among others. In the above vignette, the function of the negative behaviours were around the client's internalised identity and being accepted socially. She internalised the idea of only being socially acceptable if she embodied the thin, ideal dancer persona. Though this is a warped and negative way to achieve identity and social inclusion, it was the best solution the client could come up with given her formative years and subsequent life experience. It is the role of the occupational therapist to listen carefully, be curious and help the client identify the function of

Table 25.2 Co-morbid psychiatric conditions associated with eating disorders.

Category	Specific disorders
Mood disorders and emotional dysregulation (American Psychiatric Association 2013; Boland et al. 2021; Hambleton et al. 2022)	• Depressive episode • Mania and hypomania
Anxiety disorders (American Psychiatric Association 2013; Boland et al. 2021; Hambleton et al. 2022)	• Phobic disorders, especially social phobia • Obsessive compulsive disorder both related and unrelated to food • Panic disorder • Generalised anxiety disorder
Schizophrenia spectrum disorders, especially in those with Avoidant/ Restrictive Food Intake Disorder (American Psychiatric Association 2013; Boland et al. 2021; Hambleton et al. 2022)	• Schizophrenia • Schizoaffective disorder • Schizophreniform disorder
Suicidality and non-suicidal self-injury (Arcelus et al. 2011; Goldstein & Gvion 2019; Hambleton et al. 2022)	Suicidality and self-injury occur as part of various psychiatric disorders
Neuro-development disorders (Boland et al. 2021; Hambleton et al. 2022)	• Autism spectrum disorders • Attention deficit disorder • Attention deficit hyperactive disorder • Intellectual development disorder, especially prevalent in those with lower weight and can lead to delayed cognitive development
Substance abuse disorders (American Psychiatric Association 2013; Boland et al. 2021; Hambleton et al. 2022)	• Drug abuse • Alcohol abuse • Other substance abuse disorders
Personality disorders (Hambleton et al. 2022)	• Borderline personality disorder • Obsessive compulsive personality disorder
Trauma and stressor related disorders (Hambleton et al. 2022)	• Post traumatic stress disorder

their eating disorder. From there, we can help them find new, healthier solutions. In the above case, the occupational therapist facilitated the experience of healthy identity formation and positive social inclusion through encouraging the client to be vulnerable in the group setting and experience Yalom's curative factors (further explored later in the chapter), to contribute to her healing.

Occupational therapists can contribute to the field of eating disorders through direct treatment of clients with eating disorders, both in inpatient and outpatient settings and also by creating community resources and educating healthcare professionals and loved ones.

OCCUPATIONAL THERAPY ASSESSMENT OF CLIENTS WITH EATING DISORDERS

A comprehensive evaluation of any client presenting with disordered eating or an eating disorder is indicated. Depending on the team and setting, the occupational therapist may conduct a part of, or the whole, assessment. The objective in this chapter is to share numerous assessment tools available for utilisation. It is essential for each clinician to determine the most suitable assessment tools based on the specific context they operate within, such as inpatient, outpatient, group therapy or individual therapy settings. Occupational therapists bring a unique ability to use activity as a means for assessment to the table. We assess clients' unique strengths and challenges, tailoring specific intervention to their level of functioning.

A combination of activity observations, collateral information, comprehensive assessment interview and self-report questionnaires can be used to assess clients with eating disorders.

INTERVIEW ASSESSMENT

An interview assessment is a valuable tool to build rapport with a client, and gather information about the their functioning. It allows for observation of the client's comfort level in discussing certain symptoms, opportunity for clarification and provides understanding of the client's level of insight into their illness. In the interview, the occupational therapist will also specifically focus on daily occupations, or where poverty of occupations exists. Occupations particularly relevant to clients with eating disorders include but are not limited to food preparation, food consumption, socialisation around food, independence in self-care and social interactions.

The following topics hold significant relevance to include in an interview assessment.

The clinician needs to explore personal and family attachment patterns, dynamics and history, including familial history of eating disorders and other mental illnesses. Ask about the client's parents' relationship with food and their bodies, such as whether they ever made comments about their own appearance or talked about diets. Inquire about family meal patterns and meal preparation through questions like 'Did the family eat together or separately?', 'Who prepared the meals?' and 'Were separate meals cooked for different members of the family?'.

Assessing the client's current relationship with food and their body is crucial. Be open and non-judgemental when asking questions such as: 'How do you feel when you look in the mirror?', 'How often do you think about your body?', 'Do you spend a lot of time planning for meals or worrying about mealtimes?' One can also use the answers from self-report questionnaires to enquire further about concerning aspects.

Assessing readiness for change can be tricky as it is normal for motivation levels to fluctuate throughout the course of treatment. Remain open and curious about a client's thoughts and feelings. Questions like 'What made you seek treatment?', 'What do you think recovery will look like?' and 'What other treatment or help have you accessed before?' can help explore motivation and readiness for change. It's essential to discuss therapeutic goals and identify unrealistic of ambivalent expectations such as a client expecting recovery to look like eating normally, but staying under-weight (e.g. holding onto certain aspects of the eating disorder).

Where lack or dysfunction in certain occupational areas is identified, explore these areas further in the interview and through assessment activities where possible.

SELF-REPORT QUESTIONNAIRES

Self-report questionnaires prompt clients to consider specific eating disorder thoughts and behaviours that they may be in denial about, which can lead to increased insight into their illness. Self-report questionnaires can be given to a client prior to treatment and used to guide the initial interview, or given to clients to fill in after the initial interview or session. Below I will introduce two eating disorder specific questionnaires and then name three general mental health questionnaires the clinician may choose to utilise as part of the assessment.

SCOFF questionnaire (Morgan et al. 1999):

The acronym SCOFF refers to the five questions that the questionnaire uses, cited below. SCOFF is a five-question screening tool for anorexia and bulimia nervosa. It is user-friendly and easily memorisable for all health professionals. Despite its age, it remains effective in screening and early intervention for eating disorders, and it is free to use (Morgan et al. 1999; Evans et al. 2018; Burton et al. 2019).

Two or more positive answers to five yes/no questions in the SCOFF suggest a likely presence of an eating disorder and require further investigation (Morgan et al. 1999).

The SCOFF simply consists of the following five questions (Morgan et al. 1999):

S – Do you make yourself sick because you feel uncomfortably full?

C – Do you worry you have lost control over how much you eat?

O – Have you recently lost more than one stone (6.35 kg) in a three-month period?

F – Do you believe yourself to be fat when others say you are too thin?

F – Would you say that food dominates your life?

Eating disorder examination questionnaire (EDE-Q) (Rand-Giovannetti et al. 2020):

The EDE-Q, developed in 1993, assesses the symptoms of various eating disorders through a 28-question examination (Rand-Giovannetti *et al.* 2020). The comprehensive questionnaire evaluates specific behaviours and their severity across the following categories; restraint, eating, shape and weight concerns and is suitable for clients aged 14 years and above, and is free to use in non-commercial clinical and research settings (Rand-Giovannetti *et al.* 2020).

Screening for Co-Morbidities

Given the high incidence of psychiatric co-morbidities, screening for depression and anxiety as standard practice is recommended. In order to use The Hospital Anxiety and Depression Scale (HADS) (Snaith 2003), a license has to be purchased by the healthcare professional or facility. The Patient Health Questionnaire (PHQ-9) (Kroenke *et al.* 2009) and Generalised Anxiety Disorder Scale (Spitzer *et al.* 2006), are free to use in clinical settings.

ACTIVITY-BASED ASSESSMENT

Occupational therapists prioritise the functional and occupational aspects of illness, offering this unique perspective to the treatment team. Activity-based assessment is incredibly valuable for the evaluation of eating disorders. The following are two examples of activities the occupational therapist can use in the assessment of eating disorders.

Assessment Activity 1: Activity Log

Clients are given a blank template for a weekly schedule, broken into daily 30-minute increments, and asked to record how they spend their time over a period of two weeks. They go through the findings together with the occupational therapist. This activity can highlight the dysfunctional aspects of a client's life. One needs to curiously enquire about frequency, regularity and poverty of occupations. Analyse time spent on all areas of life: socialisation, leisure time, work, studies etc. Clients may go to great lengths to hide specific eating disordered behaviours, but this activity can help identify these behaviours as well as move clients out of denial.

The following are common behaviours that may be demonstrated in clients with eating disorders. A skilled practitioner needs to listen out for and enquire deeper into any of these behaviours:

- Fear or avoidance of eating in social groups and making spontaneous meal plans.
- Apprehension towards unfamiliar food situations, such as dining at someone else's home, consuming meals that are not self-prepared, or eating at a restaurant.
- Hiding and hoarding of food.
- Odd behaviour during meals like cutting food into very small pieces, eating very slowly and rearranging food on one's plate.
- Purging through the abuse of laxatives or diuretics, self-induced vomiting or over-exercising.
- Wearing very loose-fitting or over-sized clothing.

- Wearing warm or long-sleeved clothing on hot days, both due to cold intolerance and wanting to hide one's body.
- Anger, irritability and mood fluctuations with no other identifiable cause.
- Inflexibility and desire for control over their environment.
- Water-loading (drinking unnecessarily high amounts of water or other fluids to manipulate weight, especially when weight is monitored by caregivers or healthcare professionals).
- Withdrawal from social activities.
- Rigidity in routine, especially around meal preparation and consumption.

Assessment Activity 2: 'If . . . Then. . . .' Journaling Activity

This activity can be used to identify the level of distress around body image, as well as the deeper function of the eating disorder. As explained earlier in the chapter, the eating disorder is trying to protect the client from intolerable emotions or situations.

Clients are given the instruction, 'Please complete the following journal prompts. Try and write the first thing that comes to mind. Try and write as much as you can under each prompt'.

Journal prompts (adapt prompts for suitability to your specific client):

- If I wake up tomorrow and I've gained 5 kg, then . . .
- If I stop exercising, then . . .
- If I am no longer able to binge, then . . .
- If I can no longer purge after eating, then . . .
- If my body size changed significantly, then . . .
- If I could no longer count calories, then . . .
- If I am no longer able to weight myself, then . . .
- If I woke up tomorrow and my clothes didn't fit anymore, then . . .

One can prompt clients even further, by asking '. . . and then after that, what would happen then?'. Keep on asking '. . . and then?' a couple of times after each answer. One can do this activity with the client, or give it as homework for them to do on their own and discuss together in your next session. An example of this activity is shown in Vignette 2.

Both these activity assessments need to be adapted to the specific needs and setting of the client.

Both Vignettes 2 and 3 highlight the functional nature of an eating disorder. The exchange between Laura and the therapist helped them both understand how her eating disorder protects her from intolerable emotions like fear of rejection. Gabriella's letter illustrates how her eating disorder helped her navigate difficult situations in which she was helpless as a child.

COLLATERAL INFORMATION

Collateral information from significant others (e.g. family members, roommates and close friends) can provide valuable insight into a client's eating disorder behaviours and social/family dynamics. This information must be obtained with the client's consent and a clear explanation of the purpose. This can be challenging to navigate and the client's trust should always remain the top priority. The client may initially be reluctant to provide consent, and this may need to be revisited at a later stage as the relationship with the clinician strengthens.

Medical history and complications should also be assessed, and a medical screening is recommended for clients suspected or diagnosed with disordered eating.

Assessment should continue throughout treatment, with interview questions, activities and self-report questionnaires repeated regularly as needed.

Vignette 2: Using an Activity to Identify the Underlying Function of a Client's Restrictive Behaviour

Laura is a 15-year-old female with anorexia nervosa. Initially, she presented as motivated to change, but in subsequent sessions became resistant when challenged to increase her food intake. She described herself as 'feeling stuck between a rock and a hard place. I want to stop what I'm doing. I want to stop causing my family so much stress. But I also can't eat and gain weight. It's too scary. I can't change that'.

The occupational therapist used the activity described above in a session with Laura, using the prompt: 'If I woke up tomorrow and gained 5 kg then . . .' Here is the verbal exchange that followed:

LAURA: 'If I gained 5 kg I would be horrible. All my work to lose the weight would be for nothing. I'd be giving up.'

THERAPIST: 'What would happen then?'

LAURA: 'Everyone would see who I really am. I'm a monster inside. Everyone would see that. I won't be invited to parties anymore and no one would want to be around me.'

THERAPIST: 'That sounds like a really scary situation. Tell me more about that.'

LAURA: 'I have nothing to give. I just add drama to everyone's life. My parents. My friends. I take up too much space. I'd cause everyone drama again. If I stay sick then at least I get to be part of people's lives.'

In this example, the function of the restriction behaviour was to help Laura feel accepted socially. Her body size was linked strongly to her identity, feeling she had nothing else to contribute. This insight allowed Laura and the occupational therapist to go deeper in their work together and explore the themes of self-worth, value and social interaction, instead of just focusing on undesirable behaviour.

Vignette 3: An Example of Using a Letter-Writing Activity as a Path to Insight and Forgiveness of Self

The following is an extract from a letter a client wrote to herself, included with her consent, but with her name changed. In a session, the client and occupational therapist identified that she still held a lot of guilt and shame around, in her own words 'the drama she caused her parents' through her eating disorder. She was given homework to write a letter of forgiveness to herself for hurting those around her with her eating disorder. This activity once again offers insight into the function that her eating disorder played since childhood.

'Dear Gabriella,

You were struggling to make sense of the world and you dealt with that the only way you knew how at the time. You asked for help, you told your mother and others that you could not go on the way things were, but no one understood how much pain you were in – nor did you know how badly you were doing because you found a way to prevent yourself from acknowledging your pain. You found a way to make yourself feel okay in your world. This (the eating disorder) allowed you to continue to make your way in the world. To continue to be outwardly successful . . . You needed to protect yourself so you did it the only way you knew how . . . Even now as an adult, you never set out to hurt anyone. In fact, the method was an attempt not to hurt anyone, not even to lean on those around you, trouble them financially or trouble them emotionally'.

After reading the letter out loud to the therapist in the session, Gabriella found it interesting how the eating disorder was an attempt at taking up less space, becoming smaller and not wanting to be a burden on anyone else. During childhood, the behaviour was an attempt to protect her mother, and in adulthood an attempt to protect her husband.

This is often a theme in clients with eating disorders: the need to be overly responsible for themselves and not burden others with their emotions or problems. They find it really difficult to ask for help and have others witness what they perceive as their 'weakness' or 'imperfections'.

TEAM MEMBERS INVOLVED IN EATING DISORDER TREATMENT

As eating disorders can be complex and challenging to manage, it is important to build good relationships, and communicate closely, with the multidisciplinary team members. All team members must be knowledgeable and skilled in eating disorders, since these illnesses require specific intervention, treatment guidelines and risk management. Inadequate knowledge of eating disorders may cause more harm than good. The team needs to be cautious

Table 25.3 Team members typically involved in the treatment of eating disorders and their roles.

Team member	Role
Individual therapist (occupational therapist, psychologist, social worker or addiction counsellor)	To facilitate clients' understanding of the factors influencing their eating disorder, relational patterns, trauma intervention and gaining insight into their own thoughts and behaviours, as well as accountability and support throughout treatment.
Group therapist (occupational therapist, psychologist, social worker or addiction counsellor)	To facilitate the reduction of shame, provide a sense of community, and assist individuals in identifying their own thoughts and behaviours through observing others and offer a safe space for accountability. Yalom's curative factors play a vital role in eating disorder groups (Yalom & Leszcz 2020).
Dietetic therapist (dietician or nutritionist)	To conduct services like meal planning, nutritional education, challenge irrational food thoughts and helping clients build a healthier relationship with food. They can also monitor weight and ensure adequate nutritional intake to manage risk.
Medical practitioner (general practitioner, physician, psychiatrist or specialised nurse)	Risk management and specific medical intervention.
Physical therapist (Bio-kineticist, physiotherapist or occupational therapist)	Assists the client in re-engaging in safe physical activity, in alignment with their level of recovery.
Recovery assistant	Assist clients in the day-to-day of their recovery, offering encouragement, support, supervision and accountability on an in- or outpatient basis.

of splitting. Splitting is a defence mechanism where one views people, situations or oneself in extreme and polarised terms. For instance, a client may see the dietician as 'all bad' and the individual therapist as 'all good'. Working with splitting involves helping the client identify splitting and then to recognise the 'grey' and develop a more balanced perspective. Therefore, good communication within the team is imperative.

The roles of the multidisciplinary team typically involved in the treatment of eating disorders are described in Table 25.3.

TREATMENT OF EATING DISORDER CLIENTS

TREATMENT MODELS

This chapter highlights various models that can be used by the occupational therapist to guide the treatment of clients with eating disorders; however, many more models exist that can be used. Any occupational therapist working in the field of eating disorders must critically evaluate, and apply, the model for treatment that best suits their clients. Interven-

tions vary depending on factors like inpatient versus residential treatment, individual versus group treatment, alignment of treatment with other team members and individual presentation and risk factors of each client. When working in an inpatient facility, one often needs to align the model of treatment with the over-arching model that the facility has chosen to apply across their interventions. Eating disorder treatment is never a 'one-size-fits-all' approach. Occupational therapy is especially suited to draw on various models and frameworks.

Group therapy is one of the most commonly used interventions in the treatment of eating disorders in both in- and outpatient settings. Two group models are particularly useful in the treatment of eating disorders. Yalom's psycho-social interactive model offers us curative factors that bring about healing in a group (Yalom & Leszcz 2020). In turn, Vona du Toit's Model of Creative Ability (MOCA) offers a method of assessing the level of functioning of a group and guidelines on how to increase the level of competence according to a client or group's current capacity (Casteleijn 2014; van der Reyden et al. 2019).

In his psycho-social interactive group model, Yalom argues that there are 11 curative factors playing a crucial role in the healing power of a group (Yalom & Leszcz 2020), which are:

1. Instillation of hope
2. Universality
3. Imparting information
4. Altruism
5. The corrective recapitulation of the primary family group
6. Development of socialising techniques
7. Imitative behaviour
8. Interpersonal learning
9. Group cohesiveness
10. Catharsis
11. Existential factors

These curative factors are inter-dependent and will rarely be observed in isolation. According to Yalom, the therapist is not just a neutral observer, but instead plays a critical role in the therapeutic process (Yalom & Leszcz 2020). Occupational therapists will often be the team members running groups, and this model is widely used in treatment facilities.

The Vona du Toit MOCA (see Chapter 2 of this textbook) is a useful model to assist the occupational therapist with, among others, grouping clients for occupational group therapy and selecting appropriate activities. This model can be used in individual and group therapy.

Acceptance and commitment therapy (ACT) is part of the third wave of cognitive behavioural therapies (Fogelkvist et al. 2020). This framework conceptualises mental disorders as stemming from inflexible thought patterns, behaviours and emotions as a reaction to intolerable internal experiences (Fogelkvist *et al.* 2020). This leads to experiential avoidance and inflexible behaviours (Fogelkvist *et al.* 2020). ACT aims to increase psychological flexibility in individuals (Fogelkvist *et al.* 2020). Research indicates that emotional avoidance is a critical factor in the development of eating disorders (Manlick *et al.* 2013). ACT assists clients in tolerating uncomfortable emotions and taking value-aligned action and therefore is a good fit in the treatment of eating disorders (Fogelkvist *et al.* 2020).

ACT is a compatible treatment modality for occupational therapists because of its focus on action and behaviour change. In clients with eating disorders, the destructive behaviours are used to avoid uncomfortable emotions. ACT focuses on both the emotional regulation as well as the behaviour change aspects of this illness.

The Transtheoretical model (TTM) is a theoretical framework used to understand behaviour change (Levesque *et al.* 2001; Hasler *et al.* 2004). The model proposes that individuals move through five stages of change: precontemplation, contemplation, preparation, action and maintenance (Levesque *et al.* 2001; Hasler *et al.* 2004).

TTM offers guidelines to move from one level of motivation to the next and has successfully been used in eating disorder treatment in conjunction with other treatment modalities (Hasler *et al.* 2004). It remains a useful framework for understanding behaviour change in the context of eating disorders, but ongoing research is still needed to fully understand the specific applications of the diversity within the different eating disorders (Dray & Wade 2012). Many addiction treatment centres use the TTM as a primary model of intervention and therefore it is useful to familiarise oneself with this model.

HEALTH AT EVERY SIZE AND INTUITIVE EATING – DIETETIC MODELS INFLUENCING CURRENT DISCOURSE IN THE TREATMENT OF EATING DISORDERS

A growing body of evidence reveals that dieting is a risk factor for eating disorders and can be physically and psychologically harmful (Calogero *et al.* 2019; Brown *et al.* 2020) and can lead to weight stigma (Tomiyama *et al.* 2018) as well as create barriers in accessing health care (Mensinger *et al.* 2018). The pervasive cultural thin body ideal and perpetual pursuit of weight loss is termed as 'diet culture' (Harrison 2019; Jovanovski & Jaeger 2022). Jovanovski and Jaeger (2022, p. 9) characterise diet culture as 'a conflation of weight and health including myths about food and eating, and a moral hierarchy of bodies derived from patriarchal, racist and capitalist forms of domination'.

Health at every size and Intuitive eating are two frameworks developed by dieticians specifically in the field of eating disorders, in reaction to diet culture. Occupational therapists working with eating disorders should familiarise themselves with these emerging frameworks as they are part of the current discourse and inform the thinking and vocabulary in the treatment of eating disorders. These models are also universally applicable and highly educational to all professionals practising in this domain.

Health at every size is a public health initiative seeking to diminish weight loss as a health goal, decrease weight stigma and celebrate body diversity. The initiative seeks to honour differences in body diversity, age, race and ethnicity, dis/ability and across the gender spectrum. The movement values lived experience and body autonomy (Bacon 2010).

Intuitive Eating was developed by two dieticians, Elyse Resch and Evelyn Tribole, in the 1990s, in reaction to diet culture. It is a self-care eating framework and incorporates instinct, emotion and rational thought. The focus is on nurturing one's body, rather than the biology of starvation. It is a weight-inclusive, evidence-based model with a validated assessment scale and over 125 studies to date (Tribole & Resch 2020).

Vignette 4 highlights the complex nature of eating disorders and the impact of genetic, environmental, psychological and physical factors. It emphasises the need for individualised treatment plans and how a uniform approach is usually ineffective. It also illustrates the use of the Vona du Toit MOCA, to find a good fit and the 'just right challenge' for the client to increase their creative capacity. It also integrates principles of Health at Every Size and Intuitive Eating to decrease the shame of a person in a larger body.

Vignette 4: Illustrating the Importance of a 'Just Right Challenge' in Choosing Treatment Activities

John, a 55-year-old male, met criteria for binge eating disorder and body dysmorphia, with a history of anorexia nervosa in his twenties. He grew up in a household where food access was restricted, particularly for him and his father, who also had a larger body. His mother modelled restrictive behaviours around food and was always on a diet. John received smaller portion sizes compared to his siblings who were in smaller bodies and therefore allowed more access to food. His father also modelled certain behaviours like eating in secret and hoarding food. John's restriction became self-imposed during puberty, as a method of weight loss, impacting his physiological and psychological growth.

One of John's main treatment aims with the occupational therapist was to find sustainable exercise. It was really difficult for him to engage in consistent exercise, due to the shame that was triggered by exercising in a larger body. Healthcare professionals had previously placed him on restrictive and rigid exercise regimes, which he found impossible to sustain and only served to increase his shame and self-loathing. John engaged in all-or-nothing thinking and felt unable to implement small, sustainable steps to increase his capacity to exercise over time. He also had rigid internalised assumptions around what 'counted' as exercise and what did not. Additionally, he identified not exercising as a form of rebellion towards his deceased mother.

While seeking sustainable, enjoyable ways to exercise, we discovered that John enjoyed gardening. During the COVID-19 pandemic, his gardener was unavailable, and John started to maintain the garden himself. We started by aiming for concrete occupational outcomes, like landscaping goals such as cutting down branches from a tree. Seeing his own progress was highly motivating. He experienced a tangible improvement in his fitness when feeling less and less out of breath as he climbed his stairs to his bedroom every night. John used gardening as exercise for almost a year, and felt himself getting fitter and stronger, while loving spending time outside. Together we celebrated his success by having tea in his reformed garden!

Other themes that formed part of John's intervention included understanding his larger body as a way to feel safe in the world, especially in light of toxic masculinity and his naturally sensitive temperament. Additionally, I referred him to an eating disorder dietician who uses a Health at Every Size (HAES) approach described earlier in this chapter, to work on his rigid food rules, such as avoidance of pre-prepared meals and restriction of certain food groups, which impacted bingeing behaviour.

LEVELS OF INTERVENTION

Different levels of eating disorder intervention exist depending on factors, like severity of the illness, medical risk and availability of family support. The role of the occupational therapist may differ, depending on the setting and level of care needed. The levels of care discussed in Table 25.4 are outpatient treatment, residential treatment, medical admission or emergency care and preventative treatment.

Working with eating disorders can be challenging, but incredibly rewarding. The field is ever-growing with new research emerging around specific client groups such as transgender individuals and older individuals, as well as challenging long held beliefs around the appearance and presentation of clients with eating disorders. Occupational therapists in this field need to use inclusive, non-judgemental language and continuously examine their own relationship with food and body, being curious about unknown biases that they might hold. As clinicians, we are not immune to society's pressure on body size and appearance and may hold our own risk factors for disordered eating. In my own journey of working with eating disorders, working on my own relationship with my body and examining my own biases have been one of the key factors leading to insight and understanding not only of my clients, but myself too. I wish anyone working in this field an open heart, a curious mind and real care and compassion for your clients.

Table 25.4 Levels of eating disorder intervention and treatment aims.

Level of intervention	Indications for treatment	Occupational therapy treatment aims	General treatment aims
Outpatient treatment	• Client is medically stable and does not require extensive medical monitoring.	• Education and insight into the eating disorder for both client and loved ones.	• Weight restoration and resumption of normal eating patterns.
	• Client has fair to good motivation to recover, is cooperative in terms of treatment (shows up for appointments and implements recommendations by the team), has insight into their illness and the ability initiative behavioural change with the team's support.	• Engagement in positive daily occupations. • Understanding psychological and emotional factors underlying the eating disorder.	• Management of specific symptoms (like bingeing, purging, over-exercising etc). • Stabilisation on medication.
	• Client follows a structured meal plan with self-sufficiency or familial support, and follows the recommendations in terms of limitations around exercise, as determined by the dietician.	• Behaviour change. • Emotional insight and regulation.	
	• Client has access to professional and social/family support.		

(continued)

Table 25.4   (*Continued*)

Level of intervention	Indications for treatment	Occupational therapy treatment aims	General treatment aims
Residential treatment Residential treatment takes place in a specialised eating disorder or substance use unit. Different phases of this treatment ranging from primary care to secondary and tertiary care exist, where the client gains increasing access to the outside world like the ability to work part-time, attend social gatherings etc. while in residential care. For the purposes of this chapter, this is all described under the section on residential treatment.	• Client is medically stable to the extent that intravenous fluids, nasogastric tube feedings or multiple daily laboratory tests are not needed. • Client has poor to fair motivation to recover and is cooperative within a structured and supportive treatment environment. • Client requires extensive monitoring to prevent acting out on eating disorder behaviours like over-exercising, purging, laxative use etc. • Client experiences high levels of intrusive, repetitive eating disorder thoughts. • Client is unable to receive adequate family or social support. • Client lives too far from adequate outpatient treatment.	• Decrease of shame and moving from denial or precontemplation to contemplation, preparation/ determination and action (Levesque *et al.* 2001; Hasler *et al.* 2004). • Psycho-education, management and insight into eating disorder behaviours and underlying emotional and psychological factors. • Support and engagement in a healthy, balanced daily routine. • Psycho-education and support for families and loved ones.	• Weight-restoration and resumption of normal eating routines. • Harm reduction. • Management of specific behaviours such as bingeing, purging, laxative use etc. • Medical stabilisation if indicated, including psychiatric medication.
Medical admission or emergency care In the case of medical instability, a client may be admitted to a general hospital for specialised feeding, 72-hour emergency psychiatric assessment, or other acute medical interventions.	• The client is experiencing significant medical complications, such as reduced heart rate, changes in blood pressure, poorly controlled diabetes, low glucose, low potassium, electrolyte imbalance, low body temperature, dehydration, liver, kidney or cardiac compromise requiring acute treatment. • The client needs supervision during and after all meals or nasogastric/special feeding modality. • Client is at a very low weight and has an acute health risk. • Client is severely suicidal or experiencing a psychiatric emergency like a psychotic episode.	Occupational therapy has a limited role in emergency and medical admission, because of clients' low weight resulting in insufficient cognitive capacity to engage in therapy. In the absence of a social worker, an occupational therapist may play a role in family support and containment, and in the likely event of discharge into a residential treatment facility, may assist in the transition and/or also play a role in the development of a discharge plan. In the absence of wound specialists or physiotherapists, occupational therapists may be involved in mobilisation and wound care.	• Halting weight-loss • Harm reduction • Assessment and treatment of specific medical condition • 24-hour supervision and care

Table 25.4   (*Continued*)

Level of intervention	Indications for treatment	Occupational therapy treatment aims	General treatment aims
Preventative treatment	Preventative treatment can take place anywhere, but is especially indicated where there is a high risk for the development of eating disorders or where other health professionals need to be upskilled in the identification and treatment of clients with eating disorders.	• Education in schools to parents and teachers on eating disorder signs, symptoms and early intervention. • Education and activism roles in educating the public on body diversity, the risks of restrictive dieting and general eating disorder education. • Education in specific high-risk sectors like gyms, ballet companies, athletic coaches etc. on eating disorders. This can include warning signs of eating disorders and guidelines on harm reduction in these sports. • Educating colleagues and other healthcare professionals on eating disorders, early intervention and harm reduction through seminars, workshops and other ways of engagement. • Creating specific safe activity spaces like walking groups, social groups, yoga groups etc. where values of body diversity, inclusivity and no diet-culture talk are upheld.	

QUESTIONS

1. Name three risk factors for the development of eating disorders.

2. Is the following statement true or false? Justify your answer. 'You are presented with an overweight, Caucasian woman in her forties. It is highly likely that she has an eating disorder'.

3. Name some physical and psychiatric co-morbidities to look out for in clients with eating disorders.

4. Is the following statement true or false? Justify your answer. 'Eating disorders have a mortality rate similar to major depressive disorder'.

5. Name some of the unique risk factors and barriers to access to care that the LGBTQIA+ population experiences.

6. How would you describe the difference between an eating disorder and disordered eating?

7. Describe the role of an occupational therapist in the different levels of eating disorder care.

8. Which factors would you consider when choosing an appropriate treatment modality for a client?

9. Name three of Yalom's curative factors and describe how you might facilitate them in an eating disorder group.

10. Reflect on your own relationship with, and formative experiences around, food and your own body. How might this influence your work in this field?

REFERENCES

American Psychiatric Association (2000) Feeding and eating disorders. In: D.J. Kupfer, M.B. First & D.A. Regier (eds), *Diagnostic and Statistical Manual of Mental Disorders*, 4th edn, pp. 583–586. American Psychiatric Publishing, Arlington, Virginia.

American Psychiatric Association (2013) Feeding and eating disorders. In: B. Timothy Walsh & R.S. Weissman (eds), *Diagnostic and Statistical*

Manual of Mental Disorders, 5th edn, pp. 329–354. American Psychiatric Publishing, Arlington, Virginia.

Arcelus, J., Mitchell, A.J., Wales, J. & Nielsen, S. (2011) Mortality rates in patients with anorexia nervosa and other eating disorders: a meta-analysis of 36 studies. *Archives of General Psychiatry*, **68**(7), 724–731.

Bacon, L. (2010) *Health at Every Size: The Surprising Truth about Your Weight*, 2nd edn. BenBella Books, Dallas.

Boland, R., Verduin, M. & Ruiz, P. (2021) *Kaplan and Saddock's Synopsis of Psychiatry*, 12th edn. LWW, Alphen aan den Rijn, the Netherlands.

Brewster, M.E., Velez, B.L., Breslow, A.S. & Geiger, E.F. (2019) Unpacking body image concerns and disordered eating for transgender women: the roles of sexual objectification and minority stress. *Journal of Counseling Psychology*, **66**(2), 131–142.

Brown, T.A., Forney, K.J., Klein, K.M., Grillot, C. & Keel, P.K. (2020) A 30-year longitudinal study of body weight, dieting, and eating pathology across women and men from late adolescence to later midlife. *Journal of Abnormal Psychology*, **129**(4), 376–386.

Burton, A.L., Abbott, M.J., Norwood, S.J. & Touyz, S.W. (2019) A qualitative exploration of gendered experiences of disordered eating, body image and access to treatment in a sample of Australian transgender people. *Journal of Eating Disorders*, **7**(1), 1–11.

Calogero, R.M., Tylka, T.L., Mensinger, J.L., Meadows, A. & Danieldsottir, S. (2019) Recognising the fundamental right to be fat: a weight-inclusive approach to size acceptance and healing from sizeism. *Women and Therapy*, **42**(1/2), 22–44.

Casteleijn, D. (2014) Using measurement principles to confirm the levels of creative ability as described in the Vona du Toit model of creative ability. *South African Journal of Occupational Therapy*, **44**(1), 14–19.

Corcos, M., Taïeb, O., Benoit-Lamy, S., Paterniti, S., Jeammet, P. & Flament, M.F. (2002) Suicide attempts in women with bulimia nervosa: frequency and characteristics. *Acta Psychiatra Scandinavica*, **106**(5), 381–386.

Culbert, K.M., Racine, S.E. & Klump, K.L. (2015) Research review: what we have learned about the causes of eating disorders – a synthesis of sociocultural, psychological and biological research. *Journal of Child Psychology and Psychiatry*, **56**(11), 1141–1164.

Dray, J. & Wade, T.D. (2012) Is the transtheoretical model and motivational interviewing approach applicable to the treatment of eating disorders? A review. *Clinical Psychology Review*, **32**(6), 558–565.

Evans, E.H., Adamson, A.J., Basterfield, L. *et al* (2018) Risk factors for eating disorder symptoms at 12 years of age: a 6-year longitudinal cohort study. *Appetite*, **123**, 384–389.

Flores, L.E., Muir, R., Weeks, I., Burton Murray, H. & Silver, J.K. (2022) Analysis of age, race, ethnicity and sex of participants in clinical trials focused on eating disorders. *JAMA Network Open*, **5**(2), e220051. https://doi.org/10.1001/jamanetworkopen.2022.0051

Fogelkvist, M., Gustafsson, S.A., Kjellin, L. & Parling, T. (2020) Acceptance and commitment therapy to reduce eating disorder symptoms and body image problems in patients with residual eating disorder symptoms: a randomised controlled trial. *Body Image*, **32**, 155–166.

Frank, G.K.W. (2015) The promise of new approaches to the study of eating disorders. *Biological Psychiatry*, **77**, 602–603.

Galmiche, M., Déchelotte, P., Lambert, G. & Tavolacci, M.P. (2019) Prevalence of eating disorders over the 2000–2018 period: a systematic literature review. *The American Journal of Clinical Nutrition*, **109**(5), 1402–1413.

Garber, A.K., Cheng, J., Accurso, E.C. *et al* (2019) Weight loss and illness severity in adolescents with atypical anorexia nervosa. *Paediatrics*, **144**(6), e20192339.

Goldstein, A. & Gvion, Y. (2019) Socio-demographic and psychological risk factors for suicidal behaviours among individuals with anorexia and bulimia nervosa: a systematic review. *Journal of Affective Disorders*, **245**, 1149–1167.

Hambleton, A., Pepin, G., Le, A. *et al* (2022) Psychiatric and medical comorbidities of eating disorders: findings from a rapid review of the literature. *Journal of Eating Disorders*, **10**, 132–155.

Harrison, C. (2019) *Anti-Diet: Reclaim Your Time, Money, Well-Being, and Happiness Through Intuitive Eating*. Little, Brown Spark, New York.

Hasler, G., Delsignore, A., Milos, G., Buddeberg, C. & Schnyder, U. (2004) Application of Prochaska's transtheoretical model of change to patients with eating disorders. *Journal of Psychosomatic Research*, **57**(5), 451–457.

Hudson, J.I., Hiripi, E., Pope, H.G., Jr. & Kessler, R.C. (2007) The prevalence and correlates of eating disorders in the national comorbidity survey replication. *Biological Psychiatry*, **61**(3), 348–358.

Iannatonne, S., Cerea, S., Carraro, E., Ghisi, M. & Botessi, G. (2022) Broad and narrow transdiagnostic risk factors in eating disorders: a preliminary study on an Italian clinical sample. *International Journal of Environmental Research and Public Health*, **19**(11), 6886–6902.

Jordan, E. (2023) "If you don't lose weight, the government will take you away": an analysis of memorable messages and eating disorders in the LGBTQ+ community. *Health Communication*, **38**, 2925–2935. https://doi.org/10.1080/10410236.2022.2126695

Jovanovski, N. & Jaeger, T. (2022) Demystifying 'diet culture': exploring the meaning of diet culture in online 'anti-diet' feminist, fat activist, and health professional communities. *Women's Studies International Forum*, **90**, 2–10.

Kroenke, K., Spitzer, R.L. & Williams, J.B. (2009) The PHQ-8 as a measure of current depression in the general population. *Journal of affective disorders*, **114**(1–3), 163–173.

Latzer, Y. & Stein, D. (2016) Bio-psycho-social contributions to understanding eating disorders. In: C.G. Fairburn (ed), *Eating Disorders and Obesity: A Comprehensive Handbook*, 3rd edn, pp. 61–68. Guilford Press, New York.

Levesque, D.A., Prochaska, J.M., Prochaska, J.O., Dewart, S.R., Hamby, L.S. & Week, W.B. (2001) Organizational stages and processes of change for continuous quality improvement in health care. *Consulting Psychology Journal: Practice and Research*, **53**(3), 139–153.

Lie, S.Ø., Rø, Ø. & Bang, L. (2019) Is bullying and teasing associated with eating disorders? A systematic review and meta-analysis. *International Journal of Eating Disorders*, **52**(5), 497–514.

López-Gil, J.F., García-Hermoso, A., Smith, L. *et al* (2023) Global proportion of disordered eating in children and adolescents: a systematic review and meta-analysis. *JAMA Pediatrics*, **177**(4), 363–372. https://doi.org/10.1001/jamapediatrics.2022.5848

Manlick, C.F., Cochran, S.V. & Koon, J. (2013) Acceptance and commitment therapy for eating disorders: rationale and literature review. *Journal of Contemporary Psychotherapy*, **43**(2), 115–122.

Mensinger, J.L., Tylka, T.L. & Calamari, M.E. (2018) Mechanisms underlying weight status and healthcare avoidance in women: a study of weight stigma, body-related shame and guilt, and healthcare stress. *Body Image*, **25**, 139–147.

Morgan, J.F., Reid, F. & Lacey, J.H. (1999) The SCOFF questionnaire: assessment of a new screening tool for eating disorders. *British Medical Journal*, **319**(7223), 1467–1468.

Nagata, J.M., Ganson. K.T. & Austin, S.B. (2020) Emerging trends in eating disorders among sexual and gender minorities. *Current Opinions in Psychiatry*, **33**(6), 562–567.

National Eating Disorder Association (2022) *Eating disorders in LGBTQ+ populations.* www.nationaleatingdisorders.org. https://www.nationaleatingdisorders.org/learn/general-information/lgbtq (accessed on 25 June 2023)

Nuttall, F.Q. (2015) Body mass index, obesity, BMI, and health: a critical review. *Nutrition Today*, **50**(3), 117–128.

Parker, L.L. & Harriger, J.A. (2020) Eating disorders and disordered eating behaviours in the LGBT population: a review of the literature. *Journal of Eating Disorders*, **8**(51), 1–20.

Pennesi, J.L. & Wade, T.D. (2016) A systematic review of the existing models of disordered eating: do they inform the development of effective interventions? *Clinical Psychology Review*, **43**, 175–192.

Preti, A., de Girolamo, G., Vilagut, G. *et al* (2009) The epidemiology of eating disorders in six European countries: the results of the ESEMeD-WMH project. *Journal of Psychiatric Research*, **43**(14), 1125–1132.

Rand-Giovannetti, D., Cicero, D.C., Latner, J.D. (2020) Psychometric properties of the eating disorder examination-questionnaire (EDE-Q): a confirmatory factor analysis and assessment of measurement invariance by sex. *Assessment*, **27**(1), 54–65.

Sachs, K.V., Harnke, B., Mehler, P.S. & Krantz, M.J. (2016) Cardiovascular complications of anorexia nervosa: a systematic review. *International Journal of Eating Disorders*, **49**(3), 238–248.

Sanci, L., Coffey, C., Olsson, C., Reid, S., Carlin, J.B. & Patton, G. (2008) Childhood sexual abuse and eating disorders in females: findings from the Victorian adolescent health cohort study. *Archives of Paediatrics and Adolescent Medicine*, **162**(3), 261–267.

Smith, A.R., Zuromski, K.L. & Dodd, D.R. (2018) Eating disorders and suicidality: what we know, what we don't know, and suggestions for future research. *Current Opinion in Psychology*, **22**, 63–67.

Snaith, R.P. (2003) The hospital anxiety and depression scale. *Health and Quality of Life Outcomes*, **1**(1), 29.

Spitzer, R.L., Kroenke, K., Williams, J.B. & Löwe, B. (2006) A brief measure for assessing generalized anxiety disorder: the GAD-7. *Archives of Internal Medicine*, **166**(10), 1092–1097.

Swanson, S.A., Crow, S.K., Le Grange, D., Swendsen, J. & Merikangas, K.R. (2011) Prevalence and correlates of eating disorders in adolescents. Results from the national comorbidity survey replication adolescent supplement. *Archives of General Psychiatry*, **68**(6), 714–723.

The Trevor Project (2019) *The Trevor Project's National Survey on LGBTQ youth mental health 2019.* https://www.thetrevorproject.org/wp-content/uploads/2019/06/The-Trevor-Project-National-Survey-Results-2019.pdf (accessed on 25 June 2023)

Tomiyama, A.J., Carr, D., Granberg, E.M. *et al* (2018) How and why weight stigma drives the obesity 'epidemic' and harms health. *BMC Medicine*, **16**, 123–129.

Tribole, E. & Resch, E. (2020) *Intuitive Eating*, 4th edn (Updated edition). St. Martin's Essentials, New York.

Udo, T. & Grilo, C.M. (2018) Psychiatric and medical correlates of DSM-5 eating disorders in a nationally representative sample of adults in the United States. *International Journal of Eating Disorders*, **51**(3), 203–215.

Uniacke, B., Glasofer, D., Devlin, M., Bockting, W. & Attia, E. (2021) Predictors of eating-related psychopathology in transgender and gender nonbinary individuals. *Eating Behaviours*, **42**(1), 1–7.

Van der Reyden, D., Casteleijn, D., Sherwood, W. & de Witt, P. (eds) (2019) *The Vona du Toit Model of Creative Ability: Origins, Constructs, Principles and Application in Occupational Therapy.* Vona and Marie du Toit Foundation, Pretoria, South Africa.

White, M., Jones, S. & Joy, P. (2022) Safe, seen, and supported: navigating eating disorders recovery in the 2SLGBTQ+ communities. *Canadian Journal of Dietetic Practice and Research*, **83**(1), 1–9.

Yalom, I.D. & Leszcz, M. (2020) *The Theory and Practice of Group Psychotherapy*, 6th edn. Basic Books, New York.

Zipfel, S., Giel, K.E., Bulik, C.M., Hay, P. & Schmidt, U. (2015) Anorexia nervosa: aetiology, assessment, and treatment. *Lancet Psychiatry*, **2**(12), 1099–1111.

CHAPTER 26

Working with People with a Diagnosis of 'Personality Disorder'

Keir Harding and Hollie Berrigan

Beam Consultancy, Wrexham, United Kingdom

KEY LEARNING POINTS

- Occupational therapists focus on occupational difficulties rather than diagnosis.

- When we say 'personality disorder', we are primarily talking about people who have lived through traumatic experiences.

- The social environment around this client group has a profound impact and may require adaptions.

- Our relationships form part of the social environment and require particular focus.

- The role of the occupational therapist and the processes followed are no different than for any other client group.

- A sense of our own boundaries, ways of being and reactions to difficulties are essential for providing effective and ethical care.

INTRODUCTION

This chapter was written by people with both clinical and lived experience of the diagnosis of 'personality disorder'. In addition, we are both on the executive of the British and Irish Group for the Study of Personality Disorder and are members of the Royal College of Psychiatrists Expert Reference Group for the Labelling, Stigma and Diagnosis of Personality Disorders.

We place the term 'personality disorder' in inverted commas to recognise that many people given this diagnosis find the term offensive (Lamb *et al.* 2018). It does not require linguistic gymnastics to move from a 'personality disorder' to a disordered personality. Our experience is that many people given this diagnosis are treated as if their personalities are disordered and that this is the foundation on which the discrimination they face is built.

Occupational therapists focus on occupational difficulties rather than diagnosis. Occupational therapists do not read the diagnosis a psychiatrist has given and begin treatment. Instead, we assess what a person wants and needs to do in their life, the skills that they have to do this and the extent to which the environment supports or inhibits their ability to

function. Diagnosis gives information but not necessarily direction. This is particularly important with this client group because when we say 'personality disorder' we are primarily talking about people who have lived through traumatic experiences, which have had a significant impact on their environments, development and occupational performance. We do people a huge disservice by amputating their histories and solely viewing them through the lens of diagnosis and pathology. The social environment around this client group in particular has a profound impact and may require adaptions given the levels of stigma they experience. The relationships we have with our patients form part of their (and our) social environment and require particular focus. The role of the occupational therapist and the processes we follow are no different than for any other client group. As occupational therapists, a sense of our own boundaries, ways of being and reactions to difficulties are essential for working with people diagnosed with 'personality disorders'.

Our day-to-day work involves people who recurrently feel suicidal and use self-harm as a way of coping. We were both exasperated at how mostly cisgendered women who had

Crouch and Alers Occupational Therapy in Psychiatry and Mental Health, Sixth Edition.
Edited by Rosemary Crouch, Tania Buys, Enos Morankoana Ramano, Matty van Niekerk and Lisa Wegner.
© 2025 John Wiley & Sons Ltd. Published 2025 by John Wiley & Sons Ltd.

lived through abuse were treated within the United Kingdom healthcare system, where we are based. They are often 'detained' in institutions to 'keep them safe', ensuring that clinicians and organisations can avoid the anxiety that comes with working with people who hurt themselves (Harding *et al.* 2020). We have observed a marked proportional correlation between the level of restriction around them and the frequency and dangerousness of their self-harm. An example could be someone in a psychiatric unit who overdoses and seeks help in the community, but once access to pills is blocked on the ward, relies on self-strangulation to manage their distress. The sudden increase in risk is seen as evidence that hospitalisation in a mental health facility is required instead of recognising that hospitalisation is resulting in ways of coping becoming more lethal. In occupational therapy parlance, the environment has been adapted (compulsory admission to hospital) and the impact on functioning is severe. Those we work with receive the diagnosis of 'personality disorder' yet in our experience, they often meet few of the criteria. In our work with Beam Consultancy, we combine our clinical and lived experience to help patients and staff avoid prolonged periods of hospitalisation or 'detention in hospital' by helping patients and those who support them in the community.

We have both been a part of therapeutic and supervision processes that have required and encouraged high levels of self-awareness and introspection. As such, we recognise that this chapter represents our personal (potentially expert) perspective on what constitutes good practice in this area rather than a misleading attempt to provide a definitive account of what 'should' be done. We have opted to write in the first person to emphasise that these are our personal views, backed up by evidence and that other opinions are available.

OCCUPATIONAL THERAPY AND DIAGNOSIS

Diagnosis can be a useful shortcut in the caring professions. When a clear diagnosis is made, professionals will immediately know where to look to understand common groups of difficulties, evidence-based treatment and likely prognosis. Where the science around diagnosis is less robust, it loses a lot of its utility. Common groups become more heterogeneous. Treatments seem more generic than specific. The field of personality disorder is an area where we would argue the diagnostic label brings little and can cause harm (Klein *et al.* 2022). Our invitation in this chapter is to recognise 'personality disorder' as a flawed concept for understanding people and instead rely on core skills of occupational therapy to bring about an understanding. It is suggested that 'Rather than arriving at a label or classification of a disease, as is often the case in medicine, occupational therapists identify deficits in performance components, occupational performance or role performance' (Bennett & Bennett 2000, p. 173). The implication is that the occupational therapist will be looking outside of diagnostic criteria and lists of symptoms. While diagnostic labels can guide, they should not dictate. Our starting position

is that no one has a disordered personality, but those who are told they have one, often experience great suffering, have limited access to roles and have severe impairments in their functioning. This tends to take place in an environment that lacks compassion and understanding, where difficulties are understood as innate rather than responses to previous experiences in environments that were harmful. While we will outline the construct of the diagnosis below, we encourage occupational therapists to work outside of, or alongside, this framework, using the concepts and ideas unique to our profession.

AN OVERVIEW OF THE 'PERSONALITY DISORDER' CONSTRUCT

The fourth edition of the Diagnostic and Statistical manual contained ten different types of personality disorder (American Psychiatric Association [APA] 1994). Each type contains a number of different criteria, and hitting the threshold number implies a diagnosis of that type of personality disorder. If the requisite number of criterion are not met, one will not have that diagnosis. There has been much criticism of this binary system, with one criticism being that there is no indication of severity (Kim & Tyrer 2010). The DSM 5-TR proposed a different system based on dimensions of functioning, before reverting to the original criteria-based model (APA 2022) (see Figure 26.1). While the criteria model proposes ten different types, these types are not routinely diagnosed in practice. Additionally, comorbidity is high with people meeting the criteria for one personality disorder likely to meet the criteria for at least one other. This diagnosis thus loses some utility as it does not allow for a clear focus on a specific condition.

The ICD-11 presents a totally different model of 'personality disorder' to the DSM 5-TR. Here there are (almost) no different types, with a generic diagnosis of 'personality disorder' being

- **Cluster A** odd and eccentric
  - Paranoid personality disorder
  - Schizoid personality disorder
  - Schizotypal personality disorder
- **Cluster B** emotional/dramatic/erratic
  - Antisocial personality disorder
  - Borderline personality disorder
  - Histrionic personality disorder
  - Narcissistic personality disorder
- **Cluster C** anxious/avoidant
  - Avoidant personality disorder
  - Dependent personality disorder
  - Obsessive-compulsive personality disorder

FIGURE 26.1 Different personality disorders according to the DSM 5-TR.

Source: APA (2022)/American Psychiatric Association.

given alongside a measure of severity – mild, moderate or severe (Swales 2022). Trait descriptors of negative affectivity, dissociality, anankastia, detachment and disinhibition can also be added. The ICD-11 model recognised that the ten 'exaggerated caricatures' of the criteria-based model were not seen in practice and there was much overlap in these 'cartoonish stereotypes'. Our experience was that only Borderline and Antisocial Personality Disorder were regularly diagnosed. It remains to be seen whether the move to a more generic way of understanding aids clinical work. Figure 26.2 shows diagnostic criteria for Borderline Personality Disorder taken from the ICD-11. While these are taken from the ICD-11, they are nearly identical to the criteria in the DSM 5-TR.

One area where the DSM and ICD overlap is around the diagnosis of Borderline Personality Disorder (BPD). There was such opposition to the ICD's plan to abandon this term that it remains an option where all of the other types have been removed (Tyrer *et al.* 2019). This diagnosis again comes with many criticisms. Here, five of nine criteria (see Figure 26.2) are required for the diagnosis. This means two patients could sit next to each other with one meeting criteria one to five, and the other meeting criteria five to nine. Despite only sharing one criterion they would both have similar approaches, prognosis and treatment plans. For those with such disparate presentations, this clearly makes no sense. Given that there are 256 permutations of criteria that could be used to make a diagnosis of BPD, it is clear that it can be a term to describe a huge variety of presentations. Further criticisms recognise that around 80% of those given this diagnosis have experienced trauma such as neglect and abuse (Yen *et al.* 2002). It can be questioned how ethical it is to label those people as having what could be understood as a disordered personality. It locates the problem in them rather than the people who hurt them. In addition, this diagnosis is clinically given to three times as many women as men (APA 2022). With criteria such as 'inappropriate, intense anger' (APA 2022), we can again wonder how appropriate it is to judge the anger of survivors of abuse as inappropriate. It is widely reported by academics and survivors alike that borderline personality disorder is a diagnosis rooted in misogyny and victim blaming (Shaw & Proctor 2005). As a result, we frequently see the trauma histories and narratives of people (particularly cisgender women and transgender men and women) amputated by professionals and only seen through the lens of something being inherently wrong with the core of someone's being. Additionally, LGBTQIA+ people are also disproportionately diagnosed (Rodriguez-Seijas *et al.* 2021). It is almost as if this becomes a diagnosis applied without science and is a moral judgement of the person (Lewis & Appleby 1988). Their understanding of their sexuality or gender identity cannot be believed or trusted and can only be seen as a sign of identity or personality disturbance.

There is concern that the diagnosis of 'personality disorder' means that other conditions get missed (Warrender *et al.* 2021). While this can include physical ailments not being taken seriously, our experience is that trauma responses, post-traumatic stress disorder, complex post-traumatic stress disorder, attention deficit hyperactivity disorder and difficulties associated with living on the autistic spectrum can all be crammed into a 'personality disorder' diagnosis. It is for this reason we encourage clinicians to think of people diagnosed with 'personality disorder' as being given a label that is too often not indicative of being an accurate diagnosis.

As in every area of occupational therapy, diagnosis is not essential (Bryant *et al.* 2022). Assessment identifies what people want and need to do, the skills they have to be able to achieve this and how the environment enhances or inhibits functioning. Where diagnosis in this case brings little of value, we would encourage occupational therapists to invest particularly in the assessment process to build an understanding of the barriers to functioning independent of the diagnostic process.

THE IMPACT OF THE DIAGNOSIS ON THE SOCIAL ENVIRONMENT – STIGMA

It is commonly acknowledged that those who are given a diagnosis of 'personality disorder' experience extreme prejudice, even discrimination as a result (Klein *et al.* 2022). Sadly,

- Frantic efforts to avoid real or imagined abandonment
- A pattern of unstable and intense interpersonal relationships
- Identity disturbance, manifested in markedly and persistently unstable self-image or sense of self
- A tendency to act rashly in states of high negatice affect, leading to potentially self-damaging behaviours
- Recurrent episodes of self-harm
- Emotional instability due to marked reactivity of mood
- Chronic feelings of emptiness
- Inappropriate intense anger or difficulty controlling anger
- Transient dissociative symptoms or psychotic-like features in situations of high affective arousal.

FIGURE 26.2 Diagnostic criteria for borderline personality disorder.
Source: Swales, M. A. (2022)/Annual Reviews.

this stigma does not reside predominantly in the general public, but in the very clinicians tasked with helping people. We do see an increase in personality disorder being used as a slur in a variety of media forms and being portrayed as people who are dangerous in television and film. The recent trial of Heard versus Depp has no doubt added to this stigma (Gallaher 2022). Stigma takes many forms but includes communication being viewed as manipulative or attention seeking, reactions to injustice being viewed as inappropriate, patients having the power to break apart previously high-functioning teams, pathologising of normal human interactions such as preferring the company of one person over another, diagnostic overshadowing (where problems are missed due to the presence of the 'personality disorder' diagnosis) and therapeutic nihilism (the idea that someone cannot be helped). All the above are significant barriers to both patients engaging with the help that is on offer and that help being of any benefit. It has been argued that the difficulties resulting from the diagnosis are worse than the original problems (Berrigan 2021).

Given that applying the diagnosis of personality disorder can be viewed as an adaption to the social environment that inhibits the functioning of patients and staff, it is essential that professionals who adapt environments are alert to stigmatising attitudes and practices that impact on the patient and treating team.

COMMON MISCONCEPTIONS

Throughout our careers, we have seen a range of understandable behaviours and ways of relating described as 'just' attention seeking, manipulating, splitting or sabotaging. Rarely have we encountered a situation where this is an accurate description of what is occurring. The idea that patients do these things on purpose gets in the way of empathy and care so it is important that occupational therapists hold an awareness of these terms and some ways they can be highlighted and challenged in the social environments around people.

Just

Once people describe any behaviour as 'just' anything, it is usually an indication that they have stopped thinking about the complex nature of what drives humans to act and are making their own interpretation. This can be useful for staff groups to protect their sense of being effective practitioners but does little to ensure caring, reflective practice. As occupational therapists, we are aware of the myriad of factors that influence action and we can encourage our colleagues to be mindful of this too (Bryant *et al.* 2022).

Manipulation

With manipulation, the suggestion is that the patient is exploiting the therapist in some way. Most dictionaries describe manipulation as being artful or skilful, yet this cannot be the case if staff feel manipulated. We have heard patients being told details of staff members' lives then having the patients described as manipulating staff. We have heard of patients asking multiple members of staff for something until someone says yes and this being described as manipulative. These are never described as individuals or groups of staff having difficulty maintaining their boundaries; the problem is always located in the patient. To put this into context, if we wanted something, 50 people could give it to us and we knew one of them would say yes; at what point would it be sensible to stop asking?

The people who receive the label of 'personality disorder' have often had very poor role models of effective interactions. Staff can also be poor role models. What we are labelling as manipulative may well be ineffective communication skills that have been learned. The artful and skilful manipulation that encourages people to do things differently while maintaining good relationships with them might reside predominantly within the staff members.

Attention Seeking

The implication with attention seeking is that whatever is being witnessed is solely to attract and hold the attention of staff members. When people act in this way the attention they get is often dismissive and pejorative, so we might wonder why that is of benefit. We might wonder if there is something else going on that attracts our attention and whether the result was not the intention. We might also consider if there is something happening that cannot be expressed in words, or perhaps words have failed to elicit a helpful response in the past.

Seeking attention when in distress is a natural human behaviour. If one breaks one's leg, one seeks attention for it, but perhaps in a way that is socially acceptable. People will see the broken bone and understand that the individual is seeking relief from pain and suffering from the inability to move. No one will regard this as 'just' attention seeking. How might we regard others differently if we could understand what was motivating them?

We might also consider the impact of the environment on how people act. In under-resourced teams, do we spend the same amount of time with everyone or do we allocate time depending on how dangerous people are? If we reward the ability to regulate emotion, ask for help and accept hearing 'not now' with an absence of individual time, perhaps we should not be surprised if dangerousness and care become linked in the minds of our patients. People rarely receive 'attention' that meets a need. It is almost as if punitive, punishing and compassionless responses might increase the need for people to attempt to seek attention. People learn nothing about being worthy of care and caring for themselves if people responsible for providing care are failing to do so. There is often a sense that being human with someone will create dependency (Bornstein 2005); we would argue this is a fallacy. Compassionless services that label behaviour as attention seeking do not stop people from seeking help; they merely pathologise it.

Sabotage

With sabotage, the idea is that patients are calculating ways to destroy their recovery. We have yet to meet anyone who has articulated this. What we see described as sabotage is when staff goals and patient goals are profoundly different. Even when they are similar, the patient attending to what is important for them in the moment while potentially losing focus on long-term goals can also be described as sabotage. We would encourage occupational therapists to help patients articulate the range of motivators behind acts that are labelled as sabotage. This understanding is useful for the patient but can profoundly change how people are viewed in the environment around them. Ask 'what would "recovery" look like if the patients got to decide?' Is the reward for recovery worth it or does it involve supportive and caring relationships being withdrawn?'

Splitting

With splitting, the patient is seen as making efforts to drive apart previously high-functioning staff teams. For us this is the most damaging of all the stigmatising ideas as it pathologises and 'makes wrong' very normal and understandable human reactions. In our lives, we like some people more than others. We choose to spend time with some people more than others. For staff, this is seen as normal. For patients, this is seen as splitting. When we like people, we interact with them more and share more of ourselves than we do with others we do not warm to as much. We may be nicer to them. Again, these are normal interactions. As staff who get on well with people are resented by those who do not, disagreements and tension start to build and patients will pick up on this. We might expect our patients with difficult relationship histories to act in ways that might exacerbate these divisions. As staff, perhaps we should hold ourselves to a different standard. In his seminal article The Ailment (Main 1957), Tom Maine explained splitting with the example of a baby being brought into a room full of people. Some would try to soothe the child. Some would succeed, others might be rejected. The child might respond better to those it finds soothing. It might recoil and move away from those it did not connect with as well. People would resent this and annoyance at each other might grow. Past resentments might emerge, and people could become more antagonistic to each other. Maine's point was that the baby did not cause the split, but its distress made existing issues worse. We have often heard patients described as deliberately driving a wedge between staff. While we have met many people who intensely liked and disliked different members of staff, we have yet to meet one who had a calculated plan to sow discord. As ever, if we can think about how past interactions may play out in current ones, we are likely to see our patients in a far more empathic light.

With all the examples above, our experience is that these pejorative ways of understanding people are not used when there is a diagnosis other than 'personality disorder'. It is the stigma and prejudice in the social environment that enable this more negative interpretation.

THE IMPACT

Taking all the above into consideration, we can anticipate what care will look like if patients are seen as attention seeking, sabotaging, manipulating splitters of teams. We can also anticipate how enthusiastically patients will form relationships with us knowing this is how they are viewed. We will touch on the importance of validation in this work later, but we might consider how invalidating it might feel for staff to tell you why you have done something without any discussion or attempt to understand. We are mindful of a colleague who died who said they had self-harmed for years before someone found out and told them they were doing it for attention. Our default is that people only do things because it is better than not doing them.

People with the diagnosis of 'personality disorder' frequently perform occupations with value and meaning from which occupational therapists have traditionally shied away (Twinley 2013; Harding 2020). Where the dark side of occupation cannot be thought about, we lose all ability to help our clients. It is our job to understand that these ways of being convey this information into the environment around them. In this way, staff can understand ways of coping that have value and meaning and respond thoughtfully. The alternative is understanding behaviour in a moral or judgemental way ('it should not be done') or through a more medical lens ('self-harm is a symptom of their illness'). When we provide narratives that explain, staff can maintain the empathy and compassion they know form the foundation of effective care. The dark side of occupation is discussed further below.

THE THERAPEUTIC RELATIONSHIP AS THE MOST IMPORTANT SOCIAL ENVIRONMENT

All of the stigma covered so far would give the impression that genuine therapeutic relationships with people who have this diagnosis can be dangerous to therapists. Therapists might be manipulated, split, deceived, tricked and have their time wasted. The reality is that our therapeutic relationship will be the most useful, perhaps the only tool, we have in our work in this area of mental health. Given the high instances of traumatic and abusive experiences in the lives of people given a 'personality disorder' diagnosis, we are required to deliberately and consciously create an environment that gives the best chance of a positive therapeutic relationship being formed. While in other areas of therapy, the therapeutic relationship might develop as the work is done together; in this area, we would argue that the building of a therapeutic relationship is the work (Norcross & Lambert 2019). Our patients will have had poor experiences with those who were meant to help and protect them in the past. If we cannot create a social environment where therapeutic work can take place, it will not matter what our next goal is.

While it may sound basic, becoming someone who is genuine, honest and looking out for the agreed vision of 'best interests' of the person one is working with may be something one's patients have not experienced previously. Being consistent, reliable and someone who does what they say they will, becomes increasingly important in the lives of people who will likely have been repeatedly let down by those supposed to care for them.

While an awareness of what we bring to relationships is an important part of our therapeutic work, an understanding of the relationship patterns of those we work with is also important when attempting to maintain compassion and empathy. Our patients may well interact in ways that we would not. While there can be a tendency to judge this, it might be important to consider the idea that people interact in the way that they do because in some way, it is better than doing something different. If we can understand that, we are far more likely to react based on that understanding rather than our own interpretations. Due to people's experiences of others as being abusive, it is likely we will be interpreted as abusive at times. It can be very difficult to find you have a good relationship with someone one day but seem hated the next. It might be important to remember the role models of the people we are working with. What were their experiences of relationships where people were expected to care and where people held power over them? Due to the power we hold in our 'staff' role, we are likely to be perceived as threatening in some way. While we can work to undermine this and share power where possible, an awareness of this is again important when weighing up how to act in our relationships. We need to get rid of the idea that as professionals, we interact with people perfectly and have perfect relationships with everyone. We need to be conscious about what interactions and relationships evoke in us and process them; if we do not do this, we are likely to act them out.

BOUNDARIES, VALIDATION AND BEING HUMAN

We have frequently heard 'boundaries' and 'inappropriate' said to us and those we work with, as if there is a universally accepted code of conduct for everyone in the world. While most people would agree that staff urinating onto the beds of patients is inappropriate, there are more nuanced understandings around voice volume, personal space, questions around personal life and many other aspects of ourselves that are not immediately obvious. When working in the cultures of organisations, some boundaries will be dictated by policies and rules that can be explained. Others are communicated in more subtle ways and become more obvious generally when people are pushing against what is deemed acceptable. Here again, it is worth considering what boundaries our patients were raised with. Their past lessons on what is acceptable may well have

been literally beaten into them. Equally, they may have had little explicit or implicit instruction on how to interact with others. Care organisations tend to be less curious about the boundaries of the patient. What do they feel about physical proximity, tone of voice or an expectation to bare their soul to a stranger?

It is a useful exercise to think about the things that push our buttons in our interactions with others. They will be different to things that impact our colleagues. Sometimes it is hard to articulate where our boundaries lie, but it is obvious to us when they are being crossed. There are a variety of benefits to staff being aware of what impacts them in their relationships. Perhaps the most useful is that we can communicate our awareness to the people that we work with in order to ensure our relationships remain as therapeutic as possible. Many of our patients will have experienced relationships ending abruptly, which can have a devastating and isolating effect on them. If we cannot communicate what makes the likelihood of an ongoing positive relationship less likely, we cannot be surprised if nothing changes. Sadly, our patients will probably replay their difficulties in subsequent therapeutic relationships without ever being given the opportunity to learn and potentially change.

This invitation should not only go one way. It can be a useful discussion to help our patients express the things they find particularly difficult in relationships. It might well be the first time they have been asked. Given that people may find it difficult to describe their boundaries, it can be useful to share our experiences of being with them. It can also be useful to observe when something changes during our interactions and to be curious about what has occurred.

When discussing our boundaries, we find it useful to emphasise how our boundaries are unique to us. Others may have different ones, but if working with us is important, people may choose to take our boundaries into account. It is important to emphasise that something is not 'wrong', just how it impacts us. An example is that of a therapist who finds public criticism particularly shaming. He encourages those he works with to raise issues with him prior to criticising him in front of others. It can be useful to explain the desire to help someone and how this is affected by hearing things that are painful. Be explicit about what you would like to be different and why this is useful for your patient. There will be times when patients do wish to hurt you and keeping you away will be a priority for them. As it is difficult to help anyone without a relationship, we would encourage occupational therapists to consider the function of this, why it would make sense in terms of past experience and whether the goal of forming a relationship can still be pursued. It will always feel personal, but people's ways of defending themselves are generally aimed at anyone and everyone.

VALIDATION

In all of our work in mental health, validation has been the most useful and easily accessible tool for being helpful to people. Validation is defined as 'recognition or affirmation that a person or their feelings or opinions are valid or worthwhile' (Oxford Languages n.d.) and to us it conveys to people that they are accepted, 'normal' and understood. There are six steps to validation as outlined in Dialectical Behaviour Therapy (Linehan 1993). These are:

1. *Being present*: Doing everything to convey to the patient that you have their full attention. Not looking at your watch or trying to fill in a form.

2. *Accurate reflection*: Here we display that we are listening and summarise back to the person we are talking to. We might also check if we are getting it right by saying things like 'Have I understood correctly?' or 'Don't let me put words in your mouth but it sounds like . . .' or 'I'm wondering if . . .'

3. *Reading*: This is where we move from showing that we are listening to showing that we are thinking. We do not tell people what they felt, but we wonder, giving people the opportunity to correct us. This might involve something like 'Your breathing was fast, you wanted to get away . . . I wonder if you were frightened?' Not 'You must have been terrified'.

   The above three steps might be considered the basic tools therapists would use in their interactions with people yet we are aware of how quickly they can slip in environments with intense time pressures where staff are stressed. The following three steps add more humanity to the relationship.

4. Conveying something is normal based on past experiences: If someone tells us that they feel afraid while walking around town late at night, we might use our knowledge of their experiences to say, 'Well that makes sense, you've been hurt when in town late at night on your own'.

5. Conveying something is normal because it is normal: While this has the potential to sound dismissive, it can be hugely validating to hear that your fears and worries belong to the rest of the world too. For the above-mentioned example, we might say, 'I think lots of people feel anxious walking through town on their own late at night. You read lots of things on the news and it never seems particularly safe'. Not 'Well everyone feels like that'. It can be useful to add some of step 4 while doing step 5, for example, 'Lots of people feel frightened walking through town at night but it makes particular sense for you given what you've lived through'.

6. Conveying it is normal because you feel it too: Radical genuineness is the deliberate use of your own experiences if hearing them would be useful to the patient. Using the same example, we might say, 'I was walking through town on my own the other week and my heart was pounding, I was starting to get hot and I eventually went into a cafe and called a taxi home'. We communicate that under the same circumstances, we would have felt the same.

With all these steps there is the idea that the higher the level of validation you use, the more contained and heard your client will feel. Our experience is that patients derive much comfort from being given the message that what they feel makes sense and is not abnormal. If they feel they are 'mad', 'crazy' or 'disordered', this can be validated too without necessarily agreeing with them. While there has been a big push in mental health to challenge negative thoughts (MacLeod & Mathews 2012), our experience with this client group is that it can be a fairly humiliating experience for them if there is not a lot of validation given first. Challenging negative thoughts in a curious and sensitive way is fine, but when people have a lot of evidence to back up their thinking and we are telling people their thinking is wrong, it can be massively invalidating. When we deny and amputate people's histories, it is beyond invalidating and can feel abusive and we will be replicating the people that have harmed them.

Another benefit to using validation is that it is difficult to argue with people who agree with you. Early in our careers, we were encouraged to counter any statements we felt were personal or derogatory. We now find we can get a lot further if we validate first. If someone had said, 'You're only here because you're being paid', we might have replied that we did the job because we cared about people. These days we are likely to 'read' (use step 3) by saying, 'You seem annoyed that I'm being paid to be here, is that right?' Then be genuine, 'This isn't the same, but if I'm in a shop and I get the sense the person is just doing their job and has no interest in being kind to me I hate it. Sometimes I leave. I wonder if I am doing something that gives you the idea that I'm not interested?'

We feel that every thought and feeling can be validated. Generally, we can validate someone's urges too. We might not always validate the actions someone takes, but we can convey that the thoughts, emotions and urges behind them make sense. Even if it is not particularly grounded in reality, we can still validate the emotional experience someone has and why it is understandable they then feel what they feel.

BEING HUMAN

Part of our training and early practice was around being a professional. We have met students who told us they wanted to develop their professional persona. When we have talked more about this concept, they have described having a more formal demeanour leaving them more able to do the process of occupational therapy. Given that the quality of our therapeutic relationship is the greatest indicator of success in therapy (Stubbe 2018), it is essential to note that the relationship is the process. The relationship is the foundation upon which everything else is built. We would encourage occupational therapists to bring their real self into the work. The patients will have had lifetimes of deceit and disingenuousness. When we hide who we are, when our words and body language do not match, our patients will be aware and react in ways that are understandable. Being ultra-professional upholds a hierarchy and separation within the therapeutic relationship. It is almost impossible to feel contained by people you do not know, even if you spend lots of time with them. There is nothing therapeutic in working with a potential wolf in sheep's clothing waiting for them to come out.

THE DARK SIDE OF OCCUPATION

Those with whom we work will have lived through experiences that shape their ideas about themselves, other people and the world. These ideas will shape their behaviour, potentially leading to activities or actions of which society can disapprove. In much of mental health there can be a lack of compassion towards people who do things that cause problems for them and others. 'If only the people with anorexia would eat more; if only those with alcoholism would stop drinking'. It is essential that for us to help the people in our care, activities are things with value and meaning to be understood rather than moralised over (Twinley 2021).

People only do the thing because in that moment it is better than not doing it. In the physical realm of occupational therapy, we might perform detailed activity analysis to understand how, and to what extent, people are able to function. We need to be able to do the same with activities that are not so palatable to us. What we see as problems may not be for those with whom we are working, for example, having many sexual partners is almost always seen as a problem in a woman, but almost never in a man. A man's anger might never be questioned, a woman's may well be 'inappropriate'.

Often, people with the diagnosis of 'personality disorder' are confined to hospitals because of the dangerous things they might do to themselves. Being able to understand the different functions of self-harm and suicidal behaviour and how they apply to an individual is an essential ingredient of client-centred care. Using self-harm as an example, we might ask what was happening to someone about half an hour before they did it. What were they thinking about? What were they feeling? Did they have any urges to do anything? What did they do? What had happened that day that had impacted on them? We can then slowly take people through the different steps that led from where they were to hurting themselves. People not used to being asked about such things might find this difficult and the occupational therapist might need to keep slowing things down and taking them back. There might be a few 'I don't know's'. If that is the case, ask for their best guess or come up with the most empathic idea that you can. This process should result in a map that explains how someone moves from feeling safe to doing something dangerous. The thoughts, emotions, urges and actions will give a wealth of information that will allow the occupational therapist to target interventions that can stop or reduce self-harm, or explore less dangerous methods depending on the goals of the patient. Being able to share a coherent narrative around why self-harm makes sense is likely to be an intervention into the social environment that can inform practice and reduce anxiety in the staff team. Because it is an individual plan, it can aid decisions like 'does removing everything someone could possibly harm themselves with make them safer or more likely to do something more dangerous?' An example of us roleplaying a way of asking about self-harm can be found here: https://www.youtube.com/watch?v=WcfWh8-x4kQ&t=50s.

DIALECTICAL BEHAVIOUR THERAPY

The model of human occupation (MOHO) (Kielhofner 2008) describes occupational behaviour as being influenced by what we want to do, what we need to do, the environment around us and the skills that we have. Dialectical Behaviour Therapy (DBT), a therapy designed by someone with lived experience of self-harm and recurrent suicidality, takes the idea that many people come from environments where they were not taught skills that are useful in life (Linehan 1993). These skills are grouped into:

- *Mindfulness:* keeping your attention where you want it. Being in, and not overwhelmed by, the current moment. Not fixating on the past or future.

- *Distress tolerance:* getting through difficult situations without doing something that might make it worse.

- *Interpersonal effectiveness:* being able to keep relationships as healthy as required while getting what you want, being able to say no, ending relationships, keeping self-esteem intact, holding boundaries and negotiating.

- *Emotion regulation:* being able to feel and understand/label your emotions without shutting them off or being utterly overwhelmed by them.

We would not recommend simply teaching the above, but after assessment, if difficulties that could be addressed by learning new skills are identified, then the DBT manual has a raft of them. Many of these will be familiar to occupational therapists already, including things like problem-solving, activity engagement, self-soothing and assertiveness. DBT also takes the approach that suicidality is reduced if people have a life worth living. This is an area where occupational therapists can add days to life as well as life to days, and while we would not advocate every occupational therapist becoming a DBT therapist, there is much in the DBT training that supports people to work with potentially lethal self-harm and suicidality that is missing from our core training.

BRINGING ABOUT CHANGE

The process of occupational therapy is the same for whatever client group we are working with – assessment, intervention and evaluation of whether a change has occurred. Using the MOHO (Kielhofner 2008) as an example, we assess what people want to do, what their roles require that they do, what skills they have in order to achieve the above and how the environment supports or inhibits their ability to do this. Our assessment will lead us to areas where people want to be different or change in their lives. Our role is to help them bring about this change. When working with this client group, we may expect more occupations that bring harm to the person. We may expect difficulties in our relationship based on what staff and patients bring in terms of our ways of thinking about ourselves and others and our previous experiences of relationships. We may expect environmental pressures such as requirements to be discharged from a restrictive environment, what behaviours/interactions are considered acceptable and potentially a range of stigmatising attitudes in the team.

As discussed previously, the quality of the therapeutic alliance is the biggest indicator as to whether therapy is successful (Stubbe 2018). So long as the occupational therapist and the client have agreed what 'the problem' is, how that problem will be addressed and the occupational therapist has provided a secure, genuine relationship for the work to take place, intervention will be as good as any gold standard intervention. Hence the emphasis on the immediate social environment (the relationship) earlier in the chapter. We emphasise the importance of collaboration and the answer, not lying solely in the professional.

Once you have agreed on what you will work on, there is no one particular activity that is good for this client group, in the same way that there is no activity that is a treatment of choice for depression, schizophrenia or irritable bowel syndrome. Sometimes occupational therapists can prioritise helping a client to reach functional goals and teach skills or adapt environments to be able to do this. At other times, occupational therapists prioritise activity as the means by which therapy is delivered. There are two effective activities that can be used for this: firstly, activities that hold genuine meaning for the patient, and secondly, activities for which the therapist has a particular passion and is able to use that passion to inspire and motivate their patients.

RISK ASSESSMENT

While much has been written about risk assessment, we are always mindful of how stigma and fear can influence the environment around these clients. There can be a desire to keep sharp things away from people who self-harm, which would be a blanket approach that disregards history and context. Our experience is that there are remarkably few people who spontaneously harm themselves without warning in situations where they are focused on a specific task within the context of a collaborative relationship. We would urge occupational therapists to discuss risks, their own as well as their patient's anxieties, and how to manage them with the patient. We would always find peoples' histories and previous patterns of behaviour essential to consider when deciding how to respond to actual and perceived risks. A history of unprovoked assaults would make us wary of spending time with someone alone. A history of being violent while undergoing restraint would help

us place the risk in a different context. Equally, someone self-harming might result in leave being revoked if they are in hospital. This might make sense if the patient is dysregulated and more intense support is required. If the patient's history is such that they only self-harm severely in a hospital environment, self-harm may indicate more autonomy and freedom is required. We are not encouraging a blasé attitude to risk, but encouraging practitioners to be aware of how blanket approaches can impact by taking power away from people who will already have had power torn from them in the most painful ways. The occupational therapist should follow usual procedures but keep an awareness of how stigma and fear might be operating. Expect your clients to be able to contribute towards managing risk. The UK NICE guidelines for Self Harm provide some structure when considering risk assessment and it is important to be aware of their focus on collaboration as opposed to compelling people to live in artificial 'risk-free' environments (NICE 2022). Try to allow 'containment' to be provided by your relationship rather than locked doors and sanctions. Wonder whether you are trying to manage a risk that has never occurred before thinking, for example, 'They have a history of cutting in their bedroom during periods when they experience extreme shame; what if they jump in front of a car on the way to the shops?' We can do little to mitigate risks that are unpredictable, yet environments that are anxious and keen to avoid criticism may jettison collaborative working in order to maintain a restrictive environment that has the appearance of being safe (Veale et al. 2023). That environment may do little to foster growth and recovery.

CHOOSING THE FOCUS

The goals of client-centred occupational therapy intervention should be determined by the assessment/formulation process. This can avoid the painful situation where therapist and patient goals are different and at least lead to discussions where goals are agreed. The work environment can dictate the focus, length and method of occupational therapy and so some compromise may be required between what is possible and what is desired. Intervention that fits the patient as much as possible is encouraged.

What you agree to work on will be unique. We encourage occupational therapists to maintain their expertise in the things that people do. Traditionally, occupational therapy may have focused on things that give people pleasure and meaning. It may have been aimed at helping people fulfil roles that are required of them. It may have been developing a range of occupations that can bring pleasure, connection and texture to people's lives. It may have been teaching the skills needed to live independently. All of these are worthwhile pursuits and as mentioned previously, few people thrive if life is not worth living.

We wonder whether occupational therapists can also focus on activities that might end life or make it more painful. People tend to be detained in criminal justice and care settings due to the things that they do. Being compelled to live in an institution has a significant impact on people's functioning, dying even more so. A focus on the occupations that keep people detained – often suicidality, self-harm or violence, is entirely within our remit, fits perfectly with our focus on function and may be of more immediate concern than addressing issues that impact quality of life. In such circumstances we might delay work on quality of life to ensure there is a life to add value to. Exploring the meaning and value of violence, overdosing, standing at heights where falls will kill you and so on, may not have been the traditional focus of occupational therapy, but what other profession is better placed to examine the things people do, the environmental response and what needs to happen to ensure people are able to function? If we have nothing to say on these subjects, then we cannot be surprised if other professions become the 'go-to' people to consult about the dark side of occupation.

Potential goals of occupational therapy include being able to form trusting relationships, describe internal states of being, articulate desires and say no when required, reduce occupations that harm, learn skills that reduce difficulties which get in the way of performing certain occupations, increase activities that bring pleasure, increase activities that build mastery and to adapt environments that inhibit functioning.

The following case studies highlight some of the concepts and ideas discussed in this chapter and illustrate our work in this area.

Vignette 1: Intervention with an Individual

A patient experiences the problem that their use of potentially lethal self-harm results in them being 'detained' in hospital. Assessment indicates that self-harm, specifically cutting with a clean razor blade, is used to experience pain, bring a sense of calm and this reduces the fear that arises from being out of control. This fear is exacerbated by breathlessness, heart thumping, feeling hot and thoughts of having a heart attack and dying. These are experienced in environments where the patient either feels a sense of threat or thoughts are focused on times they have been hurt in the past. The occupational therapist validates how normal it is to experience fear at the prospect of having a heart attack. They also validate that most people feel afraid when threatened or when thinking about times they were in danger. The therapist and patient agree that if the fear around having a heart attack was not so intense, the need to cut to bring down the fear would significantly diminish. After checking with the multidisciplinary team (MDT) that the patient is at no greater risk of heart attack than the average person, the occupational therapist and patient agree to explore ways of experiencing breathlessness, increased heart rate, heat and sweating without leading to a catastrophic interpretation of what

they mean. This would then mean self-harm was not used as often.

The patient has a variety of interests that include exercise and going to the gym. The occupational therapist arranges some time to exercise together. The choice of venue is influenced by the policy of the institution, the legal framework allowing time away or not, previous risks in similar situations and a collaborative discussion with the client. As part of intense exercise in a manner that holds meaning for the client, the occupational therapist and patient have multiple experiences of being out of breath, heart thumping and being hot. They practise bringing their bodies back to baseline and relating the same physical experiences to times when the patient has hurt themselves. The occupational therapist recognises that this situation is different to the times when hurting yourself is the way to manage the discomfort, but wonders whether these bodily sensations can be experienced without the worry about heart attack. This activity was chosen purely because it had a direct relation to a problem to be worked on and had meaning for the client. The outcome would be assessed by asking the client whether increasing their ability to manage the impact of fear had had an effect on their use of self-harm. While the above would fit into a range of frames of reference, the exploration of thoughts, emotions and behaviour would fit most within a cognitive behavioural/dialectical behavioural model.

Vignette 2: Group Intervention

A community group for people who identify that relationships are difficult is held on a weekly basis. The group members have had experience of losing relationships they care about and hearing that people around them get frustrated and that it is hard to help them. These difficulties get in the way of things they would like to do, which include work, education and activities for pleasure, but also make it hard to connect with others.

The occupational therapist meets with the group and helps them decide on an activity they would all like (or at least tolerate) being part of. The occupational therapist bears in mind that it is useful to keep as much power with the group as possible and resist the urge to fill any silences or give direction. The group members eventually decide on cooking a meal together. Food is bought collaboratively, the meal prepared and the group members eat together. Once the task is completed, the group meets to reflect on the experience. If there is quiet, the occupational therapist might share some of their observations or experiences of the task. There is encouragement to hear different perspectives and to be curious about others. The activity of cooking is used to enable a discussion that can include a variety of themes. It might touch on managing the frustration of people cooking something that was not their personal choice or resentment that someone felt their task was more menial. Some people might have been more involved, whilst others may have been quiet and did not contribute. Ideally, the occupational therapist will say as little as possible, but may help people to articulate their experience in ways others can hear and reflect on.

The goal of the task was to provide a communal experience. The goal of the discussion is to help people put their experiences into words, to explore behaviour with peers, to compare their perception of others' experiences with their perceptions, and to highlight the thoughts, emotions and actions experienced in this interaction, which will also be experienced in other interactions in the wider world. The activity was chosen because that is what the group agreed to do. It could have been anything, including doing nothing. Helping people to articulate their experiences and then helping others articulate their experience of hearing them can be difficult work. Humans in general find this level of introspection difficult. While the therapist needs to be able to notice their own feelings and choose how to act, there will inevitably be conflict, anger and shame experienced by themselves and the group. The work is to help people experience the emotions that they feel and act on in other situations, in a way that allows them to be discussed and reflected on.

In all of our work, it has been the words of peers that have led to the greatest change and the validation of peers that has brought the most comfort.

SENSORY INTEGRATION AS PART OF OCCUPATIONAL THERAPY INTERVENTION

Occupational therapists find the theoretical framework of sensory integration useful when working with traumatised people, many of whom go on to receive a 'personality disorder' diagnosis. Sensory integration supports 'becoming', underpinning the development of skills and abilities, interpersonal connection and self-regulation (Ayres 2005). It is required for 'doing', supporting real-time feedforward planning and providing real-time feedback by which we fine-tune our responses to be maximally effective. Registration and perception of well-integrated sensory inputs while participating in activities enhances our 'being' in the world, connecting us via our interactions with others, supporting habits, routines, roles and place within our community and creating our 'belonging'. In essence, the ability to use and benefit from sensory inputs is essential to participation, from the idea of what to do, planning it and getting it done.

Sensory integration facilitates participation during play, learning and development in school. Adverse childhood experiences alter responses to sensation and interfere with developing early safe relationships, safety and trust within the person's body and perception of the world and others. Feelings, emotions, language, cognition, development, learning, movement and actions, connection and participation are compromised when trauma interferes with early development. Occupational therapists can consider if sensory integration and processing differences resulting from intra-uterine and/or adverse childhood events (ACEs) impact sensory registration, perception and sensory reactivity, affecting arousal (alertness), regulation and praxis. Where sensory integration and processing differences are indicated, therapy is beneficial.

Research has explored sensory integration as a model of practice for clients diagnosed with BPD and other mental health distress (Brown *et al.* 2006; Bundy *et al.* 2020). Evidence supports the idea that ACEs may adversely impact sensory integration and processing and the development of neural synchrony leading to emotional dysregulation. In childhood, medial prefrontal cortex (MPFC) lesions may impair regulation and accurate interpretation of emotion, and adults with BPD have altered frontal networks and MPFC function. Research recognises deficits in prefrontal activation for those diagnosed with early trauma and BPD. Neuroimaging provides more information recognising that BPD has a significant 'neurosensory' component. Electrophysiological and neuropsychological studies show parietal lobe difficulties in processing information, distinguishing between relevant tasks and irrelevant information. The MPFC provides top-down feedback for intentional behaviour and motivation, generating multiple options about the outcomes of particular choices.

SUPERVISION

Having a space for the therapist to be able to think about their work is essential in all forms of therapy. It is especially important when staff who get their self-worth from being helpful meet people who believe others cannot be trusted. We have described environments where even the best clinicians may feel anger, resentment, hatred, despair and/or fear about themselves, their colleagues and their patients. We encourage the patients to have help to work on their difficulties and we should role model that for ourselves. Good supervision will help us to remain empathic. It can challenge us when we have more negative ideas about people than there is evidence for. It can help us hold back when we are taking all power and autonomy away from those for whom we care. We have had supervision experiences that help us to stay effective and experiences that have validated our current emotional states without challenge. The former has been uncomfortable but allowed us to stay effective; the latter has been comforting while allowing us to stop mentalising about our patients. As in therapy, there is a need for validation and challenge, but both are essential in this work. We would recommend supervision with an intensity that reflects the intensity of the work. Thinking spaces with the MDT staff are also useful to address team splitting and can be something that occupational therapists push for as an adaption to the environment that allows staff to function effectively.

RESEARCH

Building the evidence base for occupational therapy in this area is difficult. We are not a manualised intervention and our intervention can (and should) be different for different clients and therapists. When we measure an intervention, are we measuring the effectiveness of that activity? Of doing a group regardless of its content? Of the skill of that particular therapist? Of the impact of having occupational therapists employed in general? Fortunately, there are occupational therapists developing evidence in this area (Connell 2015). There are structured programmes such as Recovery Through Activity (Parkinson 2017) and MOTION (Birken & Harper 2017) that have a strong occupational therapy component and can be researched more to build the evidence for our profession in this area, but more needs to be done. It would be unthinkable to staff a ward without nurses, but a ward can open without an occupational therapist. In the United Kingdom, the National Collaborating Centre for Health and Clinical Excellence asked professionals to contribute to updating their national guidelines around self-harm. They named almost every profession working in mental health except occupational therapists. To ensure that occupational therapists are seen as essential rather than accessories in this area, we would encourage occupational therapists and occupational therapy departments to link in with the research departments of their employer or local university. We may need to get better at describing our worth, but we certainly need to get better at proving it.

CONCLUSION

The label of 'personality disorder' can lead to greater understanding and informed treatment; however, our experience is that too often, it is used as a slur that damages care rather than makes it accessible. The World Federation of Occupational Therapy has a code of ethics that states that 'Occupational therapists approach all persons receiving their services with respect and have regard for their unique situations' (WFOT 2016, p. 1). We will certainly be working outside of this code if we brand those we work with as attention-seeking manipulators. It even becomes dubious to work within systems where survivors of abuse are labelled as having disordered personalities. We see the 'personality disorder' diagnosis being given out in a way that does not fit with a meticulous consideration of history and criteria. Our experience is that what is called 'personality disorder' is a wide-ranging spectrum of difficulties that could include diagnoses such as post-traumatic stress disorder, complex post-traumatic stress disorder, autistic spectrum disorder, attention deficit hyperactivity disorder and others. Due to the murky nature of the diagnosis, it is essential that occupational therapists maintain their focus on function as there

will be higher pressure than normal to ascribe the things people do to pathology rather than them having value and meaning. The social environment is particularly powerful around people who receive this label; thus, occupational therapists need a heightened curiosity and awareness of how the environment assists or (more likely) inhibits functioning. We would encourage occupational therapists to be particularly vigilant around terms such as manipulative, attention seeking or sabotaging as teams that understand people in this way are unlikely to be the helpful, compassionate practitioners they wish to be.

It is highly likely that the person who has the label of 'personality disorder' will have lived through some traumatic experiences. Even if it is not obvious major trauma, we can wonder or think with people about their experiences in relationships, family systems and wider society, and reflect on what they have learned from these experiences. We can explain people's difficulties without labelling them as 'disordered' and adding the subsequent stigma. These difficulties will impact their relationships. Remembering their history will help the occupational therapist to remain empathic, enabling them to expect difficulties in the relationship and respond effectively.

With those considerations in mind, the process of occupational therapy is exactly the same as it is for any client – assessment, intervention and evaluation, and through being client-centred, helping the individual and changing the environment. Occupational therapists are able to help a range of people who have difficulties in their lives. Our opinion is that the effectiveness of the work is hindered by helping people see themselves as having a disordered personality. This is an area of work where we may have been reticent to show how helpful we can be, and perhaps where we have replicated some of the more stigmatising ideas around these clients. We cannot carry on in this way. When the next edition of this chapter is written, we hope that the evidence base for occupational therapy has expanded and that we see ourselves, and are seen by others, as essential. There are a group of people who live with difficulties in what they want and need to do, difficulties with skills they have and an environment that harms them. We as occupational therapists are well placed to help these people. Let's do it.

ACKNOWLEDGEMENTS

This chapter was written with the advice and inspiration of a range of people. Without them, it would not have been written by us. We extend particular thanks to Kath Smith of ASI WISE, Dr Catriona Connell of the University of Stirling, Occupational Therapist Hattie Porter, Occupational Therapy Lecturers Alice Hortop of the University of the West of England, Ruth Hawley of the University of Derby, Kirsten Barnicot, lecturer in Mental Health at City University, London, Loraine Dryden Counselling Psychologist, Dave Atkinson psychotherapist, Nurses Sameena Akram, Dr Neil Gordon and David Willetts, Lived Experience Pioneer Kath Lovell, Occupational Therapist Leslie Kynman and Occupational Therapist Ann Nott.

REFERENCES

American Psychiatric Association (APA) (1994) *Diagnostic and Statistical Manual of Mental Disorders DSM-IV*. American Psychiatric Association, Washington, DC.

American Psychiatric Association (APA) (2022). *Diagnostic and Statistical Manual of Mental Disorders, Fifth Edition* (DSM-5-TR). American Psychiatric Association, Washington, DC.

Ayres, A.J. (2005) *Sensory Integration and the Child: Understanding Hidden Sensory Challenges*. Western Psychological Services, Torrance, California.

Bennett, S. & Bennett, J.W. (2000) The process of evidence-based practice in occupational therapy: informing clinical decisions. *Australian Occupational Therapy Journal*, **47**, 171–180.

Berrigan, H. (2021). Living with borderline personality disorder. *Mental Health Practice* **24(4)**, 8–9.

Birken, M. & Harper, S. (2017) Experiences of people with a personality disorder or mood disorder regarding carrying out daily activities following discharge from hospital. *British Journal of Occupational Therapy*, **80(7)**, 409–416. https://doi.org/10.1177/0308022617697995

Bornstein, R.F. (2005) *The Dependent Patient: A Practitioner's Guide*. American Psychological Association, Washington, DC. https://doi.org/10.1037/11085-000

Bryant, W., Fieldhouse, J., Plastow, N. (eds) (2022). Creeks Occupational Therapy and Mental Health 6th edn. Elsevier Health Sciences, London.

Brown, S., Shankar, R., Smith, K., Turner, A. & Wyndham-Smith, T. (2006) Sensory processing disorder in mental health. *Occupational Therapy News*, **14(5)**, 28–29.

Bundy, A.C., Lane, S., Murray, E.A. & Fisher, A.G. (2020) *Sensory Integration: Theory and Practice*. F.A. Davis, Philadelphia.

Connell, C. (2015) An integrated case formulation approach in forensic practice: the contribution of occupational therapy to risk assessment and formulation. *Journal of Forensic Psychiatry and Psychology*, **26(1)**, 94–106. https://doi.org/10.1080/14789949.2014.981566

Gallaher, P. (2022) *Independent*. https://inews.co.uk/news/health/johnny-depp-amber-heard-court-case-damage-people-personality-disorders-expert-1606620 (accessed 24 March 2024)

Harding, K. (2020) Enhancing the occupational therapy role around 'personality disorder' and self-harm. *British Journal of Occupational Therapy*, **83(9)**, 547–548. https://doi.org/10.1177/0308022620947642

Harding, K., Poole, R. & Robinson, C.A. (2020) The outsourcing of risk: out of area placements for those diagnosed with personality disorder in the UK. *Lancet Psychiatry*, **7(9)**, 730–731.

Kim, Y.-R. & Tyrer, P. (2010) Controversies surrounding classification of personality disorder. *Psychiatry Investigation*, **7**, 1–8.

Klein, P., Fairweather, A.K. & Lawn S. (2022) Structural stigma and its impact on healthcare for borderline personality disorder: a scoping review. *International Journal of Mental Health Systems*, **16(1)**, 48. https://doi.org/10.1186/s13033-022-00558-3

Kielhofner, G. (2008) *Model of Human Occupation: Theory and Application*, 4th edn. Lippencott Williams & Wilkins, Philadelphia.

Lamb, N., Sibbald S & Stirzacker A (2018) *"Shining lights in dark corners of people's lives"*. The consensus statement for people with complex mental health difficulties who are diagnosed with a personality disorder. https://www.mind.org.uk/media/21163353/consensus-statement-final.pdf (accessed 24 March 2024)

Lewis, G. & Appleby, L. (1988) Personality disorder: the patients psychiatrists dislike. *British Journal of Psychiatry*, **153**, 44–9.

Linehan, M. (1993) *Cognitive-behavioural Treatment of Borderline Personality Disorder*. Guilford Press, New York.

MacLeod, C. & Mathews, A. (2012) Cognitive bias modification approaches to anxiety. *Annual Review of Clinical Psychology*, **8**, 189-217.

Main, T.F. (1957) The ailment. *British Journal of Medical Psychology* **30(3)**, 129–45

NICE (2022) *Self-harm: assessment, management and preventing recurrence*. www.nice.org.uk/guidance/ng225 (accessed 24 March 2024)

Norcross, J.C. & Lambert, M.J. (2019) *Psychotherapy Relationships that Work: Vol. 1. Evidence-based Therapist Contributions*, 3rd edn. Oxford University Press, Oxford.

Oxford Languages (n.d.) *Validation*. https://www.google.com/search?q=validation+definition&oq=validation+definition&aqs=chrome.69i57j0i512l9.4942j1j4&sourceid=chrome&ie=UTF-8 (accessed on 17 September 2023)

Parkinson, S. (2017) *Recovery through Activity*, 1st edn. Taylor and Francis, London. https://www.perlego.com/book/1572611/recovery-through-activity-pdf (accessed on 14 October 2022)

Rodriguez-Seijas, C., Morgan, T.A. & Zimmerman, M. (2021) A population-based examination of criterion-level disparities in the diagnosis of borderline personality disorder among sexual minority adults. *Assessment*, **28(4)**, 1,097–1,109. https://doi.org/10.1177/1073191121991922

Shaw, C. & Proctor, G. (2005). I. Women at the margins: a critique of the diagnosis of borderline personality disorder. *Feminism & Psychology*, **15(4)**, 483–490. https://doi.org/10.1177/0959-353505057620

Stubbe, D.E. (2018). The therapeutic alliance: the fundamental element of psychotherapy. *Focus*, **16(4)**, 402–403. https://doi.org/10.1176/appi.focus.20180022

Swales, M.A. (2022) Personality disorder diagnoses in ICD-11: transforming conceptualisations and practice. *Clinical Psychology in Europe*, **4**, 1–18. https://doi.org/10.32872/cpe.9635

Twinley, R. (2013) The dark side of occupation: a concept for consideration. *Australian Occupational Therapy Journal*, **60(4)**, 301–303. https://doi.org/10.1111/1440-1630

Twinley, R. (2021) *Illuminating the Dark Side of Occupation: International Perspectives from Occupational Therapy and Occupational Science*. Routledge, London.

Tyrer, P., Mulder, R., Kim, Y.-R. & Crawford, M.J. (2019) The development of the ICD-11 classification of personality disorders: an amalgam of science, pragmatism, and politics. *Annual Review of Clinical Psychology*, **15**, 481–502. https://doi.org/10.1146/annurev-clinpsy-050718-095736

Veale, D., Robins, E., Thomson, A.B. & Gilbert, P. (2023) No safety without emotional safety. *Lancet Psychiatry*, **10(1)**, 65–70. https://doi.org/10.1016/S2215-0366(22)00373-X

Warrender, D., Bain, H., Murray, I. & Kennedy, C. (2021) Perspectives of crisis intervention for people diagnosed with "borderline personality disorder": an integrative review. *Journal of Psychiatric and Mental Health Nursing*, **28(2)**, 208–236. https://doi.org/10.1111/jpm.12637

World Federation of Occupational Therapists (2016) *Code of ethics*. https://wfot.org/resources/code-of-ethics (accessed on 16 July 2023)

Yen, S., Shea, M., Battle, C. *et al* (2002) Traumatic exposure and post-traumatic stress disorder in borderline, schizotypal, avoidant, and obsessive-compulsive personality disorders: findings from the collaborative longitudinal personality disorders study. *The Journal of Nervous and Mental Disease*, **190(8)**, 510–518.

The Occupational Therapy Approach to the Management of Schizophrenia Spectrum and Other Psychotic Disorders

CHAPTER 27

Kobela Veronica Ramodike[1], Iesrafeel Abbas[2] and Rosemary Crouch[3]

[1]School of Health Care Sciences, Faculty of Health Sciences, Sefako Makgatho Health Sciences University, Pretoria, South Africa
[2]Health and Rehabilitation Sciences, Faculty of Health Sciences, University of Cape Town, Cape Town, South Africa
[3]School of Therapeutic Sciences, Faculty of Health Sciences, University of the Witwatersrand, Johannesburg, South Africa

KEY LEARNING POINTS

- Understanding schizophrenia and its occupational implications.

- Multidisciplinary treatment approach for individuals living with schizophrenia.

- Theories underpinning the occupational therapy approach to schizophrenia.

- Management of individuals living with schizophrenia, including key points of occupational therapy intervention for:

  ◦ Acute care (short term)
  ◦ Chronic care (medium and long term)
  ◦ Community integration

INTRODUCTION

Schizophrenia spectrum and other psychotic disorders includes schizophrenia, other psychotic disorders such as schizophreniform, schizoaffective, delusional disorder, brief psychotic disorder, substance/medication-induced psychotic disorder, psychotic disorder due to another medical condition, catatonic disorder and schizotypal (personality) disorders (American Psychiatric Association [APA] 2022). The clinical presentation of this group of disorders comprises signs and symptoms such as delusions, hallucinations, disorganised thinking, grossly disorganized or abnormal behaviour, changes in cognition and negative symptoms (Ruiz 2014; APA 2022).

Schizophrenia is also described as a disorder that affects the socio-occupational functioning abilities of individuals in their daily life activities, including their roles within self-care, work, play and interpersonal relationships (Abbas & Soeker 2020).

The disorder is also described as a 'frightening illness in which intrusive "voices" (auditory hallucinations) torment the sufferer with abusive or derogatory comments, and ideas weaved together to form false beliefs (delusions), which colonise the mind' (Morrison & Murray 2012, p. 980). It is considered to be one of the most insidious, slowly progressive and disabling mental disorders that produce severe disability during the potentially most creative and productive years of life (Ruiz 2014). Therefore, schizophrenia has significant consequences on an individual's mental health status, with cognitive deficits and psychotic symptoms firmly linked to occupational and social functional impairment and performance deficits (APA 2022). This contributes to individuals living with schizophrenia having difficulty in interpreting situations and making sense of experiences; losing contact with family, friends and caregivers; becoming isolated and withdrawn; and experiencing immense challenges in engaging optimally within their respective roles (Foruzandeh & Parvin 2013).

Crouch and Alers Occupational Therapy in Psychiatry and Mental Health, Sixth Edition.
Edited by Rosemary Crouch, Tania Buys, Enos Morankoana Ramano, Matty van Niekerk and Lisa Wegner.
© 2025 John Wiley & Sons Ltd. Published 2025 by John Wiley & Sons Ltd.

The Diagnostic and Statistical Manual of Mental Disorders, fifth edition (DSM-5-TR, APA 2022) explains that most individuals with schizophrenia experience dysfunction in several areas of daily functioning, such as school or work, interpersonal relationships and self-care. Functional ability is also described as one of the diagnostic criteria for schizophrenia (Criteria B).

In recent years, the occupational functioning of individuals living with schizophrenia has become a target for innovative research and interventions. For this reason, healthcare and psychosocial rehabilitation for schizophrenia have greatly improved, with the effects of medication, for example, being less disabling on the functioning of these individuals. Of interest to the occupational therapist during intervention is the impact of negative symptoms such as diminished emotional expressions, asociality and avolition in the functioning of individuals with schizophrenia. The DSM-5-TR (APA 2022) indicates that avolition may lead to a decrease in motivation to initiate purposeful activities, with the individual also showing a lack of interest in participation in work and social activities. The individual's ability to experience pleasure from positive stimuli may lead to the reduction in their ability to function optimally in leisure and again in social participation (APA 2022).

Cultural and socioeconomic factors are some of the issues that need to be considered when treating individuals with schizophrenia. It is of utmost importance for clinicians to be culturally sensitive when assessing and treating these individuals as some of the behaviours that may appear abnormal may be acceptable in other cultures. Examples are of delusions that may form part of belief in witchcraft. Hallucinations may be interpreted as part appropriate religious content (APA 2022). On the other hand, factors such as the stigma of schizophrenia still exist globally and are particularly influential in underdeveloped and previously disadvantaged communities, thus impacting the rehabilitation of individuals living with schizophrenia and making their integration into communities challenging (Lesunyane 2010). Individuals with schizophrenia and their families/caregivers continue to suffer from 'social ostracism' due to ignorance and lack of understanding of the illness by communities and the society at large (Ruiz 2014).

To continue improving the functioning and prognosis of individuals living with schizophrenia in all areas of occupational performance, this chapter provides occupational therapists and occupational therapy students with a synopsis of schizophrenia as an illness, the occupational implications of schizophrenia and an overview of the occupational therapy process for schizophrenia and other psychotic disorders.

EPIDEMIOLOGY OF SCHIZOPHRENIA

The World Health Organisation (WHO) indicates that almost 24 million individuals are affected by schizophrenia globally, with the rate being 1 in 222 among adults. The exact cause of schizophrenia is not yet fully understood; however, there are indications that several factors may contribute to the diagnosis of schizophrenia. Ruiz (2014) indicates that the prevalence of schizophrenia is approximately 0.3–0.7%, although this may differ depending on race, ethnicity and country of origin.

Some aspects in foetal life stage (such as maternal infection, birth complications such as hypoxia, greater paternal age, maternal infections, malnutrition, stress and anxiety) may be accountable for a small percentage of incidences of schizophrenia. In addition, the rate of schizophrenia is influenced by environmental factors such as the exposure to social disadvantage and injustice, economically poor circumstances and trauma. Similarly, exposure to substances (such as cannabis and alcohol) and genetic interplay further contribute to the predisposition of schizophrenia, with the onset of the distinctive symptoms of schizophrenia typically developing in the early to mid-20s for males and late 20s for females – where the early age of onset is considered a predictor for poor prognosis. On the other hand, care should be taken that the diagnosis of schizophrenia is not based solely on mental status examination, but factors such as the history, educational level, intellectual ability, cultural and subcultural membership are also of importance (Ruiz 2014; APA 2022).

The DSM-5-TR (APA 2022) and Ruiz (2014) state that to diagnose schizophrenia, the manifestation of a minimum of one month of two or more of the following distinctive (active) symptoms is required: hallucinations, delusions, disorganised speech, catatonic or disorganised behaviour and negative symptoms. In addition, this manifestation should cause occupational and/or social dysfunction in one or more of the following areas of functioning (for a period of at least six months): self-care, work, activities of daily livings (ADLs) and interpersonal relationships. It is worthy to note that the diagnostic criteria for subtypes of schizophrenia (i.e. paranoid, disorganised, catatonic, etc.) has been omitted in DSM-5-TR (APA 2022).

To fully understand the occupational implications of schizophrenia and the focus of occupational therapy intervention, some of the core features of schizophrenia as discussed in the DSM-5-TR are highlighted below (Ruiz 2014; APA 2022).

Schizophrenia is primarily a disorganisation of thinking which can result in grossly disorganised behaviour, including inappropriate sexual behaviour, argumentativeness and an overall deterioration of functioning in all occupations, including skills in ADL such as unusual dress and a lack of hygiene.

- Positive symptoms of schizophrenia include delusions, hallucinations, disorganised thinking and grossly disorganised or abnormal behaviour (including catatonia).

- Negative symptoms of schizophrenia include reduced emotional expression, alogia, anhedonia, asociality and avolition.

- Perceptual challenges such as hallucinations are often 'responsible for profound dysfunction in all aspects of daily life. Such patients find it difficult to engage in meaningful tasks or relationships. For some patients, hallucinations are problematic only in certain situations or at specific times, such as when they are alone or in a stressful situation' (Kelkar 2002, p. 1).

- Whilst most of the hallucinations reported are auditory, they may also be olfactory, visual, gustatory and tactile.

- Abnormalities of psychomotor activity, for example, pacing, rocking and psychomotor retardation. There are often motor abnormalities such as grimacing and posturing, odd mannerisms and stereotyped behaviour.

- Impairment in concentration, attention and memory.

- Poor psychosocial functioning.

- Depersonalisation and derealisation.

- Somatic concerns such as digestive or weight challenges.

- Anxieties and phobias.

- Non-compliance with medication.

- *Suicide*: 5–6% of people living with schizophrenia die by suicide, with 20% attempting suicide on more than one occasion and many more having command hallucinations to cause harm, with the risk being high in young males than females (Ruiz 2014; APA 2022).

In a comparison of the DSM-5-TR and the International Classification of Diseases, Eleventh Revision (ICD-11) (Valle 2020), it is important for occupational therapists to note that while impaired function is a diagnostic criterion of schizophrenia in DSM-5-TR, it is not considered in ICD-11. The ICD-11 argues that 'functional deficits do not occur in all people with schizophrenia and are therefore not specific to the disorder'. The ICD-11 furthermore points out that 'mental disorders should be defined based on their symptoms and not in relation to activity limitations'. On the other hand, the DSM-5-TR uses a criterion of 'clinical significance of damage' as a threshold to identify mental disorders, and thus maintaining its use of functional impairment as a diagnostic criterion. The improvement of functional abilities of individuals living with schizophrenia and their participation in occupations are some of the aims and goals of treatment by occupational therapists during intervention.

MULTIDISCIPLINARY TREATMENT APPROACH TO SCHIZOPHRENIA

Ruiz (2014) reveals that hospitalization of individuals with schizophrenia is still a necessity despite the advanced use of antipsychotic drugs. These patients occupy 50% of mental health beds and the possibility of their readmission after two years of being discharged varies between 40 and 60%. These authors indicate that some of the reasons for hospitalization include diagnostic purposes, stabilization of medication, inappropriate behaviour, and functional impairments such as the inability to take care of oneself. Medication in the form of a new generation of neuroleptics makes it possible to alleviate the negative symptoms of schizophrenia and in doing so opens the door for the person with this illness to rehabilitation. With the use of medication and a psychosocial approach in the treatment of schizophrenia, many of those afflicted can live as normal a life as possible in the community. It is also important to note that it is during this period of hospitalisation that therapists should verify the patient's relationships and support system within the community where they live, which guides the multidisciplinary rehabilitation and discharge plans.

Three phases of treatment in schizophrenia are discussed by Ruiz (2014) namely the treatment in the acute psychotic phase, the stabilisation and the maintenance phase. The goal in the acute treatment phase is to alleviate the acute psychotic symptoms with which the patients with schizophrenia may present. During the phase of stabilisation and maintenance, patients are said to be in a remission stage with minimal psychotic symptoms, with the goal of the multidisciplinary team being to prevent a relapse and assist the patients to improve their level of functioning. For the occupational therapist, treatment may include involving the patient in educational and vocational programmes where possible to facilitate their return to work including participation in roles and effective re-integration into their communities.

Concurring with occupational therapy intervention, Ruiz (2014) states that it is during the phase of stabilisation and maintenance that the treatment plans should be directed towards the functional abilities of the patients, including self-care, employment, social relationships as well as establishing the patient's available aftercare resources. This is because these patients may still need formal or informal daily living support due to the chronic nature of the illness (APA 2022). With the advances in psychotropic medicine, there has been a trend internationally to move individuals living with chronic schizophrenia out of institutions into the community. In other countries, primary healthcare clinics are administering chronic medicines from their clinics, with some clinics doing home-based follow-ups as part of providing additional support and ensuring medication compliance. Individuals living with schizophrenia are followed up on a regular basis in this manner; however, some individuals do slip through the system and may experience relapse.

Treatment can be hospital-based or community-based depending on the severity of the first episode and on the treatment facilities available within communities. Wherever treatment takes place, occupational therapy is a vital part of the holistic approach to rehabilitation. Support groups can also be an effective medium to educate the community about schizophrenia as an illness.

A recent scoping review (Rocamora-Montenegro *et al.* 2021) indicates that occupational therapy is one of the non-pharmacological interventions, using meaningful activities, which can contribute to improvements in individuals living with severe mental illness, including schizophrenia. The study shows that four interventions are used most often, that is psychosocial intervention, followed by psychoeducation, cognitive intervention and exercise being the least used. The main objectives for psychosocial intervention were to improve symptoms of the disorder, lessen occupational imbalance and facilitate social and work reintegration. Correspondingly, psychosocial interventions resulted in improvements in the symptoms, occupational balance and socio-occupational reintegration of the patients. Psychoeducation aimed to improve the clients' ability to manage the disease and improve social abilities such as the ability to acquire a skill such as reading. Cognitive intervention aimed to improve cognitive functions and processing strategies. Exercise intervention was done by the multidisciplinary team with the aim of compensating for the patients' cognitive impairment. The principal disorder treated using these interventions was schizophrenia, and this was mainly done in group sessions (Rocamora-Montenegro et al. 2021).

OCCUPATIONAL THERAPY THEORIES AND SCHIZOPHRENIA

Considering the aforementioned symptoms of schizophrenia, the various theoretical models of occupational performance and engagement come to mind, which are the Person-Environment-Occupation Performance Model (Christiansen 2005), Model of Human Occupation (Kielhofner 2002) and the Canadian Occupational Performance Measure (COPM) (Law et al. 1998). These models contribute to occupational therapists' ability to focus on cognitive skills and their impact on functioning of individuals living with schizophrenia. Within these models, cognition is seen as a performance component or skill which contributes, along with many other performance components, to a person's ability to function competently, and to their own satisfaction, in a given occupational area (Creek 2002).

In addition to supporting treatment of performance components (or client factors) and skills such as cognition, theoretical models allow occupational therapists to facilitate clients with schizophrenia's participation in purposeful activities, which is the cornerstone and the major tool of intervention in occupational therapy. An individual with schizophrenia may have an impaired capacity for the performance of purposeful activity due to changes in cognitive functioning (Creek 1998). These changes '. . . decrease the ability to interpret and make sense of experiences that may result in a sense of detachment and ability to reflect, which is part of the occupational engagement process' (Bejerholm & Eklund 2007, p. 22). Models such as the Person-Environment-Occupational Performance Model (Law et al. 1996) also identify those factors contributing to self-identity which might be missing and thereby influence both well-being and occupational performance.

Linking to theories on the performance of purposeful activity is the research undertaken by a South African occupational therapist, Vona du Toit. She intimated that creative capacity varies from one individual to another and is influenced by factors such as intelligence, personality structure, mental health, environmental factors and security (Van der Reyden et al. 2019). The Vona du Toit Model of Creative Ability (VdTMoCA) describes volition as being central to creative theory, and this is pivotal in the illness of schizophrenia. The Model describes volition as motivation and action. The motivational component represents the energy source for occupational behaviour, and this motivation governs action. It is known that one of the central aspects of schizophrenia is loss of volition. This is the link and the critical axis at which change can occur through occupational therapy intervention. The Activity Participation Outcome Measure (APOM) has been designed in empirical research and is a reliable outcomes measurement tool emanating from the VdTMoCA (Casteleijn 2010; Casteleijn & Graham 2012) and is widely used in occupational therapy in mental health settings in South Africa.

Snowdon et al. (2002, cited in Creek 2002, p. 337) discuss the Stress-Vulnerability Model in detail in which it is suggested that 'current research is investigating a number of areas which may be indicated in the aetiology of schizophrenia'. These authors suggest that there is a vulnerability which predisposes schizophrenia that is environmentally based, like life stressors inherent in factors such as changing roles, poor coping mechanisms and stressed family relationships. See the 'Secondary Psychosocial Disabilities Model' (Snowdon et al. 2002, cited in Creek 2002, p. 338). The authors are attempting to link the psychopathology and clinical features of schizophrenia with the theory and practice of occupational therapy to provide the best possible treatment for individuals living with this illness. They conclude that 'the validity of the stress-vulnerability model continues to be strengthened as clinical evidence is amassed to support its explanation of the phenomenon of schizophrenia' (Snowdon et al. 2002, cited in Creek 2002, p. 339).

Sensory integration as a treatment for sensory modulation (SM) disorders in psychiatric illnesses has been practiced by occupational therapists for more than two decades. A systematic review conducted by Machingura et al. (2018) aimed to determine the effectiveness of sensory integration in treating SM disorders in adults with schizophrenia. The review established that SM interventions have been subjectively reported as having positive outcomes; however, that sensory integration as an intervention for SM is still evolving and that many gaps in knowledge continue to exist.

THE OCCUPATIONAL THERAPY PROCESS

Psychosocial occupational therapy is concerned with helping individuals living with schizophrenia to recover. It is also about the individual becoming occupied with experiences of events that are real, instead of being occupied with their chaotic thoughts and delusions. (Bejerholm & Eklund 2007). Purposeful activity which involves the individual living with schizophrenia in occupational engagements is a central part of occupational therapy intervention.

Several frames of references are available for the occupational therapist to use during intervention. According to Bryant et al. (2014), some of the frames of reference available for use by occupational therapist working in mental health include the Psychodynamic Frame of Reference (occupational therapy, process and understanding of interpersonal relations), occupational behaviour (Model of Human Occupation, MOHO), cognitive behavioural (cognitive therapy), occupational performance (Canadian Model of Occupational Performance and Engagement, CMOP-E), the Recovery Model and other rehabilitative approaches.

- As with all other interventions with their clients, occupational therapists follow the occupational therapy process during intervention with individuals living with schizophrenia. The occupational therapy process is used during intervention in the acute, medium term and long term, as well as during rehabilitation in the community. The occupational therapy process includes the evaluation (information gathering, the initial assessment), intervention (planning, implementation, review) and outcomes (measurement and discharge planning) (Bryant et al. 2014; AOTA 2020; Boop *et al.* 2020).

EVALUATION

All interventions by occupational therapists are based on thorough assessment methods. Prior to their commencement with intervention, occupational therapists perform an evaluation of each client to establish their needs. Bryant et al. (2014) indicates the need for a thorough assessment of all individuals to evaluate their performance and participation in different occupations, and the development and disruption of normal development. This as with all mental health care users (MHCUs), is also seen as applicable to individuals living with schizophrenia. The appropriate assessment methods for individuals living with schizophrenia (Bryant et al., 2014) include interviews, observation, review of records, projective techniques, tests and collaboration with caregivers. Occupational therapists are equipped with skills to use both standardised and non-standardised assessment methods during the evaluation process.

The aforementioned scoping review on occupational therapy interventions for adults with severe mental illness, including schizophrenia, also made findings about the use of assessment tools. The study revealed that the Positive and Negative Symptoms Scale (PANSS) was the most used measurement instrument for symptoms of the disease, while for the executive functions, the Brief Assessment of Cognition in Schizophrenia was among the tests used. Psychosocial functioning measurement instruments such as the Global Assessment of Functioning, the Personal and Social Performance or the Social Functioning Scale and quality of life such as the 36-Item Short-Form Health Survey (SF-36) questionnaire were also used (Rocamora-Montenegro *et al.* 2021).

Several other standardised assessment methods are available for use by occupational therapists. Some of the more frequently used methods include:

- The COPM (2019), a client-centred assessment of functioning – it evaluates the individual's changes in daily life participation, including satisfaction over a period.

- Assessment of ADL of Personal Life Skills (PLS): The Milwaukee Evaluation of Daily Living Skills (MEDLS):

Developed to provide a behavioural measure of the abilities of persons with long-term mental illness to do basic and complex activities of daily living (Leonardelli 1998). The Scorable Self-Care Evaluation (SCORE) (Clarke & Peters 1994) and the Klein–Bell Activity of Daily Living Scale (B–K Scale): A measure for independence in basic activities of daily living in six sub-dimensions, namely mobility, emergency communication, dressing, elimination, bathing/hygiene and eating (Klein & Bell 1979).

- ADL and some components of performance and cognitive ability: The Bay Area Functional Performance Evaluation (BaFPE): developed to measure the client's functioning task-oriented and social interactional settings (Bloomer & Williams 1986).

- Leisure and Activity Configuration (Mosey 1973): Activity Card Sort (Baum & Edwards 2001).

- Assessment of Motor and Process Skills (AMPS): An observational assessment that measures the performance quality of tasks related to activities of daily living in a natural environment (Fischer & Jones 2012).

- The Hospital Anxiety and Depression Scale (HADS): A self-assessment instrument developed to measure the depression and anxiety state of an individual (Zigmond & Snaith 1983).

- The APOM: An outcome measure for effectiveness and efficiency of the occupational therapy intervention programmes in mental health (Casteleijn 2010).

- The Functional Levels Outcome Measure (FLOM): Used to measure change in functioning after intervention (Zietsman 2011).

Non-standardised assessment methods include:

- Interviews

- Collateral information: from caregivers, friends, nursing staff, medical officers, psychologists, social workers, physiotherapists, dieticians, etc.

- Observations: within the ward, as the patients socialise, during mealtimes, during group therapy sessions etc.

- Observations during activity participation (as a means of assessment) in different occupations.

The occupational therapist uses the findings from the assessments to establish the individuals' treatment goals. These are used to guide the intervention process. The multidisciplinary team should plan intervention in consultation with the caregivers, and at a later stage with the community and employers where applicable (Boop *et al.* 2020). The initial involvement of all these stakeholders is thus of importance for a successful outcome of all clients, including individuals living with schizophrenia.

The VdTMoCA is one of the models that can be used during intervention to assess the individual's level of creative ability. Through the application of clinical reasoning during assessment, occupational therapists can establish the individual's level of creative ability. The use of the VdTMoCA can assist the therapist with further guidelines for intervention, including the individual's readiness to participate in occupational group therapy with the mentally ill clients. The guidelines are stipulated under each level of creative ability, and based on the individual's level of creative ability, activity requirements, structuring, presentation and handling principles as well as grading can be selected. Reference should also be made to the VdTMoCA for detailed assessment of the individual's level of creative ability, which will guide intervention in all phases of treatment of individuals living with schizophrenia (Van der Reyden *et al.* 2019).

SHORT-TERM HOSPITAL-BASED REHABILITATION/TREATMENT

Occupational therapists are part of the multidisciplinary team equipped to provide services to all individuals with schizophrenia and other psychotic disorders in different settings, including acute/short-term hospital-based rehabilitation, chronic/medium- and long-term care and community settings.

Even though most countries are striving to convert to community rehabilitation in psychiatry, there is still a place for the containing, acute and long-term care psychiatric units worldwide. This will remain a reality for a long time yet, until adequate community facilities are available to the affected countries. Individuals living with schizophrenia, if admitted (or committed by certification) to a hospital, are often in an acute, psychotic state and need to be hospitalised because they are a danger to themselves or others.

Short-term programmes in occupational therapy are focused on evaluating strengths, weaknesses, skills and impairments at this early stage. The occupational therapist is one of the key professionals in this process and, through skills of observation and assessment of the patient engaging in daily occupations, can contribute greatly to the diagnosis of individuals with psychotic disorders and the discharge plans. No actual rehabilitation takes place at this time, but the needs of patients must be individually assessed within the context of what they wish to do with their lives and their opportunities to fulfil this. The occupational therapy programme is usually focused on the individual patient's performance and participation in different occupations using purposeful activities. It would appear to the uninitiated and non-professionals that the purpose of this programme is to keep the patient occupied, but within these programmes the occupational performance of MHCUs can be accurately assessed by the occupational therapist whilst they are engaged in the activities. This in turn provides a vital contribution to the ongoing treatment by the multidisciplinary team. The goal of occupational therapy intervention is quality of life.

It will depend greatly on the circumstances of hospitalisation and the illness, how much the occupational therapist

will be involved in actual treatment or education about the condition at this stage, but planning must take place before the patient is discharged. It is the occupational therapy profession's belief that with the correct medication, a balanced lifestyle and support in the community, individuals living with schizophrenia can live a life of quality. It is during this acute phase, when the psychotic symptoms are under control, that the multidisciplinary team can instil hope in these patients and steer him/her towards this goal.

PRINCIPLES OF HANDLING THE PERSON WITH AN ACUTE EPISODE OF SCHIZOPHRENIA

During hospitalisation of the patient with schizophrenia, the occupational therapist is often confronted with bizarre, psychotic behaviour. The handling of the patient by the occupational therapist in a calm and consistent manner is important in bringing the patient in touch with reality:

- The patient must never be ridiculed or laughed at because of their bizarre ideas, delusions or hallucinations.

- Ideas, delusions and hallucinations must not be condoned or endorsed by the occupational therapist, and the patient should be gently reminded of reality. When psychotic thoughts and perceptions are present, the occupational therapist must not try to 'talk' the patient out of them. The best way to do this is to bring the patient back to reality by engagement in a concrete activity.

- Gently remind the patient of the time of day, date and orientation to place.

- Use touch and close proximity with care as this may become part of the delusional thought.

- Handle aggression calmly and try to channel it through the use of gross motor activities such as body movements and exercise.

- Gently correct unacceptable behaviour. Do not be punitive in approach.

OCCUPATIONAL THERAPY PROGRAMMES IN MEDIUM-TERM AND LONG-TERM HOSPITAL SETTINGS

An effective occupational therapy programme must contain '. . . elements of practicality, concrete problem-solving for everyday challenges, low-key socialisation and recreation, engagement of attainable tasks, and specific goal orientation' (Liberman *et al.* 2000, cited in Kaplan & Sadock 2000, p. 3227). Bejerholm and Eklund (2007) reveal the need to know about meaningful daily occupations of individuals with schizophrenia, which will assist the clients to set adequate life goals congruent with their abilities, interests and context.

OCCUPATIONAL THERAPY THERAPEUTIC GROUPS

Individuals living with schizophrenia are often difficult to treat in groups, particularly in the early stages of illness. This is because of their difficulty with occupational engagement. Bejerholm and Eklund (2007) describe the sense of detachment and the inability of the patient to reflect. These are factors which interfere with the socialisation process. It is therefore advisable to treat people living with schizophrenia individually at first or at least with their own activity within a group setting. In overcrowded hospitals as in many areas of the world, this may not be possible. If possible, it is best to gradually introduce them to group work. Finlay (2002, cited in Creek 2002, p. 249) states that 'In general, if a person's mental health problems are either created by or result in interpersonal difficulties, then a group offers the more relevant context in which to explore such difficulties, gain support and learn how best to cope'.

On the other hand, Crouch (2021) indicates that 'group work is the most economic and preferred method of intervention in mental illness'. The VdTMoCA has been identified as one of the occupational therapy models applicable for use in group work and occupational group therapy (Crouch 2021). Although some challenges may be encountered due to these individuals' inability to reflect during the acute phases, the use of the VdTMoCA can assist the therapist in grouping clients according to their creative ability levels, and applying the treatment principles to select, structure and handle groups for individuals living with schizophrenia. Crouch (2021) also indicates that the group leader is responsible for creating a group climate that facilitates the interaction of the members, supports and tends to the needs of individuals and the group as a whole. It is also the group leader's responsibility to select appropriate activities and structures which are suitable at the group member's level of creative ability (Crouch 2021).

Types of group work and occupational group therapy, depending on the individual's level of creative ability, may include:

- *Activities of daily living and instrumental activities of daily living:* Personal care groups and assistance in the family's daily tasks such as meal preparation, budgeting and child and home-management (where appropriate).

- Creative activity groups which should include hobby or leisure pursuits, crafts, stencilling and fabric painting, and learning a skill or developing an interest, particularly one which brings the patient into contact with other people and makes use of leisure time.

- *Sensory integration groups:* If there is no sensory integration programme, simple exercise groups, walks and sports, such as volleyball, are very important for physical fitness and health management.

- Social skills training groups which include communication skills training, when the psychotic features are diminished, are very important to counteract pervasive deficits in social functioning.

- Stress management and coping skills training. These groups are particularly relevant when there is the reintegration of the patient into the community.

The use of therapeutic groups where there is a high level of emotional involvement such as psychodrama is not suitable for these patients in the early stages of treatment due to the cognitive impairment but may be introduced when the patient's symptoms are fully controlled, and the level of creative participation is at active participation.

INDIVIDUAL SESSIONS

Individual sessions involving clients with schizophrenia in ADLs (personal hygiene and grooming), health management (personal care device management, physical activity) and Instrumental Activities of Daily Living (IADLs) (child rearing, meal preparation, home establishment and management) may be used as part of intervention to improve the patient's participation in daily activities.

Educational (formal and informal personal educational needs or interest exploration) and work (employment interest and pursuits, seeking and acquisition, job performance) assessment and rehabilitation are vitally important in returning the rehabilitated patient back to work and ensuring a balanced lifestyle across all areas of occupational performance.

Discharge planning and the plan to have continued care and support are the final and extremely important part of intervention. This is best done on an individual basis in consultation with the multidisciplinary team members and caregivers/family of the patient. As part of discharge planning, psychoeducation is used as a modality that significantly contributes to the management of the illness. The use of psychoeducation is further discussed below.

PSYCHOEDUCATION

Psychoeducation is essential for patients with schizophrenia and may make all the difference in an illness that is well managed. Psychoeducation intends to improve individuals living with schizophrenia and their caregivers' knowledge about schizophrenia as an illness (Hasan *et al.* 2015). The content of the psychoeducational intervention sessions often include topics related to general information about the epidemiology of schizophrenia, symptoms, medication management, communication skills and problem-solving skills for individuals living with schizophrenia and their caregivers. These sessions are often facilitated by an occupational therapist; however, other members of the multidisciplinary team are equipped to facilitate such sessions too, in relation to their discipline (Nasr & Kausar 2009). For example, topics such as 'understanding medication' are best presented by a psychiatrist who is an expert in this field, whilst psychosocial treatment strategies would be best presented by an occupational therapist.

These psychoeducation sessions can take place individually or in group spaces. However, caregivers often find it difficult to speak out and discuss the problems they encounter in the presence of the patient. In this instance, separate psychoeducational groups are best for patients and caregivers. Psychoeducation is also seen as an essential part of community integration.

COMMUNITY-BASED REHABILITATION FOR PERSONS WITH SCHIZOPHRENIA

Rehabilitation of the client with schizophrenia in the community is a collaborative, multidisciplinary effort. Health management is an important aspect of the holistic approach to rehabilitation, and compliance by the client in this respect must precede efforts in psychosocial rehabilitation. This is a team effort and must be addressed by every person in the rehabilitation team. Often, some of the positive symptoms of schizophrenia, such as hallucinations, remain for a long time. It has been found, however, that clients can function quite well despite this, and rehabilitation can proceed.

Today, community-based rehabilitation is recommended as the best alternative for the successful treatment of the individual living with schizophrenia. 'The goal of psychiatric rehabilitation is to teach skills and provide community support so that the individual with mental disabilities can function in the social, vocational, educational and familial roles with the least amount of supervision from the helping professionals' (Liberman et al. 2000, cited in Kaplan & Sadock 2000, p. 3218).

Rehabilitation is an essential component of the continuum of services necessary for persons served by the public sector (Sadock et al., 2015). A community-based rehabilitation programme is often an extension of the hospital programme, but some clients can join a community-based programme shortly after being diagnosed and placed on medication.

Various types of rehabilitation programmes exist in different parts of the world. Day programmes are offered by some hospitals and community centres, and in the United States, South Africa and Australia, the Life Skills/Fountain House Model of community service has proved to be very successful. In South Africa, Canada and other Western countries, occupational therapists in private and public practice can offer effective community-based programmes for individuals living with schizophrenia. Elpers (2000, cited in Kaplan & Sadock 2000, p. 3193) states that the fact that the person living with schizophrenia 'must be seen to exist in the community without being shunned or appearing bizarre, is essential to rehabilitation'.

What has come to light in community-based rehabilitation is that the individual living with schizophrenia requires a continuing, supportive and positive relationship with a suitable health professional/religious counsellor/caregiver. Often, the occupational therapist is in the position to provide this type of community care. The relationship between the occupational therapist and the client must be firm and trusting,

so that there is a possibility to correct the life skills of the client in a positive and frank way without lowering the client's self-esteem, thus building up confidence.

In a South African study, Abbas and Soeker (2020) demonstrated the effectiveness of the Model of Occupational Self-Efficacy (MOOSE) as a supported employment strategy for individuals living with schizophrenia. The use of the MOOSE was aimed at enhancing work skills and facilitating return to work. Client-centred practice, the presence of social support (from family, friends, colleagues and employers) and ongoing therapeutic support were found to be the most significant factors contributing to successful return to work experiences.

It is imperative to realise that clients require continuous rather than short-term efforts to achieve and maintain improved functioning. It is commonly understood that the cognitive influences on individuals living with schizophrenia reveal impairments in functional performance. Notably, occupational therapy is the profession well equipped to implement intervention that is focused on the rehabilitation of ADL, IADLs, social participation, leisure, work and/ education occupations for people living with schizophrenia, to enable them to function optimally within their communities. As stated by Reema et al., interventions focusing on independent living skills seem to lead to better outcomes for patients in addition to reducing burden on family and community. It is idealistic to believe that continuity of care can be the norm because it would mean that clients would have the same therapists or caregivers throughout their illness, which means their whole lives. In most cases, this is not possible, so handover to the next therapist or caregiver is necessary.

Wherever the rehabilitation takes place, the occupational therapist should focus on the client's strengths and on skills necessary for the client's survival in the community. These include:

- ADLs (toilet and toilet hygiene, dressing, feeding etc.)

- IADLs (care of others, child rearing, communication management, meal preparation and clean-up)

- Education (formal educational participation and informal personal educational needs)

- Work (employment interest and pursuits, job performance and maintenance)

- Leisure (exploration and participation)

- Health management (symptom and condition management, communication with the health system, medical management and physical activity)

- Social participation (family and community participation and friendships)

The skill of occupational therapists in the use of group work is of utmost importance because it is in groups that the person with schizophrenia learns to relate to others in the community. Occupational therapists are involved in both group work and individual treatment in community centres, day centres, early intervention programmes in schools and, in some countries, private practice.

'Without continuous attention to their psychosocial rehabilitation these individuals deteriorate over time and cost the mental health programs great sums of money' (Kaplan & Sadock 2000, p. 3190).

SUMMARY AND CONCLUSION

Both the theoretical and practical implications of the use of everyday, practical activities in the treatment and maintenance of the functioning of the individual living with schizophrenia have been highlighted. Psychoeducation has been introduced as part of intervention, demonstrating its significance in the occupational therapy process.

The recent development of the profession of occupational therapy in the mental health field and psychosocial care has provided a much more scientifically based, realistic, holistic, client-centred approach for the intervention of the individual living with schizophrenia than before. Good research and publications have supported the theories of occupational engagement, occupational performance, purposeful activity, creative ability and sensory integration of the person with schizophrenia and have provided a base for the discussion.

The chapter has covered information on intervention for the illness of schizophrenia (and other psychotic disorders) in an acute phase, during the midterm or long-term hospital stay, the reintegration of the individual into the community and their respective occupational roles. In all these stages, the role of occupational therapy has been included, and the multidisciplinary approach has been emphasised throughout.

CASE STUDY

Kelly is a 26-year-old married woman, who lives in a suburb of Cape Town, South Africa. She is an intelligent individual with a degree in oceanography, currently employed at a nearby aquarium. While she was studying at university, she met her husband, who has to this day faithfully supported her through her illness. Shortly after they were married, Kelly began to experience auditory hallucinations and delusions of a paranoid nature. She stated that she was able to hear her neighbours tapping on the walls of their flat and speaking about her and her husband. Furthermore, Kelly shared her experiences of being spied on by her neighbours, whereby they were constantly observing her in her daily tasks within her flat. Kelly's husband reported that her activities of daily living deteriorated notably, as she no longer looked after herself and her hygiene as she usually did. Kelly's behaviour was persistent for one week, after which she eventually was admitted to a psychiatric institution for further assessment and intervention. She spent two weeks in the acute ward of the hospital, where she attended group therapy sessions facilitated by an occupational therapist. She was diagnosed as schizophreniform disorder (DSM-5-TR) (APA 2022) and was placed on neuroleptic medication. Six months later, she was diagnosed with schizophrenia (APA 2022).

Upon Kelly's discharge from hospital, she was referred to a psychiatric day-clinic where she was assessed by a psychiatrist and occupational therapist. Some of the findings of this assessment included limited insight into schizophrenia as an illness, poor understanding of medication use, and anxiety related to her returning to work. As a result, realistic treatment goals in relation to the assessment findings were established, incorporating psychoeducation and occupational engagement. She was then included in an occupational therapy programme that took place at the day-clinic, where she attended groups on an outpatient basis. The psychiatrist and occupational therapist further interviewed her husband (as a form collateral), whereby guidelines

for Kelly's recovery were discussed along with the potential side effects of the medication his wife was taking.

As part of the occupational therapy programme within the day-clinic, Kelly was encouraged to attend to her appearance and start a balanced diet for herself and her husband. The occupational therapist attempted to introduce social skills training for Kelly as part of her group sessions (focussing on occupational engagement); however, the therapist soon learned that these sessions were introduced too early in the intervention process as Kelly became aggressive towards the other group members during the session, as she did not trust them. She was then included in the creative activities group, where she began to regain her confidence in her ability to engage in tasks, even though some of the positive symptoms were still present (Kelly still heard voices; however, the voices being heard were perceived as being far away and softer in volume). She was included in the psychoeducation group once a week and after the eight sessions, she could freely express herself in relation to her illness with individuals other than her husband (such as her friends and colleagues). Social skills training with Kelly was undertaken by the occupational therapist on an individual basis, so that specific challenges identified were addressed.

Kelly's intervention process has continued in occupational therapy on a part-time basis for a year and she has taken part in vocational rehabilitation as an additional intervention strategy during this time. The goal of vocational rehabilitation being to guide her return-to-work process and ensure her successful engagement within her worker roles. The occupational therapist and psychiatrist, working together, have carefully monitored her progress and assessed her regularly for decline in functioning. She has not relapsed, has remained compliant on her medication (and therefore apsychotic) and has managed to maintain optimal functioning within her various roles (worker, wife and neighbour).

QUESTIONS

1. Describe assessment methods, including standardised tests, that can be used by occupational therapist when assessing patients diagnosed with schizophrenia.

2. Discuss the importance of occupational engagement for the person with schizophrenia.

3. '. . . schizophrenia as a disorder that affects the socio-occupational functioning abilities of individuals in their daily life activities, including their roles within self-care, work, play and interpersonal relationships'. Discuss this statement with reference to the impact of schizophrenia as an illness on daily activities for individuals.

4. Occupational therapy programmes contribute significantly to the intervention process for individuals living with schizophrenia, particularly during the acute phase of the illness and whilst admitted to hospital. Discuss what a balanced occupational therapy programme may include and describe appropriate handling principles for individuals with schizophrenia.

5. Community-based programmes are preferred for the individual with schizophrenia after being discharged from hospital. Why is this the case? Briefly describe the intention of community-based rehabilitation programmes for individuals living with schizophrenia.

6. What is psychoeducation and why is it important for individuals living with schizophrenia and their carers?

REFERENCES

Abbas, I. & Soeker, M.S. (2020) The experiences of individuals with schizophrenia using the model of occupational self-efficacy in enhancing work skills and returning to work in the open labour market in Western Cape, South Africa. *South African Journal of Occupational Therapy*, **50**(**3**), 22–29.

American Psychiatric Association (APA) (2022) *Diagnostic and Statistical Manual of Mental Disorders: DSM-5-TR*, 5th edn. APA, Washington, DC.

American Occupational Therapy Association (2020). Occupational Therapy Practice Framework: Domain and Process, 4th edn. *The American Journal of Occupational Therapy*, **74**(**2**), 1–68.

Baum, C.M. & Edwards, D.F. (2001) *The Washington University Activity Card Sort*. Washington University Press, St. Louis.

Bejerholm, U. & Eklund, M. (2007) Occupational engagement in persons with schizophrenia: relationships to self-related variables, psychopathology, and quality of life. *American Journal of Occupational Therapy*, **61**(**1**), 21–32.

Bloomer, S. & William, S. (1986) *The Bay Area Functional Performance Evaluation (BaFPE)*. USCF, San Francisco.

Boop, M., Cahill, S.M., Davis, C. *et al* (2020) Occupational therapy practice framework: domain and process fourth edition. *The American Journal of Occupational Therapy*, **74**(**2**), 1–87.

Bryant, W., Fieldhouse, J., Bannigan, K., Creek, J. & Lougher, L. (2014). *Creek's Occupational Therapy and Mental Health*, 5th edn. Churchill Livingstone.

Casteleijn, D. & Graham, M. (2012) Incorporating a client centred approach in the development of occupational therapy outcome domains for mental health care settings in South Africa. *South African Journal of Occupational Therapy*, **42**(**2**), 8–13.

Casteleijn, J.M.F. (2010) *Development of an Outcome Measure for Occupational Therapists in Mental Health Care Practice*. Unpublished Doctoral Thesis. University of Pretoria, Pretoria. http://upetd.up.ac.za/thesis/available/etd-02102011-143303/ (accessed on 30 June 2012)

Christiansen, C. (2005) Time use and patterns of occupations. In: C. Christiansen, C. Baum & J. Bass-Haugen (eds), *Occupational Therapy: Performance, Participation, and Well-Being*, 3rd edn, pp. 71–91. SLACK Inc, Thorofare, New Jersey.

Clarke, E. & Peters, S. (1994) *The Scorable Self-Care Evaluation (SCORE)*. SLACK Inc., Thorofare, New Jersey.

Creek, J. (1998) *Occupational Therapy: New Perspectives*. Whurr Publishers, London.

Creek, J. (2002) *Occupational Therapy and Mental Health,* 3rd ed. Churchill Livingstone, Edinburgh.

Crouch, R. (2021) *Occupational Group Therapy*, 1st edn. Wiley Blackwell, UK.

Finlay, L. (2002) Groupwork. In: J. Creek (ed), *Occupational Therapy and Mental Health*, 3rd edn, pp. 245–264. Churchill Livingstone, Edinburgh.

Fisher, A.G. & Jones K.B. (2012) *Assessment of Motor and Process Skills, Volume 2*, 7th revised edn. Three Star Press, Fort Collins, Colorado.

Foruzandeh, N. & Parvin, N. (2013) Occupational therapy for inpatients with chronic schizophrenia: a pilot randomized controlled trial. *Japan Journal of Nursing Science*, **10**(**1**), 136–141.

Hasan, A.A., Callaghan, P. & Lymn, J.S. (2015) Evaluation of the impact of a psycho-educational intervention for people diagnosed with schizophrenia and their primary caregivers in Jordan: a randomized controlled trial. *BMC Psychiatry*, **15**(**72**), 1–10.

Kaplan, B.J. & Sadock, V.A. (2000) *Comprehensive Textbook of Psychiatry*, 7th ed. Lippincott Williams & Wilkins, New York.

Kelkar, R.S. (2002) Occupational therapy intervention in hallucinations. *The Indian Journal of Occupational Therapy*, **34**(**2**), 1–6.

Kielhofner, G. (2002) *A Model of Human Occupation: Theory and Application*, 3rd ed. Lippincott Williams & Wilkins, Baltimore.

Klein, R.M. & Bell, B. (1979) *Klein-Bell Activity of Daily Living Scale*. Seattle University of Washington, Division of Occupational Therapy, Seattle.

Law, M., Baptiste, S., Carswell, A., McColl, M.A., Polatajko, H. & Pollack, N. (1998) *Canadian Occupational Performance Measure (COPM)*, 3rd ed. CAOT Publications ACE, Ottawa.

Law, M., Cooper, B., Strong, S., Stewart, D., Rigby, P. & Letts, L. (1996) The person-environment-occupation model: a transactive approach to occupational performance. *Canadian Journal of Occupational Therapy*, **63**(**1**), 9–23.

Leonardelli, C. (1998) Milwaukee evaluation of daily living skills (MEDLS). In: B. Hemphill (ed), *Mental Health Assessment in Occupational Therapy*, pp. 151–162. SLACK Inc., Thorofare, New Jersey.

Lesunyane, A. (2010) Psychiatry and mental health in Africa: the vital role of occupational therapy. In: V. Alers & R. Crouch (eds), *Occupational Therapy: An African Perspective*, pp. 206–231. Sarah Shorten Publishers, Johannesburg.

Liberman, R.P., Kopelwicz, A. & Silverstein, M. (2000) Psychiatric rehabilitation. In: B.J. Kaplan & V.A. Sadock (eds), *Comprehensive Textbook of Psychiatry*, 7th edn, pp. 3218–3245. Lippincott Williams & Wilkins, New York.

Machingura, S.D., Molineux, M. & Lloyd, C. (2018) Effectiveness of sensory modulation in treating sensory modulation disorders in adults with schizophrenia: a systematic literature review. *International Journal of Mental Health and Addiction*, **16**(3), 764–780.

Morrison, P.D. & Murray, R.M. (2012) Schizophrenia. *Current Biology*, **15**(24), 980–984.

Mosey, A.C. (1973) *Activities Therapy*. Rana Press, New York.

Nasr, T. & Kausar, R. (2009) Psychoeducation and the family burden in schizophrenia: a randomized controlled trial. *Annals of General Psychiatry*, **8**(17), 1–6.

Rocamora-Montenegro, M., Compañ-Gabucio L.M. & Garcia de la Hera M. (2021) Occupational therapy interventions for adults with severe mental illness: a scoping review. *British Medical Journal Open*, **11**(10), 1–11.

Ruiz, P. 2014 *Kaplan and Sadock's Synopsis of Psychiatry: Behavioral Sciences/Clinical Psychiatry*. Lippincott Williams and Wilkin, Philadelphia.

Sadock, B. J., Sadock, V. A. & Ruiz, P. (2015). *Kaplan and Sadock's Synopsis of Psychiatry: Behavioral Sciences/Clinical Psychiatry*, 11th edn. Wolters Kluwer Health, 1460 pages.

Snowdon, K., Molden, G. & Dudley, S. (2002) Long-term illness. In: J. Creek (ed), *Occupational Therapy and Mental Health*, 3rd edn, pp. 335–352. Churchill Livingstone, Edinburgh.

Valle, R. (2020) Schizophrenia in ICD-11: comparison of ICD-10 and DSM-5. *Revista de Psiquiatria y Salud Mental (English Ed.)*, **13**(2), 95–104.

Van der Reyden, D., Casteleijn, D., Sherwood, W. & de Witt, P. (2019) *The Vona du Toit Model of Creative Ability: Origins, Constructs, Principles and Application in Occupational Therapy*. The Marie and Vona du Toit Foundation, Pretoria.

World Health Organization. (2019/2021). *International Classification of Diseases*, Eleventh Revision. [online]. World Health Organization. Available at: https://icd.who.int/browse11 (accessed 13 September 2023).

Zietsman, K. (2011) *The Functional Levels Outcomes Measure (FLOM) for Large Numbers of Mental Health Care Users*. Workshop presentation on May 2011, University of the Free State, Bloemfontein.

Zigmond, A.S. & Snaith, R.P. (1983) The hospital and anxiety and depression scale. *Acta Psychiatrica Scandinavica*, **67**(1), 361–370.

CHAPTER 28

Substance Use Disorders and Occupational Therapy

Lisa Wegner[1], Zarina Syed[2] and Rosemary Crouch[3]

[1]Department of Occupational Therapy, Faculty of Community and Health Sciences, University of the Western Cape, Bellville, South Africa

[2]Division of Occupational Therapy, Faculty of Health Sciences, University of Cape Town, Cape Town, South Africa

[3]School of Therapeutic Sciences, Faculty of Health Sciences, University of the Witwatersrand, Johannesburg, South Africa

KEY LEARNING POINTS

- Overview of substance use disorders and dual diagnosis.

- Impact of substance use on individuals, families, communities and society.

- Influence of substance use on occupational engagement and performance.

- Models of intervention for treatment planning and implementation.

- Occupational therapy intervention for persons with substance use disorders.

- Importance of follow-up, aftercare and family.

- Prevention and community-based intervention programmes.

OVERVIEW OF SUBSTANCE USE DISORDERS AND DUAL DIAGNOSIS

Substance use is the harmful or hazardous use of psychoactive substances, including alcohol and illicit drugs, and is a major, global health concern that has negative consequences for individuals, families, communities and society (World Health Organisation 2023). In dealing with substance use, the use of precise, non-stigmatising language and terminology is encouraged to avoid negatively impacting the quality of care; therefore, in this chapter, we use terms such as 'a person with substance use' or 'substance user' instead of 'addict', 'substance abuse', 'abuse' or 'dependence'.

Substance use occurs on a continuum (Figure 28.1) from low-risk use (experimentation or consumption below what is considered physically or psychosocially hazardous) to unhealthy use (which includes at-risk/hazardous use, harmful use, substance use disorder (SUD) or addiction) (Saitz et al. 2021). Substance use typically starts on an experimental basis, and may escalate to frequent or regular use. According to The Diagnostic and Statistical Manual-5 (DSM-5 TR), SUD refers to an individual's continued use of a substance over time despite the negative effects, which results in a pattern of symptoms (American Psychiatric Association [APA] 2022). A SUD is diagnosed by considering a number of criteria (or symptoms) that fall into four broad categories: impaired control, physical dependence, social problems and risky use (Hartney 2023). According to the DSM-5 TR (2022), psychiatrists consider the number of presenting symptoms to make a diagnosis of either at-risk, mild, moderate or severe SUD. Symptoms include the use of substances despite knowing that the effects are harmful to mental and physical health, using more of a substance than intended or using it for longer than intended, trying to cut down or stop using the substance but being unable to, experiencing

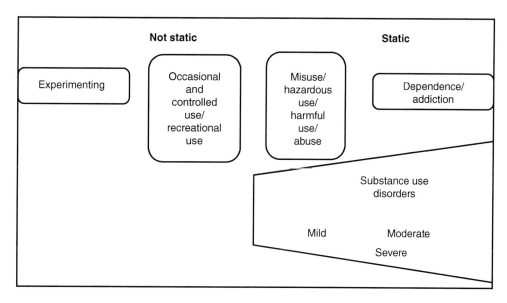

FIGURE 28.1   Spectrum of substance use disorder.

intense cravings or urges to use the substance, needing more of the substance to get the desired effect (tolerance), developing withdrawal symptoms when not using the substance, spending more time getting and using substances and recovering from substance use, neglecting responsibilities, continuing to use substances despite relationship problems, giving up important or desirable social and recreational activities, and using substances in risky settings.

Dual diagnosis (DD) or comorbidity are terms used to describe the presence of both a mental illness as well as a SUD in a person (Thylstrup & Johansen 2009). The combination of these co-occurring diagnoses influences occupational functioning and places a burden on families and communities due to the complexity of the interactions (Stevens *et al.* 2003). The presence of DD in a client requires specific assessment, diagnosis and intervention that includes an effective continuum of care in the form of follow-up post-discharge. Mental health and SUD interventions need to be specifically planned but at the same time, flexible and in accordance with the complex, multifaceted needs of clients (Stevens *et al.* 2003). Programme planning takes into consideration comprehensive assessment, problem identification and treatment planning. The psychosocial issues associated with a lack of purposeful engagement in occupations are prioritised in occupational therapy intervention (Stevens *et al.* 2003). The occupational therapist should consider dysfunction associated with poor participation in purposeful activities in relation to age and stage, poor social skills and other cognitive and emotional component deficits such as problem-solving, motivation, emotional regulation and difficulties in maintaining roles and routine as a result of substance use (Stevens *et al.* 2003).

Interventions offered by the multidisciplinary team are integral to address the multifaceted needs of clients with DD. Cognitive behavioural therapy enables clients to focus on problem-solving by managing their activating triggers, beliefs around the triggers and subsequent behaviours. This process reduces anxiety, aggression and low mood symptoms. Motivational interviewing is a counselling style that allows clients to explore their ambivalence when considering behavioural changes and has the potential to enhance treatment adherence. Family interventions are important in providing holistic care to not only the person but others in their social environment as well. Dual diagnosis is often associated with family disruptions; therefore, addressing the needs of the family has the potential for more positive outcomes. An interdisciplinary approach to intervention that includes occupational therapists, psychiatrists, psychologists, social workers and nurses harnesses the best of each profession to ensure quality care is provided to clients with DD (Borge *et al.* 2013).

IMPACT OF SUBSTANCE USE ON INDIVIDUALS, FAMILIES, COMMUNITIES AND SOCIETY

IMPACT OF HUMAN ECOSYSTEM DISRUPTIONS

Human ecosystem disruptions such as natural disasters, socio-economic crises and pandemics threaten the health and well-being of individuals and societies. A recent human ecosystem disruption is the COVID-19 pandemic, which resulted in an increase in mental health problems including substance use (Kumar *et al.* 2022). While the focus of the impact of the pandemic was on the physical effects of the virus on populations, the long-lasting psychosocial influence on people will magnify for years to come. Those struggling with SUDs particularly remain a vulnerable group due to the complexities of the impact of the diagnosis on functioning (Zaami *et al.* 2020).

The psychological impact of the COVID-19 pandemic potentially exacerbated already existing symptoms of mental illness, SUDs being an example of this. While the world ground to a halt during the pandemic, populations worldwide were in the throes of an insidious, invisible substance use pandemic. Struggles with substance use within the confines of the pandemic brought changes in the way people engaged in activities, the environments they engaged in, and age-appropriate role performance. Approximately 35 million individuals around the world struggle with SUDs and when viewed through the lens of occupational therapy, it was evident that the pandemic resulted in worsening the deficit in functioning (Wei & Shah 2020). Therefore, clinicians need to be alert to the risk behaviours associated with human ecosystem disruptions.

VULNERABLE POPULATIONS AND SUBSTANCE USE

Vulnerable (at-risk) populations fall along a continuum of severity that varies depending on context. Vulnerable populations refer to those already with impairment, or at risk for the development of impairment due to social, biological and economic disadvantages (Sussman & Sinclair 2022). The complexity of vulnerability in health care considers the various dimensions in which contextual factors are situated (Sussman 2017). At the intrapersonal level are neurobiological factors such as mental and physical illness. At the microlevel are issues associated with adverse childhood experiences, parental substance use, and domestic violence. Issues of culture and history are positioned within the macrosocial layer, for example discrimination regarding racial and religious minorities; gender; lesbian, gay, bisexual, transgender, queer/questioning, intersex and asexual (LGBTQIA+) communities; historical trauma experienced by indigenous people; as well as asylum seekers and refugees (Sussman & Sinclair 2022).

Low- to middle-income countries are particularly vulnerable to the challenge of substance use due largely to limited resources to manage the issue. For example, in South Africa, which is classified by the World Bank as an upper-middle income country, 10.3% of the adult population consumes harmful levels of alcohol while 8.6% uses illicit drugs including cannabis, mandrax and stimulants like methamphetamine as well as opiates (Myers *et al.* 2022). Given that 13.3% of the South African population meets the diagnostic criteria for a SUD with alcohol-use disorder being the most prevalent, it is unsurprising that South Africa's burden of disease attributable to alcohol is amongst the highest in the world; however, only around 5% of the population has access to treatment resources (Myers *et al.* 2022).

Most countries have laws governing substance use, and it is essential that occupational therapists understand the legislation and policies applicable to SUD in the country where they practice. Approaches to substance use intervention should be considered within the context of the added complexity of users being from vulnerable populations. Cognisance should be given to how both dynamic and static precipitating and perpetuating factors influence the development and continuation of substance use. With these issues at play, occupational therapists should consider how the occupational risk factors are associated with vulnerable populations' experiences of substance use.

INFLUENCE OF SUBSTANCE USE ON OCCUPATIONAL ENGAGEMENT AND PERFORMANCE

The Occupational Therapy Practice Framework (OTPF-4) (American Occupational Therapy Association [AOTA] 2020) provides a useful theoretical base for understanding the influence of substance use on occupational engagement and performance, and for assessment and intervention planning for persons with SUDs. In addition, occupational therapists may consider their clients from an occupational injustice approach that examines how social and cultural determinants of health influence choices and opportunities (Helbig & McKay 2003). Three risk factors are significant when it comes to contextualising addictive behaviours: occupational imbalance, deprivation and alienation (Wilcock & Hocking 2015). With occupational imbalance, individuals struggle with life role commitments as a result of unmet physical, social and mental needs. This causes a lack of harmony between internal bodily systems of the person and the environment. There is an inability to engage in balanced occupations because substance use becomes the predominant focus of daily life. With occupational deprivation, there are limited opportunities to make use of physical, mental and social capacities, as external forces restrict engagement in occupations. The risk factor of occupational alienation speaks to the larger scale of society that influences individuals, where the occupational nature of the culture or individual is not congruent with the lived experiences. Loneliness as a result of lack of connection may force individuals into a retreat into self that transitions into substance use to alleviate the isolation experienced.

MODELS OF INTERVENTION FOR TREATMENT PLANNING AND INTERVENTION

Effective practice should be based on sound theoretical models. Therefore, making use of various theories to contextualise substance use as an occupation is important to occupational therapists working in the field of SUD care. An SUD affects the user's occupational narrative as well as those who share their environments. As a result of these interactions, the user's roles and subsequent engagement in occupations are affected. Substance use is considered an occupation, as users engage in what they consider to be meaningful activity as part of daily living (Rojo-Mota *et al.* 2017). Twinley and Addidle (2012, p. 203) referred to substance use as a 'dark occupation' because it can be detrimental to health and frequently antisocial in nature despite having meaning for the user.

It is pertinent to consider the biological, social and cultural aspects that negatively influence the trajectories of people using substances. The field of substance use and the care of users is an evolving and dynamic practice that requires interaction from various facets of society and a multidisciplinary health approach. In order to understand the person who becomes dependent on substances, one needs to have a holistic and empathetic clinical reasoning process. Only concentrating on one model to conceptualise the populations we serve results in a distorted outlook. There is, however, no definitive model to use, and an integrated approach that addresses the bio-psycho-social-spiritual domains simultaneously is effective in SUD intervention. Each person is unique and the avenues used to remediate their difficulties with substance use should be developed in a way that is person- or client-centred. The following models are applicable to SUD intervention.

STAGES OF CHANGE MODEL

The Stages of Change Model postulates that persons using substances move through six stages in their efforts to change their behaviour (Prochaska *et al.* 2013). The stages include precontemplation, contemplation, preparation, action, maintenance and termination. The Stages of Change Model assists the multidisciplinary team to understand clients' behaviour according to which stage they are in, and select appropriate treatment goals and activities according to that stage. The client can be an active participant in the process of identifying their stage and setting realistic goals.

BIOLOGICAL MODEL

The biological model investigates the pathological changes that occur at a neurobiological level (Volkow & Li 2004). The suggestion is that exposure to substances causes neural pathways to be distorted. The influence of neurobiology on motivation and subsequent drug-seeking behaviour is situated by considering genetic vulnerability and pharmacology involved in psychological processes (Volkow & Li 2004). Sustained drug use results in chemical changes at a neurological level.

LEARNING MODELS

Learning models conceptualise SUDs based on the premise that substance-seeking behaviour is learnt and can therefore be unlearnt through specific modalities of intervention. Associated learning theory such as classical conditioning theory suggests that patterns and cues are established with exposure in any circumstance resulting in correlation (West & Brown 2013). With application to SUDs, these learnt patterns become linked to substance seeking and use in order to derive satisfaction. Pavlov's theory of classical conditioning is an example of such learning theory (Rescorla & Wagner 1972).

When individuals use and become addicted to substances, a specific decision-making process is followed based on certain bio-behavioural processes.

ENVIRONMENT MODELS

The role of social and cultural environments on the initiation and development of SUDs is the focus of environment models. The impact that certain settings have and the circumstances within those settings on the user are brought to the forefront and unpacked in order to reason behaviour. Certain factors influence the process of substance use and how users will experience the effect of substances (Orford 2001). Identified factors include the pharmacological factors, the substance itself and the user's expectation of substance use. The setting is also considered pivotal in controlling how a substance will affect users. Furthermore, the cultural considerations of a user's environment need to be contemplated. One needs to gain clarity on the ideal norms of a society versus the behavioural norms and identify the norm conflict where divergence occurs. This results in an understanding of the possibility of likely pathological substance use.

LEGAL MODEL

This model considers harsh disciplinary action as the means to resolve the substance use problem. This type of model is very confrontational and ostracising, resulting in the user feeling shamed and undeserving of the potential to improve and seek help. This type of model is based on judgements about negative eventualities of substance use that are laid on users (West 2013). Within this model, the likeliness of negative outcomes is compounded by events like incarceration. Suggesting some sort of mandate for intervention during the time of incarceration is a more productive remedy than punishment alone (Kerrison 2018).

OCCUPATIONAL THERAPY INTERVENTION FOR PERSONS WITH SUBSTANCE USE DISORDERS

Intervention for people with SUDs is a complex and lengthy process. Individuals may be admitted to inpatient or outpatient treatment at government or private medical facilities, where the length of treatment may range from two weeks to six months, or even longer in some cases. Developing insight into the condition, skills training, lifestyle change, treatment of underlying conditions such as depression, counselling and ongoing support are essential components of 'therapeutic' or 'rehabilitative' treatment. Recovery for people struggling with SUDs is not merely about resisting the temptation to use substances, but about lifestyle changes to avoid relapse. Recovery is a process of change where individuals improve their health and wellness, live a self-directed life, and attempt to reach their full potential (Rawat *et al.* 2021).

REFERRAL

Individuals who are using substances often tend to have limited insight into the damaging effects of substances on their occupational performance. This may be combined with a desire to conceal the substance use from families and employers. Often, an individual gets referred for treatment after an incident such as an accidental overdose, or a warning from the school or employer triggers the individual or a family member to seek help. Clients can be referred for treatment by doctors, social workers, occupational therapists, psychologists, nurses, educators, employers and family members. The courts may also refer people who have been involved in criminal activities associated with their use of substances.

ASSESSMENT

Detoxification is considered a stabilisation method required in medical emergencies and should only take place under close medical and nursing supervision. The period of detoxification depends on the substances used and what the context offers. Assessment by the multidisciplinary team starts at this time. The occupational therapist's role is to assess the influence of substance use on the client's occupational performance and the extent of the dysfunction in their life. Assessment should be client centred, where the occupational therapist assists the individual to identify the level of dysfunction within their performance areas and role fulfilment. The OTPF-4 (AOTA 2020) can be used to guide assessment and intervention planning. This entails assessment of the client's occupations (activities of daily living [ADL], instrumental activities of daily living [IADL], work, leisure and social participation), contexts (environmental and personal), performance patterns (habits, routines, roles and rituals), performance skills (motor, process and social interaction) and client factors (values, beliefs, body function and structures). The assessment of clients should be quick and efficient and can take place during both group and individual sessions. Assessment continues during treatment. The occupational profile (AOTA 2020) can be compiled by means of the following methods of assessment, which should be adapted according to the time available for assessment and the intervention context:

1. *Interviewing the client:* The Occupational Performance History Interview (OPHI) (Kielhofner 2002) enables the occupational therapist to obtain information about the client's past and present occupational functioning:

   - Organisation of daily living routines
   - Life roles
   - Interests, values and goals
   - Perceptions of ability and responsibility
   - Environmental influences

The Canadian Occupational Performance Measure (COPM) (Law *et al.* 1998) enables the occupational therapist to assess which aspects of the performance areas are important to the client and the level of satisfaction with their task performance. This facilitates the establishment of meaningful goals for intervention.

2. *Observation of occupational performance:* Insight into performance can be obtained by observing the client's participation in structured settings such as groups, as well as in unstructured settings such as mealtimes. The client's self-presentation, social interaction and ability to carry out tasks can be observed.

3. *Self-assessments and checklists:* The client completes these independently; therefore, they are a useful tool for promoting insight and self-awareness and eliciting discussion. Examples are the Role Checklist and the Modified Interest Checklist (Kielhofner 2002).

4. *Activity participation:* Through the client's engagement and performance of structured and unstructured activities, the occupational therapist is able to make a variety of assessments regarding performance skills. This includes the client's strengths and problems with all aspects of cognition, affect, self-concept, volition, body concept, insight, judgement and interpretation, decision-making and problem-solving. The occupational therapist should also assess physical factors such as gross and fine motor coordination, noting difficulties and problems, for example tremor, poor balance and gait, muscular weakness, emaciation or obesity and peripheral neuritis.

5. *Specific screening and assessment tools:* The following are commonly used:

   - Addiction Severity Index (ASI) (American Addiction Centers n.d.)
   - Alcohol, Smoking and Substance Involvement Screening Test (ASSIST) (World Health Organisation 2010)
   - ASSIST-Youth for children and adolescents aged 10–17 years (Humeniuk *et al.* 2016)
   - Alcohol Use Disorders Identification Test (AUDIT) (World Health Organisation 2001)
   - CRAFFT (a substance use screening tool for adolescents aged 12–21 years) (Knight *et al.* 2002)
   - Drug Use Disorders Identification Test (DUDIT) for adults (European Monitoring Centre for Drugs and Drug Addiction 2002)

Common problems experienced by individuals using substances are:

- Lack of emotional insight. Intellectual insight may be present and the client may be proficient at describing the effects of their substance of choice, yet lack emotional (or true) insight into the consequences of the substance use. This may be attributed to the defence mechanism of intellectualisation. The occupational therapist should recognise this (and other) defence mechanisms and realise that the client has no real understanding of their illness.

- Preoccupation with the substance.

- Temporary short-term memory and concentration loss.

- Inability to make decisions and solve problems.

- Poor self-concept and self-esteem, which are major precipitating factors in SUDs and also a result of the illness.

- Free-floating anxiety or situation-based anxiety and an inability to cope with stress.

- High-risk situations that trigger relapse for individuals with a dual diagnosis of mental illness and substance use disorder include psychological symptoms, positive and negative affect, reminders of substance use, being around people who use drugs and alcohol, interpersonal conflict, offers of drugs or alcohol, experiencing loss, receiving money, loss of appetite, and being abstinent (Bradizza & Stasiewicz 2003). It is a vicious circle since individuals use the substance to cope with their problems. Often the substance is a central nervous system depressant and thus has a sedative effect, which increases the depression (Bradizza & Stasiewicz 2003).

- Passive or active underlying aggression, and poor emotional regulation.

- Poor frustration tolerance and an inability to delay gratification.

- Poor social skills, assertiveness skills and conflict management.

INTERVENTION

Establishing Intervention Aims

Occupational therapy intervention should aim to support re-engagement in occupations that move away from the dysfunctional impact of addictive behaviours (Ryan & Boland 2021). The occupational therapist provides the forum to explore various forms of productivity to engage in age-appropriate roles and untap the client's potential for skills development.

For substance users with low to moderate risk, it is recommended to do a brief intervention as part of the Screening, Brief Intervention and Referral to Treatment (SBIRT) model (Office of Addiction Services and Supports n.d.). This can also take the form of outpatient sessions. For substance users with moderate to high risk, the intervention needs to be more specialised and may require inpatient treatment.

The overall aim or focus of intervention is on changing behaviour and lifestyle. This is achieved by enabling the client to recognise the problem and its consequences, admit the need for help and concentrate on learning to live with the

problem in a constructive manner, identify the changes that need to be made in lifestyle and behaviour, and translate this into action by making the necessary changes in order to develop a new way of life (Bekker 2003). Occupational therapists use their knowledge of the transactional relationship between the client, their engagement in meaningful occupations, and the context, to design occupation-based interventions (AOTA 2020). Therefore, intervention aims and strategies are directed at the person, their occupations and context in the following ways.

- *Promoting a new lifestyle, way of living and engagement in occupation:* To do this, the occupational therapist engages the client in purposeful therapeutic activities and occupations, which are graded to promote competency, mastery and self-esteem. The treatment plan might include ADL and IADL such as self-care, home management, meal preparation, budgeting and childcare. It is extremely important to encourage constructive use of free time and leisure activities to promote a balanced lifestyle, alleviate leisure boredom (Wegner 2011) and replace periods where substances were used. Vocational rehabilitation may be used where appropriate to prepare the client for work.

- *Establishing prosocial, constructive performance patterns:* By assisting the client to establish new roles and reconnect with previous roles which might have been neglected or delayed through the substance use, and develop constructive habits, rituals and routines.

- *Improving performance skills:* Gaining emotional insight into the illness and its consequences is essential. Individual counselling and group work, which can include psycho-education, are important to develop emotional (or true) insight. Techniques such as role play enhance the client's insight into situations and ability to perform new behaviours. The client's self-concept can be improved by encouraging a feeling of self-worth through skills development, for example, learning how to handle stress effectively to reduce anxiety. Treating specific difficulties such as depression, poor memory and concentration and building up physical fitness are important. Socialisation and the encouragement of long-lasting, mature interpersonal relationships may also be a focus of treatment.

- *Context – planning for ongoing support within the environment post-discharge:* Counselling or educating relevant people within the community, work, school or home setting is essential to support clients as they reintegrate into their communities post-discharge.

Principles for Activity Requirements and Structuring of Treatment Sessions

Initially, short, creative activities with a successful end product should be used. This raises the client's self-esteem and caters for poor frustration tolerance and lack of concentration. The cost of creative activities must be taken into consideration and will depend on the context. There should be a good balance of activities incorporating both work and leisure activities. Leisure activities that are appropriate and meaningful, and that can be continued post-discharge should be introduced, which will assist in the replacement of the substance use. Importantly, all activities should be culturally appropriate and relevant.

Both individual and group activities should be planned although, it is highly likely that most treatment will take place in groups due to their cost-effectiveness. The occupational therapist is ethically responsible for all substances and tools in the department, and must take the necessary precautions to ensure the safety of the clients and staff. As a precautionary measure, all noxious substances and alcohol-based substances such as methylated spirits, thinners, glue and leather dyes should be used under supervision, carefully monitored and locked away after use. Sharp knives and implements/tools should be well controlled by the occupational therapist.

Harm Reduction Intervention

Traditional treatment approaches suggest total abstinence in an 'all or nothing' approach with only sobriety as the key to successful substance use treatment. This approach has been criticised as it contributes to the stigma associated with the user and ignores the fact that the recovery process is non-linear. The complexity of substance use means that change happens in increments, with new behaviours evolving within the change process (Prochaska et al. 2013). Harm reduction intervention addresses risk behaviour like substance use by reducing the negative effects of these behaviours without eliminating the substance use completely (Hawk et al. 2017). Harm reduction principles are formulated with the understanding that people are autonomous in decision-making, even if there is the potential for harm (Denning 2010). The following harm reduction principles are commonly used in intervention:

- Accepting that drugs and risky behaviours are a part of society that will never be eliminated.

- Placing the focus on reducing the harm associated with risky behaviours rather than reducing or eliminating the behaviour itself.

- Meeting the individual where they are at, and working with them to minimise the effects of harmful behaviour.

- Honouring individual choices, resisting condemnation and refraining from judgement.

- Setting practical goals by focusing on immediate, achievable objectives rather than abstinence or other unrealistic expectations.

OCCUPATIONAL THERAPY AND HARM REDUCTION

When considering the interventions associated with SUDs, harm reduction is often overlooked as a key strategy to alleviate occupational dysfunction. Integrating harm reduction strategies in occupational therapy practice to affect change in occupational performance areas and components while addressing contextual limitations ensures a holistic approach to intervention. One of the core principles of occupational therapy practice is the client-centred approach that emphasises the primary directive of the profession – to respect the autonomy of the client and include and support them in the decision-making process around their well-being. This is necessary even if decisions appear to be unconventional at times. It should be kept in mind that the engagement in the occupation of substance use is meaningful for clients for a variety of reasons and therefore the restructuring that occurs within the recovery process needs to include consideration of a strategy like harm reduction. Harm reduction strategies that are implemented in health-promoting programmes and interventions spanning a variety of professions are received often with uncertainty by both professionals and the general public. One of the leading causes of this ambiguity in the implementation of harm reduction strategies is 'intervention stigma'. Intervention stigma refers to the experience of being in receipt of a particular type of harm reduction service that may subject individuals to mistreatment since the prominent viewpoint held generally is that sobriety is the ultimate goal (Sulzer et al. 2022).

Occupational therapy intervention makes use of harm reduction strategies by understanding the various occupations that clients engage in, and using them to address the issues associated with substance use and the effect on occupational engagement (Clarke 2019). Therefore, intervention is aimed at improving engagement in occupations associated with age and stage, when total sobriety is not the option that the client is able to commit to at a particular time. Areas of occupation that could be looked at include home management, self-care, money management and care of others. The overall goal in the use of harm reduction as a strategy in occupational therapy intervention is to facilitate the development of realistic choices that honour the clients' autonomy in an empathetic manner without judgement.

CO-DEPENDENCY

Co-dependency is a noticeable characteristic assigned to people within the recovery process. Both the user and the people within their social environment are at risk for this behaviour. Understanding co-dependency is instrumental to dissect the underlying problems experienced by the user and those who engage with them in social environments known as significant others. These significant other individuals may develop their whole identity around the well-being of the user, which results in maladaptive rescuing behaviour. The manifestation of this is often hypervigilance and controlling actions as a result of difficulty expressing emotions and mistrust. While co-dependent behaviour is associated with protecting and even enabling the user, significant others' failure to prioritise self-care is often observed and overall ambivalence is also present (Beattie 2022). Significant others are at risk of developing negative coping strategies related to occupational performance. Wegner *et al.* (2014) described mothers' roles of enabling addiction in their substance-using children, which negatively influenced their own mental health and well-being. As health professionals, it is important that we view co-dependency as a parallel factor that influences the long-term recovery of clients. Interventions therefore need to be geared towards being aware of, and addressing, these behaviours from the perspective of both the user and their significant others, which once again highlights the importance of family interventions (Denning 2010; Wegner *et al.* 2014).

ACTIVITIES USED IN OCCUPATIONAL THERAPY

OCCUPATIONAL GROUP THERAPY

Occupational therapy intervention with SUDs occurs predominantly by means of occupational group therapy in both the community and treatment centre environment (Table 28.1). Fouchè in Crouch (2021, p. 25), states that 'Groups are a generic technique/medium/skill used by many professionals, but occupational therapists all over the world should be clear as to the unique contributions which they bring to groups used as intervention in treatment'. The occupational therapist should make use of the therapeutic factors inherent in groups, such as instillation of hope, universality, imparting information, developing social skills, altruism and interpersonal learning (Yalom 1995) to shape

Table 28.1 Occupation-based group therapy and objectives.

Occupation-based group	Examples of activities	Objectives
Work	Craft activities such as woodwork, jewellery making, paper crafts, fabric painting and beadwork. Ward chores such as gardening, meal preparation and cleaning rooms.	Develop worker role Develop work habits Develop work skills Improve cognitive components (frustration tolerance, delay of gratification, memory, concentration) Develop responsibility Improve self-esteem
Leisure	Sports such as volleyball, aerobics, soccer, walking, yoga, swimming and jogging, creative activities, hobbies and games.	Identify and explore personal leisure interests, skills, activities and opportunities Opportunity for relaxation Improve self-esteem and self-concept Improve socialisation and physical health
ADL and IADL	Meal preparation, shopping, budgeting, parenting, grooming, hygiene.	Develop and practice skills in relevant areas Improve self-confidence and self-concept

desired behaviour. Members of the multidisciplinary team can be invited to co-facilitate occupational group therapy and contribute their unique perspectives.

WARM-UP AND ICEBREAKER TECHNIQUES

These techniques are a distinguishing feature of typical occupational group therapy. Usually, they are employed at the beginning of a group and assist in helping group members to relax, get to know one another and begin to participate in the group interaction. These techniques are described in detail elsewhere (see, e.g. Remocker & Storch 1992; Crouch 2021).

ORIENTATION GROUPS

During the orientation phase, new clients are introduced to the environment of the facility and to other clients and staff members. Orientation groups enable new clients to become familiar with the approach and goals of the programme, the rules of the facility, clients' rights and expectations. These groups are an opportunity for clients to commit to the treatment process. It is useful to get the group members to establish their own set of norms and sign a group contract. Clients who have been in the facility longer can take responsibility for certain aspects of these groups.

OCCUPATION-BASED ACTIVITY GROUPS

These are groups which focus on the therapeutic use of work, leisure and ADL. A variety of treatment goals can be achieved by facilitating clients' participation in occupation-based groups and altering the handling, structuring and grading principles for each client. It is not so much the type of activity, but more the expectations inherent within the objectives of the activity that are important.

INTRAPERSONAL SKILLS GROUPS

Intrapersonal skills groups focus on self-awareness, insight, values, goals, self-esteem and self-concept. People who have been using substances for a long time often experience a delay in personal development. By considering the client's chronological and developmental stage, the occupational therapist can select appropriate activities to facilitate the client's ability to deal with developmental issues. As part of the process, clients need to become aware of their intrapersonal strengths and weaknesses. They need to understand why they use substances and become aware of the destructive effects of their substance use behaviour on relatives, friends and their lives in general. It is important that client identify their values and set realistic short-term and long-term goals. Achievement of these goals will boost their self-esteem. Activities should enable clients to create a new personal identity as non-substance users and develop their self-concept. Of particular value to achieve these goals, is evocative/projective occupational group therapy using art, mandalas, poetry, music, creative writing, role play and psychodrama (Crouch 2021).

PSYCHODRAMA

For many years projective techniques such as drama, art and music have been used in group therapy as well as with individual clients. Psychodrama is a group approach used by occupational therapists trained in the technique. According to Blatner (1992, 1996), psychodrama is a valuable technique for assisting clients gain insight into their problems. With a skilled occupational therapist, psychodrama is a dynamic and powerful technique. Crouch (2021, p. 104) describes psychodrama as '. . . an enactment involving emotional problem-solving and is essentially a system-ised method of acting out within the confines of a close, cohesive group'. Group members develop spontaneity, creativity and self-disclosure through action in the group. In this way, clients gain insight regarding self, behaviour, relationships and consequences of substance use. They are also able to experiment with new behaviours and plan for the future.

INTERPERSONAL SKILLS GROUPS

Interpersonal skills groups aim to develop effective communi-cation, assertiveness and conflict resolution skills, thereby improving interpersonal relationships. The groups should be carefully graded, taking clients through a process of identify-ing their difficulties, learning effective skills and methods, practicing these in the relatively safe environment of the group as well as in real life and receiving feedback. Social skills training should include training in both verbal and non-verbal communication. Special emphasis should be placed on assertiveness training so that the substance user can learn to be assertive without the use of a drug/alcohol. Clients should be encouraged to practice their new skills whilst participating in other aspects of the programme. Fouchè in Crouch (2021, p. 24) discusses a psychosocial approach to group work, which also emphasises interpersonal relationships particularly in individuals with a substance use problem. Emphasis is on learning to understand the use of harmful substances and become aware of the destructive effects on interpersonal rela-tionships with family and friends.

COPING SKILLS GROUPS

According to the needs of the client population, the occupational therapist may implement relevant coping skills groups including anger, stress and anxiety management. Relaxation groups can be held daily to expose clients to differ-ent methods of relaxation and enable them to practise their relaxation skills. Stress management is an integral part of the treatment of the substance user (Crouch 2008). The stress management programme may include the following subjects:

- Identifying stressors and triggers of stress
- How stress affects the body and mind and the influence on a person's functioning
- Learning to balance the lifestyle and control stress

- Stress and substance use
- Relaxation and breathing

FAMILY GROUPS

The family can be a vital support mechanism for the client as they reintegrate into the community. Family relationships have often been affected, and attention should be given to working with the client and the family members. The occupational therapist may counsel the family about issues such as structuring the daily routine, encouraging the client to find and maintain work, dealing with stigma and the value of engaging in leisure pursuits.

LEISURE ACTIVITIES

The substance user needs to adapt to a new lifestyle, and developing an interest in leisure activities can provide a mean-ingful replacement for substance use. A certain amount of time, every day, should be devoted to being actively involved in an enjoyable, leisure activity other than work. Clients with families should be encouraged to undertake activities that would be suitable to share with the family. Not only does this support the client in their endeavour, but it will improve fam-ily relationships too. The culture of the client should always be considered. Examples of leisure activities are:

Creative activities such as candle making, beadwork, jewel-lery making, art, pottery, woodwork, sewing and painting.
Gardening and horticulture, for example vegetable gardening or bonsai.
Physical activity such as walking or hiking.
Sport which may involve both active and passive participa-tion. Sport however is often associated with substance use, particularly alcohol, and the client must be cautioned.
Involvement in social clubs, religious groups, community support groups such as Alcoholics and Narcotics Anony-mous (AA, NA) and voluntary work.

PHYSICAL FITNESS

Physical fitness training should be an integral part of the programme and should ideally take place early in the morning. Exercise in the form of walking, yoga or exercise groups is effec-tive. Correct breathing and posture should be encouraged and if necessary, attention given to weight loss or gain. General fitness and improved circulation will be achieved. Exercise on a regular basis has been proven to improve mood and motivation, so it is extremely important to encourage appropriate exercise.

VOCATIONAL REHABILITATION

Occupational therapists should use their expertise in voca-tional rehabilitation to assist the substance user to stay at, or return to, work whether in the home or open labour market, as this is an important achievement in the whole rehabilitation process. The attitude of the employer towards substance use should be evaluated and if possible, the occupational therapist should work with the employer. Employers are encouraged to keep a client's job open whilst they are in rehabilitation. The occupational therapist must take care that the employer understands the illness and that the contact does not place the client's job in jeopardy.

FINANCIAL MANAGEMENT AND BUDGETING

Many clients have financial difficulties. Group sessions which deal with budgeting and financial control are extremely helpful. It may be useful to bring in an expert on the subject, so that clients can work out their own budgets and pinpoint difficulties. Working with the social worker where major problems occur is essential.

IMPORTANCE OF FOLLOW-UP, AFTERCARE AND FAMILY

Rehabilitation is a long process for the substance user and it is essential for the occupational therapist to help the client plan realistically. The multidisciplinary team needs to collaborate with the client and their family to discuss follow-up and support options for the period following discharge. In preparation, the occupational therapist should run psychoeducation and goal-setting groups where clients consider their future plans regarding issues such as relapse prevention and goals associated with various relevant age-appropriate occupations. Referral to support groups should be implemented, and other resources that the client can approach should be identified. Most importantly, clients should make realistic plans to structure their time with constructive, meaningful activities and occupations.

Community approaches are crucial in being a catalyst for the connection that people seek within the recovery process; therefore, occupational therapists need to provide a space for collaboration with communities. The following are examples of integrating community practice into SUD interventions.

Psychosocial rehabilitation as well as health promotion incorporate principles that when implemented, can enable clients to attain optimal functioning and add value in creating supportive environments (Rasmus *et al.* 2021). Occupational therapists can apply principles such as actively involving clients in intervention and improving client competencies to effect change in unearthing the potential people possess to grow and develop skills in an environment of hope. Additionally, education and skills development go hand in hand in terms of continuum of care and ongoing support to those

in communities. Empowering people in communities to take ownership and take back lost autonomy as a result of substance use is an important step.

Contingency management is traditionally based on positive reinforcement and extrinsic reward systems. Occupational therapists can make use of the concept of engagement in occupation as the means or the reward when considering lifestyle changes that are necessary in the process of recovery from substance use (Sarsak 2018). The fulfilment of engaging in meaningful occupation can then be interpreted as the tangible reward associated with contingency management.

Risk assessment needs to be integrated into community approaches to identify the risk factors associated with vulnerable groups within the context. An example of making use of resources within the community is to tap into the potential offered by community rehabilitation workers. Upskilling this critical group of workers to be able to perform risk assessments to identify susceptibilities in the community also has the advantage of strengthening interprofessional collaboration (Syed *et al.* 2022).

Strategies that consider gender analysis as part of response efforts result in improved effectiveness of interventions and the equitable promotion of health equality. Other strategies that include culture and spirituality as well as family interventions within communities need to be represented in planning community-based interventions.

PREVENTION AND COMMUNITY-BASED INTERVENTION PROGRAMMES

Prevention intervention focuses on increasing awareness about substances and their harmful effect and supports people to stay substance-free. Prevention programmes may be offered in various community settings such as community clinics, religious and non-governmental organisations, libraries and schools. Support and advice are available from Narcotics Anonymous and Alcoholics Anonymous, which are non-profit fellowships of recovering substance users who meet regularly to help each other 'stay clean'. Nar-Anon Family groups provide support for family and friends affected by substance use.

As part of their health promotion role, occupational therapists are involved in establishing community-based intervention programmes aimed at decreasing substance use in communities. These programmes are often directed at children and adolescents but could involve parents, educators and other stakeholders in the community. Community intervention programmes can be based on the framework and principles provided by the World Health Organisation's Ottawa Charter for Health Promotion (1986). The Community Process (Vermeulen *et al.* 2015) is a useful guide for developing community-based intervention programmes.

CASE STUDY 1 — Substance-Induced Psychotic Disorder

Thabo is a 17-year-old IsiXhosa/English-speaking male. He was born in Cape Town (South Africa), but spent most of his early childhood in the rural Eastern Cape with his grandmother. At the age of 14 years, Thabo returned to Cape Town to live in an informal settlement with his mother, older sister and younger brother. His parents are divorced. His father does not live with them and is employed as a bus driver. Since no-one in Thabo's home is employed, the family relies on his father for financial support as well as a government, child care social grant. Thabo is a learner in Grade 10 at a local high school. Thabo experimented with smoking cannabis on his return to Cape Town three years previously. Over time, he began smoking cannabis every day. Recently, he has been acting strangely, for example shouting at educators, staring at other learners for prolonged periods, saying he can heal people and singing loudly during class despite being asked to stop. After his educator found him smoking cannabis in the school toilets during break, the school informed his mother who took Thabo to the local district hospital. Thabo was diagnosed with substance-induced psychotic disorder (SIPD). Thabo tells the admitting doctor that he hears voices inside his head which order him to carry out certain actions.

Indication/referral for occupational therapy: Thabo was admitted to the Male Psychiatric Observation Unit. He was referred for occupational therapy to assess his functioning, facilitate his engagement in age-appropriate occupations through various modalities and prepare for discharge planning.

Assessment: It was clear that the SIPD hindered his ability to fulfil his primary age and stage-appropriate role as a learner. The assessments used and the reason for their use are summarised in Table 28.2.

Disability experience: Thabo does not think that he has a mental illness but believes that he has a calling to be a sangoma (traditional healer). He believes that the voices he hears are the ancestors having a conversation with him and testing his obedience. He believes if he accepts the calling to be a sangoma, the voices will stop.

OCCUPATIONAL PERFORMANCE AND ROLE COMPETENCE

Activities of daily living: Pre-admission, Thabo neglected his ADL, including eating, bathing, brushing teeth and dressing as his engagement in smoking cannabis was the primary focus of his routine. He is now able to engage in ADL independently. He is assisted by nurses in the occupation of medication management.

Schooling/learning performance: A few weeks before admission, Thabo's learning performance deteriorated in that he was hearing voices when he was in class, which ordered him to behave bizarrely. He was often removed from class as a result of what was considered disruptive behaviour, which impacted his learning. The findings of the WHO Disability Assessment Scale 2.0 (WHODAS 2.0) revealed that he had difficulty performing his school tasks. This hindered his ability to have a positive experience at school and made it difficult for him to make friends in his class, highlighting his learning performance and social participation as barriers.

Leisure performance: Thabo indicated smoking cannabis as his primary leisure occupation.

Role performance: Thabo's role performance as a learner, son, brother and friend had deteriorated as a result of his diagnosis, and led to his admission as an inpatient.

OCCUPATIONAL THERAPY PLAN

Long term aim: By the end of six months, Thabo will have an improved quality of life to the extent that he will be able to fulfil his roles as a son, brother, friend and learner within his home and school context.

Negotiated main aims: At the end of five weeks, Thabo will have gained intellectual and emotional insight into his diagnosis as well as its cause to the extent that he will adhere to the medication/treatment of his diagnosis with maximum assistance from the occupational therapist. He will understand how his use of cannabis has negatively influenced his roles and occupational performance and the consequences for his future plans.

Table 28.2 Assessment methods and reason for use.

Assessment methods	Reasons for use
Interview	To get general information about Thabo such as his personal history, medical history, social and personal habits and educational history.
Mental state examination	To assess his mental state by looking at the various psychosocial and cognitive performance components.
Mini-mental state examination	To assess whether Thabo has any cognitive impairments related to his immediate memory.
Role checklist	To assess Thabo's occupational roles and the importance of those roles to him.
Occupational Self-Assessment Daily Living Scale	To assess Thabo's ability to complete daily living skills and the importance to him of being able to perform those skills.
Occupational Therapy Task Observational Scale (OTTOS)	To assess Thabo's ability to interact and socialise with therapist and peers during engagement in a game of Jenga.
	To determine Thabo's task behaviour and general behaviour.
World Health Organisation Disability Assessment Schedule 2.0 (WHODAS 2.0)	To assess Thabo's functioning and whether he had any difficulties in cognition, mobility, self-care, getting along with others and participation in life activities during the previous 30 days as a result of his drug problem and mental or emotional problems.
Collateral	Mother
	Medical file

PRINCIPLES FOR INTERVENTION

Humanistic Frame of Reference (Rogers 1951)

Treatment should encourage discussion and social interaction to facilitate gaining intellectual and emotional insight through feedback about impact of behaviour on others and own health and functioning.

Give individual feedback to facilitate appropriate judgement and insight, and incorporate training regarding alternative options for behaviours.

Treatment process should enhance and promote Thabo's unique potential, creativity and independence to flourish.

Treatment aims should be client-centred and allow Thabo to set his own agenda.

Cognitive Behavioural Frame of Reference (Duncan & Fletcher-Shaw 2020)

Make client aware how thinking patterns affect behaviour.

Learning should occur in a social context through imitation and modelling.

People choose to imitate behaviours where a positive consequence is anticipated.

These principles should be incorporated into intervention activities.

PLAN OF ACTION

Select activities based on the following criteria:

Elicit creativity and participation.

Promote autonomy.

Align with the client's uniqueness and individuality.

Educate the client about his condition, help him understand his behaviour and thoughts.

Facilitate experiential learning in applying cognitive restructuring in action.

Enable acquisition of alternative, functional cognitive behaviours.

Role of therapist (handling principles to ensure client-centred practice):

Provide reinforcement that shapes functional, adaptive thinking patterns.

Focus on the client's thinking.

Display unconditional positive regard.

Be non-judgemental and value individuality.

Be warm and genuine.

Encourage autonomy and self-awareness.

Assist the client to identify and reshape negative and inaccurate thinking.

Provide modelling on how to stop negative thinking.

Optimising the environment (structuring principles):

Structure the environment to:

Offer a range of choices to allow free expression and decision-making.

Provide optimal antecedent clues for the desired cognitive behaviour to occur.

Provide negative reinforcement if dysfunctional behaviour has occurred.

Ensuring change (grading / adapting / modifying principles):

Increasing the duration of activity/session.

Increase the demand for behavioural control.

Decrease the amount of structure and support.

Increase expectation for compliance to rule and regulations.

Make client aware of compliant/non-assertive behaviour.

Downgrade the amount of encouragement and support given to the client.

Grade from therapist-directed to patient-directed problem-solving.

Grade from generic to personal problem-solving.

CASE STUDY 2   Substance Use Disorder

Jack (28 years) was referred to a therapeutic substance rehabilitation unit by his doctor after being diagnosed with SUD (moderate). He has been admitted to a public psychiatric hospital as an inpatient for a period of four weeks. He will be able to go home for weekends. Jack previously lived with his girlfriend and their three-year-old daughter, but his girlfriend broke up with him because of his drug use. He admits being verbally abusive towards her because he *'could not handle her nagging him to stop drugging and get a job'*. He moved in with his parents, but conflict soon arose as his drugging habit escalated and he stole money from his parents. His mother insisted that he see the family doctor.

During his interview and assessment, the occupational therapist builds a therapeutic relationship with Jack by engaging him in a conversation about his life. Jack started drinking alcohol and smoking cigarettes when he was 14 years old, then progressed to smoking cannabis in later adolescence, and in his twenties started using cocaine. Jack says, *'Looking back on things now, the reason I didn't study further after finishing school was probably because of my drugging. My girlfriend supported me financially, which made me feel less of a man'*. The occupational therapist notices Jack's feelings of guilt. She asked him what talents he possessed. He replies, *'I think I am quite creative and I use this talent to make jewellery. I like using wire, beads and natural*

(continued)

materials like shells and feathers. I've even made a bit of money selling some of my jewellery – but then I just use the money to buy drugs'.

Observations by the multidisciplinary team reveal Jack to be a quiet, passive person who does not interact much with the other patients in the unit, preferring to keep to himself. On occasion, Jack gets frustrated easily and loses his temper, becoming verbally abusive. Following a full assessment, the occupational therapist draws up Jack's occupational profile (Table 28.3).

On admission to the unit, Jack is identified as being in the *Contemplation stage* according to the Stages of Change model (Prochaska *et al.* 2013). The priority goal of intervention at this stage is to resolve Jack's ambivalence about giving up drugs and motivate him to stay in the substance rehabilitation unit. In week 1, Jack participates in the following programme:

Orientation group: In the first group, he is orientated to the unit programme and introduced to other clients and staff.

Self-awareness: In group 2, he engages in activities that aim to develop self-awareness about his drug problem. This could be done through concrete activities such as art therapy, for example, collage of my inner self and outer self.

Building insight: In group 3, Jack starts to develop awareness of the problems caused by his addiction and resulting behaviour toward himself and others. He is involved in a structured role-play scenario about how drugs dominate and control users' lives. The occupational therapist uses the handling principles of support and encouragement at this stage.

A few days after his admission, Jack verbalises his decision to commit himself to the process of stopping his drug use and seeking an alternative lifestyle. The team regards this as a sign that Jack is in the *Preparation stage*. Now the goal of intervention is to facilitate the *Action stage* by empowering Jack with the skills needed to overcome his drug addiction, thus boosting his self-esteem. At the same time, Jack will need to gain insight into the reasons for his addiction and the consequences of his drugging behaviour. As he does this, his self-concept will develop. Jack will be involved in the following types of occupational group therapy:

Values clarification

Insight building

Occupational groups (e.g. work – developing his jewellery making as a potential means of generating an income, leisure – exploring various leisure activities, ADL – self-care, and IADL – parenting, budgeting and meal preparation)

Interpersonal skills groups (e.g. social skills and communication skills)

Coping skills (anger, anxiety and stress management)

Team members remain supportive in their handling of Jack, but increase their expectations of performance and goal achievement. They also encourage Jack to take more responsibility in the unit. He returns home over weekends, where he has the opportunity to try out newly learned skills and behaviours.

Table 28.3 Occupational performance profile for Jack using the OTPF-4 (AOTA 2020) framework.

Occupations

ADL: Jack neglects aspects of his basic ADL.

IADL: Limited parenting, home management and budgeting skills.

Work: Jack is unemployed and shows poor work habits. However, he is creative and can be encouraged to develop his talent for making jewellery as a potential source of income/work.

Leisure: Jack has limited leisure interests as drugs have been his only interest for many years. Occasionally, he spends time designing jewellery in his free time and watches sports on television.

Social participation: Jack has strained relationships with his girlfriend, daughter and his parents. He has no friends apart from his drug acquaintances. He avoids social interaction and has poor social skills becoming verbally abusive in conflict situations.

Contexts

Environment: Jack lives at home with his parents, although he would prefer to be living with his girlfriend and daughter.

Personal: He is at a stage when he should be establishing his roles as partner, father and worker. He has recognised the need to stop using drugs.

Performance patterns

Habits and routines: Jack's use of time is not constructive. His days have lacked structure and planning and are characterised by disorganisation. Most of his time is spent getting and using drugs or recovering from the effects of drugs.

Roles: Jack's significant life roles are father, boyfriend, son, friend and worker. He has neglected these roles and has had difficulty performing the tasks associated with role expectations; therefore, his role experience has been limited.

Performance skills

Motor: Jack is physically unfit and has low endurance.

Process: Jack shows poor self-esteem and awareness and lacks a consolidated self-concept and personal identity. His belief in his own capabilities (self-efficacy) is poor. He regards himself as a failure and feels that his problems are insurmountable. He shows poor coping skills, poor time management and he struggles to handle conflict, stress and anxiety. He has some intellectual insight but no emotional insight. He has poor memory, a limited attention span and difficulties with problem-solving and decision-making.

Social interaction: Poor interpersonal skills affect his ability to conduct himself appropriately in social situations. He has difficulty expressing his thoughts, feelings and needs resulting in conflict in relationships with girlfriend and parents. He has difficulty with self-control/regulation and anger management.

Client factors

Values: Jack has not been able to adhere to his value system as his need to obtain and use drugs has dominated his life. He feels very guilty about stealing money from his family and verbally abusing his girlfriend.

Beliefs and spirituality: Jack identifies with the drug/alcohol subculture. He has no strong spiritual or religious beliefs.

He is also faced with challenges which he needs to negotiate, such as communicating with his parents and rekindling his relationships with his girlfriend and daughter. On Monday mornings, he reflects on his progress in the occupational group therapy.

As Jack nears discharge, the occupational therapist focuses on the *maintenance stage* through goal setting and planning for reintegration into his life – this entails resumption of roles, considering work opportunities and identifying a place to stay. Follow-up and support resources in the community are also explored.

CONCLUSION

Recovery from a SUD is a complex, dynamic process and clients are likely to move through various stages depending on their contextual stressors. The occupational therapist plays an important role in the rehabilitation of the substance user, basing intervention on theoretical perspectives to assess and treat the occupational dysfunction associated with substance use. By drawing up an occupational profile, the occupational therapist assesses the impact of substance use on the client's occupational performance and the extent of the dysfunction in their life. Assessment and treatment take into account the individual's roles, tasks, values, interests, goals, performance areas and components, within a temporal, social, cultural and physical context. The focus of intervention with SUDs is on changing behaviour and lifestyle, and this occurs through intervention in an integrated programme that typically involves a multidisciplinary team approach.

QUESTIONS

1. Discuss the diagnosis of SUD by highlighting how occupational performance may be affected. Use the Occupational Therapy Practice Framework-4 (AOTA 2020) to assist you.

2. Brainstorm relevant questions for an initial interview with a client who is diagnosed with SUD. Role-play your interview with a partner and then discuss how it felt to be in the roles of the interviewer and the client.

3. Describe a treatment session for a group of clients who are in the contemplation stage of the Stages of Change model, where the aim is to improve their emotional (or true) insight about how substance use has affected significant people in their lives.

4. Describe three types of groups which could be used in the treatment of the substance user nearing discharge. Explain how you would grade the sessions.

5. Discuss the importance of follow-up occupational therapy groups after discharge. Think about challenges regarding this type of group and suggest strategies to overcome challenges. Outline a structure for the monthly follow-up groups and suggest possible topics.

REFERENCES

American Addiction Centers (n.d.) *Addiction severity index.* https://americanaddictioncenters.org/rehab-guide/asi-addiction-severity-index-assessment (accessed on 23 May 2023)

American Occupational Therapy Association (2020) The occupational therapy practice framework (OTPF-4). *American Journal of Occupational Therapy,* **74 (Supplement_2)**, 7412410010p1–7412410010p87. https://doi.org/10.5014/ajot.2020.74S2001

American Psychiatric Association (APA) (2022) *Diagnostic and Statistical Manual of Mental Disorders: DSM-5 TR,* 5th edn, Text Revision. American Psychiatric Association, Washington, DC.

Beattie, M. (2022) *Codependent No More: How to Stop Controlling Others and Start Caring for Yourself.* Hazeldon Publishing, Center City.

Bekker, C. (2003) *What to expect.* http://www.stepping-stones.co.za (accessed on 19 March 2014)

Blatner, A. (1992) *Foundations of Psychodrama: Theory and Practice,* 3rd edn. Springer Publishing Co., New York.

Blatner, A. (1996) *Acting-in: Practical Applications of Psychodramatic Methods.* Springer Publishing Co., New York.

Borge, L., Angel, O.H. & Røssberg, J.I. (2013) Learning through cognitive milieu therapy among inpatients with dual diagnosis: a qualitative study of interdisciplinary collaboration. *Issues in Mental Health Nursing,* 34(4), 229–239.

Bradizza, C. M. & Stasiewicz, P. R. (2003). Qualitative analysis of high-risk and alcohol use situations among severely mentally ill substance abusers. *Addictive Behaviors,* **28**(1), 157–169. https://doi.org/10.1016/S0306-4603(01)00272-6

Clarke, C. (2019) Can occupational therapy address the occupational implications of hoarding? *Occupational Therapy International,* **2019**, 5347403.

Crouch, R.B. (2008) A community-based stress management programme for an impoverished population in South Africa. *Occupational Therapy International,* **915**(2), 71–86.

Crouch, R.B. (2021) *Occupational Group Therapy.* Wiley Blackwell, Oxford.

Denning, P. (2010) Harm reduction therapy with families and friends of people with drug problems. *Journal of Clinical Psychology,* **66**(2), 164–174.

Duncan, E. & Fletcher-Shaw, S. (2020) The cognitive-behavioural frame of reference. In: E. Duncan (ed), *Foundations for Practice in Occupational Therapy,* 6th edn, pp. 141–151. Elsevier Science & Technology, Edinburgh.

European Monitoring Centre for Drugs and Drug Addiction (2002) *Drug use disorders identification test (DUDIT) for adults.* https://www.emcdda.europa.eu/drugs-library/drug-use-disorders-identification-test-extended-dudit-e_en (accessed on 23 May 2023)

Fouchè, L. (2021) The occupational therapy interactive group model (OTIGM). In: R. Crouch (ed), *Occupational Group Therapy*, pp. 21–64. Wiley Blackwell, Oxford.

Hartney, E. (2023) *DSM-5 criteria for substance use disorders.* https://www.verywellmind.com/dsm-5-criteria-for-substance-use-disorders-21926 (accessed on 17 July 2023)

Hawk, M., Coulter, R.W., Egan, J.E. *et al* (2017) Harm reduction principles for healthcare settings. *Harm Reduction Journal*, **14**, 1–9.

Helbig, K. & McKay, E. (2003) An exploration of addictive behaviours from an occupational perspective. *Journal of Occupational Science*, **10**(3), 140–145, https://doi.org/10.1080/14427591.2003.9686521

Humeniuk, R., Holmwood, C., Beshara, M. & Kambala, A. (2016) ASSIST-Y V1.0: first-stage development of the WHO alcohol, smoking and substance involvement screening test (ASSIST) and linked brief intervention for young people. *Journal of Child & Adolescent Substance Abuse*, **25**, 384–390. https://doi.org/10.1080/1067828X.2015.1049395

Kerrison, E.M. (2018) Exploring how prison-based drug rehabilitation programming shapes racial disparities in substance use disorder recovery. *Social Science & Medicine,* **199**, 140–147.

Kielhofner, G. (ed) (2002) *A Model of Human Occupation: Theory and Application*, 3rd edn. Lippincott Williams & Wilkins, Baltimore.

Knight, J.R., Sherritt, L., Shrier, L.A., Harris, S.K. & Chang, G. (2002) Validity of the CRAFFT substance abuse screening test among adolescent clinic patients. *Archives of Pediatrics & Adolescent Medicine*, **156**(6), 607–614.

Kumar, N., Janmohamed, K., Nyhan, K. *et al* (2022) Substance use in relation to COVID-19: a scoping review. *Addictive Behaviors*, **127**, 107213.

Law, M., Baptiste, S., Carswell, A., McColl, M.A., Polatajko, H. & Pollock, N. (1998) *Canadian Occupational Performance Measure*, 3rd edn. CAOT Publications ACE, Toronto.

Myers, B., Koch, J.R., Johnson, K. & Harker, N. (2022) Factors associated with patient-reported experiences and outcomes of substance use disorder treatment in Cape Town, South Africa. *Addiction Science & Clinical Practice*, **17**(1), 8.

Office of Addiction Services and Supports (n.d.) *Screening, brief intervention and referral to treatment (SBIRT) model.* https://oasas.ny.gov/sbirt (accessed on 23 May 2023)

Orford, J. (2001) Addiction as excessive appetite. *Addiction,* **96**, 15–31. https://doi.org/10.1046/j.1360-0443.2001.961152.x

Prochaska, J.O., Norcross, J.C. & DiClemente, C.C. (2013) Applying the stages of change. *Psychotherapy in Australia,* **19**(2), 10–15.

Rasmus, P., Lipert, A., Pękala, K. *et al* (2021) The influence of a psychosocial rehabilitation program in a community health setting for patients with chronic mental disorders. *International Journal of Environmental Research and Public Health*, **18**(8), 4319.

Rawat, H., Petzer, S.L. & Gurayah, T. (2021) Effects of substance use disorder on women's roles and occupational participation. *South African Journal of Occupational Therapy*, **51**(1), 54–62.

Remocker, A. & Storch, E.T. (1992) *Action Speaks Louder: A Handbook of Structured Group Techniques.* Churchill Livingstone, Canada.

Rescorla, R.A., Wagner, A. (1972) A theory of Pavlovian conditioning: variations in the effectiveness of reinforcement and nonreinforcement. *Classical Conditioning II: Current Research and Theory*, **2**, 64–99.

Rogers, C.R. (1951) *Client-centered Therapy: Its Current Practice, Implications and Theory.* Houghton Mifflin, Boston.

Rojo-Mota, G., Pedrero-Pérez, E.J. & Huertas-Hoyas, E. (2017) Systematic review of occupational therapy in the treatment of addiction: models, practice, and qualitative and quantitative research. *American Journal of Occupational Therapy*, **71**(5) 7105100030p1–7105100030p11.

Ryan, D.A. & Boland, P. (2021) A scoping review of occupational therapy interventions in the treatment of people with substance use disorders. *Irish Journal of Occupational Therapy*, **49**(2), 104–114.

Saitz, R., Miller, S.C., Fiellin, D.A. & Rosenthal, R.N. (2021) Recommended use of terminology in addiction medicine. *Journal of Addiction Medicine*, **15**(1), 3–7. https://doi.org/10.1097/ADM.0000000000000673

Sarsak, H.I. (2018) Overview: occupational therapy for psychiatric disorders. *Journal of Psychology and Clinical Psychiatry*, **9**(5), 518–521.

Stevens, H., Redfearn, S. & Tse, S. (2003) Occupational therapy for people with dual diagnosis: a single case study. *British Journal of Therapy and Rehabilitation*, **10**(4), 166–173.

Sulzer, S.H., Prevedel, S., Barrett, T., Voss, M.W., Manning, C. & Madden, E.F. (2022) Professional education to reduce provider stigma toward harm reduction and pharmacotherapy. *Drugs: Education, Prevention and Policy,* **29**(5), 576–586. https://doi.org/10.1080/09687637.2021.1936457

Sussman, S. (2017) *Substance and Behavioral Addictions: Concepts, Causes, and Cures*, 1st edn. Cambridge University Press, Cambridge.

Sussman, S. & Sinclair, D.L. (2022) Substance and behavioral addictions, and their consequences among vulnerable populations. *International Journal of Environmental Research and Public Health*, **19**(10), 6163.

Syed, Z., De Bastos, M., Pindela, C. *et al* (2022) A rapid review of the roles of community rehabilitation workers in community-based mental health services in low-and middle-income countries. *Disability, CBR and Inclusive Development*, **33**(2), 108–128. https://doi.org/10.47985/dcidj.537

Thylstrup, B. & Johansen, K.S. (2009) Dual diagnosis and psychosocial interventions—introduction and commentary. *Nordic Journal of Psychiatry*, **63**(3), 202–208.

Twinley, R. & Addidle, G. (2012) Considering violence: the dark side of occupation. *British Journal of Occupational Therapy*, **75**(4), 202–204.

Vermeulen, N., Bell, T., Amod, A., Cloete, A., Johannes, T. & Williams, K. (2015) Students' fieldwork experiences of using community entry skills within community development. *South African Journal of Occupational Therapy*, **45**(2), 51–55. https://dx.doi.org/10.17159/2310-3833/2015/V45N2A8

Volkow, N.D. & Li, T.K. (2004) Drug addiction: the neurobiology of behavior gone awry. *Nature Reviews Neuroscience,* **5**(12), 963.

Wegner, L. (2011) Through the lens of a peer: understanding leisure boredom and risk behaviour in adolescence. *South African Journal of Occupational Therapy*, **41**(1), 18–24.

Wegner, L., Arend, T., Bassadien, R., Bismath, Z., Cross, L. (2014) Experiences of mothering drug-dependent youth: influences on occupational performance patterns. *South African Journal of Occupational Therapy*, **44**(2), 6–11.

Wei, Y. & Shah, R. (2020) Substance use disorder in the COVID-19 pandemic: a systematic review of vulnerabilities and complications. *Pharmaceuticals*, **13**(7), 155. https://doi.org/10.3390/ph13070155

West, R. & Brown, J. (2013) *Theory of Addiction.* Wiley Blackwell, London.

Wilcock, A.A. & Hocking, C. (2015) *An Occupational Perspective of Health*, 3rd edn. SLACK Incorporated, Thorofare, NJ.

World Health Organisation (2001) *Alcohol Use Disorders Identification Test (AUDIT)*. https://www.who.int/publications/i/item/WHO-MSD-MSB-01.6a (accessed on 23 May 2023)

World Health Organisation (2010) *The Alcohol, Smoking and Substance Involvement Screening Test (ASSIST)*. https://www.who.int/publications/i/item/978924159938-2 (accessed on 23 May 2023)

World Health Organisation (2023) *Substance abuse*. https://www.afro.who.int/health-topics/substance-abuse (accessed on 17 July 2023)

World Health Organisation, Health and Welfare Canada, Canadian Public Health Association (1986) *Ottawa Charter for Health Promotion*. WHO, Ottawa.

Yalom, I.D. (1995) *The Theory and Practice of Group Psychotherapy*. Basic Books, New York.

Zaami, S., Marinelli, E. & Varì, M.R. (2020) New trends of substance abuse during COVID-19 pandemic: an international perspective. *Front Psychiatry*, **16**(**11**), 700. https://doi.org/10.3389/fpsyt.2020.00700

CHAPTER 29

Gerontology, Psychiatry and Occupational Therapy

Susan Beukes[1], Rosemary Crouch[2], Zaakirah Haffejee[3] and Matty van Niekerk[4]

[1]Division of Occupational Therapy, Stellenbosch University, Tygerberg, South Africa
[2]School of Therapeutic Sciences, Faculty of Health Sciences, University of the Witwatersrand, Johannesburg, South Africa
[3]Occupational Therapy Department, Kingston Hospital NHS Trust, London, United Kingdom
[4]Department of Occupational Therapy, School of Therapeutic Sciences, Faculty of Health Sciences, University of the Witwatersrand, Johannesburg, South Africa

KEY LEARNING POINTS

- Understand the terminology used in this field such as gerontology, neurocognitive disorders, genomics and geriatrics.

- Understand the ageing process and its impact on behaviour and cognition.

- Understand what is entailed in the direct services to a person with a neurocognitive disorder/person who is ageing.

- Understand the depth and variety of services that can be implemented by the occupational therapists through indirect services to the elderly, both in prevention and intervention.

- Understand the process of managing the indirect services.

INTRODUCTION

It is reported worldwide that the elderly population is on the increase (World Health Organisation [WHO] 2022). There is, therefore, a growing need for occupational therapy interventions as a combination of direct and indirect services within the fields of gerontology and geriatrics. Gerontology is 'the study of the aging processes and individuals as they grow from middle age through later life' (University of Alaska Anchorage 2012). The term 'geriatrics' is viewed as 'the study of health and disease in later life' (Association for Gerontology in Higher Education 2012).

In order to determine which clinical services will be most effective for older persons, it is important to understand three broad areas: first, information on the ageing process and its impact on function; second, age-related diseases and disabilities (including how they affect health and well-being); and finally, current treatments and interventions of ageing people along with the specific clinical issues involved in working with older persons (Barney & Perkinson 2016). The occupational therapist is required to be knowledgeable in the theories and models of the profession of occupational therapy and how intervention is best implemented in this very rewarding area of practice.

The relatively new subject of genomics and its influence on neuropsychiatric conditions in the 21st century has implications for occupational therapy practice, for example the study of the genetic components of diseases such as Alzheimer's disease, which improves health through earlier diagnosis (thus improved prognosis) and more rational management of illness (Medical News.net 2014).

Theories and models of occupational therapy are important in the study of gerontology. This chapter discusses the

Crouch and Alers Occupational Therapy in Psychiatry and Mental Health, Sixth Edition.
Edited by Rosemary Crouch, Tania Buys, Enos Morankoana Ramano, Matty van Niekerk and Lisa Wegner.
© 2025 John Wiley & Sons Ltd. Published 2025 by John Wiley & Sons Ltd.

psychiatric disorders of later life and the mental health of the elderly, against the backdrop of holism and the bio-psycho-social model (BPSM), which is described below.

HOLISM

Since the establishment of occupational therapy as a profession, its philosophical basis has been rooted in a holistic approach. 'The holistic approach emphasises the organic and functional relationship between the parts of, and the whole, being. This approach maintains that a person is a whole – an interaction of biological, psychological, sociocultural and spiritual elements' (Hussey *et al.* 2007, p. 41). When relating these concepts to human beings, the authors refer to the interaction of all the different body structures and functions that contribute towards occupational performance, which is the aim of occupational therapy intervention.

The term 'holistic' is 'an approach that deems that each individual should be seen as a complete and unified whole rather than a series of parts or problems to be managed' (Hussey *et al.* 2007, p. 288). The concept of 'holism' is embedded in the paradigm and philosophy of the occupational therapy profession and is particularly pertinent to practice in the field of geriatrics and in particular psychogeriatrics. 'Holistic evaluation and assessments that explore participation (or barriers to participation) in meaningful occupations important to the caregivers (and clients), and subsequent interventions that caregivers deem as important to their life situation, are essential in the practice of occupational therapy' (Scaffa *et al.* 2010, p. 566). The following section illustrates how 'holism' is integrated into the BPSM.

Bio-Psycho-Social Model (BPSM)

In 1977, George Engel introduced the BPSM (Engel 1992, p. 317). The motivation he gave for developing the model was:

> To provide a basis for understanding the determinants of disease and arriving at a rational treatment and patterns of health care, a medical model must also take into account the patient, the social context in which he lives and the complementary system devised by society to deal with the disruptive effects of illness, that is, the physician role and the health care system. This requires a biopsychosocial model. (Lakham 2006, p. 1)

The BPSM, as proposed by Engel, was used as the basis for compiling an occupational therapy BPSM. This model can be viewed as a generic and practical model for occupational therapy interventions as it takes into account body functions and structures (biological and psychological) and environmental factors (social), which form the basis of the model and serve as building blocks for the execution of activities within various occupations. From an occupational therapy perspective, the BPSM may be used as a basic, but holistic model to understand the various components which may affect occupational performance throughout the ageing process. In this way, the occupational performance within various roles in relation to

the developmental level of the person, which ultimately determines the lifestyle of a person, can be established.

The occupational therapist working within a team needs to be able to communicate effectively with all team members; thus, using universally known and understood models and classification systems is important. Figure 29.1 takes into the consideration the BPSM in conjunction with the World Health Organisation's (WHO) International Classification of Functioning, Disability and Health (ICF) (WHO 2001). The ICF is a more global classification/framework and can be used across professions. It can be used in conjunction with the BPSM because it takes into consideration that functioning and disability exist within a context. Additionally, the ICF can be used for individuals and/or populations, making it appropriate for use in areas of occupational therapy which require group classifications. The ICF assigns a code to a group of disabilities or functional components where 'b' codes relate to body functions, 's' codes relate to body structures, 'd' codes describe activity and participation and 'e' codes relate to environmental components. The codes are allocated to a person or group of people based on their current presentation of functioning and disability. Table 29.1 summarises the ICF codes as of 2023.

'There is an increasing interest in various disciplines about the types and configurations of lifestyles that lend themselves to higher levels of satisfaction and general well-being; this, in turn, is health promoting through their opportunities for enjoyment, socialisation, challenge, rest, and recreation, personal growth and self-expression' (Scaffa *et al.* 2010, p. 537). Occupational therapy is situated in a prime

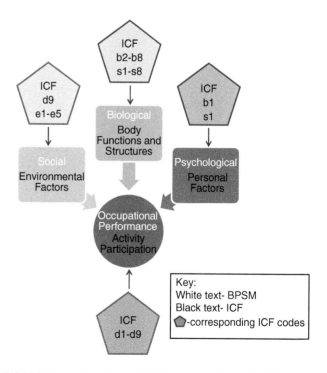

FIGURE 29.1 Depiction of BPSM in conjunction with ICF.
Source: WHO (2001)/WHO.

Table 29.1 Summary of ICF codes (WHO 2001).

Factor	Body functions (b)	Body structures (s)	Environmental (e)	Activity and participation (d)
Codes	b1: mental functions	s1: nervous system	e1: products and technology	d1: learning/knowledge application
	b2: sensory and pain functions	s2: eye/ear and related structures	e2: natural environment/man-made environment	d2: general tasks and demands
	b3: voice and speech	s3: voice and speech structures	e3: support and relationships	d3: communication
	b4: cardiovascular/haematological/immunological/respiratory functions	s4: cardiovascular/immunological/respiratory structures	e4: attitudes	d4: mobility
	b5: digestive, metabolic and endocrine functions	s5: digestive, metabolic and endocrine structures	e5: services, systems, policies	d5: self-care
	b6: genitourinary/reproductive functions	s6: genitourinary/reproductive structures		d6: domestic life
	b7: neuromusculoskeletal and movement functions	s7: structures related to movement		d7: interpersonal interactions
	b8: skin and related functions	s8: skin and related structures		d8: major life areas
				d9: community/social/civic life

position to provide this by presenting elderly persons with opportunities for occupational engagement whereby they can experience health-promoting lifestyles. An example includes planning and organising activity programmes for the elderly in various settings.

The ageing process affects all biological and psychological body functions, which directly affects occupational performance and fulfilment of various roles. 'A specific occupation may also be carried out in different roles and contexts, which will influence how that occupation is performed' (Hussey *et al.* 2007, p. 44). The ageing person is most likely to have major changes in the occupations of work (they may retire or change work roles) and/or Personal Activities of Daily Living (PADLs) and Instrumental Activities of Daily Living (IADLs) (as physical and psychological abilities change). Changes in, or loss of, roles are realities for persons in late adulthood and in later life and occur due to changes in the activity profiles as a result of ageing. Duration of performing different roles varies depending on the developmental stage of a person. However, opportunities should be created for people to participate in various age-related activities that can result in the fulfilment of new roles in new communities where they may be relocated. Examples include homes for the aged or psychogeriatric wards in hospitals. Both areas can be viewed as communities on their own. Social structures, in this case the communities, have four features, namely, 'values, norms, collective groups and roles' (Jones 2002, p. 42).

Occupational therapists must assess whether these features, specifically opportunities for role fulfilment, are present in the environment where the people live – this can be in homes for the aged, in their own homes or in a psychogeriatric ward in a hospital. Some international guidelines suggest that a range of group and one-to-one activities should be provided to older people, largely due to their risk of decline in independence and mental well-being (NICE 2016). In other situations, the occupational therapists can organise activity programmes that include age-appropriate activities to create social structures providing opportunities for a variety of roles to be performed, such as team member, participant and chairperson. Participation in activities generates opportunities to fulfil roles, which can result in individuals who find themselves in a process of role transition because of ageing performing new roles. New roles arising from ageing may include that of a retiree and/or grandmother/grandfather.

New roles go hand-in-hand with the concept of 'role making' as described by Jones (2002, p. 16): 'Roles are created, moulded and modified by individuals themselves, according to their own interpretation, and is therefore more in concert with an interactionist perspective'. Role fulfilment varies according to each stage of development. It is very important to emphasise the importance of providing the elderly with choices related to role fulfilment: 'Roles are a source of identity and are the framework for everyday life' (Jones 2002, p. 16).

Environmental factors influence occupational performance within various roles. It is necessary to identify the different effects each environmental factor has on occupational performance for the appropriate actions to be taken, therefore minimising negative effects. 'The Model of Occupational Role Performance' as described by Hillman and Chapparo (in Jones 2002, p. 51) confirms that the interaction between persons and their environments is interdependent and determines the person's occupational role performance.

DIRECT INTERVENTION BY OCCUPATIONAL THERAPY WITH PSYCHOGERIATRICS

This section is based on the chapter by Rae Labuschagne in Crouch and Alers (2005).

Persons with psychogeriatric disorders are found in a hospital setting in most countries; however, in the rural areas of South Africa and elsewhere in the Global South, there are sometimes severely mentally and physically disabled elderly members of a family/community tucked away in isolated rooms or dwellings. Very few services are available to these individuals (and their caregivers), putting the disabled elderly community members at risk of occupational deprivation. Older adults exposed to occupational deprivation may be at a greater risk for physical and mental decline. Decreased ability to participate in occupations can lead to physical and mental comorbidities such as increased frailty or depression. Additionally, faster rates of mental decline may be seen in older adults with dementia resulting from occupational deprivation (Zinger & Roche 2020). The BPSM can enable the occupational therapist to identify the areas in which direct intervention will be required when assessing a person.

Occupational therapists play an important role in combatting occupational deprivation. In the field of psychogeriatrics, occupational therapists can play a direct role, for example by identifying those who are at risk of deterioration, among others by considering the individual's recent life events (loss of a partner, retirement, driving cessation, illness and living alone/loneliness) (NICE 2016). Occupational therapists will encounter two main diagnostic areas where intervention is required, namely, minor and major neurocognitive disorders (APA 2022) and affective disorders. Both categories offer unique challenges to the occupational therapist and their patients. In addition, occupational therapists need to be aware of the fact that conditions such as Alzheimer's disease and depression do not exist as isolated conditions and there may well be concomitant illnesses in ageing patients.

CHANGES IN THE ELDERLY

As people age, various stressors occur that are specifically related to the ageing process. If a person is undergoing a process of neurocognitive decline and impairment, there are specific changes related to this process which, if the person is aware of in the early part of the illness, are very distressing. These changes include memory loss, disorientation, deterioration in physical health and, very importantly, the possible relocation of the person to another environment. These changes can often result in challenges and stressors for the patient, family and carers.

This section of the chapter is mostly concerned with the changes caused by ageing which may result in stress to the elderly person. These include financial issues, physical health issues, cognitive changes, changes in the ability to perform occupations, relocation from environments often to a retirement village or to the family, family relationships, loss of a partner and other circumstances which affect elderly people in different ways depending on the culture and socio-economic status of the person.

PHYSICAL DETERIORATION

While ageing may cause various forms of physical deterioration, some of the most common changes are visual deterioration (including conditions such as cataracts), hearing loss, muscle weakness and decreased mobility. Balance may also be significantly affected. Elderly patients also tend to have a higher prevalence of bone disorders such as osteoporosis and joint disorders like arthritis. Because of the physical deterioration that comes with ageing, this population tend to experience more falls, leading to hospital admissions, fractures and other health complications. Because of the societal notion that older people should 'rest', many ageing individuals will experience general physical deconditioning.

COGNITIVE CHANGES/DETERIORATION

'Normal aging is accompanied by alterations in brain structure and function, and associated cognitive changes' (Kirk-Sanchez & McGough 2014, p. 51). In the ageing adult, atrophy of the brain is a common occurrence and atrophy in the temporal, frontal and parietal regions of the brain and in individuals with mild cognitive impairment and Alzheimer's disease showing atrophy of the hippocampus too. The atrophy in these parts of the brain can easily explain the difficulties this population has with memory, attention, executive functions (including multi-tasking), behavioural changes and a slowed reaction speed. These cognitive changes result in difficulty performing occupations to the same standard and efficiency as the individual did prior.

CHANGE IN OCCUPATIONAL PERFORMANCE

Because of the various changes (biological, psychological and possible social) associated with ageing, the BPSM can be used to explain the likelihood of changes in the ability to perform occupations. Many elderly persons become activities unhealthy because they lack participation in some occupations (work, home management, meal preparation etc.) and replace that time with excessive time spent on passive activities, for example sleeping or watching television.

One of the most significant changes to occupational performance in early ageing is work. Once the individual retires, new occupational roles may replace the role of a worker for some people; however, this is not the case with all individuals. In many countries in the Global South taking on hobbies or additional leisure tasks may be too costly for people whose main aim is financially supporting their families even post-retirement. Retirement may also result in social isolation and/or a lack of purpose, which could have negative effects on psychological well-being. The occupational therapist who is in contact with individuals reaching retirement may include aspects of retirement planning in their interventions. This may include financial management skills, goal setting and future planning, and the possibility of other roles that may replace the worker role.

Another important occupation which should be considered is community mobility in the elderly population as this could have major impacts on their ability to attend social/leisure groups, medical appointments or maintain social interaction with family and/or friends. Driving is a component of community mobility which is considered important in order to maintain independence. With age comes muscle weakness, visual changes and cognitive changes (including slowed reaction times and thought processing), all of which could have potentially negative impacts on driving ability. Older persons are often reluctant to stop driving, especially those who live alone and who do not have good support systems (nearby). In countries, often in the Global South, where public transport systems are either poorly developed or inaccessible to people with disabilities (or both), elderly people may be even more resistant to driving cessation due to the significant impact on their community mobility and ability to perform chores and tasks that cannot be done without driving. However, occupational therapists must recognise the ethical and legal implications for an elderly person who continues to drive and the risks to the community (e.g. fellow road users) and to the elderly person's financial future that arise from accidents and related lawsuits (Carr & Ott 2010). Recurrent minor dings and scratches and small repairs at the panel beater are indications that the elderly person may no longer be safe to drive, but elderly people often hide these incidents from their families and other support systems. The loss of driving ability and resulting loss of independence or participation in other occupations have been shown to have an adverse impact on mood (causing depression) and causing decreased quality of life of individuals who are already vulnerable to occupational deprivation. The cessation of driving in older adults also places more responsibility on their families or carers, who often need to meet transportation needs for their elderly relatives or find alternative transport for them (Connell et al. 2013). Driving cessation planning must be part of retirement planning that should occur by the latest when a person reaches their 50s – retirement planning is about more than just having enough money to live out one's old age: it is also about maintaining a productive activity profile post-retirement, and making decisions about transitions towards driving cessation and assisted living.

STRESS IN THE ELDERLY

Stress is not a concept that is difficult to define but does influence both the body and the mind. Stress relies on the coping mechanisms of a person, and it is known that stress for one person is not necessarily the same for another. It also depends on how well the individual can cope and the environmental factors surrounding the elderly person. Parkview Health (2021) states that stress is a normal part of everyday life, but it can be debilitating for older adults. 'Stress for seniors often manifests in more physical ways, including health problems. Warning signs of stress could include frequent headaches, sleep problems, insomnia, fatigue (physical and mental), difficulty concentrating, change in appetite, muscle tension, pain, chest pain, stomach upset and more' (Parkview Health 2021, pp. 2–4).

An occupational therapist can play an important role in assisting the elderly person recognise and accept that stress is a normal part of life and that there are ways to deal with it. An occupational therapist treating an elderly person should note that:

> '. . . one thing the senior community has in their favour is that they have lived. They have undoubtedly gone through many different forms of stress and change in their lifetime. They have developed resilience, which is the ability to bounce back from difficult situations'. (Parkview Health 2021, pp. 1–4)

DEPRESSIVE DISORDERS

Unfortunately, depression is a common disorder in the elderly. Whether older people become more susceptible to depression as they age is questionable, but the losses which occur during the ageing process, which may range from changes in health status to loss of the family home, spouse, income or friends often precedes a depressive episode. It is likely that similar losses would adversely affect younger individuals in the same way, but for many older people, these losses may be experienced in a condensed period of time, and the individual may feel highly vulnerable. It is unfortunate that depression in the elderly often goes untreated by doctors and unrecognised by friends, families and carers who assume that old age is a depressing time. The elderly themselves may resist seeking help from health professionals for a number of reasons such as denial, not wanting to be a 'nuisance' and lack of knowledge of such illnesses. Importantly, acute, as well as mild, depression in

the aged generally reacts well to therapy and medication (American Psychiatric Association [APA] 2022).

MINOR AND MAJOR NEUROCOGNITIVE DISORDERS (PREVIOUSLY CALLED DEMENTIA)

Neurocognitive disorders (commonly known as dementias) are the global impairment of the higher cortical functions including memory, the capacity to solve problems of day-to-day living, the use of perceptual motor skills and the control of emotional reactions. It occurs in the absence of gross clouding of consciousness. The condition is often irreversible and progressive (APA 2022). These disorders present a different kind of challenge to depression, particularly when gross deterioration has taken place. Of all the neurocognitive disorders, Alzheimer's disease is the most prevalent among the aged. It is described as a subtype of a neurocognitive disorder characterised by problems with learning, memory, behaviour, emotion and reasoning (Aderinwale et al. 2010). It is now among the top ten leading causes of death (WHO 2012). It causes high health care costs; therefore, facilitating the preservation of participation in occupations and the ability to stay in the community is a priority for occupational therapy intervention (Voigt-Radloff et al. 2011).

With the deficits that occur with Alzheimer's disease and other neurocognitive disorders such as vascular neurocognitive disorder, caregivers, particularly in facilities where 24-hour care is provided, tend to concentrate on the basic physiological needs of the individual. These needs, as well as those of security, are generally fulfilled. However, the more esoteric needs of the individual, such as a sense of belonging and acceptance, opportunities that foster feelings of self-esteem and self-actualisation and achieving a sense of integrity, may be ignored. These needs are often less tolerated and considered to be too much of a challenge or are simply considered by caregivers to be impossible to meet. To complicate matters, the pathology present and the demands of an effective programme often lead to stress in the carers, burnout and a quick turnover of staff.

It is these higher needs that embody the uniqueness of the individual and acknowledge the fact that, despite gross deterioration in many areas, both cognitive and functional, the needs are real and present. Satisfying these needs, in the face of an inexorable passage of the illness and of the life course itself, becomes the challenge to occupational therapists.

Erikson (1997) said of the last phase of life that the individual strives to achieve a sense of integrity versus despair. The elderly person without dementia can express their preferences and needs and may be given the opportunity to realise them and achieve a sense of integrity and self-actualisation. Where possible, it is important for the occupational therapist to offer choices to the client with dementia as well, even if it is difficult.

In this very important area of occupational therapy intervention, the services of occupational therapy assistants

(OTAs) and occupational therapy technicians (OTTs) can be employed. They work closely with the nursing staff and nursing assistants. All work within the multidisciplinary team but have more hands-on experience.

Before commencing any type of intervention, however, a thorough assessment must take place.

ASSESSING COGNITIVE AND PHYSICAL LEVELS INCLUDING PRINCIPLES OF PRESENTING ACTIVITIES

Thorough assessments of the cognitive and physical abilities must be done on an on-going basis and should be complemented by on-going observation and reporting. These assessments form the basis of any planned activities. *The Diagnostic and Statistical Manual of Mental Disorders, Fifth Edition, Text Revision* (DSM-5-TR) (APA 2022) does not recommend the use of the Mini-Mental State Examination (MMSE) or the Montreal Cognitive Assessment screening tools for formal diagnosis. Formal testing by a psychometrist is recommended.

Clinical observations and the use of both creative activities and occupation-based tasks (including PADLs and IADLs) are excellent tools used by the occupational therapist to determine the level at which the patient is functioning, for example, the Activity Participation Outcome Measure (APOM) (Casteleijn & Graham 2012) and Functional Levels Outcome Measure (FLOM) (Zietsman 2011). An understanding of the Vona du Toit Model of Creative Ability (VdTMoCA) in relation to the assessment of the elderly is needed in order to use these assessments effectively, since they are all based on the VdTMoCA (see Chapter 2).

An awareness of the symptoms of the illness and their manifestation is extremely important for any assessment to be done. The guidelines in the following section outline the problematic abilities of the patient with a neurocognitive disorder, as well as the influence these have on possible activities.

NEUROCOGNITIVE DISORDER PROBLEMS

Orientation

Many patients will have difficulty keeping track of the date and time of day, and during advanced stages of the neurocognitive disorder, they may perform activities at incorrect times of the day because of this. They may also be disorientated to person and place, which will cause them distress. It is important to structure the environment in a way that facilitates orientation and encouraging routine activities during appropriate times of the day.

Abstract Thought

The patient will have problems with logic, insight and abstract concepts and ideas. Activities are more likely to be successful when the occupational therapist breaks them down into their simplest and most concrete steps and demonstrates one step at a time.

Concentration and Attention

Sustained concentration and attention become problematic, and to initiate and sustain an activity and bring it to its logical conclusion is difficult. Activities should be tailored to the attention and concentration span of individual patients. If even just one step of an activity is completed and enjoyed by the patient, then it could be said that it has been successful. The fact that activities are short and may not occupy the major part of the day is very often problematic for families who are concerned about their family members not being busy all day. Education of families about the illness and about the ageing process is important.

Executive Functioning

This is primarily divided into four components:

- **Volition** refers to 'the complex process of determining what one needs or wants and conceptualising some kind of future realisation of that need or want' (Lezak 1995, p. 651).

- **Planning** refers to 'the identification and organisation of the steps and elements (e.g. skills, materials, other persons) needed to carry out an intention or achieve a goal' (Lezak 1995, p. 655).

- **Purposeful action** is 'the translation of an intention or plan into productive, self-serving activity requires the actor to initiate, maintain, switch, and stop sequences of complex behaviour in an orderly and integrated manner' (Lezak 1995, p. 658).

- **Effective performance** means that 'a performance is as effective as the performer's ability to monitor, self-correct, and regulate the intensity, tempo, and other qualitative aspects of delivery' (Lezak 1995, p. 674).

Given the complex components of executive functioning, the occupational therapist needs to take care not to set the patient up for failure, but rather set the patient up to achieve. This is only possible if assessments are accurate and sensitive and if activities are broken into their simplest steps. The occupational therapist needs to often demonstrate and act as the initiator for those patients who have no volition or are not able to initiate an idea, movement or action themselves. For example, if the patient demonstrates apraxia, the occupational therapist may hold their hand and demonstrate the movement or action needed. Often, the patient may not be able to complete all the steps of the activity, but whatever they can do should be encouraged, and the occupational therapist should offer help and support throughout the activity.

Activities with the aged are more likely to succeed if they fall within the field of reference and experience of the patient. The occupational therapist once again needs to have an accurate history of the patient as a tool for planning meaningful activities.

INTERACTING WITH PEOPLE WHO HAVE COGNITIVE IMPAIRMENTS

In their seminal work, Nissenboim and Vroman (2000, pp. 34, 35) recommend the following four steps when planning interactions with people who have cognitive impairments: familiarising, naming, demonstrating, encouraging and rewarding.

FAMILIARISING

The occupational therapist describes the object while the patient familiarises themself with it and is encouraged to use all appropriate senses in the familiarisation process such as hearing, feeling and touching.

NAMING

In this step, the occupational therapist names the object(s) being handled and encourages the person to do so. Nissenboim and Vroman (2000) stress that no pressure should be placed on the person and that they need to receive approbation and recognition for any attempt to respond.

DEMONSTRATING

Visual, tactile and auditory focus is provided by the occupational therapist. Occupational therapists need to remember that executive functioning is a problem with cognitively impaired people, so that any activity should be broken down into its simplest steps and be performed as discrete activities.

ENCOURAGING AND REWARDING

We all need encouraging and rewarding for efforts made. Recognition of a person's attempt to participate is essential for self-esteem. The occupational therapist should consider the individual's feelings, and this forms a bond and creates a feeling that the interaction has been a participatory one and satisfying to both the client and the occupational therapist.

CREATING AN APPROPRIATE THERAPEUTIC ENVIRONMENT

By providing a calm, relaxed atmosphere where there is a consistent routine, which is geared to the habits and strengths of the individuals in the unit, the occupational therapist is able to encourage the individual to function optimally with self-respect in an atmosphere of trust and security. If the routine is staff- and not patient-orientated, it may well defeat the purpose.

Cognisance of the normal sensory deficits of ageing is important, and attention should be given to the fact, for example, that more lighting is needed for the older eye and that older eyes are sensitive to bright sunlight and flickering florescent lights. However, the physical environment should compensate not only for sensory deficits and losses but for cognitive ones as well. An appropriate environment should be:

- Consistent and predictable
- Unambiguous, with discrete areas clearly defined for various activities and functions (e.g. furniture may give clues as to the use of the space)
- One that provides neither too much nor too little stimulation
- Sensitive to the declining abilities of the individual and make an attempt to compensate for these
- Small rather than large
- One in which the individual is able to function optimally
- One which preserves skills
- One which encourages optimal use of skills and abilities
- One which will compensate for cognitive deficits by providing cues (e.g. for special orientation)
- One in which the person feels safe (this should include aspects of psychological and physical safety)
- One which allows for habits and customs of a lifetime
- One which encourages and preserves long-term memories and relationships
- Appropriate for adults, as patients should continue to function as such
- Reflective of the experience of the particular cohort and cultures
- One that encourages the residents to want to participate in familiar activities such as bed making (use duvets which are simple to pull up), setting tables, removing dishes, dusting and sweeping

PROMOTION OF AWARENESS AND ORIENTATION

It is also important for the therapeutic environment to promote orientation and maximise awareness. Possible techniques are to:

- Use simple unambiguous signs, as residents may not be able to comprehend complex language.
  - Signs should make use of fonts that are easy to read (block letters) and large enough for the elderly person to see.
- Place signs at eye level.
- Use bright contrasting colours
- Create personalised doors to make each patient's room more relevant and understandable to the residents, for example hang favourite photographs or personal moments

on the bedroom door and make sure that they are securely attached to the door or wall.

- Follow a regular schedule by doing the same activities in the same location. Routine and familiarity are important.

- Create purpose-specific rooms if possible so that residents always know what to expect when they enter, for example, do not have the dining room doubling as an activity room.

- Make areas such as the bathrooms and lounges easily visible.

- Disguise exits and underplay the visibility of rooms that the residents should not use. This may be done by attaching mirrors, and hanging curtains or posters in front of the doors.

- All furniture and bathroom equipment such as beds, easy chairs, toilets and showers should be so designed that they promote the physical independence of the patient.

- Environmental accessories should be carefully considered such as having dementia-friendly clocks on walls (large numbers, contrasting colours, date and day visible).

SENSORY STIMULATION

Another area to note is that of sensory stimulation, and the occupational therapist should be sensitive to over- and under-stimulation of clients' sensory processes. By in-depth assessments of the patients, occupational therapists can determine each person's particular threshold level. It is a challenge to provide a balance so that the individual is not subjected to overload or, conversely, sensory deprivation. Loud noises, be it music, talk or housekeeping sounds; untidy and disorderly rooms; and materials and equipment that are not stored neatly, or not stored at all, can distract the resident who may already have a short attention span. Make sure that only the materials and equipment for that specific activity are visible. Limit the extraneous distractions, both auditory, visual and other, as far as possible. Occupational therapists should consider integrating daily occupations and physical exercise into the daily routine of adults with neurocognitive diseases (such as Alzheimer's disease) to enhance occupational performance and delay functional decline (Smallfield & Heckenlaible 2017).

DIRECT SERVICE DELIVERY TO THE ELDERLY COMMUNITY

Occupational therapists mainly encounter groups of elderly people in areas such as community centres where senior citizens may spend time during the day or at homes for the aged. The reality is that nowadays, elderly people utilise the option of living in their own homes rather than retiring into centres of care due to the development of support systems within the arena of service delivery. This is termed as 'ageing in place' and is one of six areas identified by Baum (2007, p. 53 in Hussey *et al.*) as emerging practice areas for occupational therapy. The occupational therapist can offer a variety of services that enable the elderly person to live in their own homes for longer. These services include:

- Modifications in the home whereby independent functioning in self-care activities can be possible

- Considerations for and assessment of community mobility, be it the continuation of driving (with or without adaptations), driving cessation or alternative transportation options, which may be considered with family

- The provision of assistive devices to compensate for functional decline or loss

- Establishment of support systems in communities that provide the necessary support to elderly who wish to stay or are able to stay at home

- Retirement planning which may include retirement from work and driving, and be done in conjunction with older persons and their families

Collaboration with the family or caregiver of the elderly person aids the occupational therapist to assess whether staying at home is a viable option. Collaboration with family may also be useful in order to establish means for the elderly to remain socially active. Many elderly persons will have adult children who may be able to drive them to meet transportation needs and assist with maintaining community mobility if the elderly person should cease to drive (Connell *et al.* 2013). Family may also be able to supervise driving and ensure the elderly person is following recommendations such as only driving at specific times, shorter distances or driving at slower speeds. These considerations and affordances are a new area for investigation for direct occupational therapy intervention.

Occupational therapy interventions at the level of body functions or at the level of participation in occupations are dependent on the problem areas and needs of each person. These interventions, at the basic and integrated psychological level, can be related to a specific psychiatric diagnosis. Simultaneously, interventions to the basic and integrated biological functions may also be necessary; for example a person diagnosed with Alzheimer's disease may also suffer from rheumatoid arthritis. Direct occupational therapy services at this level will be therapeutic or compensatory in nature and will be aimed at treating certain body functions or compensating for permanent loss of body functions with the objective of employing activities to improve or adapt to the body functions in order to ultimately enhance occupational performance.

Once body functions and structures are restored to their optimal level, the focus shifts to restoring the three abilities, namely, knowledge, skill and attitude. Consequently, these abilities permit execution of occupations like PADLs, leisure time and work/productivity activities and also IADL, that is, financial management, transport and participation in community activities. Once the person participates in these activities, a level of occupational performance is established that enables the person to perform age-related roles and have their own lifestyle.

The occupational therapist plays a pivotal role in the continued planning, organising and presentation of activity programmes in homes for the aged and/or in communities. Volunteers and other team members often present activities as well. The following should be taken into account by the occupational therapist:

- The environment – physical layout of the home, facilities and the accessibility. This should not limit participation in activities, and services should be accessible to a population who may have varying physical accessibility needs.

- A safe environment for the elderly can be obtained by establishing a fall prevention team that will monitor on a regular basis all the risk areas in the home where falls may occur. Nonetheless, one of the key problems in relation to falls is that individuals do not report falling due to the fear of being moved to other areas, for example the care unit in the home. For elderly people living in their own homes, pendant alarms may sometimes be a safety net in countries that can support this.

- Another factor that may prevent participation in activities is a hearing problem. Individuals may not hear announcements of available activities, which limits their participation and can ultimately lead to isolation. Therefore, it is necessary to post and update information regularly on notice boards that are accessible to all.

- Memory impairments of the elderly person may result in the individual forgetting that they have an appointment or group to attend or how to get to the community centres. Being disorientated to day and time may cause elderly people to attend activities on the wrong day. The occupational therapist should routinise activities, have consistent days and times for certain activities and provide this population with appropriate reminders.

- A vitally important factor for the occupational therapist to consider is consent. The elderly population with neurocognitive disorders who have poor memory, decision-making, judgement and reasoning skills may have difficulty consenting to interventions or remembering that they have consented. Capacity to consent may also be affected. The occupational therapist should consider written consent so that documents serve as a reminder for the individual, gaining consent prior to each session or gaining consent from family. When presenting information to this group of individuals, the occupational therapist may provide both written and verbal information so that written information can be kept by the elderly person as a reminder. Ideally, retirement planning should include identifying a suitably qualified professional, or appropriate family member such as an adult child/grandchild, to act as administrator

when the elderly person no longer can make decisions, both in the health care context and regarding managing their finances. Depending on the context, this may need to be a formal process through the courts, which can be costly, and thus appropriate funding should be set aside for it.

By adapting activity processes and materials, the occupational therapist can ensure participation in spite of limitations that the elderly may experience. The following activities or programmes can provide opportunities for meaningful occupational engagement of the elderly person.

ORIENTATION PROGRAMME FOR NEW INHABITANTS IN A HOME FOR THE AGED

It is important to establish a welcoming committee that will accept the responsibility to orientate and integrate the new inhabitants in the home. This can aid the success of the orientation programme. Programmes may be presented over a two-week period during which individuals are familiarised with the facilities, activities, programmes and the community where homes are situated. Once a month, a welcoming party can, depending on the arrival of new inhabitants, conclude the orientation programme.

CAREGIVER GROUP

A healthy population within a home can serve as caregivers to other groups. Examples include visits to patients in sickbays and accompanying people diagnosed with Alzheimer's disease for walks to maintain their physical fitness.

Groups for caregivers can also be run to educate and empower caregivers with knowledge and strategies on how to deal with various aspects of the ageing person, for example how to manage behaviour changes and how to facilitate engagement in activity.

PROJECT GROUPS

Group projects are run in relation to needs identified in the communities. These may include knitting baby jerseys for the maternity section of a nearby hospital and cooking for a soup kitchen at a shelter or for a school in a sub-economic area.

ADOPT-A-GRANNY

A group of active elderly individuals can be responsible for preparing and serving refreshments on a weekly basis to fellow elders in frail care or sickbays. This provides the more active elderly individuals with the opportunity to serve a meaningful purpose and be able to make a valuable contribution to their community. This presents people in sickbays with something to look forward to, to participate in a meaningful activity and thus be less isolated from the rest of the home.

EXCURSIONS

Voluntary workers or service groups can organise monthly excursions to places or shows in the community. Participating in such activities may provide topics for discussion and stimulate interest in what is happening outside the home. For some residents, completing their own toiletry or snack shopping may be a means of expressing their individuality, independence and choice. This could be facilitated through bi-monthly shopping outings, which may be supervised and transport provided. This also maintains orientation of cost of living and IADL performance in financial management and shopping.

HELPING THE ELDERLY MANAGE STRESS

First, the older person must be made aware of what is causing the debilitating stress. To overcome the daily challenges, the occupational therapist can 'help patients learn how to perform exercises and rehabilitation techniques that make it easier for patients to perform ADLS: These activities of daily living include walking, dressing, eating, and toileting' (Liberty Health Care and Rehab 2023, pp. 4–8). Discussions on family relationships and methods of communicating with them can help too. Behavioural issues such as continually complaining about everything and 'how it is not like it used to be in the old days', including angry responses and general aggression can be discussed in a very diplomatic way.

Involving the elderly person in positive activity is essential. Becoming involved in activity groups and discussions, participating in events in the local environment such as attending visiting therapy dog sessions, interesting talks and music presentations and learning new skills such as painting, woodwork and carving, baking demonstrations, playing memory enhancing activities including puzzles and crosswords. Some may be fit enough to attend Tai Chi, Pilates or line dancing sessions, if available to them.

What if an old person lives in a community where facilities such as those mentioned above do not exist? In South Africa and other parts of the Global South a number of occupational therapists work in this type of environment, and old people are encouraged to be inactive and to sit and be wise. Activities, however, are available, such as vegetable gardening, (often in containers for easy access), feeding the chickens, taking regular walks, attending 'indabas' (community talks on local subjects), being asked to cook a favourite meal and attending religious meetings. It is important to talk to the family and encourage them to include and activate the elderly person. In some contexts, teachers involve elderly community members in activities with junior primary school children linked to significant cultural or national events. This provides the children with a link to their cultural roots, as well as a sense of belonging and value to the elderly community members, after all, 'community participation is integral in wellness' (Mulry *et al.* 2017, p. 7).

REGARDFUL HANDLING OF THE OLDER PATIENT

Some older people can be difficult as regards their behaviour. Often this is because the person is aware of their lack of faculty in various areas, or possibly they have always been difficult personalities and age is not improving the situation. How an occupational therapist handles an elderly person is extremely important. There is a tendency worldwide, however, for people generally to belittle old people – Hello dearie, hello granny, how are you *Gogo* [granny], or *Madala* [old man] (Zulu), how are you today old girl/man, or calling a person by their first name but changing it to a child's name, for example Barbie instead of Barbara. It must be borne in mind by the occupational therapist that a person is entitled to their correct name and status and that this should be recognised. In this way, a lot of stress will be relieved for both the occupational therapist and the elderly person. Furthermore, it is important to call the person by their proper name that they are accustomed to, for example, Mrs Evans or Dr Jones. It depends a lot on the culture. This assists with orientating the person to their identity and also shows respect for the individual, which might make them more cooperative with occupational therapy interventions.

As many older people may experience anxiety when doing things and may be more fearful to move around because of their physical deterioration, it is important that the occupational therapist recognises this anxiety and fear and is able to converse with the patient in a calm, comforting and encouraging manner. Older individuals who are anxious to mobilise should be provided with physical and psychological support and reassurance when mobilising initially, and this support can be decreased as their confidence improves.

LEARNING TO BALANCE AND CONTROL STRESS

Just identifying the cause of stress is not enough. The occupational therapist must work with the patient on learning to both balance and control the stress. Looking at the causes of the stress will help in advising and involving the older person in activities that will help control the stress. It is often difficult to change an elderly person's way of running their life, but it can be done. A good relationship with the person is imperative. Gently persuading them to participate in activities already discussed, making a programme (which includes exercise and other activities so many times a week) and regular conversations and discussions go a long way towards ensuring that the client follows the programme. Group activities such as those described in Crouch (2021, pp. 126–128), are relevant, for example 'to learn how to recognise and cope with stress in the best possible way. How to balance one's lifestyle, change how things are accomplished and adapt to being older without causing unhappiness. In other words, how to control stress' (Crouch 2021, p. 127).

OCCUPATIONAL GROUP THERAPY

- *Discussion groups:* 'Health talks' on various health- and age-related topics, reminiscence groups where topics identified by the elderly themselves can be discussed.

- *Weekly activity/game groups:* By presenting various weekly activity/game groups, a daily activity programme can be created. Activities that can be completed in one session may include the making of birthday cards. Besides the aforementioned, on-going activities, such as knitting or patchwork groups, can be presented. Inhabitants can act as chairpersons of reading groups, of bridge club or of committees such as a social activity committee. A weekly bingo group where prizes can be won is a popular and much-enjoyed activity.

- *Exercise groups:* Simple stretching and breathing exercises are a good start to the day and motivate the elderly person to participate in daily activities. They are particularly important for those who are depressed as movement lifts the mood. Exercise reduces cardiovascular risk factors and improves fitness, both of which have correlated with improved cognitive performance and brain health in older adults. Programs should be structured well, have multiple components (aerobics, resistance exercises and cardiovascular exercises) and be of longer duration (two days a week for multiple weeks) to be most effective (Kirk-Sanchez & Mcgough 2014).

VALIDATION THERAPY

'Validation therapy' is an interesting approach to managing the institutionalised disorientated elderly person. Validation has been described as 'a helping method that restores dignity and well-being to disorientated old people by accepting them the way they are. Validation respects their intuitive wisdom. What they do and what they say has meaning' (Feil 1993). The actions of a disorientated elderly person are often misinterpreted as being meaningless. Validation therapy offers an alternative perspective to the communication and actions by meeting the person in their space and point in time and acknowledging the reality offered by the person. This is in direct contrast to reality orientation, where the aim is to orientate the person to the here and now. Validation therapy underlines the principle of not ignoring what a person offers during a conversation, but rather to meet the individual where they are at a particular point in time by acknowledging the information communicated and to then steer the communication to the present time and situation.

INDIRECT OCCUPATIONAL THERAPY SERVICES

The indirect occupational therapy services are described by Reed and Sanderson (1980, p. 142) as 'those which do not involve the consumer directly but provide dimensions to improve and augment the delivery of direct services'. The indirect service implies that no direct personal contact with the patients/clients is made by the occupational therapist.

Patients/clients benefit as the indirect services create the platform for the effective and efficient delivery of direct services to an individual or groups of persons.

The contribution of indirect services towards creating structures for the execution of direct services is often not given the acknowledgement they deserve as the focus tends to only be on direct service delivery. This often limits the contribution of the occupational therapist to groups and communities as the direct interventions are mostly geared towards individual persons.

The indirect services include (Reed & Sanderson 1980):

- Education, including educating the broader community and community leaders about retirement planning

- Management and supervision

- Cooperation with team members

- Record-keeping and reporting

- Consultation

- Research

- Advocacy

- Networking, that is with community and/or religious leaders to enhance opportunities for elderly community members' community engagement

In the following section, each of the indirect services will be discussed in relation to service delivery to groups of elderly persons.

EDUCATION

A primary aim of education is to impart knowledge, skills and attitudes to team members and caregivers on how to make activity participation possible for elderly persons. This includes handling principles and adaptations to activities and to the environment. An essential aspect when working in a home for the aged is to develop competencies by providing education about physical handling principles to the nursing staff or caregivers who physically manage elderly persons who need care. Examples of other stakeholders to whom education can be provided that will benefit the elderly persons indirectly are:

- Family members – education on handling principles in relation to the diagnosis and its progression. Scaffa *et al.* (2010, p. 409) state that 'Assisting caregivers who are coping with caregiving challenges, whether chronic or acute, can be of enormous benefit to enhancing the life and quality of life of both the caregiver and the client'.

- Voluntary workers – providing information on basic handling principles in relation to specific problems the elderly persons may experience.

- Management committee of a home for the aged or community centres on the programmes and activities that will contribute to promoting occupational performance resulting in healthy lifestyles of the inhabitants/attendees. Occupational therapists can also propose structural adaptations to the environment to enable participation in activities (Nelson 1997, p. 12).

- Community members – provide education to community groups about the needs of the elderly and which resources can be provided to enable the elderly to participate in the community. The general community should also be educated on the importance of community integration for the ageing population. Community initiatives should encourage the participation of ageing individuals.

- Government departments – provide information about actions that can be taken by different government departments to accommodate the elderly population and aspects such as providing safe and accessible transportation, community mobility and special help desks to assist elderly persons who have queries related to their functioning as community members. This encompasses advocacy to the government departments.

MANAGEMENT

Continuity in presenting activity programmes to groups in settings such as homes for the aged is dependent on effective and efficient performance of the administrative activities and management functions by the occupational therapist. This implies that programmes and activities must be planned according to the needs of the persons in a specific situation. To compile a suitable activity programme, a planning process has to be followed. This includes:

- *Gathering information*: information about the persons, the activities and the environment

- Predicting what is possible based on the information obtained

- Deciding on long- and short-term goals to be achieved

- Identifying all the actions that will be needed to achieve the aims

- Placing the actions in the order that they will be performed

- Scheduling the time when and the duration of each activity

- Compiling the budget – people, finances, space and time

The plan has to be discussed at the management level to obtain support to progress to the next step of organising the programmes and putting in place the policies, procedures, manpower, physical resources and materials needed for the programme. Voluntary workers are often recruited as a manpower resource to present activities and assist with the on-going presentation of activity programmes in various settings. The programmes and activities are only of value if they regularly take place within a set routine. Continuity of volunteer participation in presenting activity programmes can be supervised by the occupational therapist using motivation and delegation principles. The motivation factors proposed by Herzberg cited in Braveman (2006) provide clear guidelines that can be used to motivate people. Factors such as recognition, responsibility, personal growth and development can be utilised to motivate volunteers, junior staff or OTTs (Braveman 2006). As supervisor, the occupational therapist has to provide educational, administrative and supportive supervision, thereby making it possible for staff to perform satisfactorily. Compiling duty sheets and accompanying procedure descriptions ensures that all tasks will be executed on a regular, on-going basis.

Coordination of the planned actions with all the team members in a facility to ensure smooth running of the programmes is an essential management function to be performed.

Monitoring the execution of activities and programmes is needed to ensure that the long-term goals will be achieved. Identifying aspects that can be improved upon and taking corrective action is also vital.

The execution of the various management functions and using the management skills, namely, decision-making, delegation, motivation, creative thinking and communication, enable the occupational therapist to create the structures for the direct service delivery to take place (Nelson 1997, p. 12).

COOPERATION WITH TEAM MEMBERS

It is important to identify the type of team cooperation is needed in the work environment, be it in the home for the aged or in a hospital ward for geriatric patients. Multidisciplinary, interdisciplinary or trans-disciplinary teams have different dynamics, methods of communication and leadership styles. Multidisciplinary teams are more likely to function in private hospitals, where the knowledge and expertise of each team member is valued, but everyone stays in 'their own lane' (Choi & Pak 2006). The interdisciplinary team operates more often in health care environments like hospitals, whereas the trans-disciplinary teams are operational in community settings, and 'members cross over professional boundaries and share roles and functions' (Choi & Pak 2006; Hussey *et al.* 2007, p. 84). Braveman (2006, p. 89) is of the opinion that interdisciplinary and trans-disciplinary teams are preferable as the dynamics in these two team types allow equal participation by all team members. The team members of any team are determined by the type of problems and/or needs of the elderly persons that have to be addressed as well as the policy of the governing body regarding the funding of posts. The dynamics in teams that have fewer health professionals in the team, as in management teams at homes for the aged, can be different to the dynamics within a team consisting of various health professions in a hospital setting. Interactions amongst the team members within different settings will each have a unique pattern. 'The understanding of these patterns allows the occupational therapy practitioner to guide and direct the interactions in positive, goal-orientated directions' (Hussey *et al.* 2007, p. 238).

The profession-specific contribution of each team member has to be discussed to prevent duplication of interventions and to clarify what each member can offer in the different settings. The combination of team members and type of team may change over time. Open and honest communication is the basis for effective functioning of a team. Braveman (2006, p. 86) suggests that 'Each member shares in the responsibility and accountability for outcome, the meetings involve collaboration, communicating, and consolidating knowledge that changes the treatment plan as appropriate'.

Voluntary workers need to be acknowledged as team members and can, from time to time, be included in team discussions. Optimal inputs by voluntary workers are only possible if they are given the knowledge and skill to execute the tasks delegated to them by the occupational therapist. This aspect refers back to the Indirect Service of Education. The challenge is to have a stable core of voluntary workers who will take responsibility for presenting activities on a regular basis. The motivation to do voluntary work must be nurtured.

Braveman (2006, p. 86) states that at the beginning, 'Functional roles are established, team relies on facts and data, a strong sense of team cohesiveness develops, trust in each other is high, and much work is accomplished'.

Last, but not least, it is important to acknowledge the elderly persons as team members. They must be given the opportunity to participate in discussions pertaining to them and the circumstances where they live. Where possible, their decision-making should be facilitated and encouraged.

RECORDS AND REPORTS

It is suggested that the following question should be answered before recording of data commences: 'What do want to know and what will this data help me learn in order to improve performance of my department?' (Braveman 2006, p. 136). Record-keeping has to be comprehensive and accurate when used as a management tool to gather information as the first step in the planning function of management. Personal data pertaining to age groups, male/female ratios, education levels as well as the number of persons who attend activities gives background information which can be used when choosing activities and compiling activity programmes that will be presented in a specific environment.

Reporting can be verbal as in ward rounds or team meetings or written as a report or sessional notes and be filed/saved in patient folders. Reports provide a longitudinal record of a person's occupational performance and monitoring thereof over time. It is a communication tool whereby information about the occupational performance of elderly persons is shared with other team members. Reports on assessments, interventions and the evaluation thereof have to be available throughout the occupational therapy process: 'The habits of good planning and regular documentation make record keeping easier, whatever the demands, and ultimately, lead to better quality treatment' (Hussey *et al.* 2007, p. 190).

While reporting is an important aspect of communication within the team, occupational therapists should still maintain relevant aspects of confidentiality when sharing information about their clients. Considerations such as the elderly person who may not always want all family members to know about their condition may need to be respected if this is still within the elderly person's best interest. Only necessary and relevant information should be shared with relevant or authorised people, particularly in countries with legislation about data privacy, such as the European Union's General Data Protection Regulations and the Protection of Personal Information Act of South Africa.

CONSULTATION

Consultation is defined as 'giving advice, assistance, or an opinion based on professional knowledge, skill or judgement' (Punwar & Peloquin 2000, p. 190). Jaffe and Epstein define a consultant 'as a professional who has specialised training in the basic principles of consultation and who provides indirect rather that direct service' (Jaffe & Epstein 1992, p. 18). A consultant can be from within an organisation or can be a person from outside who acts as an external consultant.

If the person who acts as a consultant is from outside the organisation, then they can only advise and recommend as the team has to decide whether they accept the advice and it is their responsibility to implement any proposed actions or changes on occasion. Homes for the aged request consultation input from occupational therapists from time to time to enhance the occupational performance of residents, regarding the activities and programmes, adaptations to the environment or assistive devices that can be considered. The cycle of the consultation process that the external consultant must negotiate and follow is described by Jaffe and Epstein (1992) and includes:

- Entry into system
- Negotiation of contract
- Diagnostic analysis leading to problem identification
- Goal setting and planning through establishment of trust
- Maintenance phase of intervention and feedback
- Evaluation
- Termination
- Possible renegotiation (Jaffe & Epstein 1992, p. 136)

Successful consultation is dependent on the cycle being negotiated before actions pertaining to consultation are considered. There are advantages and disadvantages to having an internal or external consultant. The needs of the organisation will determine which one is preferred at a specific point in time, but as a general rule, the advantages of contracting an external consultant outweigh the disadvantages. The most important advantages are the objectivity and the negotiation skills the consultant has and the contract to deliver a 'product'. Due to the aforementioned consultation process, the status of the external consultant creates opportunities to address the area for which the consultation is required and to be objective in making recommendations to address the problem area(s) identified. Advocacy and mediation with the authorities by the consultant can follow that could benefit the direct service delivery component provided by the occupational therapists employed in the situation. It could be that the problem that the consultant was contracted for is not actually the real problem, but by the external consultant having the negotiated contract, he/she can ask questions that may identify the real problem and thus be able to assist in addressing the real issue that precipitated the need to contract an external consultant.

An aspect that is recognised as a measurement of the severity of ill health is a person's occupational performance or the functional performance level of the elderly person. The occupational therapist who acts as a consultant to a team has the opportunity to make recommendations not only pertaining to occupational therapy but also to all the facets that should be addressed in a situation that will improve the functional performance status of the elderly persons.

Jaffe and Epstein (1992) indicate that the consultant can fulfil the following roles in a situation such as in a psychogeriatric ward in a hospital:

- Diagnostician – identifies problems and formulates hypotheses about possible causes for the person's functional deficit.

- Clinician – provides intervention for identified problems.

- Advocate – persuades consultee to accept particular values, goals, objectives or actions.

- Collaborative problem solver – works with consultee to solve problems.

- Information specialist – provides knowledge and technical expertise.

- Educator/trainer – teaches consultee attitudes, knowledge and skill (Jaffe & Epstein 1992, p. 300).

The consultant can, from the perspective of each of the aforementioned roles, provide the consultee with a range of possible options for actions from which the individual, the group and/or the situation can benefit. An important advantage of engaging an external consultant is that a larger group of persons will benefit from the recommendations made by the consultant as opposed to the delivery of direct services to individual persons. Due to the limited number of occupational therapists working in the psychogeriatric field, along with the limited resources in certain settings and the limited awareness of services in this field, particularly in countries of the Global South, consultants can provide an efficacious model of service delivery. If the consultee does not act on the recommendations made by the consultant, the situation can be disadvantaged.

RESEARCH

In recent years there has been more research on the role of occupational therapy in the field of gerontology and geriatrics with evidence on the effectiveness of occupational therapy interventions. Clinicians doing research specifically in the practice field of geriatrics in the Global South are, however, more the exception rather than the rule. This can be changed by planned recording of the data pertaining to interventions in these two service fields in a predetermined way. Recording the everyday occupational therapy interventions according to set data sheets will contribute to providing evidence for the interventions, whether it is to confirm or discard the value of such an intervention. The ideal situation is to establish a partnership between a clinician and a researcher to perform the activity of research in the course of everyday clinical practice performed in the fields of gerontology and geriatrics. Research results are needed to motivate the creation of posts to serve the elderly population, particularly in countries of the Global South where resources and access to services may be different from those of the Global North. Much research exists in the Global North regarding the care, treatment and safeguarding of the elderly with clearly defined guidelines, yet this is not the case for the Global South (NICE 2016). A systematic review published in 2004 revealed the benefits of occupational therapy interventions for the elderly living in the community (Steultjens et al. 2004). This systematic review showed that comprehensive occupational therapy can be effective in maintaining quality of life, functional ability and social participation for elderly people and that a home assessment conducted by the occupational therapist was found to be effective for improving functional ability. The systematic review further found that occupational therapists played an important role in falls prevention; however, further research was needed on efficacy of occupational therapy for individuals with dementia living in the community (Steultjens et al. 2004). Research should be aimed at the needs of this population in countries with lower socio-economic and pluralistic demographics and how these countries can meet these needs. Occupational therapy research should focus on the occupational changes of this population and how to overcome/cope with these changes using both direct and indirect services in various contexts.

ADVOCACY AND NETWORKING

In order to ensure that this possibly vulnerable population's needs are met, it is important that the team looking after the elderly are able to advocate for their needs to be met. This may include providing evidence to obtain funding, resources or environmental adjustments. This may also consist of activities that advocate for the integration of older people into communities. Keeping good records, reports and research can be used as evidence when performing the advocacy role.

In the 21st century, networking has become a major role in all professions. While the health profession may be slightly lacking in this regard, largely due to the already known need for healthcare services in general, this role is vital in the development of awareness of the elderly population and of new services. Networking is important to integrate the healthcare systems with social and corporate awareness systems as well as to obtain awareness of projects, funding for services and community engagement and support.

EXTERNAL FACTORS AFFECTING THE ELDERLY

The COVID-19 pandemic elicited worldwide changes that have seriously affected the lives of elderly people. Loneliness due to the mandatory covid lockdowns was a serious stress factor. Elderly people were isolated, unable to shop, socialise and run their lives as before. Many elderly people died at the beginning of the pandemic. Pozzi *et al.* (2020) state that 'The aging population requires new innovative approaches to improve the quality of life'. The COVID-19 pandemic meant that many individuals were reliant on technology, including video calling and social media, to maintain social interaction.

Elderly people, particularly those with neurocognitive changes, may not always be privy to these resources, or have the ability to adapt to this change and new learning. Occupational therapists can play a role is assisting the elderly person with these external factors by keeping them orientated to current world events, adaptation groups and skill development groups.

The other change that has occurred, particularly in South Africa, is a surge in the development of retirement homes (old age homes), some with frail-care facilities and some without. Some even have a mid-care facility. The reason in South Africa is largely a security one as the crime rate is escalating and older people are particularly vulnerable to attack. This means that more elderly people have access to occupational therapy and other services such as physiotherapy and social work, if they can afford residency in these facilities. This is an important factor in dealing with ageing and stress. Residents are assessed and assisted in many ways including counselling about challenges regarding relationships with family and carers, physical difficulties, mental health, modifications to homes and self-care issues. Occupational therapists also encourage independence, maintain range of motion, maintain and stimulate cognitive skills, develop coping mechanisms for pain and improve the overall quality of life within this population.

CASE STUDY

The director of a home for the aged requested the occupational therapist to propose contributions that an occupational therapist can make within a home for the aged. They do not have the funds to appoint a full-time occupational therapist, but can appoint an occupational therapist for 20 hours a week. Fifty elderly persons – 10 men and 40 women – live permanently in the home. Fifteen of them are in the special care unit for person diagnosed with Alzheimer's disease. The home is situated in a low socio-economic residential area. Four of the bedrooms accommodate married couples and the rest accommodate two persons per room. Other facilities available are a dining room, a recreational area with a television and one other room that can accommodate 15 persons and can be used for various activities.

A small component of the nursing staff is permanently employed at the home and the rest of the nursing services are provided on a contract basis by an outside nursing agency. There is no regular weekly activity programme presented and the inhabitants spend their time mostly in their rooms or watching television.

The occupational therapy process provides a sound point of departure to identify which direct and indirect occupational therapy services are indicated. As a point of departure, the occupational therapist must screen all persons, the micro and macro environments and the activities that take place in the home. The Person-Environment-Occupational Model (Law 1996,

p. 9) gives a comprehensive overview of what should be assessed. The BPSM described earlier in this chapter can also be used. In this case, the social aspects of clients may be similar as they are all in the same home with access to the same facilities; however, the biological and psychological components will differ. An example of this is demonstrated below (Figures 29.2 and 29.3).

DIRECT OCCUPATIONAL THERAPY SERVICES

Completed activity profiles, activity histories and the Canadian Occupational Performance Measure (Law *et al.* 1990, p. 82) of all residents provide information to make a functional diagnosis, identify existing personal and environmental assets and provide a reference point for planning direct and indirect service delivery. In addition, the occupational therapist can ascertain what motivates the resident to participate in their activities and whether modifications to these activities (or the environments in which they take place) are necessary (Cantor 1981, p. 638), to further guide interventions.

The occupational therapist may also do a complete initial assessment of residents at the home to establish their baseline functioning of body functions and structures such as muscle strength, range of motion, balance and cognitive abilities. This allows the occupational therapist to monitor progress, or provide further input if a resident's functioning or abilities decline with further ageing. This also assists the occupational therapists

(continued)

CASE STUDY　*(Continued)*

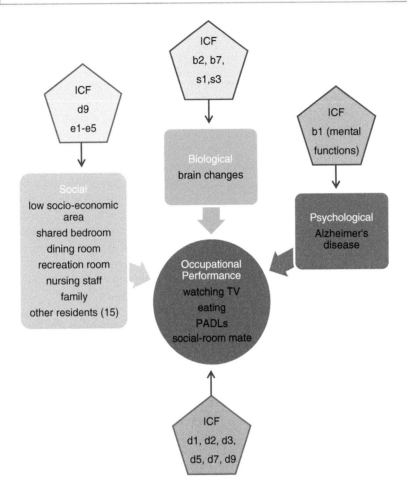

FIGURE 29.2　Example of BPSM and ICF for resident in special care unit for Alzheimer's disease.

to allocate residents to appropriate groups and make individualised recommendations. It is important to note that this may be the most time-consuming aspect of the direct occupational therapy services initially; however, it is vital that residents are still provided with appropriate recommendations and not a one-size-fits-all group therapy program.

Once this is completed, the occupational therapist will implement the appropriate direct interventions described above such as provision of assistive devices if needed, suggestions of environmental modifications, assessment of community mobility, retirement planning and group therapy in the available space. Because the occupational therapist is only contracted for 20 hours a week, group therapy will be the most efficient way to provide interventions to most residents within a limited time frame, even while recruitment for volunteers and OTTs is still underway (Figures 29.2 and 29.3).

INDIRECT SERVICE DELIVERY

Due to the limited time available for direct occupational therapy interventions, indirect services such as management, education, cooperation with team members and consultation will enable the

occupational therapist to create structures in the home whereby the needs of a large group of the elderly can be addressed.

The occupational therapist will take on the role of manager to plan, organise, coordinate, guide and monitor the interventions proposed, but the interventions may be implemented by other persons, such as voluntary workers, OTTs, family members or nursing staff. The type and frequency of the interventions will be planned so as to provide a weekly activity programme in the home.

The occupational therapist will educate the voluntary workers to enable them to provide on-going activities within a weekly programme that will be developed in the home. They will be educated on topics such as handling elderly persons with specific problems, the practice of validation, how to manage groups, presenting a variety of activities and games. Presenting an on-going weekly programme can provide the structure whereby the elderly persons will be given the opportunity to develop satisfactory lifestyles and perform various roles within the home.

The permanent nursing staff will be educated regarding the physical handling of elderly persons. Topics such as how to transfer a person from the bed to the wheelchair, caregiver back

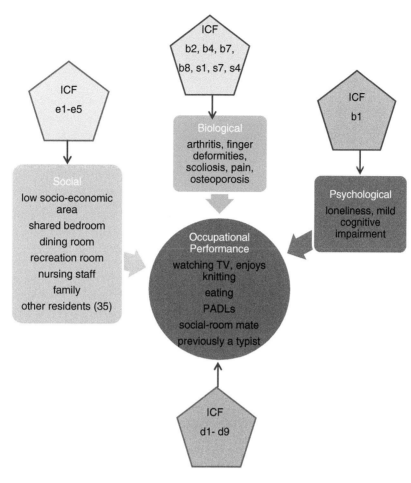

FIGURE 29.3   Example of BPSM and ICF of resident in home for the aged.

saving principles when lifting, stress management and relaxation techniques can be covered. The occupational therapist may also stress the importance of facilitating engagement in ADLs rather than just doing it for residents. If this is done effectively, the staff will not hurt themselves and there will be continuity in the delivery of care in the home. Cooperation within the team in the home will be developed. The occupational therapist can contribute to establishing interdisciplinary teamwork whereby common goals will be set, and all team members will work towards realisation of these goals, whereby the elderly persons will benefit.

If the occupational therapist can become a member of the management committee of the home, it will present the opportunity to fulfil the role of consultant and advocate. As consultant and advocate, the occupational therapist will act as a resource to provide information to the committee to enhance the quality of life for the residents. Information for assistive devices needed for independent functioning in the home, inputs pertaining to structural changes that may be planned in the home, health promotion and preventative actions to be implemented, are a few examples about which the occupational therapist can provide information.

On-going formative evaluation of all the above will take place and the occupational therapist will adapt direct and indirect services based on the result of the evaluation. Summative evaluation will take place every six months as to give feedback to the director about the results of the occupational therapy service delivery. Recommendations will be included in the six monthly reports that will be presented to the director and the management committee of the home for the aged.

CONCLUSION

The holistic approach prevalent within the BPSM ensures that the elderly person will be viewed as an individual within a context influenced by various environmental factors.

Knowledge of what each direct or indirect service entails empowers the occupational therapist to collaborate on a managerial level to create structures for service delivery within various environments. The indirect service delivery allows many more people to have the advantage of occupational therapy services and should be considered by all service delivery departments dealing with the psychogeriatric population in homes, care centres and in the community at large.

QUESTIONS

1. Describe the type of deterioration the occupational therapist is likely to see in the patient with Alzheimer's disease.

2. Describe the important treatment principles to be observed by the occupational therapist who is working in a direct service to the patient with a neurocognitive disorder.

3. List the indirect occupational therapy services and discuss how each one can contribute to effective direct service delivery to elderly patients in a long-term psychogeriatric ward.

4. Explain how the concept of 'holism' is represented in the BPSM.

5. List the steps of the consultation process and discuss the actions to be performed under each step if you are contracted to act as an external consultant to propose an activity programme for a home for the aged.

6. Discuss how the occupational therapist can, by implementing indirect services, enable an elderly person to stay at home for longer.

REFERENCES

Aderinwale, O.G., Ernst, H.W. & Mousa, S.A. (2010) Current therapies and new strategies for the management of Alzheimer's disease. *American Journal of Alzheimer's Disease & Other Dementia,* 25(5), 414–424.

American Psychiatric Association (APA) (2022) *Diagnostic and Statistical Manual of Mental Disorders: DSM-5-TR,* 5th edn, Text Revision. APA, Washington, DC.

Association for Gerontology in Higher Education (2012) *What is gerontology? Geriatrics?* www.aghe.org/500217 (accessed on 31 January 2014)

Barney, K.F. & Perkinson, M.A. (2016) *Occupational Therapy with Aging Adults: Promoting Quality of Life through Collaborative Practice.* Elsevier, St. Louis.

Baum, C. (2007) Emerging practice areas. In: S.M. Hussey, B. Sabonis-Chafee & J.C. O'Brien (eds), *Introduction to Occupational Therapy* Elsevier Mosby, St. Louis, p. 53.

Braveman, B. (2006) *Leading & Managing Occupational Therapy Services: An Evidence-Based Approach.* F.A. Davis Co., Philadelphia.

Cantor, S. (1981) Occupational therapists as members of preretirement resource teams. *American Journal of Occupational Therapy,* 35(10), 638–643.

Carr, D.B. & Ott, B.R. (2010) The older adult driver with cognitive impairment: "it's a very frustrating life". *JAMA,* 303(16), 1632–1641. https://doi.org/10.1001/jama.2010.481

Casteleijn, D. & Graham, M. (2012) Incorporating a client-centred approach in the development of occupational therapy outcome domains for mental health care settings in South Africa. *South African Journal of Occupational Therapy,* 42(2), 8–13.

Choi, B.C.K. & Pak, A.W.P. (2006) Multidisciplinarity, interdisciplinarity and transdisciplinarity in health research, services, education and policy: 1. Definitions, objectives, and evidence of effectiveness. *Clinical and Investigative Medicine,* 29(6), 351–364.

Connell, C.M., Harmon, A., Janevic, M.R. *et al* (2013) 'Older adults' driving reduction and cessation: perspectives of adult children. *Journal of Applied Gerontology,* 32(8), 975–996. https://doi.org/10.1177/0733464812448962

Crouch, R.B. (2021) *Occupational Group Therapy.* John Wiley & Sons, Oxford.

Engel, G.L. (1992) The need for a new medical model: a challenge for biomedicine. *Family Systems Medicine,* 10(3), 317–331.

Erikson, E.H. (1997) *The Life Cycle Completed.* Norton, New York.

Feil, N. (1993) *The Validation Breakthrough: Simple Techniques for Communicating with People with "Alzheimer's-Type Dementia".* Health Professions Press, Baltimore.

Hillman, A. & Chapparo, C.J. (2002) What is sociology. In: D. Jones (ed), *Sociology and Occupational Therapy: An Integrated Approach.* Churchill Livingstone, Edinburgh, p. 51.

Hussey, S.M., Sabonis-Chafee, B. & O'Brien, J.C. (eds) (2007) *Introduction to Occupational Therapy.* Elsevier Mosby, St. Louis.

Jaffe, E. & Epstein, C.F. (1992) *Occupational Therapy Consultation: Theory, Principles, and Practice.* Mosby-Year Book, St. Louis.

Jones, D. (2002) *Sociology and Occupational Therapy: An Integrated Approach.* Churchill Livingstone, Edinburgh.

Kirk-Sanchez, N.J. & McGough, E.L. (2014) Physical exercise and cognitive performance in the elderly: current perspectives. *Clinical Interventions in Aging,* 9, 51–62. https://doi.org/10.2147/CIA.S39506

Labuschagne, R. (2005) Gerontology, psychiatry and occupational therapy. In: R.B. Crouch & V.M. Alers (eds), *Occupational Therapy in Psychiatry and Mental Health,* 4th edn, pp. 552–567. Whurr Publishers, London.

Lakham, S.E. (2006) *The biopsychosocial model of health and illness.* http://cnx.org/content/m13589/latest/# (accessed on 31 February 2014)

Law, M. (1996) The person-environment-occupation model: a transactive approach to occupational performance. *Canadian Journal of Occupational Therapy,* 63(1), 9–23.

Law, M., Baptiste, S., McColl, M. *et al* (1990) The Canadian occupational performance measure: an outcome measure for occupational therapy. *Canadian Journal of Occupational Therapy,* 57(2), 82–87.

Lezak, M.D. (1995) *Neurological Assessment.* Oxford University Press, New York.

Liberty Healthcare and Rehab Blog (2023) *Benefits of occupational therapy for seniors.* https://libertycareandrehab.com/benefits-of-occupational-therapy-for-Seniors/# (accessed on 2 September 2023)

Medical News.net (2014) *What is genomics.* http://www.news-medical.net/health/What-is-Genomics.aspx (accessed on 19 March 2014)

Mulry, C.M., Papetti, C., De Martinis, J. *et al* (2017) Facilitating wellness in urban-dwelling, low-income older adults through community mobility: a mixed-methods study. *The American Journal of Occupational Therapy,* 71(4), 1–7.

Nelson, D.L. (1997) Why the profession of occupational therapy will flourish in the 21st century. *The American Journal of Occupational Therapy*, **51**(**1**), 11–24.

NICE (2016) *Mental Well-Being and Independence for Older People.* National Institute for Health and Care Excellence, Manchester, United Kingdom. https://doi.org/10.7748/ns.31.24.15.s16

Nissenboim, S. & Vroman, C. (2000) *The Positive Interactions Program of Activities for People with Alzheimer's Disease.* Health Professions Press, Baltimore.

Parkview Health (2021) *Stress and its effect on older adults.* www:Parkview.com/community/dashboard/stress-and-its-effect-on-older-adults.# (accessed on 3 July 2023)

Pozzi, C., Lanzoni, A., Graff, M.J.L. *et al* (2020) *Occupational Therapy for Older People.* SpringerLink, Switzerland.

Punwar, A. & Peloquin, S. (2000) *Occupational Therapy: Principles and Practice.* Lippincott Williams & Wilkins, Philadelphia.

Reed, K.L. & Sanderson, S.N. (1980) *Concepts of Occupational Therapy.* Lippincott Williams & Wilkins, Baltimore.

Scaffa, M.E., Reitz, S.M. & Pizzi, M. (2010) *Occupational Therapy in the Promotion of Health and Wellness.* F.A. Davis Co., Philadelphia.

Smallfield, S. & Heckenlaible, C. (2017) Effectiveness of occupational therapy interventions to enhance occupational performance for adults with Alzheimer's disease and related major neurocognitive disorders: a systematic review. *The American Journal of Occupational Therapy*, **71**(**5**), 7105180010p1–7105180010p9. https://doi.org/10.5014/ajot.2017.024752

Steultjens, E.M.J., Dekker, J., Bouter, L.M. *et al* (2004) Occupational therapy for community dwelling elderly people: a systematic review, *Age and Ageing*, **33**(**5**), 453–460. https://doi.org/10.1093/ageing/afh174

University of Alaska Anchorage (2012) *Gerontology.* www.uaa.alaska.edu/gerontology (accessed on 31 January 2014)

Voigt-Radloff, S., Graff, M., Leonhart, R. *et al* (2011) A multicentre RCT on community occupational therapy in Alzheimer's consultation. *British Medical Journal Open*, **1**, e000096.

World Health Organisation (2001) *International classification of functioning, disability and health.* https://www.icf-elearning.com/wp-content/uploads/articulate_uploads/ICF%20e-Learning%20Tool_English_20220501%20-%20Storyline%20output/story_html5.html (accessed 22 July 2023)

World Health Organisation (2012) *Dementia: A Public Health Priority.* World Health Organisation, Geneva.

World Health Organisation (2022) *Ageing and Health.* World Health Organisation, Geneva.

Zietsman, K. (2011) *The functional levels outcome measure (FLOM) for large numbers of mental health care users.* Workshop presentation on 27 May 2011, University of the Free State, Bloemfontein.

Zinger, A. & Roche, E. (2020) *Using meaningful leisure activities in OT to decrease occupational deprivation in older adults.* Critically Appraised Topics, 10. https://commons.und.edu/cat-papers/10 (accessed 2 July 2023)

Care, Treatment and Rehabilitation Programmes for Large Numbers of Long-Term Mental Health Care Users

CHAPTER 30

Daleen Casteleijn[1] and Kobie Zietsman[2]

[1]Occupational Therapy Department, School of Health Care Sciences, Faculty of Health Sciences, University of Pretoria, Pretoria, South Africa

[2]Glenmore, South Coast, South Africa

KEY LEARNING POINTS

- Global and national trends in provision of mental health care for severe mental illness.

- The legal context that regulates mental health care for occupational therapists.

- De-institutionalisation and the move towards community-orientated care.

- Comprehensive rehabilitation in long-term settings.

- Specific programme planning with appropriate activities for different levels of activity participation.

INTRODUCTION

People suffering from severe mental disorders and who need long-term care are often marginalised (Knaak *et al.* 2017; Li *et al.* 2022; Gamieldien *et al.* 2023). The marginalisation is a complex issue that stems from a combination of societal attitudes, systemic barriers and a lack of resources (Kapadia 2023). Societal attitudes such as stigmatisation and stereotyping aggravate the marginalisation, which increases the risk of social and occupational injustice for this population (Madlala *et al.* 2020; Kapadia 2023). Systemic barriers such as a struggle to access adequate mental health care due to financial constraints, lack of specialised facilities, or geographical barriers lead to inadequate treatment, exacerbating the condition and hindering the service users' ability to participate fully in society. The inadequate availability of resources exacerbates the challenges faced by individuals with severe mental illnesses, as there is an imbalance between the financial resources allocated for mental health care and those designated for physical health care. All the marginalisation factors impede the service user's right to meaningfully engage in desired occupations and to experience well-being and therefore are in dire need of rehabilitation provided by occupational therapists.

This chapter starts with a summary of the global and national trends in provision of mental health care for severe mental illnesses, with emphasis on the move from institutionalisation to community mental health care and residential care facilities outside of traditional healthcare institutions. This section is followed by an explanation of the legal context and how the South African Mental Health Care Act (MHCA) No. 17 of 2002 (MHCA nr 17 2002) (as an example) positions occupational therapists as one of the vital mental health care providers for those in need of care, treatment and rehabilitation. The latter half of this chapter is devoted to specific

Crouch and Alers Occupational Therapy in Psychiatry and Mental Health, Sixth Edition.
Edited by Rosemary Crouch, Tania Buys, Enos Morankoana Ramano, Matty van Niekerk and Lisa Wegner.
© 2025 John Wiley & Sons Ltd. Published 2025 by John Wiley & Sons Ltd.

programme planning for large numbers of mental health care users who need long-term stays in residential care facilities.

GLOBAL AND NATIONAL TRENDS IN PROVISION OF MENTAL HEALTH CARE

The World Health Organization (WHO) emphasises the importance of comprehensive and person-centred mental health interventions for people with severe mental illnesses. In their Comprehensive Mental Health Care Plan of 2013–2030, they refer to a number of principles which all healthcare care providers should take note of (WHO 2021):

- The WHO emphasises that people with severe mental illnesses have the same human rights as anyone else. They should be treated with dignity, respect and without discrimination. In occupational therapy terms, occupational justice for all people, including mental health, is supported (WFOT 2019; Morrow & Hardie 2023). Informed consent, privacy and autonomy are important considerations in their care and are captured in all heathcare professionals' codes of ethical conduct.

- Community-based care over institutionalisation is another principle that has been globally adopted by developed and developing countries (Madlala *et al.* 2020; Cano Prieto *et al.* 2023). People with severe mental illnesses should have access to quality mental health services in their local communities, which can enhance social inclusion and reduce stigma. Efforts to reduce stigma around mental illness are essential. Public awareness campaigns and education can help create more supportive and understanding communities (Kapadia 2023).

- Mental health care for severe mental illnesses should be integrated into the broader healthcare system. This includes collaboration between mental health professionals and primary care providers to address both physical and mental health needs (Lake & Turner 2017).

- The focus of comprehensive and person-centred mental health interventions should be on recovery and rehabilitation rather than just symptom management. Individuals with severe mental illnesses should be empowered to regain functional skills, engage in meaningful activities and participate in their communities. Treatment should consider the individual's physical, psychological and social needs. This might involve addressing housing, employment/work, family support and other factors that impact mental health and well-being (de Wet & Pretorius 2022; Kastrup 2023).

- Families and caregivers play an important role in the care and support of individuals with severe mental illnesses. Involving them in treatment planning and providing them with education and support is crucial (de Wet & Pretorius 2022). One of the top three strategies to strengthen the provision of mental health care is to empower families, carers and patients (Mapanga *et al.* 2019).

Overall, the WHO advocates for a holistic and human-rights-centred approach to mental health interventions for people with severe mental illnesses. The goal is to promote recovery, improve quality of life, and support individuals in achieving their full potential within their communities. The goals of occupational therapy in mental health align well with the WHO principles as their focus is on helping individuals engage in meaningful activities, develop skills and reintegrate into their communities.

In South Africa, the National Mental Health Policy Framework and Strategic Plan 2023–2030 (NMHP) mirrors the principles of the WHO. However, more emphasis is given to the move of mental health care services to community care and a staging model of promotion, primary, secondary and tertiary prevention. The practical implication of this is that mental health care users should have access to care close to home and receive the least restrictive form of care within the legal prescriptions. Both the present (2023–2030) and past (2013–2020) NMHPs provide a sound framework that spans all sectors and healthcare personnel, guiding them toward achieving effective and efficient mental health care services. However, due to significant budget limitations and a shortage of human resources, it will require additional dedication and effort to fully implement the action plans outlined by the current NMHP.

The move towards community mental health services has been a global challenge (Thornicroft *et al.* 2016; Li *et al.* 2022). In South Africa, most services are still delivered in district and tertiary hospitals (Docrat *et al.* 2019; de Wet & Pretorius 2022). Although some integrated care plans are already in place at selected primary healthcare centres in South Africa (de Wet *et al.* 2019), the majority of clinics and community hospitals are not yet equipped to deal with mental health care needs. Docrat *et al.* (2019) reported that almost 25% of mental health care are re-admitted within three months after a previous discharge, and this can be attributed to a lack of community mental health services.

South Africa has suffered dire consequences from neglected mental health interventions. The Life Esidimeni tragedy, which occurred in South Africa in 2016, involved the improper and poorly managed relocation of mental health patients from the Life Esidimeni health care facilities to various non-governmental organisations (NGOs) and other facilities. The decision was made by the Gauteng Department of Health as a cost-cutting measure. The tragedy resulted in the deaths of at least 144 patients, who experienced neglect, inadequate care, and harsh living conditions at the new facilities. The incident highlighted serious flaws in the planning, coordination, and execution of the relocation process, and it sparked widespread outrage, condemnation and calls for accountability. Families of the victims, civil society organisations, and the public demanded justice and proper care for individuals with mental health conditions. The Life Esidimeni tragedy exposed systemic failures within the healthcare system, led to a public inquiry and underscored the need for improved mental health care policies, oversight, and human rights protections in South Africa (Ferlito & Dhai 2018; Robertson & Makgoba 2018).

Regardless of past failures, the recently introduced South African mental health policy (Republic of South Africa 2023) provides a chance for everyone involved in mental health initiatives in South Africa to unite, draw insights from past encounters and reaffirm healthcare workers' dedication to enhancing mental health care. This involves enhancing mental health services, safeguarding the rights of individuals facing mental health difficulties, and preventing mental health disorders within our communities.

The next section highlights aspects of the MHCA of 2002 (Republic of South Africa 2002) and the importance of occupational therapy interventions.

LEGAL CONTEXT THAT GUIDES THE OCCUPATIONAL THERAPY PROCESS

The legal framework for mental health care differs significantly from one country to another. Some countries have comprehensive mental health laws that cover various aspects of mental health care, including involuntary hospitalisation, treatment and patients' rights. Others may have more general healthcare laws that touch on mental health as part of overall healthcare provision. In some countries, the regulation of mental health care may vary by region or state, leading to different legal frameworks within the same country. Several countries adhere to international agreements and guidelines that address mental health care, such as those set forth by the WHO. Generally, mental health legislation recognises and involves a range of healthcare professionals in the care and treatment of individuals with mental illnesses, including psychiatrists, psychologists, nurses and occupational therapists. When setting up occupational therapy programmes for residents in long-term facilities, it is recommended to screen the mental health care legislation to provide interventions within the relevant frameworks of the country.

The South African MHCA No. 17 of 2002 (Republic of South Africa 2002) is used as an example to highlight significant implications for service delivery for occupational therapy. With the advent of democracy in South Africa, the focus of mental health care has shifted from a legally driven process to a human rights approach. This shift was welcomed by occupational therapists as the profession is grounded in a client-centred and holistic approach to care that values individuals' rights, dignity and well-being.

Chapters V and VI in the South African MHCA stipulate four categories of mental health care users, namely voluntary (a person gives consent to intervention), assisted (person unable to make informed decisions but does not refuse intervention) and involuntary (person unable to make informed decisions and refuses care but requires intervention). The fourth category is a state patient (where a person has been classified by a court directive due to a criminal offence while having a mental illness). All four categories of mental health care users need occupational therapy in the form of care, treatment and rehabilitation. In the act, care, treatment and rehabilitation are never separated and no specific definitions have been offered for each term (Republic of South Africa 2002). In general, care involves providing a supportive and nurturing environment, treatment involves targeted interventions to manage symptoms, and rehabilitation focuses on building skills and restoring functioning. All three concepts are integral to a holistic approach to mental health support, and they often work together to improve the overall well-being and quality of life of individuals with mental health conditions.

The fundamental provisions of the act are to provide the best mental health care for the population and to provide community-based care. It also stipulates the need to provide care, treatment and rehabilitation in the least restrictive manner. The implication of this is that occupational therapists in primary healthcare and community clinics need to receive referrals from the discharging hospitals to continue with treatment and rehabilitation programmes. In some provinces, this is already happening, but where mental health care users and families live in remote areas, other problems such as transport may impede the continuation of care.

Another important provision of the act is to establish review boards to oversee, monitor and regulate processes (Republic of South Africa 2002). Review boards investigate appeals from families and service users, the appropriateness of involuntary and assisted admissions, compliance monitoring and protecting the human rights of mental health care users and their families. Occupational therapists should follow all necessary procedures and complete documentation as required by their employers and assist review boards with the necessary information in the level of functioning of their clients.

Under Chapter IX of the Act (Republic of South Africa 2002), regulations are established to authorise and licence health establishments, non-governmental organisations, or private entities that offer care, treatment and rehabilitation to mental health care users who lack independent living capabilities (Republic of South Africa 2017). In certain provinces, occupational therapists are tasked with assessing these establishments to ensure the adequacy of care and the implementation of treatment and rehabilitation programs. This responsibility accentuates the vital role of occupational therapists within community settings, guaranteeing the provision of high-quality care to mental health care users.

The next section describes the provision of long-term residential care to address the needs of mental health care users who need support in the community with independent living.

LONG-TERM RESIDENTIAL CARE FOR MENTAL HEALTH CARE USERS WITH SEVERE MENTAL ILLNESSES

Long-term residential care for people with severe mental illness serves as a critical support system that aims to provide individuals with a safe and structured environment where they can receive ongoing care, treatment, and assistance. The South African NMHP (2023) urge healthcare workers to explore all possible outpatient and community-based residential care options explored before inpatient care is undertaken. The essence of such care is to offer a comprehensive and holistic approach to addressing the complex needs of individuals with severe mental illness. The advantages of long-term residential care include:

- *Safe and supportive environment:* Residential care offers a stable and secure living environment that minimises risks and provides round-the-clock supervision. This is particularly important for individuals with severe mental illness who may be vulnerable to self-harm, neglect or exploitation (Sun *et al.* 2023).

- *Continuity of care:* Long-term residential care ensures consistent access to medical, psychiatric, and therapeutic services. Regular assessments and treatment adjustments are possible, promoting better management of symptoms and overall well-being (Biringer *et al.* 2017).

- *Structured daily routine:* Establishing a structured daily routine helps individuals with severe mentalillnessess maintain stability. Activities such as group sessions, recreational activities and self-care practices are integrated into their daily lives (Iseselo & Ambikile 2020; Ramafikeng *et al.* 2020).

- *Medication management:* Effective monitoring and administration of medications are crucial for individuals with severe mental illness. Residential care provides a controlled setting for managing medication regimens, ensuring adherence and minimising potential side effects (Loots *et al.* 2021).

- *Social interaction:* Residential care settings encourage social interaction and peer support among residents. Engaging in social activities helps combat isolation, build relationships, and improve overall mental health (Höhl *et al.* 2017; Rocamora-Montenegro *et al.* 2021).

- *Skill development:* Long-term care programs often focus on skill development tailored to an individual's needs. This includes teaching daily living skills, vocational training, and strategies for managing symptoms and stressors (Tungpunkom *et al.* 2012; Gamieldien *et al.* 2023).

- *Community integration:* While individuals reside in a care facility, the goal is to promote their eventual integration into the community. This involves preparing them for eventual reintegration, including teaching social skills and offering opportunities for supervised outings (Gamaldien *et al.* 2021; Gamieldien *et al.* 2023).

- *Family and caregiver involvement:* In many cases, family members or caregivers play a role in the care process. Residential care facilities often encourage family involvement through counselling, education and support programs (Ong *et al.* 2021).

- *Quality of life:* The ultimate goal of long-term residential care is to improve the overall quality of life for individuals with severe mental illness. This includes enhancing their emotional well-being, independence and ability to engage in meaningful activities (Gamieldien *et al.* 2023).

In summary, long-term residential care for people with severe mental illness is designed to provide a comprehensive, supportive and structured environment that addresses their unique needs and supports their journey towards recovery, stability and improved quality of life. For many mental health care users, this is the only option to have quality of life. Occupational therapists play a vital role in designing and implementing programmes that will promote health and well-being of mental health care users with severe mental illnesses of a chronic nature.

AN OCCUPATIONAL PERSPECTIVE ON MENTAL HEALTH CARE USERS IN RESIDENTIAL CARE FACILITIES

Occupational therapists believe that engagement and participation in meaningful activity and occupation are key to health and well-being (Rebeiro & Cook 1999; Kielhofner 2008; Wright-St Claire & Hocking 2018; van der Reyden *et al.* 2019). When a person needs healthcare and admission to a residential care facility, the normal patterns of engagement in daily life and culturally defined occupations are disrupted. The individual is constantly facing factors that create occupational injustice in the form of occupational alienation, deprivation and imbalance (Townsend & Wilcock 2004; Govender *et al.* 2015; Pizarro *et al.* 2018).

When admitted to a residential care facility, far removed from home and community life, disconnected and isolated from usual ways of engaging in life, the individual is alienated, and faces unknown and new encounters with fellow users with different values, beliefs and habits. The staff in the institution might expect the person to perform tasks that he/she has never done before, for instance, taking part in group activities that are not part of his/her culture. Occupational alienation is similar to loss of contact with the outside world, family, friends and personal events and can lead to a lack of identity and a sense of meaninglessness (Townsend & Wilcock 2004).

Occupational deprivation happens when the individual is deprived of opportunities to engage in preferred occupations according to his/her cultural values and beliefs. For example, the routine in the ward is structured to manage large numbers of users, and the person is being washed, fed and dressed by staff in a predetermined manner. The structure of the facility often requires users to go to bed at an early hour of the evening, depriving users of evening occupations such as reading, conversations with others or religious routines. Occupational deprivation is similar to enforced idleness often observed in persons in long-term care (Govender *et al.* 2015).

Occupational imbalance occurs when the occupational needs of individuals are not met. People have needs in social, physical, rest and mental areas (to name a few), and when these needs are not met, an imbalance in role performance happens (Govender *et al.* 2015). In an institution with large numbers of individuals with different cultural values and needs, clearly some needs would not be fulfilled.

A client-centred approach combined with an occupational justice framework that provides opportunities for engagement in preferred occupations to improve feelings of accomplishment, success and well-being becomes imperative in long-term care for mental health care users. It is the role of the occupational therapist to provide a programme that will compensate for the loss of engagement in known occupations.

The next section describes an occupation-based theoretical framework that could guide occupational therapists in the development of programmes for large numbers of users in long-term care.

A THEORETICAL FRAMEWORK TO GUIDE CARE, TREATMENT AND REHABILITATION

The American Occupational Therapy Association (AOTA) has released multiple editions of the Occupational Therapy Practice Framework (OTPF). This is a comprehensive document that emphasises the holistic nature of occupational therapy practice and the importance of client-centred care. When planning programmes to promote occupational justice and create chances for meaningful participation in activities within residential care facilities, the OTPF-4 (AOTA 2020) is a valuable resource.

The OTPF-4 describes the domain of the occupational therapy profession in areas of occupation, client factors, performance skills, performance patterns, context and environment and activity demands. This framework recognises the classification of client factors from the International Classification of Functioning, Disability and Health (ICF) published by the WHO (2001). The ICF provides a common language for body functions and structures as well as domains for activity and participation. Values, beliefs and spirituality are also viewed as client factors as they, together with body functions and structures, affect and are affected by performance in occupational areas, performance skills, performance patterns, activity demands and environmental factors.

Performance skills is the domain that explains the skills that a person needs to perform certain occupations, while the domain of performance patterns includes habits, routines, roles and rituals (AOTA 2020). These patterns capture the essence of the occupational nature of a person and allow occupational therapists to view the individuality of a person performing occupations. The influence of the environment or context that a person lives in is another vital domain to consider and further influences occupational behaviour. The last aspect included in the domain is the demands that activity participation requires from a person. This domain captures the activity analysis process that occupational therapists do before selecting activities and occupations as a therapeutic medium in evaluation or intervention of occupational performance.

THE PROCESS OF OCCUPATIONAL THERAPY

The process of occupational therapy is well described in the OTPF-4 and comprises three main components: evaluation, intervention and outcomes (AOTA 2020). After the evaluation phase is completed, the occupational therapist should use an outcome measure to determine the baseline functioning of the client. The aims of intervention should then be negotiated with the client or the family or other involved people. Regular intervention reviews should then follow to determine progress. A final assessment using the outcome measure should be complete to decide whether the client has reached all the aims or if he/she is sufficiently prepared for discharge.

MODELS OF PRACTICE

Each version of the OTPF was created with the intention of advocating for and conveying the role of occupational therapy. This was achieved by emphasising the enhancement of health and well-being of individuals, organisations, and communities through active participation in meaningful occupations. The framework is not prescriptive of specific theories or models of occupational therapy. It is intended to be used in conjunction with appropriate theories, models and practice guidelines in the occupational therapy process. Practitioners have many options for theoretical frameworks to guide the occupational therapy process. Examples of theoretical frameworks and practice models include the Model of Human Occupation (Kielhofner 2008), the Canadian Model of Occupational Performance and Engagement (Davis 2017), the Person-Environment-Occupation model of Occupational Performance (Turpin 2017), the Kawa model

(Teoh & Iwama 2015), the Vona du Toit Model of Creative Ability (VdTMoCA) (van der Reyden *et al.* 2019) and many more.

THE Vona du Toit MODEL OF CREATIVE ABILITY

A popular model in South Africa is the VdTMoCA. It has been developed by Vona du Toit and colleagues during the 1960s and 1970s. Vona du Toit's thinking was influenced by existentialism, phenomenology and developmental theories (van der Reyden *et al.* 2019).

Du Toit believed that the concept of occupational therapy is substantiated by two basic principles. She presented these two principles in a dissertation which she submitted in 1962 (only published later in 1991). She stated the first principle as follows: 'Man, through the use of his body (which is himself) in purposeful activity can, and indeed must influence the state of his own physical and mental health, and spiritual well-being' (du Toit 2009, p. 2). This principle is almost identical to the hypothesis postulated by Mary Reilly: 'that man, through the use of his hands, as energised by mind and will, can influence the state of his own health' (Reilly 1961, p. 81). du Toit emphasised from a phenomenological perspective that 'living man pre-reflectively is his body, although reflectively he also has a body' (du Toit 2009, p. 2). This means that people are alive because life is 'energised, vitalised and given qualitative dimension and direction by his inner Spiritual Living Force' (du Toit 2009, p. 2). This force is expressed in the world we live in and therefore man is indubitably linked to the environment and in communication with his world. People are responding to the demands of everyday life and, in this process, determining the quality of their being and becoming themselves (du Toit 2009). People are constantly 'creating' themselves.

Du Toit's second principle accentuates the patient's personal decision to participate (du Toit 2009, p. 2), and according to Du Toit, this decision to participate presupposes man's spiritual preparedness to be occupied and fulfil his need to contribute to the world (du Toit 2009). The preparedness to be occupied is expressed in different levels of being motivated to be occupied, and it is observed through actions and behaviours.

In Du Toit's opinion, a person goes through different stages of motivation and action in the psychical recovery process. Motivation is the inner force that initiates or directs all behaviour and results in the creation of a tangible or intangible product. The different actions, which a person displays and which are observable, express his motivation. Motivation governs action and action is the manifestation of motivation. Thus, through the assessment of action, the occupational therapist is able to measure the strength of motivation (du Toit 2009). Readers are referred to van der Reyden *et al.* (2019) for comprehensive information on the characteristics of the levels of creative ability, the assessment and intervention thereof.

The assessment and intervention principles of the VdTMoCA have been valuable in practice settings dealing with large numbers of users in long-term mental health care institutions. This resulted in the development of assessment guidelines and outcome measurement tools. One such a tool is the Functional Levels Outcome Measure (FLOM) (Zietsman & Casteleijn 2014), which has been developed and refined over many years by different clinicians. The latest version of this outcome measurement has been refined by Zietsman and Casteleijn (2014) and has been implemented routinely in a long-term healthcare facility with great success.

The next section highlights the importance of using outcome measures to track change in mental health care users who receive long-term care. The functional levels derived from the first five levels of the VdTMoCA and how they are measured with the FLOM (Zietsman & Casteleijn 2014) are described in the next section.

AN OUTCOME MEASURE FOR LONG-TERM MENTAL HEALTH CARE USERS

Occupational therapists need to provide systematic objective evidence of the therapeutic outcomes of their services to gain respect from the clients they serve as well as the funder of the service. Outcome measurement seeks to measure change as a result of intervention (Laver Fawcett 2013; Casteleijn 2014). Clinicians should use a specific outcome measure routinely for this purpose. Measurement of outcomes facilitates a number of management functions, for example, predicting recovery; calculating efficiency, effectiveness and efficacy of services; allocating resources; and determining critical pathways of professional conduct, to name a few (Jette 1995; Kwan & Rickwood 2015; Barbalat *et al.* 2019). If outcome measurement is routinely part of clinical practice, trends may be evident, for example, identifying clients who are making poor progress.

Functional levels are well described by Du Toit (2009) and Van der Reyden *et al.* (2019) according to the levels of creative ability and ideal for measuring change in mental health care users (Casteleijn 2014). Zietsman and Casteleijn (2014) used the levels and added typical observations of behaviours in patients as seen in users in long-term healthcare facilities. Ten domains were identified, namely, mental illness, orientation, self-care, appearance, continency, social behaviour, activity participation, domestic activity, responsibility and employment potential. Each domain is described in five levels of function. The five levels correlate with the first five levels of creative ability as described by du Toit (2009, pp. 23–26) and Casteleijn and Holsten (2019, pp. 110–134). These descriptions are typical behaviours simply observed by mental health care practitioners. Table 30.1 is an example of the domain of activity participation with the descriptions of observable behaviour.

Table 30.1 Descriptions of observable behaviour in the domain of activity participation of the FLOM (Zietsman 2011).

Level 1 – tone	Automatic reflex action
	Action is haphazard, is unplanned and has no purpose
Level 2 – self-differentiation	Incidentally unconstructive action through contact with materials and objects
	Follows one to two step instructions/demonstrations/movements
	Unproductive, aimless action, unable to plan or follow what is expected
	Persistent danger of hurting self or others
Level 3 – explorative	Making an effort, explorative action results in incidental product
	Product is poor, needs constant supervision to complete any task
	Seems to understand the task partially
	Explores with materials and tools – will try out – skill is poor
	Follows three to four steps/needs constant supervision to do so
Level 4 – norm awareness	Aware of expectations, knows more or less what is expected but hesitant to engage
	Realises when the product is of poor quality, can identify obvious errors of poor quality
	Is aware of norms and rules but needs an example to follow
	Attempts to comply with norms, but external motivation is needed
	Uses tools and materials reasonably well
	Follows instruction for tasks with five to seven steps
Level 5 – norm compliance	Aware and able to comply with norms of behaviour and task performance
	Good pre-vocational and vocational skills are present
	Understands and follows seven- to ten-step instructions, handles tools well
	Action is product-centred
	Wants to achieve a certain standard
	May show initiative

REHABILITATION

Every individual undergoes growth and development in the spheres of occupational performance from birth. However, this progression can be disrupted when a person exhibits signs of mental illness. In cases of severe mental illness, each instance of a psychotic episode or relapse results in a decline in their engagement in meaningful activities and occupations. The occupational therapist's role involves assessing the extent of this functional decline, which may be temporary. Yet, it's rare for the person to fully revert to their initial level of functioning. Hence, it's vital for mental health care users to partake in rehabilitation programs that match their current functional abilities. These programs should introduce activities at a suitable level, facilitating the individual's gradual re-engagement and growth.

The occupational therapist is responsible for devising practical interventions that are well structured and ensure the user experiences a sense of accomplishment. The overarching aim of rehabilitation is to guide the individual towards achieving an optimal level of independent functioning.

ASSESSMENT

The members of the multidisciplinary team administer independent admission assessments of the users admitted to long-term care facilities. A month should be allowed for this process. This allows the users to adapt to the new environment and for medication to take effect.

All new users are involved in balanced programmes, and this allows the occupational therapy and nursing staff to observe behaviour in the different areas of occupational performance. Observations of responses in terms of self, others, materials, objects and the environment are made.

Observations are recorded by means of the FLOM as illustrated in Figure 30.1. Comments to justify the level of functioning are extremely important as these comments are useful for writing periodical reports for review boards (as stipulated in the MHCA). Behaviours with serious consequences should be noted, for example, the content of delusions and hallucination and acts of destruction to self or others.

The admission assessment forms the baseline assessment. The FLOM graph (Figure 30.1) is used to plot the baseline data for each item of the FLOM, which is displayed on the y-axis. The score for each item is shown on the y-axis of the graph. Once the score per item is summed, the programme level is determined according to the score out of 50. A score between 1 and 10 refers to programme level 1, a score between 10 and 25 to programme level 2, a score between 25 and 35 to programme level 3, a score of 35–42 to programme level 4, while a score between 42 and 50 to programme level 5. Reassessments of the items are recorded on the same graph to track the change in the functional levels. The final assessment is recorded when discharge is indicated. The graph of the FLOM shows change from admission to discharge, and progress or decline is easily visible. Figure 30.1 is an example of a FLOM of a user who was admitted and progressed well, but placement after discharge was not successful. He was readmitted on a much lower level but gradually improved again. The case study of this user is described in the shaded box and serves as an example of the clinical application of the FLOM.

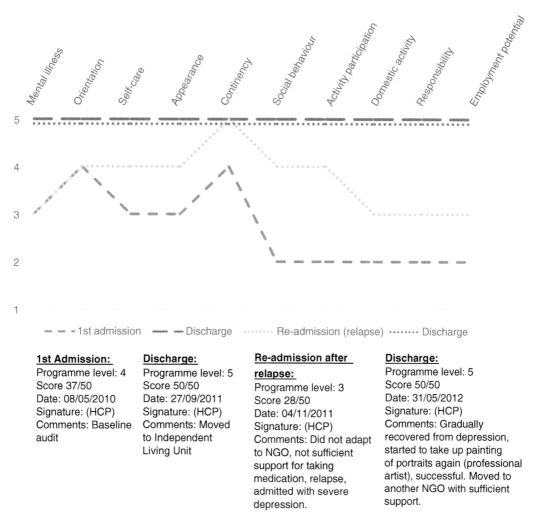

FIGURE 30.1   Example of a completed FLOM record.

MULTIDISCIPLINARY TEAM AND MEETINGS

Members of the multidisciplinary team should all contribute to the common purpose of rehabilitation, that is, to attain the optimal level of independent functioning for each user. On admission, all members of the team do assessment and present their findings at a multidisciplinary meeting. The user should be interviewed during this meeting. The meeting should confirm the DSM-5 diagnosis (APA 2013). An individual biopsycho-social plan for each user should be recorded including programme level, planned input by each team member and possible reintegration options into the community.

Reassessments are recorded on the same FLOM form using different colours. The FLOM is a useful outcome measure to determine the programme level but it also provides valuable information to assist in writing periodical reports to the review board. It is therefore recommended that the FLOM is completed prior to completion of a periodical report and when there is change in the level of function.

REHABILITATION PROGRAMMES

The role of the occupational therapist, particularly within residential care facilities with large numbers of users, is often that of manager, planner and organiser of programmes and services for the entire population of patients. Occupational therapists therefore make extensive use of auxiliary staff, for example, occupational therapy assistants and technicians, to implement many aspects of direct service provision within the psychosocial field of practice (van der Reyden 2014 in Crouch & Alers p. 165).

The occupational therapist must develop well-structured rehabilitation programmes to achieve the aforementioned. The population can be between 500 and 1000 users. Users are grouped according to the same functional level preferably not in groups larger than 25. Each group should have a full-day programme representing the eight areas of occupational performance. These areas should include play, leisure, social participation and education for all levels; personal management, survival skills and work-related activities for levels 3, 4 and 5; and multimodal sensory stimulation (MMSS) for levels 1 and 2.

CASE STUDY

Peter (49) was admitted from the psychiatric ward of a tertiary care government hospital. He was diagnosed with schizo-affective disorder and had a history of several admissions to psychiatric facilities. He displayed verbal and physical aggression and was roaming the streets when the police picked him up and took him to hospital.

Peter was transferred to a long-term psychiatric facility. On admission, he was psychotic and aggressive. He presented with disorganised thinking, hallucinations and delusions.

After a few weeks, he became very quiet and withdrawn, and his baseline assessment indicated that he was functioning on level 4 (norm awareness; see Figure 30.1). He was referred to occupational therapy and placed in the candle workshop. The occupational therapy technician took care to get to know Peter as an individual. She focused on restoring his self-esteem and assessing his strengths. He mentioned to her that he is an artist but has lost his talent. The question was whether this was a delusion or whether he was really talented. The occupational therapy technician provided him with art materials. Initially, he copied pictures of birds and then he did a watercolour of an elephant. Eventually, he made paintings that appeared to be self-portraits reflecting his emotions. His art was of good quality and later displayed at a psychiatric convention in Cape Town.

At this stage, Peter was transferred to the independent living unit in the facility. He mentioned that he had a new hope for the future and his pictures portrayed joy. He actively took part in discussion groups and social and recreational activities and continued to work in the candle workshop. He would paint when he had a 'picture in his brain'. It was recorded that he was functioning on level 5 (norm compliance; see Figure 30.1).

Peter was discharged to a non-governmental organisation but suffered a relapse due to insufficient support and non-compliance to medication. He was readmitted suffering severe depression, and his functional level was recorded as level 3 (explorative; see Figure 30.1). Initially, he was very quiet and displayed no interest to participating in any activities. He gradually recovered from the depression, and the occupational therapy technician started to involve him in the activities he engaged in before. The occupational therapist provided him with quality art materials and created a special quiet area where he could paint. He mentioned that he had pictures in his head again. The Mental Health Society requested him to make a painting of Nelson Mandela. The society had the picture framed and presented it to Nelson Mandela on his birthday. Peter received a personal thank you letter from the Nelson Mandela Foundation. At this stage, his functional level was recorded as level 5, and he was discharged to a different non-governmental organisation. He was allowed to take his art materials with him.

The occupational therapy department forms an integrated part of the ward programme in the sense that it has facilities to provide opportunities for engaging in meaningful occupations like cooking, sport, laundry, hair salon, barbershop, income generating workshops, boutique and gardening. These opportunities are vital to counteract the negative effects of occupational injustice.

SPECIFIC PLANNING OF ACTIVITIES

The incorporation of auxiliary staff is critical to the successful implementation of rehabilitation programmes (van der Reyden 2014).

The specific planning of activities for each programme level should be done by the staff allocated to the specific group. The occupational therapist should, in consultation with the auxiliary staff, continually develop a list of activities listed under the occupational performance areas. Continued training in presenting these activities on the different levels must take place. The relevant staff should plan specific activities on a regular basis. If education is indicated in the programme, they should decide on a relevant topic, for example, insight into mental illness. This list of activities should be updated regularly. The users should also be given an opportunity to express their choice of activities. Institutionalised individuals are involved in a routine programme and should be given the opportunity to think and plan wherever possible.

The facility should plan an annual programme of monthly social events taking into consideration what is happening in the community, public holidays and the health calendar. It is advisable to have different committees for different events.

Care, treatment and rehabilitation programmes for groups at the five levels of function.

Programmes are developed with the assumption that group interventions will be executed mainly by auxiliary and nursing staff. SMART aims (specific and simple, measurable, attainable and realistic with a time frame) should be available in the group file for each specific group. Staff is trained to choose two to three aims for each activity session, and records are kept of observations made in terms of the chosen aims. Care, treatment and rehabilitation aims are presented for each level with a brief discussion of the programme.

Level 1: Tone (Unplanned Action)

Users on this level are mostly unresponsive and similar to patients who are unconscious. Bizarre behaviour may be present.

The approach on level 1 would be very similar to the stimulation given to an individual who is unconscious. One sense at a time would be stimulated, and the occupational therapist would observe whether there was any reaction.

The MMSS principles described for level 2 are also applicable for this level.

Level 2: Self-differentiation (Destructive Action or Incidental Constructive Action)

The behaviour that is described on the self-differentiation level can be attributed to many years of mental illness, institutionalisation and the lack of sensory stimulation. The result is that the senses are intact but that the thalamus is not processing information from senses adequately and inappropriate behaviour is displayed. The users do not understand what they hear, they are often considered to be mute, their behaviour is unpredictable and they are incontinent because they do not register that the bladder is full. These users are considered to be a heavy burden of care, and occupational therapy is often challenged to provide evidence that the intervention is indeed making a difference.

Sensory stimulation has been successfully implemented on this level, and the main objective is to reconnect pathways in the brain with past experiences. The brain should be stimulated in such a way that the thalamus will start processing information received from the senses. The result would be that behavioural response and reaction can be observed.

The MMSS programmes have been developed for users on levels 1 and 2 and showed promising results (Longhorn 1993; Lotan & Gold 2009). The principles and practical tips for MMSS are provided in the following text as levels 1 and 2 with their challenges are often forgotten, but this programme might be able to address these challenges.

Principles of MMSS: The What, Why and How of the Seven Senses Longhorn (1993) has largely influenced the development of the MMSS programmes and was instrumental in providing training to staff. The programmes that include MMSS are based on the principles provided by Longhorn (1993) to stimulate the seven senses. These principles are summarised in the following texts.

Vision is the main coordinating sense. The brain is stimulated by light and dark, contrast and movement. There are 45 areas in the brain that deal with vision. Movement promotes visual tracking, and it is more useful if the tracking crosses the midline. Vision is linked to the vestibular system and has an effect on balance.

Always make eye contact when speaking to a person. Always approach the person from the front.

Tactile/touch is the second most important sensation. The whole body is covered with skin, which has millions of touch receptors. These sensory messages from the skin send information to the brain with regard to temperature, texture, pain and pressure. Deep, firm pressure is perceived as safe and calming by the brain. Without touch, humans do not grow and flourish emotionally.

Warm, cosy temperature is comforting. Rather stimulate the dorsal parts of the body since the frontal parts are more sensitive and personal. Stimulation should be done with the direction of hair growth. Be aware that some people, for instance, people with schizophrenia, might be sensory defensive.

Auditory/sound: The ears and eyes work together to locate sounds. The different components of sound determine the sensory response, for example, pitch (high and low), volume, rhythm or speed of voices. Sound is linked to the vestibular system. Sound also links to emotions and memories. One needs to understand what is said to respond appropriately.

The human voice is a powerful therapeutic tool to orientate, stimulate, reassure, explain and confirm. The use of music can be calming and relaxing, yet lively rhythmic music can stimulate physical movement. Music often allows for spiritual stimulation, while background music could be contained.

Smell is the only sense that links directly with the smell area of the brain without passing through the thalamus; therefore, it provides the quickest brain response. The smell receptors at the upper end of the nose carry odours directly to the hippocampus, which controls emotions and memory. Pleasant smell can elicit happy memories. Smell can also set the tone for what is coming. The use of pleasant smells can encourage self-care activities. The use of lavender oil is especially useful.

Taste is closely linked with smell and perhaps one of our most pleasant senses. Taste is mostly linked to food and eating. Strong flavours like liquorice or peppermint elicit immediate responses and could be incorporated with food activities. Favourite dishes or food often triggers the memory of the past, for example, remembering Christmas after tasting a piece of ginger biscuit.

Proprioception is awareness of the whole body and knowing where it is in space. It is also awareness of movement through receptors in the joints. Any body movement provides proprioceptive input. Lively rhythmic music that stimulates body movements could stimulate proprioceptive input. Combining the movements with scarves, hula hoops or ribbon sticks usually elicits more interest and motivation to participate.

Vestibular sense is important for balance and sensing of speed of movement. Rhythmic vestibular movement has a calming effect on the central nervous system. People with chronic schizophrenia are often observed to be rocking. A mother instinctively rocks her crying baby. Swinging in a swing or hammock has a calming effect. Bumping on a large ball or inner tube also provides vestibular input.

Stimulating as many senses as possible in treatment sessions and using the aforementioned principles with unresponsive users were found to be very beneficial. Orientation to reality and awareness of others improved and behaviour became less destructive. This improvement relieved the burden of care on the nursing staff. It is important to distinguish between unconstructive or destructive action, and incidentally constructive action on level 2 as the sensory stimulation programme includes different techniques and principles for the two different actions. Following are examples of a typical MMSS routine for users with unconstructive or destructive action and incidental constructive action.

A Sensory-focused Approach for Destructive Action The suggested frequency of this routine is two times per week in the morning. Greet each person individually, make eye contact, call the person by name and shake hands. Use name tags if necessary.

Observe any reaction after the stimulation. Analyse how many senses are stimulated right through the exercise. Change the smell of the room by spraying lavender spray and play cool, calm music. The therapist must switch between lively and calming music. It is easier to change music if a CD/tape player is used. Encourage physical movement by changing the music to rhythmic and lively and provide ribbon sticks, scarves and flags.

Play lively music and do a firm shoulder massage from the back through the clothing. Apply deep pressure. Play familiar music from the past and provide bits of pleasant taste and drink. Provide a pleasant smell of food or drink. Change the music to calming music and do a firm hand massage using lavender oil. Provide materials and objects with rough and smooth textures. Use partially see-through fabric and play peek-a-boo with each individual. Blow bubbles in the air.

Use the person's name as often as possible. Say or sing goodbye to each person. A mirror can be used when you say goodbye, encouraging the person to look in the mirror when the name is said.

It is useful to have all materials in a large container and to display the routine and aims on top of the lid of the container. Students, helpers or even visitors can follow what is done and can join in. This becomes part of the ward routine, and it was found that users who could not be grouped would recognise the container with anticipation and would eventually join the group spontaneously.

A Sensory-focused Approach for Incidentally Constructive Action As the user starts responding to the sensory stimulation and one can observe reaction and even boredom with the routine, it is an indication that progress was made within the level.

On this level, the focus must shift from providing total care to providing a balanced programme but bearing the sensory stimulation principles in mind.

Ideas for incidentally constructive activities can be lacing activities, handling of different types of dough and clay, matching of two to four pieces, tearing paper or sponge and finger-painting. Present one-step food preparation activities using one verb, like dip: dipping a piece of fruit on a toothpick in melted chocolate and then tasting it.

Self-care and grooming sessions are ideal for impactful MMSS sessions. Firm head and shoulder massages can be included with hair care sessions.

Use lavender soap, cream and oil when doing hand and nail care. Mix five drops of lavender oil with 50 mL cooking or olive oil. Apply oil whilst doing a firm hand massage, make eye contact, greet the user by name, identify oneself and continue verbalising what you are doing. Verbalise colour, shape, smell and name of objects. Calming background music can be played.

The same principles could be used for physical movement sessions and spiritual sessions, for example.

The sensory-focused approach shifts the provision of care from merely going through the procedure to a therapeutic experience. Every activity experience should be a sensory experience to stimulate maximally to elicit a positive response.

Level 3: Self-presentation (Constructive Explorative Action)

Users on this level have a desire to present themselves but cannot yet achieve self-directed participation. Behaviour is therefore impulsive and explorative in nature.

Activity participation in all the occupational performance areas is about trying out and not about a product. A keyword would be to say, 'Let's see what will happen if . . .'. The user should be given the opportunity to explore the properties of materials and start to develop basic skills in all the areas of occupational performance. They could start to assist with food preparation in a group setting and explore tool-handling skills as well as social contact.

Level 4: Passive Participation (Norm Awareness Experimental Action)

Users on this level show interest in product-centred activities but are hesitant to initiate participation in activities and situations. The chronic user has a long history of failure, and anxiety levels are high when exposed to new activities, situations and people. The action is experimental as they are willing to follow rules and judge the quality of the product but need regular supervision and verbal guidance for task completion.

The multidisciplinary team should start to consider placement options for the user. The user can now move to an independent living area in the facility. One of the benefits of placement in an independent living unit is to observe the effect of reduced supervision on the user's anxiety levels. Site visits should be done to community-based placements. The admission criteria to an independent living unit should be similar to those of community-based centres. It will be necessary to determine which survival skills are necessary if placement at home is an option. An example would be to determine the mode of food preparation. It could be an open fire, paraffin stove, liquid gel stove, gas stove or electric stove. Establish whether there are workshops at the community-based centre and what skills the user might need to adapt easily to the new environment.

Level 5: Imitative Participation (Norm-compliant Action)

Users on this level are usually on a pre-discharge programme, and skills for independent living are consolidated. They find satisfaction and security in imitating activities.

Determine if transfer to an independent living unit would be successful. Education in terms of community survival skills will include the following topics: insight into mental illness, compliance with medication and substance abuse. Financial management should include making a shopping list, drawing money like a disability grant at an automated teller machine, money handling and shopping. Community mobility, for example, making use of public transport, should be practised. Arrange visits to public places like the local clinic, recreational facilities and religious places.

Family members will often require a day programme. It is a good idea to prepare information on the skills the user has acquired, a suggested day programme, instructions of craft activities and even recipes, information with regard to mental illness as well as a checklist for signs of a pending relapse. Family must have information regarding realistic performance expectations, and they should not keep their family member in a sick role.

The rehabilitation programme presented here covers the first five levels of creative ability as these levels have been admitted to long-term stay facilities. Users above these levels are able to manage their mental disorder and have sufficient support to fulfil the demands and expectations of everyday living.

CONCLUSION

This chapter described the care, treatment and rehabilitation programmes for long-term mental health care users. It gave an overview of global and national trends in mental health care services and the trend to move towards community-based mental health care and residential care was presented. The South African MHCA of 2002 is included since this act provides a clear direction for the role of occupational therapy in the provision of healthcare services. Occupational therapy plays a vital role in delivering residential care, treatment and rehabilitation programmes and should aim to alleviate occupational injustice that may be caused by residential care facilities where a user is only a number.

A theoretical framework to guide practice, the OTPF-4, was briefly presented. A popular model of practice in South Africa, the VdTMoCA, introduced practical guidelines for implementation of rehabilitation in long-term residential care facilities. The use of the multidisciplinary team in assessment, programme planning, implementation and evaluation of the effect of intervention was discussed.

Although providing care, treatment and rehabilitation to long-term mental health care users is sometimes extremely challenging, well-designed programmes and auxiliary staff who are trained and empowered to deliver the programmes make the difference to those in need of care and to the morale of the staff.

QUESTIONS

1. Discuss the global and national trends in mental health care.

2. Explain how legislation guides occupational therapy intervention in long-term facilities.

3. Describe the need to move to community-based mental health care and away from institutionalised care.

4. Argue the effect of long-term residential care facilities on individuals' occupational performance.

5. Explain the phenomenon of occupational injustice in the long-term mental health care user.

6. Explain the concept of rehabilitation and discuss how this will influence the planning of programmes for the long-term users.

7. Give examples for activities in an MMSS programme for the incidental constructive level as well as the incidental destructive level.

8. Discuss the major differences between the stimulation programmes for the incidental constructive level and the incidental destructive level.

9. Formulate objectives for treatment for the five levels of function.

REFERENCES

American Psychiatric Association. (2013) Anxiety disorders, In: *Diagnostic and statistical manual of mental disorders*, 5th edn. https://doi.org/10.1176/appi.books.9780890425596.dsm05

AOTA (2020) The occupational therapy practice framework: domain and process – fourth edition. *The American Journal of Occupational Therapy*, **74 (Suppl 2)**, 7412410010p7412410011–7412410010p7412410087. https://doi.org/10.5014/ajot.2020.74S2001

Barbalat, G., van den Bergh, D. & Kossakowski, J.J. (2019) Outcome measurement in mental health services: insights from symptom networks. *BMC Psychiatry*, **19(1)**, 202. https://doi.org/10.1186/s12888-019-2175-7

Biringer, E., Hartveit, M., Sundfør, B., Ruud, T. & Borg, M. (2017) Continuity of care as experienced by mental health service users - a qualitative study. *BMC Health Services Research*, **17(1)**, 763. https://doi.org/10.1186/s12913-017-2719-9

Cano Prieto, I., Simó Algado, S. & Prat Vigué, G. (2023) Peer interventions in severe mental illnesses: a systematic review and its relation to occupational therapy. *Occupational Therapy in Mental Health*, **39(2)**, 99–136. https://doi.org/10.1080/0164212X.2022.2085645

Casteleijn, D. (2014) Using measurement principles to confirm the levels of creative ability as described in the Vona du Toit model of creative ability. *South African Journal of Occupational Therapy*, **44**, 14–19. http://www.scielo.org.za/scielo.php?script=sci_arttext&pid=S2310-38332014000100004&lng=en (accessed 18 September 2023)

Casteleijn, D. & Holsten, E.A. (2019) Creative ability – its emergence and manifestation. In: D. van der Reyden, D. Casteleijn, W. Sherwood &

P. de Witt (eds), *The Vona du Toit Model of Creative Ability: Origins, Constructs, Principles and Application in Occupational Therapy*. Vona and Marie du Toit Foundation.

Davis, J.A. (2017) The Canadian model of occupational performance and engagement (CMOP-E). In: M. Curtin, J. Adams & M. Egan (eds), *Occupational Therapy for People Experiencing Illness, Injury of Impairment: Promoting Occupation and Participation*, 7th edn. pp. 148–168. Elsevier.

de Wet, A., Parker, J. & Pretorius, C. (2019) The spring foundation: a recovery approach to institutional public mental health services in South Africa. *Perspectives in Public Health*, **139**(3), 123–124. https://doi.org/10.1177/1757913919838767

de Wet, A. & Pretorius, C. (2022) From darkness to light: barriers and facilitators to mental health recovery in the South African context. *International Journal of Social Psychiatry*, **68**(1), 82–89. https://doi.org/10.1177/0020764020981126

Docrat, S., Besada, D., Daviaud, E. & Crick, L. (2019) Mental health system costs, resources and constraints in South Africa: a national survey. *Health Policy and Planning*, **34**(6), 706–719. https://doi.org/10.1093/heapol/czz085

du Toit, V. (2009) *Patient Volition and Action in Occupational Therapy*, 4th edn. Vona & Marié du Toit Foundation, Pretoria.

Ferlito, B.A. & Dhai, A. (2018) The life esidimeni tragedy: some ethical transgressions. *South African Medical Journal*, **108**(3), 157. https://doi.org/10.7196/SAMJ.2018.v108i3.13012

Gamaldien, F., Galvaan, R. & Duncan, M. (2021) The perspectives of males with serious mental disorders on their community integration following a residential-based rehabilitation programme in South Africa: "it's a catch-22 situation". *South African Journal of Occupational Therapy*, **51**(1), 63–71. https://dx.doi.org/10.17159/2310-3833/2021/vol51n1a9

Gamieldien, F., Galvaan, R., Myers, B. & Sorsdahl, K. (2023) Mental health service users and their caregivers perspectives on personal recovery from severe mental health conditions in Cape Town, South Africa: a qualitative study. *Journal of Psychosocial Rehabilitation and Mental Health*, 1–19. https://doi.org/10.1007/s40737-023-00341-8

Govender, P., Boyd, J., Hassim, A., Jordaan, T., Mahomed, N. & Straeuli-Paul, D. (2015) Life within chronic care: is this a service or sentence? *African Health Sciences*, **15**(2), 665–672. https://doi.org/10.4314/ahs.v15i2.46

Hocking, C., Townsend, E. & Mace, J. (2022) World Federation of Occupational Therapists position statement: Occupational Therapy and Human Rights (Revised 2019) – the backstory and future challenges. *World Federation of Occupational Therapists Bulletin*, **78**(2), 83–89. https://doi.org/https://doi.org/10.1080/14473828.2021.1915608

Höhl, W., Moll, S. & Pfeiffer, A. (2017) Occupational therapy interventions in the treatment of people with severe mental illness. *Current Opinion in Psychiatry*, **30**(4), 300. https://www.proquest.com/scholarly-journals/occupational-therapy-interventions-treatment/docview/1937394961/se-2?accountid=14717 (accessed 18 September 2023)

Iseselo, M.K. & Ambikile, J.S. (2020) Promoting recovery in mental illness: the perspectives of patients, caregivers, and community members in Dar es Salaam Tanzania. *Psychiatry Journal*, **2020**, 3607414. https://doi.org/10.1155/2020/3607414

Jette, A.M. (1995) Outcomes research: shifting the dominant research paradigm in physical therapy. *Physical Therapy*, **75**(11), 965–970.

Kapadia, D. (2023) Stigma, mental illness & ethnicity: time to centre racism and structural stigma. *Sociology of Health & Illness*, **45**(4), 855–871. https://doi.org/10.1111/1467-9566.13615

Kastrup, M. (2023) Global aspects of psychosocial rehabilitation. *World Social Psychiatry*, **5**(1), 47–50. https://doi.org/10.4103/wsp.wsp_3_23

Kielhofner, G. (2008) *Model of Human, Theory and Application Occupation*. Lippincott Williams & Wilkins.

Knaak, S., Mantler, E. & Szeto, A. (2017) Mental illness-related stigma in healthcare: barriers to access and care and evidence-based solutions. *Healthcare Management Forum*, **30**(2), 111–116. https://doi.org/10.1177/0840470416679413

Kwan, B. & Rickwood, D.J. (2015) A systematic review of mental health outcome measures for young people aged 12 to 25 years. *BMC Psychiatry*, **15**, 279. https://doi.org/10.1186/s12888-015-0664-x

Lake, J. & Turner, M.S. (2017) Urgent need for improved mental health care and a more collaborative model of care. *The Permanente Journal*, **21**, 17–024. https://doi.org/10.7812/tpp/17-024

Laver Fawcett, A. (2013) *Principles of Assessment and Outcome Measurement for Occupational Therapists and Physiotherapists: Theory, Skills and Application*. Wiley.

Li, C., Yang, F., Yang, B.X., Chen, W., Wang, Q., Huang, H., Liu, Q., Luo, D., Wang, X.Q. & Ruan, J. (2022) Experiences and challenges faced by community mental health workers when providing care to people with mental illness: a qualitative study. *BMC Psychiatry*, **22**(1), 623. https://doi.org/10.1186/s12888-022-04252-z

Longhorn, F. (1993) *Planning a Multisensory Massage Programme for Very Special People*. Catalyst Education Resources Limited.

Loots, E., Goossens, E., Vanwesemael, T., Morrens, M., Van Rompaey, B. & Dilles, T. (2021) Interventions to improve medication adherence in patients with schizophrenia or bipolar disorders: a systematic review and meta-analysis. *International Journal of Environmental Research and Public Health*, **18**(19). https://doi.org/10.3390/ijerph181910213

Lotan, M. & Gold, C. (2009) Meta-analysis of the effectiveness of individual intervention in the controlled multisensory environment (Snoezelen) for individuals with intellectual disability. *Journal of Intellectual and Developmental Disability*, **34**(3), 207–215.

Madlala, S.T., Miya, R.M. & Zuma, M. (2020) Experiences of mental healthcare providers regarding integration of mental healthcare into primary healthcare at the iLembe health district in KwaZulu-Natal province. *Health SA Gesondheid*, **25**, a1143. https://doi.org/10.4102/hsag.v25i0.1143

Mapanga, W., Casteleijn, D., Ramiah, C., Odendaal, W., Metu, Z., Robertson, L. & Goudge, J. (2019) Strategies to strengthen the provision of mental health care at the primary care setting: an evidence map. *PLOS ONE*, **14**(9), e0222162. https://doi.org/10.1371/journal.pone.0222162

Morrow, M. & Hardie, S. (2023) Intersectionality. In: W. Bryant, J. Fieldhouse & N. Plastow (eds), *Creek's Occupational Therapy in Mental Health*, 6th edn, pp. 200–220. Elsevier.

Ong, H.S., Fernandez, P.A. & Lim, H.K. (2021) Family engagement as part of managing patients with mental illness in primary care. *Singapore Medical Journal*, **62**(5), 213–219. https://doi.org/10.11622/smedj.2021057

Pizarro, E., Estrella, S., Figueroa, F., Helmke, F., Pontigo, C. & Whiteford, G. (2018) Understanding occupational justice from the concept of territory: a proposal for occupational science. *Journal of Occupational Science*, **25**(4), 463–473. https://doi.org/10.1080/14427591.2018.1487261

Ramafikeng, M., Beukes, L., Hassan, A., Kohler, T., Mouton, T. & Petersen, S. (2020) Experiences of adults with psychiatric disabilities participating in an activity programme at a psychosocial rehabilitation centre in the Western Cape. *South African Journal of Occupational Therapy*, **50**(2), 44–51. https://dx.doi.org/10.17159/2310-3833/2020/vol50no2a6

Rebeiro, K.L. & Cook, J.V. (1999) Opportunity, not prescription: an exploratory study of the experience of occupational engagement. *Canadian Journal of Occupational Therapy*, **66**(4), 176–187. https://doi.org/10.1177/000841749906600405

Reilly, M. (1961) Occupational therapy can be one of the great ideas of 20th century medicine – Eleanor Clarke Slagle lecture. *American Journal of Occupational Therapy*, **16**(1), 1–9.

Republic of South Africa (2002) *Mental health care act, no. 17 of 2002. Government Gazette, 2002:79*. Cape Town

Republic of South Africa (2017) *Guidelines for the licensing of residential and day care facilities for people with mental and/or intellectual disabilities*. Government Gazette no. 50847 Retrieved from https://www.gov.za/sites/default/files/gcis_document/201705/40847gon441.pdf (accessed 18 September 2023)

Republic of South Africa (2023) *National mental health policy framework and strategic plan 2030–2030*.

Robertson, L. & Makgoba, M.W. (2018) Mortality analysis of people with severe mental illness transferred from long-stay hospital to alternative care in the Life Esidimeni tragedy. *South African Medical Journal*, **108**(10), 813–817. https://www.ajol.info/index.php/samj/article/view/178532 (accessed 18 September 2023)

Rocamora-Montenegro, M., Compañ-Gabucio, L.-M. & Garcia De La Hera, M. (2021) Occupational therapy interventions for adults with severe mental illness: a scoping review. *BMJ Open*, **11**(10), e047467. https://doi.org/10.1136/bmjopen-2020-047467

Sun, X., Zhang, X., Liu, L., Zhang, L., Zhan, T. & Chen, Y. (2023) A qualitative of stable symptomatology for patients with schizophrenia: do they have adequate post-discharge rehabilitative resources? *Schizophrenia*, **9**(1), 29. https://doi.org/10.1038/s41537-023-00358-9

Teoh, J.Y. & Iwama, M.K. (2015) *The Kawa Model Made Easy: A Guide to Applying the Kawa Model in Occupational Therapy Practice*, 2nd edn. www.kawamodel.com

Thornicroft, G., Deb, T. & Henderson, C. (2016) Community mental health care worldwide: current status and further developments. *World Psychiatry*, **15**(3), 276–286. https://doi.org/10.1002/wps.20349

Townsend, E. & Wilcock, A. (2004) Occupational justice. In: C.H. Christiansen & E.A. Townsend (eds), *Introduction to Occupation: The Art and Science of Living*, pp. 243–273. Prentice Hall.

Tungpunkom, P., Maayan, N. & Soares-Weiser, K. (2012) Life skills programmes for chronic mental illnesses. *Cochrane Database Systematic Reviews*, **1**(1), Cd000381. https://doi.org/10.1002/14651858.CD000381.pub3

Turpin, M. (2017) Occupational therapy practice models. In: M. Curtin, J. Adams & M. Egan (eds), *Occupational Therapy for People Experiencing Illness, Injury of Impairment: Promoting Occupation and Participation,* 7th edn. pp. 115–133. Elsevier.

van der Reyden, D. (2014) Auxiliary staff in mental health care. In: R. Crouch & V. Alers (eds), *Occupational Therapy in Psychiatry and Mental Health,* 5th edn, pp. 162–174. Wiley. https://doi.org/10.1002/9781118913536.ch11

van der Reyden, D., Casteleijn, D., Sherwood, W. & de Witt, P. (2019) *The Vona du Toit Model of Creative Ability: Origins, Constructs, Principles and Application in Occupational Therapy*. The Vona and Marié du Toit Foundation.

WHO (2001) *International classification of functioning, disability and health*. https://icd.who.int/dev11/l-icf/en (accessed 12 April 2023).

WHO (2021) *Comprehensive mental health action plan 2013–2030*. Geneva. https://www.who.int/publications/i/item/9789240031029 (accessed 18 September 2023)

Wright-St Claire, V. & Hocking, C. (2018) Occupational science: the study of occupation. In: B. Schell & G. Gillen (eds), *Willard and Spackman's Occupational Therapy*, 13th edn. pp. 348–374. Wolters Kluwer Health.

Zietsman, K. (2011) Background to FLOM. 2011. Unpublished presentation at Workshop Bloemfontein.

Zietsman, K. & Casteleijn, D. (2014) Care, treatment and rehabilitation programmes for large numbers of long-term mental health care users. In: R. Crouch & V. Alers (eds), *Occupational Therapy in Psychiatry and Mental Health,* 5th edn. pp. 148–161. Wiley. https://doi.org/10.1002/9781118913536.ch10

Index